Neural Microelectrodes

Neural Microelectrodes: Design and Applications

Special Issue Editors

Joseph J. Pancrazio
Stuart F. Cogan

MDPI • Basel • Beijing • Wuhan • Barcelona • Belgrade

MDPI

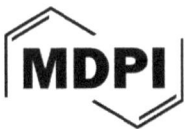

Special Issue Editors
Joseph J. Pancrazio
University of Texas at Dallas
USA

Stuart F. Cogan
University of Texas at Dallas
USA

Editorial Office
MDPI
St. Alban-Anlage 66
4052 Basel, Switzerland

This is a reprint of articles from the Special Issue published online in the open access journal *Micromachines* (ISSN 2072-666X) from 2018 to 2019 (available at: https://www.mdpi.com/journal/micromachines/special_issues/neural_microelectrodes)

For citation purposes, cite each article independently as indicated on the article page online and as indicated below:

LastName, A.A.; LastName, B.B.; LastName, C.C. Article Title. *Journal Name* **Year**, *Article Number*, Page Range.

ISBN 978-3-03921-319-1 (Pbk)
ISBN 978-3-03921-320-7 (PDF)

Cover image courtesy of Stuart F. Cogan.

Contents

About the Special Issue Editors

Joseph Pancrazio earned a B.Sc. in electrical engineering from the University of Illinois followed by a M.Sc. and Ph.D. in biomedical engineering from the University of Virginia. He has a 30-year career spanning academia and federal government, working in the fields of biosensors and neural engineering. He currently serves as the vice president for research and a professor of bioengineering at UT Dallas. Prior to joining UT Dallas in 2015 as associate provost, he served as the founding chair of bioengineering at George Mason University in Fairfax, VA. Before arriving at Mason in 2008, he served in the US federal government as a material scientist at the US Naval Research Laboratory and as the program director for Neural Engineering at the National Institutes of Health (NIH) in Washington, DC. Dr. Pancrazio's research focuses on the development of novel neural interface technology, which is used to understand and influence the brain and nervous system for the purposes of improving human health. In 2011, Dr. Pancrazio was elected to the College of Fellows in the American Institute for Medical and Biological Engineering, a distinction reserved for the top 2% of professionals in the field.

Stuart Cogan is a professor of bioengineering at the University of Texas at Dallas, conducting research on neural stimulation and recording electrodes, the electrode–tissue interface, implantable materials, and vision prostheses. His current research focuses on multielectrode arrays based on amorphous silicon carbide and the application of ultra-microelectrodes for chronic applications in the central and peripheral nervous systems. He received B.Sc. and M.Sc. degrees in mechanical engineering and materials science from Duke University and a Sc.D. in materials science from the Massachusetts Institute of Technology. Prior to joining UT Dallas in 2014, Dr. Cogan spent 30 years at EIC Laboratories, departing as vice-president and the head of materials research. Besides neural devices, his research interests have included superconductivity, thin-film optical switching, crystal growth, and thin-film deposition processes. Dr. Cogan is an elected member of the College of Fellows in the American Institute for Medical and Biological Engineering.

micromachines

MDPI

Editorial

Editorial for the Special Issue on Neural Electrodes: Design and Applications

Joseph J. Pancrazio * and Stuart F. Cogan *

Department of Bioengineering, The University of Texas at Dallas, 800 W. Campbell Road, BSB 13.633, Richardson, TX 75080, USA
* Correspondence: Joseph.Pancrazio@utdallas.edu (J.J.P.); sxc149830@utdallas.edu (S.F.C.)

Received: 9 July 2019; Accepted: 9 July 2019; Published: 12 July 2019

Neural electrodes enable the recording and stimulation of bioelectrical activity from the nervous system. This technology provides neuroscientists and clinicians with the means to probe the functionality of neural circuitry in health and modulate activity in disease states. In their simplest forms, neural electrodes can be viewed as collections of wires or exposed electrical contacts in an insulating substrate. The exposed electrical contact can vary in size depending on the application. For conventional therapeutic devices, the neural electrode sites are relatively large, allowing the electrical stimulation of a volume of tissue to effect neuromodulation. For example, neural electrodes can deliver therapeutic stimulation for the relief of debilitating symptoms associated with Parkinson's Disease, a disorder characterized by a deficit in dopaminergic neurons, via deep brain stimulation (DBS). The neural electrodes for DBS consist of a relatively small number of metallic contacts along a single shaft.

In comparison, microelectrode and even ultramicroelectrode-based devices, which offer the opportunity for a more intimate interface with the nervous system tissue, are 1–3 orders of magnitude smaller in dimension, and the field is driving towards high spatial densities of electrode sites. Indeed, from a historical standpoint, basic and applied neuroscience has made significant strides from insights derived from small, yet fragile and unstable neural electrodes. At small dimensions, neural electrodes can stimulate relatively small tissue volumes to provide selectivity or allow the measurement of activity from a single "unit" or presumptive individual neuron for decoding purposes. While the performance consistency of the microelectrode–tissue interface has been problematic, the experimental results have inspired efforts to develop motor and sensory neuroprosthesis as well as provided fundamental insights into brain circuitry. Commercially available arrays of microelectrodes include bundled microwires, multi-shank silicon-based Utah (or Blackrock) arrays, and the Michigan (or Neuronexus) single and multi-shank devices. A significant obstacle to large-scale implementation is the "many wire problem", i.e., how many wires can one logistically implement across the skull? Consider, for example, a mouse skull with a surface area of approximately 100 mm^2. For the smallest Omnetics connector, often used in basic science and pre-clinical neuroscience studies, the pitch between electrical contacts is 0.635 mm. The largest number of connection points for the entire 100 mm^2 surface area would be 225, far fewer than the 75 million neurons in a mouse brain. While multiplexing and wireless transmission will likely ameliorate or avoid altogether cabling and connector issues in future devices for clinical applications and long-term behavioral studies, robust cabling is non-trivial, and stresses created by cable bundles remain a major limitation for high density microelectrode devices, affecting positioning and stability.

Furthermore, there are failure mechanisms that include both biotic and abiotic processes. As reviewed by Campbell and Wu [1], the biotic mechanism is believed to originate from the chronic foreign body response following initial implantation, and downstream processes that have features consistent with CNS trauma and neurodegeneration. There is evidence implicating the mechanical mismatch between the nervous system tissue and the neural electrodes as a source of the tissue response [2]. The Young's modulus for brain tissue is approximately 7 orders of magnitude softer than silicon, a common neural microelectrode structural material. Neural probes that either consist of materials that soften on implantation [2,3] or have extremely small cross-sectional areas resulting in device flexibility [4] show diminished tissue response. From an abiotic perspective, electrical connectors, never intended by design for biological experiments, are prone to fail due to repeated plugging and unplugging, a problem that plagues neural recordings in animal models. The combination of optogenetics with neural recording and stimulation paradigms creates new challenges for ensuring that heat dissipation during illumination is minimized to reduce the likelihood of tissue damage. Lastly, the age of bioelectronic medicines has brought the realization that the viscera are subject to neuromodulation and that new electrode technologies will be required to unravel functional neural connectivity. Multidisciplinary approaches are the key, and so this Special Issue on "Neural Microelectrodes: Design and Applications" showcases 22 research papers and review articles that leverage new perspectives from fields including tissue biomechanics, material science, and biological mechanisms of inflammation and neurodegeneration that are critical to advancing the technology. The papers in this Special Issue explore the following aspects of neural electrodes design and application in the following theme areas: (1) biomaterials, (2) enabling technology and fabrication, and (3) the biology of the interface.

1. Biomaterials. Hess-Dunning and Tyler [3] report that neural probes can be fabricated from a mechanically-adaptive polymer that is stiff prior to insertion, but rapidly transitions in vivo to an extremely compliant state (~10 MPa). These devices are fabricated from a nanocomposite derived from a soft poly(vinyl acetate) (PVAc) matrix polymer with a percolated network of high-aspect-ratio cellulose nanocrystals harvested from tunicate mantles. The nanocomposite supports embedded Parylene-C-coated Au leads to produce stable electrochemical properties in vivo and well-resolved single units from probes implanted chronically for 4 months in rat cortex. Stiller et al. [5] describe the chronic recording and electrochemical performance of fully encapsulated shape memory polymer (SMP) microelectrode arrays in rat cortex. These single shank devices, fabricated from conventional thin film polymer processing, are based on thiol-ene/acrylate SMP that softens by an order of magnitude once implanted. After 4 months in vivo, single units were prominent, and the neuroinflammatory profile determined by immunohistochemistry was modest, suggesting the feasibility of SMP-based devices. Shoffstall et al. [6] describe a comprehensive analysis of the neuroinflammatory response of SMP-coated silicon structures and compare the surface properties to uncoated silicon structures. After 4 months in rat cortex, the non-softening thiol-ene SMP devices appeared to produce a histological profile similar to the silicon controls, although astrocytic scarring was reduced for the SMP-coated probes. Rihani et al. [7] present early stage work showing that another smart polymer, specifically liquid crystal elastomer with shape-changing characteristics, may be a promising neural interface material. Based on in vitro studies, they report that the material is neither cytotoxic nor likely to affect neuronal electrophysiologic behavior. Furthermore, they demonstrate that functional multi-layer devices consisting of arrays of electrodes can be fabricated and are electrically stable under in vitro conditions.

Rather than having a device consist of material that changes its modulus, Kil et al. [8] demonstrate that dextran can be used to temporarily stiffen flexible probes fabricated from Parylene-C to enable insertion into rat somatosensory cortex without buckling. They characterized the rapid dissolution rate as a function of molecular weight and probe surface area, showing that a 37 µm thick coating of 40 kDa dextran provides a dissolution time of approximately 4 min, well within the typical time period needed to insert a cortical probe. Histological analyses of dextran-coated probes implanted for 4 months demonstrated little or no neuroinflammatory response, indicating that dextran is a practical option for temporarily stiffening ultrasmall and highly flexible probes for insertion. Deku et al. [4] describe the fabrication and in vivo performance of ultrasmall microelectrode arrays that leverage amorphous silicon carbide (a-SiC), an insulating material known to be non-corrosive and fracture-resistant. Prototype a-SiC intracortical implants fabricated containing 8–16 single shanks with a thickness of 6 µm penetrated rat cortex without an insertion aid or transient coating, and single unit recordings were well-resolved from sputtered iridium oxide-coated electrode sites. Recognizing that delamination is one of the means by which implanted multi-layer devices fail, Bernardin et al. [9] report on the early stage development of a monolithic probe that makes use of a crystalline form of silicon carbide (SiC). Capitalizing on SiC as a chemically inert semiconductor, the device structure was micromachined from p-type SiC with conductors created from n-type SiC, simultaneously providing electrical isolation through the resulting p-n junction. Electrical characterization of the electrode sites showed high-performance p-n diode behavior, with typical turn-on voltages of ~2.3 V and reverse bias leakage below 1 nA$_{rms}$ with impedances suitable for extracellular recording.

2. Enabling Technology and Fabrication. Sridharan et al. [10] show that rat peripheral nerve can be wirelessly stimulated using volume-conducted AC fields directed towards implanted Schottky microdiodes coupled to cuff electrodes. Muscle twitches monitored by electromyography could be elicited by 500 kHz AC fields for as brief as 1 ms in duration. While there may be limitations in terms of the number of selective channels, this approach is promising for a range of "bioelectronics medicines" applications. Straka and colleagues [11] report that electrochemical impedance spectroscopy (EIS) performed in vivo can provide insights into degradation kinetics and mechanisms associated with implanted Utah arrays in peripheral nerve. Capitalizing on electrode-electrolyte equivalent circuit representation for Pt and Pt/Ir. microelectrodes based on the Randles circuit model, distinct classes of EIS become apparent that implicate the emergence of a glial scar from the neuroinflammatory response, parasitic capacitance pathways, lead-wire breakage or loss of electrode tip metallization, or electrode insulation degradation. While DBS systems typically operate in an open loop, always on mode, Vajari et al. [12] describe the design of a hybrid DBS probe, comprised of glassy carbon electrodes on a polyimide substrate, which couples electrical stimulation and local field potential recording with fast scan cyclic voltammetry (FSCV). FSCV offers the possibility of real time measurements of dopamine for use as a feedback signal for a closed loop DBS system. In vitro characterization of the prototype device showed sub micromolar sensitivity to dopamine and minimal artifacts during magnetic resonance imaging. Future preclinical work will be necessary to characterize the stability of glassy carbon electrode measurements in vivo.

Nicolai et al. [13] provide a characterization of motion artifacts associated with real world, in vivo use of ultra-small, flexible 7-μm diameter carbon fiber electrodes. They show that motion artifacts generated by the movement of electrodes during electrophysiological recordings and fast-scan cyclic voltammetry are difficult to distinguish from the characteristic action potential and neurochemical signals. They hypothesize that motion alters the electrode/electrolyte interface by affecting the electric double layer to trigger the artifacts. Sharma et al. [14] address the "many wire" problem with the design and testing of a novel electronic architecture for intracortical neural recording. By integrating mixed-signal feedback, windowed integration sampling, and a successive approximation analog-to-digital converter, they show promising results from a 180 nm CMOS integrated circuit prototype capable of multiplexing high channel count microelectrode arrays. Xu et al. [15] offer a technological solution to the problem of simultaneous recording and stimulation. They propose a novel bidirectional neuromodulation system-on-chip, which includes a frequency-shaping neural recorder and a fully integrated neural stimulator with charge balancing capability. A prototype device was fabricated and shown to be capable of achieving simultaneous electrical stimulation and recording on the same nerve preparation in vivo.

To provide enhanced control during optogenetic studies, Goncalves et al. [16] describe a hybrid device combining optical stimulation and neural recording, which is capable of monitoring the heat generated during light exposure. A proof-of-concept device, with double-sided function: on one side, an optrode with LED-based stimulation and Pt recording sites on one side of the probe and with a Pt-based thin-film thermoresister for temperature measurement on the opposite side, was fabricated and characterized. The silicon-based device showed good recording and optical features with suitable optical power delivery and a high-resolution temperature monitoring, indicating that this optrode approach may be useful for limiting tissue damage from excessive heating. Scholvin et al. [17] report on a scalable, modular strategy for fabricating high-density 3D neural probes. They demonstrate a 3D probe constructed from individual 2D components where there are arrays of shanks consisting of densely packed, at a 40 μm pitch, electrode sites. The probes are assembled using mechanical self-locking and self-aligning techniques followed by electroless nickel plating to establish electrical contact. By combining scalable 3D design and high-density recording sites, this fabrication approach may enable new classes of devices capable of large-scale neural recording to elucidate the functional connectivity of the brain. Hoch et al. [18] address the problem associated with neural probe connector failure, which is triggered by excessive forces generated by repeated plugging/unplugging between recording sessions. They developed a new magnetic connector system that uses multiple magnet pairs and spring-suspended electrical contact pads realized using micro-electromechanical systems technologies to achieve reliable self-alignment of the connector parts at ±50 μm with negligible connection forces.

3. Biology of the Interface. Campbell and Wu [1] provide a comprehensive review of the tissue response to devices implanted within the brain and illustrate how both biotic and abiotic processes result in failure in bioelectrical performance. They discuss the tissue response to electrode implantation and the associated molecular pathways that act on acute and chronic timescales. In addition, they review current strategies to minimize the tissue response to enhance device reliability. Genetic tools offer an opportunity to target critical proteins that may have pivotal roles in neuroinflammatory response at the tissue–device interface. Winter et al. [19] characterize three different approaches for modifying gene expression at the tissue–device interface: viral-mediated overexpression, siRNA-enabled knockdown, and cre-dependent conditional expression. By making use of an implantable neural probe that incorporates microfluidics, they successfully delivered the vectors along the length of the device based on protein expression levels, indicating that this approach can be used to modulate various molecular pathways. In a meta-analysis derived from the published literature, Stiller et al. [2] explore the relationships between the neuroinflammatory responses to implanted devices that vary with respect to structural device stiffness, which is a function of both material modulus and cross-sectional area. By incorporating data from nine published studies, spanning a wide range of implant dimensions and materials, it was determined that the severity of the immune response, within the first 50 μm of the device, is highly correlated with device stiffness, as opposed to either the device modulus or cross-sectional area independently.

To complete the Special Issue, three papers provide insight into the past and future of neural electrodes. Shokoueinejad et al. [20] provide a historical perspective on the use and evolution of electrocorticography for a wide range of experimental and clinical applications. These grids, especially those that are 10–100 s of microns in dimension, offer the advantage of high-density neural signal acquisition and stimulation capabilities. In addition, this approach is considered relatively minimally invasive based on a muted neuroinflammatory response, at least compared to penetrating microelectrode arrays. Similar to electrocorticography arrays, devices suitable for recording the activity of the gut have been recently considered to shed light on the enteric nervous system. Barth et al. [21] describe the opportunity for advancing enteric neuroscience offered by single-unit recording capabilities in awake animals, using flexible conformal grids, and identify the primary design challenges for such devices. Finally, Kozai [22] provides a historical perspective on the progress and challenges for implantable neural electrodes, arguing that understanding the complexities associated with reliable chronic neural interfaces requires simultaneous proficiency in multiple scientific and engineering disciplines.

We extend our appreciation to all of the authors for their excellent contributions to this Special Issue of Micromachines. We also thank the peer referees who provided in depth, thoughtful, and rapid reviews of all of the manuscripts. Lastly, we acknowledge the dedicated journal staff of the editorial office who professionally and gracefully kept the entire process on track.

Conflicts of Interest: The authors declare no conflict of interest.

References

1. Campbell, A.; Wu, C. Chronically Implanted Intracranial Electrodes: Tissue Reaction and Electrical Changes. *Micromachines* **2018**, *9*, 430. [CrossRef] [PubMed]
2. Stiller, A.M.; Black, B.J.; Kung, C.; Ashok, A.; Cogan, S.F.; Varner, V.D.; Pancrazio, J.J. A Meta-Analysis of Intracortical Device Stiffness and Its Correlation with Histological Outcomes. *Micromachines* **2018**, *9*, 443. [CrossRef] [PubMed]
3. Hess-Dunning, A.; Tyler, D.J. A Mechanically-Adaptive Polymer Nanocomposite-Based Intracortical Probe and Package for Chronic Neural Recording. *Micromachines* **2018**, *9*, 583. [CrossRef] [PubMed]
4. Deku, F.; Frewin, C.L.; Stiller, A.; Cohen, Y.; Aqeel, S.; Joshi-Imre, A.; Black, B.; Gardner, T.J.; Pancrazio, J.J.; Cogan, S.F. Amorphous Silicon Carbide Platform for Next Generation Penetrating Neural Interface Designs. *Micromachines* **2018**, *9*, 480. [CrossRef] [PubMed]
5. Stiller, A.M.; Usoro, J.; Frewin, C.L.; Danda, V.R.; Ecker, M.; Joshi-Imre, A.; Musselman, K.C.; Voit, W.; Modi, R.; Pancrazio, J.J.; et al. Chronic Intracortical Recording and Electrochemical Stability of Thiol-ene/Acrylate Shape Memory Polymer Electrode Arrays. *Micromachines* **2018**, *9*, 500. [CrossRef] [PubMed]
6. Shoffstall, A.J.; Ecker, M.; Danda, V.; Joshi-Imre, A.; Stiller, A.; Yu, M.; Paiz, J.E.; Mancuso, E.; Bedell, H.W.; Voit, W.E.; et al. Characterization of the Neuroinflammatory Response to Thiol-ene Shape Memory Polymer Coated Intracortical Microelectrodes. *Micromachines* **2018**, *9*, 486. [CrossRef] [PubMed]
7. Rihani, R.T.; Kim, H.; Black, B.J.; Atmaramani, R.; Saed, M.O.; Pancrazio, J.J.; Ware, T.H. Liquid Crystal Elastomer-Based Microelectrode Array for In Vitro Neuronal Recordings. *Micromachines* **2018**, *9*, 416. [CrossRef]
8. Kil, D.; Carmona, M.B.; Ceyssens, F.; Deprez, M.; Brancato, L.; Nuttin, B.; Balschun, B.; Puers, R. Dextran as a Resorbable Coating Material for Flexible Neural Probes. *Micromachines* **2019**, *10*, 61. [CrossRef]
9. Bernardin, E.K.; Frewin, C.L.; Everly, R.; Ul Hassan, J.; Saddow, S.E. Demonstration of a Robust All-Silicon-Carbide Intracortical Neural Interface. *Micromachines* **2018**, *9*, 412. [CrossRef]
10. Sridharan, A.; Chirania, S.; Towe, B.C.; Muthuswamy, J. Remote Stimulation of Sciatic Nerve Using Cuff Electrodes and Implanted Diodes. *Micromachines* **2019**, *9*, 595. [CrossRef]
11. Straka, M.M.; Schafer, B.; Vasudevan, S.; Weller, C.; Rieth, L. Characterizing Longitudinal Changes in the Impedance Spectra of In-Vivo Peripheral Nerve Electrodes. *Micromachines* **2018**, *9*, 587. [CrossRef] [PubMed]
12. Vajari, D.A.; Vomero, M.; Erhardt, J.B.; Sadr, A.; Ordonez, J.S.; Coenen, V.A.; Stieglitz, T. Integrity Assessment of a Hybrid DBS Probe that Enables Neurotransmitter Detection Simultaneously to Electrical Stimulation and Recording. *Micromachines* **2018**, *9*, 510. [CrossRef] [PubMed]
13. Nicolai, E.N.; Michelson, N.J.; Settell, M.L.; Hara, S.A.; Trevathan, J.K.; Asp, A.J.; Stocking, K.C.; Lujan, J.L.; Kozai, T.D.Y.; Ludwig, K.A. Design Choices for Next-Generation Neurotechnology Can Impact Motion Artifact in Electrophysiological and Fast-Scan Cyclic Voltammetry Measurements. *Micromachines* **2018**, *9*, 494. [CrossRef] [PubMed]
14. Sharma, M.; Gardner, A.T.; Strathman, H.J.; Warren, D.J.; Silver, J.; Walker, R.M. Acquisition of Neural Action Potentials Using Rapid Multiplexing Directly at the Electrodes. *Micromachines* **2018**, *9*, 477. [CrossRef] [PubMed]
15. Xu, J.; Guo, H.; Nguyen, A.T.; Lim, H.; Yang, Z. A Bidirectional Neuromodulation Technology for Nerve Recording and Stimulation. *Micromachines* **2018**, *9*, 538. [CrossRef] [PubMed]
16. Goncalves, S.B.; Palha, J.M.; Fernandes, H.C.; Souto, M.R.; Pimenta, S.; Dong, T.; Yang, Z.; Ribeiro, J.F.; Correia, J.H. LED Optrode with Integrated Temperature Sensing for Optogenetics. *Micromachines* **2018**, *9*, 473. [CrossRef] [PubMed]
17. Scholvin, J.; Zorzos, A.; Kinney, J.; Bernstein, J.; Moore-Kochlacs, C.; Kopell, N.; Fonstad, C.; Boyden, E.S. Scalable, Modular Three-Dimensional Silicon Microelectrode Assembly via Electroless Plating. *Micromachines* **2018**, *9*, 436. [CrossRef]
18. Hoch, K.; Pothof, F.; Becker, F.; Paul, O.; Ruther, P. Development, Modeling, Fabrication, and Characterization of a Magnetic, Micro-Spring-Suspended System for the Safe Electrical Interconnection of Neural Implants. *Micromachines* **2018**, *9*, 424. [CrossRef]
19. Winter, B.M.; Daniels, S.R.; Salatino, J.W.; Purcell, E.K. Genetic Modulation at the Neural Microelectrode Interface: Methods and Applications. *Micromachines* **2018**, *9*, 476. [CrossRef]

20. Shokoueinejad, M.; Park, D.W.; Jung, Y.H.; Brodnick, S.K.; Novello, J.; Dingle, A.; Swanson, K.I.; Baek, D.H.; Suminski, A.J.; Lake, W.B.; et al. Progress in the Field of Micro-Electrocorticography. *Micromachines* **2019**, *10*, 62. [CrossRef]
21. Barth, B.B.; Huang, H.I.; Hammer, G.E.; Shen, X. Opportunities and Challenges for Single-Unit Recordings from Enteric Neurons in Awake Animals. *Micromachines* **2018**, *9*, 428. [CrossRef] [PubMed]
22. Kozai, T.D.Y. The History and Horizons of Microscale Neural Interfaces. *Micromachines* **2018**, *9*, 445. [CrossRef] [PubMed]

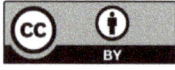

micromachines

MDPI

Review

Chronically Implanted Intracranial Electrodes: Tissue Reaction and Electrical Changes

Andrew Campbell [1,*] and Chengyuan Wu [2]

1   Sidney Kimmel Medical College, Thomas Jefferson University, Philadelphia, PA 19107, USA
2   Department of Neurological Surgery, Vickie and Jack Farber Institute for Neuroscience, Thomas Jefferson University Hospital, Philadelphia, PA 19107, USA; chengyuan.wu@jefferson.edu
*   Correspondence: andrew.campbell@jefferson.edu

Received: 18 July 2018; Accepted: 22 August 2018; Published: 25 August 2018

Abstract: The brain-electrode interface is arguably one of the most important areas of study in neuroscience today. A stronger foundation in this topic will allow us to probe the architecture of the brain in unprecedented functional detail and augment our ability to intervene in disease states. Over many years, significant progress has been made in this field, but some obstacles have remained elusive—notably preventing glial encapsulation and electrode degradation. In this review, we discuss the tissue response to electrode implantation on acute and chronic timescales, the electrical changes that occur in electrode systems over time, and strategies that are being investigated in order to minimize the tissue response to implantation and maximize functional electrode longevity. We also highlight the current and future clinical applications and relevance of electrode technology.

Keywords: intracranial electrodes; foreign body reaction; electrode degradation; glial encapsulation

1. Introduction

The brain-electrode interface is one of the most exciting topics in modern neuroscience. Progress in this field represents the culmination of research in separate collaborating disciplines including materials science, neural engineering, and neurosurgery among others. We are now able to record from and stimulate the brain at the level of individual neurons, termed single-units, which holds great promise for future research, and clinical applications.

In humans, advances in recording and neuromodulation technology have led to new medical devices that use electrodes for neural recording, stimulation, or both in the central nervous system (CNS) and peripheral nervous system (PNS). Examples of these breakthroughs include stereo electroencephalography (sEEG), where implanted recording depth electrodes have enhanced our ability to detect and localize epileptogenic foci in the brain (see Figure 1A); deep brain stimulation (DBS), which involves the placement of stimulating electrodes into brain areas for therapeutic effect in conditions like Parkinson's disease or essential tremor; and responsive neurostimulation (RNS), which aims to both detect seizure activity and respond with electrical stimuli that essentially stops seizures before they start (see Figure 1B). Spinal cord and vagal nerve stimulators as well as cochlear implants are additional examples of neuromodulation devices capable of providing patients relief from back pain, control of drug-resistant epileptic seizures, and even the ability to hear, respectively.

Although these technologies exemplify remarkable medical achievements, further work in this field has involved the incorporation of brain-computer interfaces (BCIs) and neuroprosthetics in humans, which rely on the precision that can be achieved through the implantation of chronic microelectrode arrays into the brain parenchyma. However, there are a number of obstacles that must be overcome before long-term stability of the tissue-electrode interface can be achieved. While the issues of glial encapsulation and electrode degradation remain at the forefront of current thinking, a precise and complete understanding of the mechanisms underlying electrode failure over time has yet to be attained. In this review, we will explore the tissue-electrode interface, with particular focus on the acute and chronic inflammatory reactions, changes that occur in electrodes, and strategies being investigated to mitigate these issues.

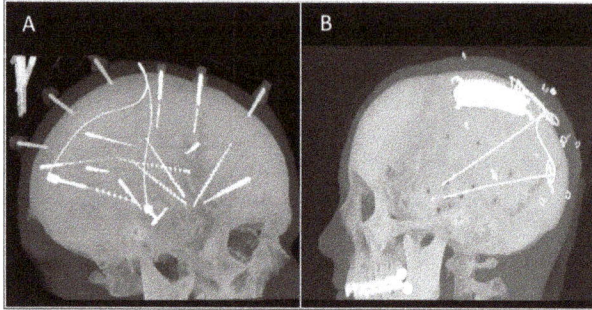

Figure 1. Computed tomography (CT) reconstruction images of patients after implantation of (**A**) sEEG electrodes and (**B**) RNS system.

2. Contemporary Recording and Stimulation Systems

Overview

While a nuanced discussion about electrode hardware is beyond the scope of this review, we will address the basic electrode types in this section. In recent years, there have been numerous electrode systems manufactured for use in scientific and clinical applications. These applications range from recording and stimulation studies in basic neuroscience animal research to deep brain stimulation (DBS) in Parkinson's disease or intracranial electroencephalography (iEEG) recording for investigating drug-resistant epilepsy. After traditional scalp EEG electrodes, progressively more invasive placement options include epidural, subdural, intracortical, and depth electrodes (see Figure 2). This increased invasiveness puts the electrodes in closer proximity to the neurons producing the signals of interest, which allows for improved detection and stimulation. For example, iEEG using a grid of subdural electrodes, or electrocorticography (ECoG), has distinct advantages over traditional scalp EEG including an increased signal-to-noise ratio, superior spatial resolution, and greater spectral frequency [1].

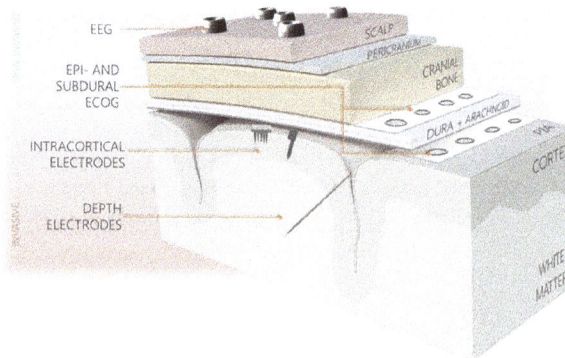

Figure 2. Types of brain interfacing electrodes and their locations in reference to the brain. Reproduced with permission from Creative Commons open access policy from [2].

Intracortical electrodes, such as the popular Utah microelectrode array, and depth electrodes are even more invasive and are placed within the brain parenchyma, next to the nuclei or even individual neurons of interest (Figure 2). They allow for an even greater spatial and temporal resolution than subdural electrodes and are capable of single-neuron recording. In contrast with subdural grid placement, depth electrodes in DBS for Parkinson's disease or sEEG in epilepsy do not require an extensive craniotomy for implantation and can instead be implanted through a small burr hole.

3. Tissue Reaction and Histopathologic Observations Due to Electrode Implantation

3.1. Overview

Understanding the neural tissue response to device implantation is pivotal for achieving long-term stability and viability of neuroprosthetics and neurostimulation systems. On shorter timescales, recording and stimulating electrodes are able to achieve impressive functionality. But for chronic implants, the body's response at the tissue-microelectrode interface eventually leads to mechanical failure and signal degradation [3–9]. Despite extensive investigations into the inflammatory response and numerous trials investigating strategies to mitigate it, clearing this hurdle has remained elusive [5,6,10–37]. It is consequentially one of the most important obstacles to overcome in order for neural interface technology to be fully realized. In this section we will review current understanding of the tissue reaction to implanted devices.

Microglia, astrocytes, and oligodendrocytes are the three main glial cell types in the brain. The actions of microglia and astrocytes after electrode implantation are key in both short and long-term responses to injury [3]. Microglia function as immunologic surveillance in the CNS by monitoring neuronal health and responding to injury [38]. They function as cytotoxic cells, killing pathogenic organisms and phagocytes that secrete proteolytic enzymes to degrade cellular debris and damaged extracellular matrix during regular turnover or after injury [3]. Microglia exist in an inactivated or "ramified" state, exhibiting a branched morphology, sampling the microenvironment until a stimulus, such as injury, leads to activation [3,38]. Once activated, they begin proliferating and undergo a morphology change to a more compact, "amoeboid" state [3,38]. In this state, the activated microglia phagocytose foreign material, upregulate cell-surface receptors, increase secretion of reactive oxygen species, and produce more lytic enzymes, pro-inflammatory cytokines, and cytotoxic factors [3,38]. Activated microglia have many of the same markers as macrophages, including ED1, which is used for immunohistochemical staining to visualize and quantify microglia in tissue sections [5].

Astrocytes, so named due to their star-like set of cytoplasmic extensions, have many roles in the CNS [3]. These functions include providing mechanical support to circuits of neurons, aiding in control of the neuronal chemical microenvironment, providing growth cues during development, and modulating the firing patterns of neurons [3]. They have a pivotal role in nutrient transfer across the blood brain barrier (BBB), regulating this process via specialized extensions, called end feet, which interface with the capillary walls [3]. After tissue injury, astrocytes become reactive and undergo hypertrophy, proliferation, and upregulate the expression of glial fibrillary acidic protein (GFAP), which is a common target for astrocyte detection in immunostaining [3,5,10,38,39].

Oligodendrocytes have the key role of electrically insulating axons projecting from neurons in the CNS. These cells extend their cytoplasm to form sheaths of myelin that surround axons, greatly increasing the conduction velocity of signals propagating down axons [3].

3.2. Initial Injury and Acute Tissue Response to Intraparenchymal Electrode Insertion

When an electrode is inserted into the brain, it first passes through the meninges, consisting of the dura mater (which is usually reflected prior to implantation), the arachnoid, and pia mater. Arteries and veins on the pial surface must be avoided [40]. The cortex below has the highest vascular density in the brain, consisting of numerous capillaries and small-caliber arteries [40]. As the electrode is inserted, these vessels are ruptured, severed, and pulled, leading to bleeding, serum protein leakage, and infiltration of neutrophils, blood-borne macrophages, and T-lymphocytes [3,4,40]. In addition to vascular damage, during insertion, the electrode tears the extracellular matrix, ruptures neuronal and glial cell bodies and processes, and causes tissue displacement [3,4,40]. The electrode pushes progressively more tissue aside as it travels deeper, creating a high-pressure region around it [3].

Immediately following electrode insertion, microglial cells in the vicinity of the probe become activated, and respond to the injury by sending long projections toward the injury site [11]. Although the mechanism for microglial activation is unknown, the rapidity of this response suggests that a chemical gradient is immediately generated and may be related to cellular debris, messenger molecules released from dying cells, and leaking plasma contents [11,40]. After approximately 12 h, the microglial cells begin to migrate towards the implant; and by 24 h post implantation, the tissue around the implant is surrounded by a greater density of microglial cells (see Figure 3) [4,10,11].

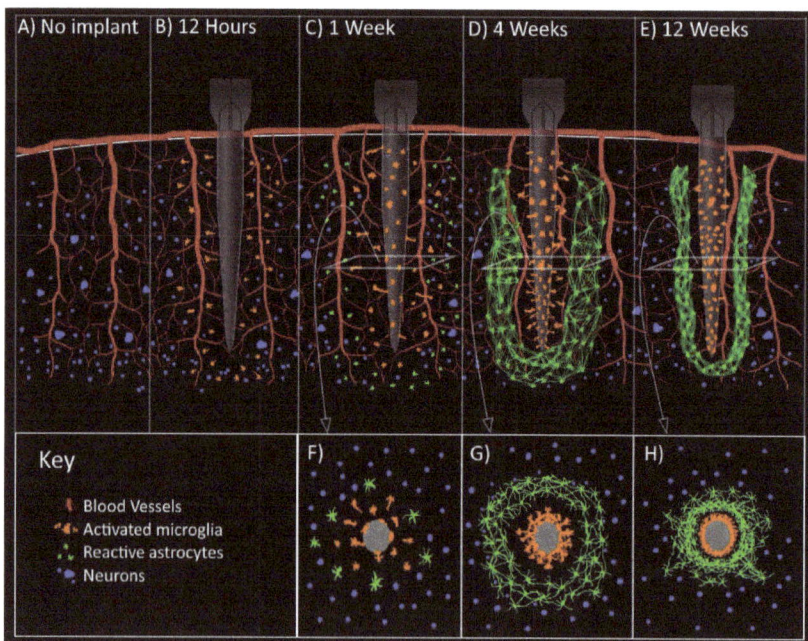

Figure 3. Illustration of the glial encapsulation response (**A**) prior to implantation, (**B**) 12 h post-implantation, (**C**) 1 week post-implantation, (**D**) 4 weeks post-implantation, and (**E**) 12 weeks post-implantation. Panels (**F**), (**G**), and (**H**) represent cross sectional views of (**C**), (**D**), and (**E**), respectively.

Astrocytes appear to have a more varied and slower reaction than microglia to tissue injury, with a response that becomes robust over several days rather than almost immediately. Results from histochemical analysis and live imaging studies reveal that at least three distinct types of astrocytes react to stab wound injury [10,39]. One study demonstrated significant heterogeneity of astrocyte behavior, where certain subsets of astrocytes proliferated or became polarized and extended processes to the site of injury [39]. It was also shown that astrocytes do not migrate after tissue injury and that increases in detected GFAP immunostaining after injury are due primarily to upregulation of GFAP expression rather than astrocyte proliferation (although some proliferation does occur, particularly in astrocytes close to blood vessels near the injury site) [39].

Release of blood and plasma contents from the disrupted BBB post implantation contributes to the recruitment of activated microglia and astrocyte activation [3,4,6,10,12,40]. Specific plasma proteins that deposit into CNS tissue following vascular disruption include albumin, globulins, fibrin/fibrinogen, thrombin, plasmin, complement, and hemosiderin [4,40]. In particular, thrombin has been implicated in triggering astrogliosis and microglial activation [40]. The cellular effects due to thrombin are mediated by proteinase-activated receptors (PARs) [40]. Thrombin activates the PAR-1 receptor on astrocytes, inducing morphological changes, proliferation, and the release of inflammatory mediators [40]. Mice deficient in PAR-1 were noted to have reduced astrocyte activation after a cortical stab wound, supporting the role of thrombin in astrogliosis [40]. Additionally, thrombin induces microglial proliferation and activation via the action of PAR-1 and PAR-4 receptors, respectively [40].

Albumin binds to transforming growth factor beta (TGF-beta) receptors in astrocytes, inducing upregulation of myosin light chain kinase (MLCK) expression [4]. MLCK phosphorylates myosin light chain (MLC), which leads to contractions, weakening of endothelial cell-to-cell adhesion, and ultimately increased BBB permeability [4]. Inhibition of MLCK has been shown to reduce edema following traumatic brain injury in mice, although this did not improve neurologic outcomes or significantly alter lesion histology [41]. Albumin also leads to astrocyte and microglial activation via the mitogen-activated protein kinase (MAPK) pathway, resulting in increased IL-1β and nitric oxide levels in astrocytes [4]. Fibrinogen is polymerized in the perivascular space to fibrin in the CNS leading to the activation of microglia [4]. Depletion of fibrin is associated with inhibition of microglial activation and attenuated inflammatory demyelination of neurons [4].

Many inflammatory mediators are part of the brain tissue response to injury during electrode implantation. Some of the most prominent chemical mediators we will consider are TNF-α, IL-1, IL-6, MCP-1, and TGF-β. TNF-α expression appears to be caused by the initial implantation injury with elevated mRNA levels present around the electrode-tissue interface at one week following implantation that diminish by four weeks [40,42]. Activated macrophages that infiltrate from the breached BBB and activated microglia are significant early sources of TNF-α [40]. IL-1 has many effects on glial cells and neurons, with particularly strong effects on astrocytes, including the promotion and modulation of astrogliosis [40]. IL-1 exists in both a membrane bound (IL-1α) and secreted form (IL-1β) [40]. IL-1β is one of the most significantly upregulated cytokines in the response to implantation, and it is rapidly produced by activated microglia within 15 min of cortical injury [4,40]. It is a major pro-inflammatory cytokine with important roles in inflammation and apoptosis [4].

While TNF-α and IL-1 tend to exert mainly pro-inflammatory effects, IL-6 has both pro-inflammatory and anti-inflammatory properties [40]. IL-6 is produced by microglia, astrocytes, and endothelial cells as part of the downstream sequence of IL-1 and TNF-α signaling, and it has been shown to downregulate the expression of TNF-α and promote neuronal survival and neurite outgrowth [40,43]. Its overexpression causes a pathologic response, leading to reactive gliosis, neurodegeneration, breakdown of the BBB, and angiogenesis [44]. This suggests that tight regulation of IL-6 is necessary in order to promote its beneficial effects [43]. TGF-β is similarly both pro-inflammatory and anti-inflammatory, and it has been shown to inhibit glial cell proliferation as well as expression of IL-1 and TNF-alpha [40,42]. It is normally present in the brain at low levels, but, after injury, appears to be upregulated in astrocytes around the site of tissue damage [40,42]. At these higher concentrations, it plays a role in reactive astrogliosis and scar formation, with studies demonstrating attenuation of the scarring response when TGF-β function is blocked with antibodies [40].

Proteases, such as matrix metalloproteases (MMPs), are expressed in activated glial cells and have been shown to have both beneficial and harmful effects [40]. MMPs may contribute to neuronal cell death by degrading the extracellular matrix protein laminin, but could also facilitate removal of debris after injury via this same process [40]. After a cortical stab wound or electrode implantation, the expression of MMPs is increased within 24 h in the tissue around the site of injury [4,40]. This includes MMP-9 which is known to degrade gap junctions of BBB endothelial cells, and therefore disrupt the BBB [4].

Reactive oxygen species (ROS) are oxygen free radicals that can exert oxidative stress on cells when produced in excess [40]. Following injury, as red blood cells are being broken down, there is an increase in hemoglobin that leads to an increase in ROS [4]. In this context, production of the

ROS nitric oxide (NO), which is normally neutralized by cellular antioxidants, can overpower the antioxidants, resulting in cellular damage [39]. In addition, ROS downregulate tight junction proteins, which increases BBB permeability [4]. This setting of increased oxidative stress leads to activation and upregulation pro-inflammatory cytokines [4].

3.3. Foreign Body Reaction and Sustained Inflammatory Response

Long-term application of intraparenchymal electrodes is limited partly by a chronic tissue response that consists of the foreign body reaction and sustained inflammation. This leads to the formation of a glial encapsulation or sheath that interferes with the recording and stimulating of neurons. Factors that contribute to this persistent response are initial tissue injury, micromotion of the electrode, persistent BBB leakage, and mechanical compliance mismatch between electrodes and brain tissue. The sustained response appears to be dependent on continual interaction between the electrode and the surrounding tissue. Conversely in stab wound studies, the inflammatory response has been shown to steadily decrease to resolution after the initial injury reaction [13,45]. Similar to the inflammatory response, neuronal cell death that occurs in the space around the electrode also appears to be greatly influenced by the tissue response associated with its continued presence rather than just the initial stab injury [13].

One week after implantation, an increased density of ED1 staining microglia can be seen, extending around the injury site covering an area approximately 3–4 times the size of the stab wound void left after electrode explantation (Figure 3) [10]. The ED1 positive microglia closest to the injury site send out short, thick processes, while those further away exhibit a highly elongated morphology [10]. Similarly, an increase in number and intensity of GFAP staining astrocytes is also seen around the wound void [10]. A number of these cells possess cytoplasmic processes that extended to the injury site [10].

At two weeks, the density of ED1 staining microglia immediately around the electrode increases and reactive astrocytes begin forming a GFAP staining sheath that surrounds this space [5,10,13,45]. The cellular distribution appears to represent distinct, segregated layers of ED1 and GFAP staining cells [5,13]. These layers of immunoreactivity suggest a structure characterized by an inner microglial core in contact with the electrode, which drops off by about 50 µm, and a shell of surrounding astrocytes, which predominately occupy the 50–150 µm space surrounding this core [5,10,13]. Neurons in the vicinity of the implant site have died off at this point, indicated by the significantly decreased number of NeuN staining neuronal cell bodies in the 50 µm surrounding the electrode [5,13].

After four weeks, the density of ED1 staining microglia directly around the electrode continues to increase, while the overall amount of ED1 reactivity in the vicinity around the electrode is not significantly different compared to two weeks (Figure 3) [5,13]. The microglia appear to form a more compact structure around the electrode with increasing time [5,13]. In contrast with microglia, statistically significant increases in GFAP reactivity within 100 µm of the electrode at four weeks compared to two weeks have been observed [5]. This suggests that astrocytes play a role in the core region of the glial sheath as the sustained tissue response develops.

At six and 12 weeks, both the ED1 and GFAP staining layers of microglia and astrocytes are more compact and localized (Figure 3) [5,10,45]. Overall the layers become thinner but stronger and denser, with less ED1 and GFAP reactivity found outside of these layers [5,10,45]. This coincides with the peak of GFAP intensity shifting closer to the implant site, suggesting contraction of the reactive astrocytes over time [5]. At this point, the glial sheath has effectively walled the implant off from the rest of the brain tissue with minimal extension of the inflammatory response into the surrounding area. It should be noted that at these later time points, there is significant variability in the degree of these immunohistochemically visualized cellular responses, which tend to coincide with similar variability in the changes occurring in individual electrodes [5,46,47].

3.4. Tissue Response to Subdural Electrodes

While the above discussion has been focused mainly on the tissue response to intraparenchymal electrode insertion, a chronic foreign body reaction occurs due to subdural electrode implantation as well. There is a growing interest in the use of chronic subdural electrodes in brain machine interfaces and neuroprosthetics; but, to the best of our knowledge, there is a paucity of literature describing the chronic inflammatory changes associated with subdural ECoG systems [48]. Therefore, long-term studies evaluating tissue response and subdural electrode function are necessary to determine viability and feasibility for extended use.

Histological studies that have been conducted thus far in humans involve shorter timescales, as they are limited to patients receiving invasive monitoring for epilepsy who subsequently undergo surgical resections. In one study, tissue samples were examined on the order of days to several weeks after subdural electrode implantation, and have shown chronic meningeal and perivascular inflammation consisting of lymphocytes and macrophages to be the most common histopathologic finding [49]. Longer investigations have been performed in animals, with recent studies involving the use of micro-ECoG subdural implants in rats revealing vascular growth through holes in the electrode substrate material and moderate tissue reactivity at 25 weeks post implantation on histopathologic analysis [50,51]. Similarly, a nearly two-year case study of a rhesus monkey implanted with a subdural ECoG array demonstrated minimal inflammatory response, with fibrous encapsulation surrounding the grid following explantation [48]. The cortex below the implant appeared to be unaffected by the grid and was consistent with the contralateral hemisphere where no grid had been placed [48]. These results, as well as the success of long term RNS systems in human patients, are encouraging for the prolonged application of subdural electrodes.

4. Changes in Electrode Signaling Over Time

Factors Influencing Electrode Function

There are many factors that contribute to the changing function of electrodes. With time, the common endpoint of these changes is a diminished ability to record neurons and elicit responses through stimulation [4,6–8]. The metric most often correlated with changes in electrode function is electrical impedance at the tissue-electrode interface. Impedance refers to the resistance to the flow of charged particles, or current, in a circuit or circuit component. At the tissue-electrode interface, impedance is inversely related to the volume of tissue activated by stimulating electrodes and the listening sphere of recording electrodes [52,53]. If the impedance is low, current can flow more freely in the volume around the tissue-electrode interface, resulting in a larger stimulation and recording radius. In addition to measurement of the magnitude of impedance, some groups have used complex impedance spectroscopy as a method of detecting more specific changes at the tissue-electrode interface [46,47,54,55].

In the first few weeks after implantation, impedance rises quickly and then begins to stabilize [47,54–56]. The initial rise is thought to be due to the tissue reaction and this is supported by histological studies correlating the degree of tissue encapsulation with the magnitude of impedance increases [47,55]. Glial scarring and the attachment of molecular and cellular species to the electrode surface increase impedance, but these components are not considered to be sufficient to hinder electrode function or cause failure [56,57]. This finding has led some groups to suggest that eliminating the glial scar may not be required in order to achieve long term electrode stability [56].

While the precise interplay is not currently understood, several influences may contribute to the impedance changes that occur at the tissue-electrode interface. These factors can be roughly differentiated by biotic effects and abiotic effects [53,58,59]. Biotic effects refer to tissue reactions such as glial encapsulation, BBB disruption, and macrophage recruitment to the implant site [53,58,59]. Abiotic effects refer to causes of electrode degradation including electrode corrosion, insulation delamination, and cracking (See Figure 4) [53,58,59]. Insulation delamination of the electrode, caused by the corrosion and degradation secondary to the persistent inflammatory response, can result in a lower impedance than the original reference impedance of an electrode [58,59].

In a long term study in non-human primates, one group showed that, for silicon-based intracortical microelectrode arrays (MEAs), the most common type of electrode failure was acute mechanical failures, accounting for 48% percent of the failures in the study, while biological causes accounted for about 24% of failures [8]. They found that most failures occurred in the first year after implantation and that, after an initial increase, impedance slowly declined along with signal quality, suggesting that insulation material degradation is one of the most important factors in long term viability of silicon MEAs [8]. This same group also performed scanning electron microscopy (SEM) on silicon MEAs with platinum electrode tips implanted for long durations in non-human primates, and revealed that progressive corrosion occurs over time at the electrode tips as well as cracking and delamination of the parylene insulation [9]. In addition, the tissue encapsulation response was shown to grow into defects formed in the platinum and parylene over time [9].

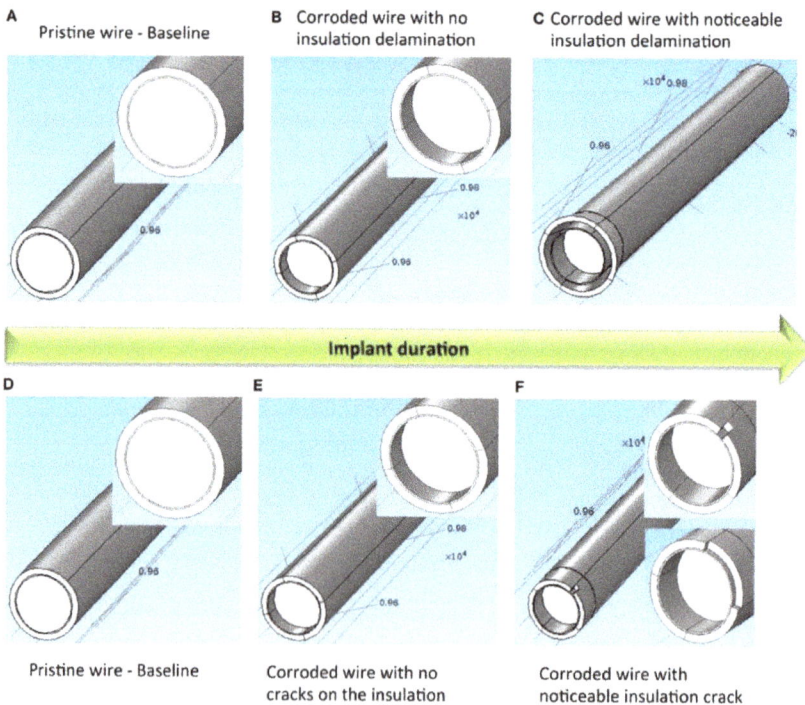

Figure 4. Two models of electrode degradation. (**A**) Pristine electrode with intact metal and insulation, (**B**) electrode with corroded metal and no insulation delamination, and (**C**) electrode with corroded metal and noticeable insulation delamination. (**D**) Pristine electrode with intact metal and insulation, (**E**) electrode with corroded metal and no insulation crack, and (**F**) electrode with corroded metal and noticeable insulation crack. Inset on the left, middle and right images shows a closer view of the gold layer around the tungsten. Illustration and caption reproduced with permission from Creative Commons open access policy from [58].

Interestingly, clinically-relevant stimulation in DBS electrodes has been associated with rapid and reversible changes in impedance [54]. Immediately following the cessation of stimulation, impedance begins to rise and eventually reaches pre-stimulation levels within a few days, revealing the dynamic nature of the foreign body reaction [54]. It is thought that stimulation temporarily "cleans off" adherent molecules and cells that are attached to the electrode, but it does not clear away the encapsulation sheath surrounding the electrode [54,60]. This "rejuvenation" stimulation has also been shown to decrease impedance and increase the signal to noise ratio at the electrode-tissue interface, and it has been suggested that this could be used as treatment to improve the quality of stimulation and recording in chronically implanted microelectrodes [60]. As such, both short term and long term factors appear to effect electrode impedance [53]. Electrode functionality can be predicted with impedance measurements, and actively controlling impedance over time may be a possible strategy to improve long term performance and neuronal yield [53].

5. Strategies for Reducing Chronic Tissue Reaction

5.1. Overview

Many strategies to reduce the foreign body reaction have been investigated that focus on different factors involved in the generation of the response. The main types of approaches can be broken down into mechanically based and biologically based, with some degree of overlap existing. These strategies range from adjusting material properties of the electrodes to delivering anti-inflammatory drugs to the implant site. Minimizing neuronal loss, promoting neural regeneration, and limiting the formation of the glial sheath are the end goals of these different strategies. A combined approach will likely be necessary due to the multiple mechanisms involved in the inflammatory and regenerative responses.

5.2. Insertional Approaches

If we start from the beginning of the electrode implantation process, planning the insertional trajectory is one way to potentially reduce the tissue response. Avoiding damage to major blood vessels can lessen the overall BBB disruption, minimizing this contribution to the overall post-implantation inflammation [12]. Large intracortical blood vessels do not penetrate perpendicularly into the brain, but instead deviate slightly from the normal axis [12]. Inserting electrodes on the normal axis at a distance greater than 49 μm from a major blood vessel greatly reduces the likelihood of disrupting the penetrating segment of these vessels deeper in the brain [12]. Interestingly, neuronal nuclei lie further away from blood vessels than would be expected in a random distribution, which suggests that avoiding major blood vessels would also allow for better recording and stimulation [12]. In addition to trajectory, the insertional velocity and implant diameter has also been studied, with evidence showing fast insertions (2000 μm/s) and sharp implants to be superior at minimizing tissue strain and vascular injury [14].

5.3. Mechanical Approaches

Mechanical considerations such as the size, flexibility, and material density of electrodes relative to the tissue density are important factors in the foreign body reaction. Compliant electrodes can be made using ultra-thin geometries or very soft materials [15]. Newer generations of electrodes have become considerably smaller and thinner, and it has been shown that smaller implants lead to less initial tissue damage, decreased neuronal loss in the vicinity of the electrode, and reduced chronic tissue responses [15,16]. Similarly, implanted ultrasoft microwire electrodes consisting of elastomers and conducting polymers mechanically similar to brain tissue display a reduced inflammatory response compared to tungsten electrodes [17].

The thinking behind flexible and density matched electrodes is that they exhibit less micromotion related trauma and inflammation over time and therefore increase electrode longevity. Flexible microwire electrodes implanted into rabbit cortex displayed diminished foreign body response and increased neuronal density around the electrode relative to conventional microwire over 26–96 weeks indwelling periods [18]. This is despite the insertional method for the flexible microwire electrode being inherently more traumatic than conventional microwire, due to the requirement of a stiff, sharp carrier to guide it into place [18]. The densities of stainless steel (8 g/cm^3), tungsten

(19.25 g/cm^3), and platinum (21.45 g/cm^3) and iridium (22.6 g/cm^3) are much greater than that of brain tissue (0.99 g/cm^3) [19]. Significantly reduced astrocytic and microglial reactions have been observed at 6 weeks post implantation around 500 μm diameter low density electrodes more analogous to that of brain tissue (1.16–1.48 g/cm^3) relative to high density electrodes of the same size (22.45 g/cm^3) [19].

In one study, mechanically-adaptive implants were introduced into the brain that were rigid at first but became compliant after implantation [20]. Interestingly, while the acute tissue response was comparable to stiff control implants, the chronic inflammatory response was significantly reduced and the BBB was more stable [20]. Another interesting strategy being investigated involves promoting integration of the surrounding brain tissue with electrodes by structuring the surface topography of electrodes on the microscale or nanoscale level, with some results indicating increased neuronal survival in the 100 μm surrounding the implant [21].

Of note, it has been shown that implants tethered to the skull have a significantly increased inflammatory response [22]. This is thought to be due to the migration and colonization of fibroblasts from the meninges to the electrode-tissue interface [22]. Finally, these tissue reactions appear to occur independently; when multiple electrodes were separately implanted onto rat cortex, they did not aggravate the tissue reactions occurring at the other implant sites [23].

5.4. Biological Approaches

Biologically based strategies focus on attenuating the inflammatory response and promoting neuronal regeneration. Dexamethasone, a synthetic glucocorticoid, has been infused intramuscularly, coated on electrodes, and perfused through microdialysis probes, with all methods diminishing the reactive tissue response [24–26]. Probes coated with neural adhesion molecule L1 have been shown to have a reduced early microglial response, completely diminished loss of neuronal cell bodies, increased axonal density in the electrode vicinity relative to the background tissue, and significantly lowered activation of microglia and reactive astrocytes relative to uncoated probes [27,28]. A recent study showed that an astrocyte-derived extracellular matrix coating reduced the degree of astrogliosis surrounding a chronically implanted electrode [29].

Peptide-based coatings are also being explored with promising preliminary in vitro results [30]. In addition, silicon-based probes seeded with neural progenitor cells have been implanted into rat brains with early results showing that the cells can be successfully be implanted and may diminish the surrounding astrocytic response [31]. Probes capable of both drug delivery and electrophysiology recordings have also been designed and implanted with early success [32].

Targeting CD14 in circulating myeloid cells and not brain-derived microglia has been shown to improve chronic microelectrode recording, measured by the number of single neuron units detected per electrode channel and the percentage of electrode channels detecting single neurons [33]. The role of CD14 activity in microglia may be neuroprotective as complete knockout of CD14 in mice did not produce as a strong an improvement in microelectrode recordings as CD14 inhibition in macrophages [33]. This group also demonstrated that complete knockout of CD14 resulted in microelectrode improvement in acute but not chronic time periods, while inhibition of CD14 using a small molecule inhibitor called IAXO-101 improved both acute and chronic performance [34]. Together, these results suggest that therapies do not necessarily need to cross the BBB to benefit the quality of microelectrode recording after implantation [33,34].

Anti-oxidant therapy using resveratrol has been investigated as a potential therapeutic agent for mitigating the inflammatory response to electrode implantation [35–37]. Resveratrol is an anti-oxidant molecule derived from grapes that can suppress the accumulation of ROS [35]. In one study, resveratrol was incorporated onto intracortical implants consisting of physiologically responsive mechanically adaptive nanocomposites [35]. The materials in this device are initially stiff, allowing for placement, but then soften after implantation, becoming mechanically compliant with the brain tissue [35]. This material combined with the film of resveratrol, allowing for three days of localized delivery, resulted in reduced microglial activation and improved neuronal density at two weeks post implantation [35]. Another group studied the effects of intraperitoneal resveratrol injections in rats administered both 16–24 h before and immediately following implantation of single-shank Michigan style electrodes [36,37]. The results suggest that initial suppression of reactive oxygen species leads to chronic improvement in neuronal viability [36,37]. Decreased expression of toll-like receptor 4 was identified at week 2 post implantation, but not at later time points, and likely contributes to these beneficial effects [36]. However, intraperitoneal administration of resveratrol was also associated with some side effects in this study, including increased BBB permeability and adhesions [37].

6. Conclusions

The current progress toward achieving stable, long term electrode implantation is promising, but additional improvements still need to be made. A complete understanding of the tissue response to electrodes and mastery of implant materials and biocompatibility will enhance our ability to manipulate the foreign body reaction and lead to electrodes that do not degrade over time, allowing for the realization of chronic viability. These are challenging problems that have been investigated for decades, testing the creativity and intuition of several scientific and engineering disciplines, but incremental progress has been made and is poised to continue.

Author Contributions: A.C. primarily authored this review article. C.W. edited and contributed to the organization and scope of the article.

Funding: The APC was funded by the Department of Neurological Surgery of the Vickie and Jack Farber Institute for Neuroscience at Thomas Jefferson University.

Conflicts of Interest: The authors declare no conflict of interest.

References

1. Adewole, D.O.; Serruya, M.D.; Harris, J.P.; Burrell, J.C.; Petrov, D.; Chen, H.I.; Wolf, J.A.; Cullen, D.K. The Evolution of Neuroprosthetic Interfaces. *Crit. Rev. Biomed. Eng.* **2016**, *44*, 123–152. [CrossRef] [PubMed]
2. Szostak, K.M.; Grand, L.; Constandinou, T.G. Neural Interfaces for Intracortical Recording: Requirements, Fabrication Methods, and Characteristics. *Front. Neurosci.* **2017**, *11*, 665. [CrossRef] [PubMed]
3. Polikov, V.S.; Tresco, P.A.; Reichert, W.M. Response of brain tissue to chronically implanted neural electrodes. *J. Neurosci. Methods* **2005**, *148*, 1–18. [CrossRef] [PubMed]
4. Kozai, T.D.Y.; Jaquins-Gerstl, A.S.; Vazquez, A.L.; Michael, A.C.; Cui, X.T. Brain Tissue Responses to Neural Implants Impact Signal Sensitivity and Intervention Strategies. *ACS Chem. Neurosci.* **2015**, *6*, 48–67. [CrossRef] [PubMed]
5. Winslow, B.D.; Tresco, P.A. Quantitative analysis of the tissue response to chronically implanted microwire electrodes in rat cortex. *Biomaterials* **2010**, *31*, 1558–1567. [CrossRef] [PubMed]
6. Nolta, N.F.; Christensen, M.B.; Crane, P.D.; Skousen, J.L.; Tresco, P.A. BBB leakage, astrogliosis, and tissue loss correlate with silicon microelectrode array recording performance. *Biomaterials* **2015**, *53*, 753–762. [CrossRef] [PubMed]
7. Thomas, G.P.; Jobst, B.C. Critical review of the responsive neurostimulator system for epilepsy. *Med. Devices* **2015**, *8*, 405–411. [CrossRef]
8. Barrese, J.C.; Rao, N.; Paroo, K.; Triebwasser, C.; Vargas-Irwin, C.; Franquemont, L.; Donoghue, J.P. Failure mode analysis of silicon-based intracortical microelectrode arrays in non-human primates. *J. Neural Eng.* **2013**, *10*, 066014. [CrossRef] [PubMed]
9. Barrese, J.C.; Aceros, J.; Donoghue, J.P. Scanning electron microscopy of chronically implanted intracortical microelectrode arrays in non-human primates. *J. Neural Eng.* **2016**, *13*, 026003. [CrossRef] [PubMed]
10. Szarowski, D.H.; Andersen, M.D.; Retterer, S.; Spence, A.J.; Isaacson, M.; Craighead, H.G.; Turner, J.N.; Shain, W. Brain responses to micro-machined silicon devices. *Brain Res.* **2003**, *983*, 23–35. [CrossRef]
11. Kozai, T.D.Y.; Vazquez, A.L.; Weaver, C.L.; Kim, S.-G.; Cui, X.T. In vivo two-photon microscopy reveals immediate microglial reaction to implantation of microelectrode through extension of processes. *J. Neural Eng.* **2012**, *9*, 066001. [CrossRef] [PubMed]

12. Kozai, T.D.Y.; Marzullo, T.C.; Hooi, F.; Langhals, N.B.; Majewska, A.K.; Brown, E.B.; Kipke, D.R. Reduction of neurovascular damage resulting from microelectrode insertion into cerebral cortex using in vivo two-photon mapping. *J. Neural Eng.* **2010**, *7*, 046011. [CrossRef] [PubMed]

13. Biran, R.; Martin, D.C.; Tresco, P.A. Neuronal cell loss accompanies the brain tissue response to chronically implanted silicon microelectrode arrays. *Exp. Neurol.* **2005**, *195*, 115–126. [CrossRef] [PubMed]

14. Bjornsson, C.S.; Oh, S.J.; Al-Kofahi, Y.A.; Lim, Y.J.; Smith, K.L.; Turner, J.N.; De, S.; Roysam, B.; Shain, W.; Kim, S.J. Effects of insertion conditions on tissue strain and vascular damage during neuroprosthetic device insertion. *J. Neural Eng.* **2006**, *3*, 196–207. [CrossRef] [PubMed]

15. Pancrazio, J.J.; Deku, F.; Ghazavi, A.; Stiller, A.M.; Rihani, R.; Frewin, C.L.; Varner, V.D.; Gardner, T.J.; Cogan, S.F. Thinking Small: Progress on Microscale Neurostimulation Technology. *Neuromodulation* **2017**, *20*, 745–752. [CrossRef] [PubMed]

16. Kozai, T.D.; Langhals, N.B.; Patel, P.R.; Deng, X.; Zhang, H.; Smith, K.L.; Lahann, J.; Kotov, N.A.; Kipke, D.R. Ultrasmall implantable composite microelectrodes with bioactive surfaces for chronic neural interfaces. *Nat. Mater.* **2012**, *11*, 1065–1073. [CrossRef] [PubMed]

17. Du, Z.J.; Kolarcik, C.L.; Kozai, T.D.Y.; Luebben, S.D.; Sapp, S.A.; Zheng, X.S.; Nabity, J.A.; Cui, X.T. Ultrasoft microwire neural electrodes improve chronic tissue integration. *Acta Biomater.* **2017**, *53*, 46–58. [CrossRef] [PubMed]

18. Sohal, H.S.; Clowry, G.J.; Jackson, A.; O'Neill, A.; Baker, S.N. Mechanical Flexibility Reduces the Foreign Body Response to Long-Term Implanted Microelectrodes in Rabbit Cortex. *PLoS ONE* **2016**, *11*, e0165606. [CrossRef] [PubMed]

19. Lind, G.; Linsmeier, C.E.; Schouenborg, J. The density difference between tissue and neural probes is a key factor for glial scarring. *Sci. Rep.* **2013**, *3*, 2942. [CrossRef] [PubMed]

20. Nguyen, J.K.; Park, D.J.; Skousen, J.L.; Hess-Dunning, A.E.; Tyler, D.J.; Rowan, S.J.; Weder, C.; Capadona, J.R. Mechanically-Compliant Intracortical Implants Reduce the Neuroinflammatory Response. *J. Neural Eng.* **2014**, *11*, 056014. [CrossRef] [PubMed]

21. Bérces, Z.; Tóth, K.; Márton, G.; Pál, I.; Kováts-Megyesi, B.; Fekete, Z.; Ulbert, I.; Pongrácz, A. Neurobiochemical changes in the vicinity of a nanostructured neural implant. *Sci. Rep.* **2016**, *6*, 35944. [CrossRef] [PubMed]

22. Biran, R.; Martin, D.C.; Tresco, P.A. The brain tissue response to implanted silicon microelectrode arrays is increased when the device is tethered to the skull. *J. Biomed. Mater. Res. A* **2007**, *82*, 169–178. [CrossRef] [PubMed]

23. Lind, G.; Gällentoft, L.; Danielsen, N.; Schouenborg, J.; Pettersson, L.M.E. Multiple Implants Do Not Aggravate the Tissue Reaction in Rat Brain. *PLoS ONE* **2012**, *7*, e47509. [CrossRef] [PubMed]

24. Zhong, Y.; Bellamkonda, R.V. Dexamethasone Coated Neural Probes Elicit Attenuated Inflammatory Response and Neuronal Loss Compared to Uncoated Neural Probes. *Brain Res.* **2007**, *1148*, 15–27. [CrossRef] [PubMed]

25. Spataro, L.; Dilgen, J.; Retterer, S.; Spence, A.J.; Isaacson, M.; Turner, J.N.; Shain, W. Dexamethasone treatment reduces astroglia responses to inserted neuroprosthetic devices in rat neocortex. *Exp. Neurol.* **2005**, *194*, 289–300. [CrossRef] [PubMed]

26. Kozai, T.D.Y.; Jaquins-Gerstl, A.S.; Vazquez, A.L.; Michael, A.C.; Cui, X.T. Dexamethasone retrodialysis attenuates microglial response to implanted probes in vivo. *Biomaterials* **2016**, *87*, 157–169. [CrossRef] [PubMed]

27. Eles, J.R.; Vazquez, A.L.; Snyder, N.R.; Lagenaur, C.; Murphy, M.C.; Kozai, T.D.Y.; Cui, X.T. Neuroadhesive L1 coating attenuates acute microglial attachment to neural electrodes as revealed by live two-photon microscopy. *Biomaterials* **2017**, *113*, 279–292. [CrossRef] [PubMed]

28. Azemi, E.; Lagenaur, C.; Cui, X.T. The Surface Immobilization of the Neural Adhesion Molecule L1 on Neural Probes and its Effect on Neuronal Density and Gliosis at the Probe/Tissue Interface. *Biomaterials* **2011**, *32*, 681–692. [CrossRef] [PubMed]

29. Oakes, R.S.; Polei, M.D.; Skousen, J.L.; Tresco, P.A. An astrocyte derived extracellular matrix coating reduces astrogliosis surrounding chronically implanted microelectrode arrays in rat cortex. *Biomaterials* **2018**, *154*, 1–11. [CrossRef] [PubMed]

30. Righi, M.; Puleo, G.L.; Tonazzini, I.; Giudetti, G.; Cecchini, M.; Micera, S. Peptide-based coatings for flexible implantable neural interfaces. *Sci. Rep.* **2018**, *8*, 502. [CrossRef] [PubMed]

31. Azemi, E.; Gobbel, G.T.; Cui, X.T. Seeding neural progenitor cells on silicon-based neural probes. *J. Neurosurg.* **2010**, *113*, 673–681. [CrossRef] [PubMed]

32. Rohatgi, P.; Langhals, N.B.; Kipke, D.R.; Patil, P.G. In vivo performance of a microelectrode neural probe with integrated drug delivery. *Neurosurg. Focus* **2009**, *27*, E8. [CrossRef] [PubMed]

33. Bedell, H.W.; Hermann, J.K.; Ravikumar, M.; Lin, S.; Rein, A.; Li, X.; Molinich, E.; Smith, P.D.; Selkirk, S.M.; Miller, R.H.; et al. Targeting CD14 on blood derived cells improves intracortical microelectrode performance. *Biomaterials* **2018**, *163*, 163–173. [CrossRef] [PubMed]

34. Hermann, J.K.; Ravikumar, M.; Shoffstall, A.J.; Ereifej, E.S.; Kovach, K.M.; Chang, J.; Soffer, A.; Wong, C.; Srivastava, V.; Smith, P.; et al. Inhibition of the cluster of differentiation 14 innate immunity pathway with IAXO-101 improves chronic microelectrode performance. *J. Neural Eng.* **2018**, *15*, 025002. [CrossRef] [PubMed]

35. Nguyen, J.K.; Jorfi, M.; Buchanan, K.L.; Park, D.J.; Foster, E.J.; Tyler, D.J.; Rowan, S.J.; Weder, C.; Capadona, J.R. Influence of resveratrol release on the tissue response to mechanically adaptive cortical implants. *Acta Biomater.* **2016**, *29*, 81–93. [CrossRef] [PubMed]

36. Potter, K.A.; Buck, A.C.; Self, W.K.; Callanan, M.E.; Sunil, S.; Capadona, J.R. The effect of resveratrol on neurodegeneration and blood brain barrier stability surrounding intracortical microelectrodes. *Biomaterials* **2013**, *34*, 7001–7015. [CrossRef] [PubMed]

37. Potter-Baker, K.A.; Stewart, W.G.; Tomaszewski, W.H.; Wong, C.T.; Meador, W.D.; Ziats, N.P.; Capadona, J.R. Implications of Chronic Daily Anti-Oxidant Administration on the Inflammatory Response to Intracortical Microelectrodes. *J. Neural Eng.* **2015**, *12*, 046002. [CrossRef] [PubMed]

38. Karumbaiah, L.; Norman, S.E.; Rajan, N.B.; Anand, S.; Saxena, T.; Betancur, M.; Patkar, R.; Bellamkonda, R.V. The upregulation of specific interleukin (IL) receptor antagonists and paradoxical enhancement of neuronal apoptosis due to electrode induced strain and brain micromotion. *Biomaterials* **2012**, *33*, 5983–5996. [CrossRef] [PubMed]

39. Bardehle, S.; Krüger, M.; Buggenthin, F.; Schwausch, J.; Ninkovic, J.; Clevers, H.; Snippert, H.J.; Theis, F.J.; Meyer-Luehmann, M.; Bechmann, I.; et al. Live imaging of astrocyte responses to acute injury reveals selective juxtavascular proliferation. *Nat. Neurosci.* **2013**, *16*, 580–586. [CrossRef] [PubMed]

40. He, W.; Bellamkonda, R.V. A Molecular Perspective on Understanding and Modulating the Performance of Chronic Central Nervous System (CNS) Recording Electrodes. In *Indwelling Neural Implants: Strategies for Contending with the In Vivo Environment*; Reichert, W.M., Ed.; CRC Press/Taylor & Francis: Boca Raton, FL, USA, 2008; Chapter 6.

41. Luh, C.; Kuhlmann, C.R.; Ackermann, B.; Timaru-Kast, R.; Luhmann, H.J.; Behl, C.; Werner, C.; Engelhard, K.; Thal, S.C. Inhibition of myosin light chain kinase reduces brain edema formation after traumatic brain injury. *J. Neurochem.* **2010**, *112*, 1015–1025. [CrossRef] [PubMed]

42. Ghirnikar, R.S.; Lee, Y.L.; Eng, L.F. Inflammation in traumatic brain injury: Role of cytokines and chemokines. *Neurochem. Res.* **1998**, *23*, 329–340. [CrossRef] [PubMed]

43. Van Wagoner, N.J.; Oh, J.W.; Repovic, P.; Benveniste, E.N. Interleukin-6 (IL-6) production by astrocytes: Autocrine regulation by IL-6 and the soluble IL-6 receptor. *J. Neurosci.* **1999**, *19*, 5236–5244. [CrossRef] [PubMed]

44. Campbell, I.L.; Abraham, C.R.; Masliah, E.; Kemper, P.; Inglis, J.D.; Oldstone, M.B.; Mucke, L. Neurologic disease induced in transgenic mice by cerebral overexpression of interleukin 6. *Proc. Natl. Acad. Sci. USA* **1993**, *90*, 10061–10065. [CrossRef] [PubMed]

45. Turner, J.N.; Shain, W.; Szarowski, D.H.; Andersen, M.; Martins, S.; Isaacson, M.; Craighead, H. Cerebral astrocyte response to micromachined silicon implants. *Exp. Neurol.* **1999**, *156*, 33–49. [CrossRef] [PubMed]

46. Williams, J.C.; Hippensteel, J.A.; Dilgen, J.; Shain, W.; Kipke, D.R. Complex impedance spectroscopy for monitoring tissue responses to inserted neural implants. *J. Neural Eng.* **2007**, *4*, 410–423. [CrossRef] [PubMed]

47. Cody, P.A.; Eles, J.R.; Lagenaur, C.F.; Kozai, T.D.Y.; Cui, X.T. Unique electrophysiological and impedance signatures between encapsulation types: An analysis of biological Utah array failure and benefit of a biomimetic coating in a rat model. *Biomaterials* **2018**, *161*, 117–128. [CrossRef] [PubMed]

48. Degenhart, A.D.; Eles, J.; Dum, R.; Mischel, J.L.; Smalianchuk, I.; Endler, B.; Ashmore, R.C.; Tyler-Kabara, E.C.; Hatsopoulos, N.G.; Wang, W.; et al. Histological Evaluation of a Chronically-implanted Electrocorticographic Electrode Grid in a Non-human Primate. *J. Neural Eng.* **2016**, *13*, 046019. [CrossRef] [PubMed]

49. Fong, J.S.; Alexopoulos, A.V.; Bingaman, W.E.; Gonzalez-Martinez, J.; Prayson, R.A. Pathologic findings associated with invasive EEG monitoring for medically intractable epilepsy. *Am. J. Clin. Pathol.* **2012**, *138*, 506–510. [CrossRef] [PubMed]

50. Schendel, A.A.; Thongpang, S.; Brodnick, S.K.; Richner, T.J.; Lindevig, B.D.B.; Krugner-Higby, L.; Williams, J.C. A cranial window imaging method for monitoring vascular growth around chronically implanted micro-ECoG devices. *J. Neurosci. Methods* **2013**, *218*, 121–130. [CrossRef] [PubMed]

51. Henle, C.; Raab, M.; Cordeiro, J.G.; Doostkam, S.; Schulze-Bonhage, A.; Stieglitz, T.; Rickert, J. First long term in vivo study on subdurally implanted micro-ECoG electrodes, manufactured with a novel laser technology. *Biomed. Microdevices* **2011**, *13*, 59–68. [CrossRef] [PubMed]

52. Butson, C.R.; Maks, C.B.; McIntyre, C.C. Sources and effects of electrode impedance during deep brain stimulation. *Clin. Neurophysiol.* **2006**, *117*, 447–454. [CrossRef] [PubMed]

53. Prasad, A.; Sanchez, J.C. Quantifying long-term microelectrode array functionality using chronic in vivo impedance testing. *J. Neural Eng.* **2012**, *9*, 026028. [CrossRef] [PubMed]

54. Lempka, S.F.; Miocinovic, S.; Johnson, M.D.; Vitek, J.L.; McIntyre, C.C. In vivo impedance spectroscopy of deep brain stimulation electrodes. *J. Neural Eng.* **2009**, *6*, 046001. [CrossRef] [PubMed]

55. Mercanzini, A.; Colin, P.; Bensadoun, J.C.; Bertsch, A.; Renaud, P. In vivo electrical impedance spectroscopy of tissue reaction to microelectrode arrays. *IEEE Trans. Biomed. Eng.* **2009**, *56*, 1909–1918. [CrossRef] [PubMed]

56. Malaga, K.A.; Schroeder, K.E.; Patel, P.R.; Irwin, Z.T.; Thompson, D.E.; Nicole Bentley, J.; Lempka, S.F.; Chestek, C.A.; Patil, P.G. Data-driven model comparing the effects of glial scarring and interface interactions on chronic neural recordings in non-human primates. *J. Neural Eng.* **2016**, *13*, 016010. [CrossRef] [PubMed]

57. Merrill, D.R.; Tresco, P.A. Impedance characterization of microarray recording electrodes in vitro. *IEEE Trans. Biomed. Eng.* **2005**, *52*, 1960–1965. [CrossRef] [PubMed]

58. Sankar, V.; Patrick, E.; Dieme, R.; Sanchez, J.C.; Prasad, A.; Nishida, T. Electrode impedance analysis of chronic tungsten microwire neural implants: Understanding abiotic vs. biotic contributions. *Front. Neuroeng.* **2014**, *7*, 13. [CrossRef] [PubMed]

59. Prasad, A.; Xue, Q.S.; Dieme, R.; Sankar, V.; Mayrand, R.C.; Nishida, T.; Streit, W.J.; Sanchez, J.C. Abiotic-biotic characterization of Pt/Ir microelectrode arrays in chronic implants. *Front. Neuroeng.* **2014**, *7*, 2. [CrossRef] [PubMed]

60. Otto, K.J.; Johnson, M.D.; Kipke, D.R. Voltage pulses change neural interface properties and improve unit recordings with chronically implanted microelectrodes. *IEEE Trans. Biomed. Eng.* **2006**, *53*, 333–540. [CrossRef] [PubMed]

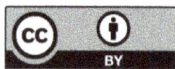

micromachines

MDPI

Article

A Meta-Analysis of Intracortical Device Stiffness and Its Correlation with Histological Outcomes

Allison M. Stiller *, Bryan J. Black, Christopher Kung, Aashika Ashok, Stuart F. Cogan, Victor D. Varner and Joseph J. Pancrazio

Department of Bioengineering, The University of Texas at Dallas, 800W. Campbell Rd., Richardson, TX 75080, USA; bjb140530@utdallas.edu (B.J.B.); christopher.kung@utdallas.edu (C.K.); aashika.ashok@utdallas.edu (A.A.); sxc149830@utdallas.edu (S.F.C.); vdv@utdallas.edu (V.D.V.); joseph.pancrazio@utdallas.edu (J.J.P.)
* Correspondence: allison.stiller@utdallas.edu; Tel.: +1-972-883-2138

Received: 31 July 2018; Accepted: 30 August 2018; Published: 6 September 2018

Abstract: Neural implants offer solutions for a variety of clinical issues. While commercially available devices can record neural signals for short time periods, they fail to do so chronically, partially due to the sustained tissue response around the device. Our objective was to assess the correlation between device stiffness, a function of both material modulus and cross-sectional area, and the severity of immune response. Meta-analysis data were derived from nine previously published studies which reported device material and geometric properties, as well as histological outcomes. Device bending stiffness was calculated by treating the device shank as a cantilevered beam. Immune response was quantified through analysis of immunohistological images from each study, specifically looking at fluorescent markers for neuronal nuclei and astrocytes, to assess neuronal dieback and gliosis. Results demonstrate that the severity of the immune response, within the first 50 μm of the device, is highly correlated with device stiffness, as opposed to device modulus or cross-sectional area independently. In general, commercially available devices are around two to three orders of magnitude higher in stiffness than devices which induced a minimal tissue response. These results have implications for future device designs aiming to decrease chronic tissue response and achieve increased long-term functionality.

Keywords: intracortical implant; microelectrodes; stiffness; immunohistochemistry; immune response; neural interface response; neural interface

---

1. Introduction

Paralysis and limb loss pose significant personal, financial, and health burdens. Each year in the U.S. alone, there are over 17,500 cases of spinal cord injury where less than 1% achieve complete recovery [1]. The nationwide prevalence of amputees is even higher at 185,000 new cases each year [2]. To address this issue, engineers and scientists are developing a range of technologies with the intent of bypassing the damaged component of the peripheral or central nervous system, to replace or restore lost motor function [3]. State-of-the-art devices are implanted intracortically, or directly into the brain, where they can record biopotentials associated with voluntary movement [4]. Neural data can then be decoded and used to drive the movement of assistive devices and prosthetic limbs, or control stimulation for functional restoration of paralyzed limbs [5,6].

While many groups have demonstrated success resolving neural signals with intracortical probes for periods of about one year [7,8], these devices tend to lose their ability to record neural signals for longer time periods [4,8,9], limiting more widespread clinical use. While there are multiple factors influencing device performance, one prominent hypothesis for device failure pertains to a chronic immune response characterized by glial encapsulation of the device, as well as local neuronal death [10,11]. Both of these compromise stable neural recordings over time. It has been suggested that a drastic mismatch in mechanical properties between the soft brain tissue and stiff neural implant may regulate the immune response [12–14]. Commercially available devices are fabricated using materials with a high elastic modulus, resulting in stiff devices that create concentrations of mechanical stress at the tissue interface [15], and provoke a significant, persistent immune response.

A common goal in the neuroengineering community is the development of more biocompatible implants, which elicit a decreased tissue response, with the intent of increasing their functional lifetime. These efforts are largely divided into two groups: (1) creating devices that are significantly smaller than the state-of-the-art [16,17], or (2) fabricating devices from softer materials to bridge the mechanical mismatch at the brain-device interface [18,19]. Both approaches have yielded promising results, such as decreased neuronal death and glial encapsulation, raising the possibility that a common link exists between both approaches. Our hypothesis is that these outcomes may be attributed to a single underlying parameter hereafter referred to as stiffness (k_b), a function of both the material properties and geometric dimensions of the device.

Based on the mechanics of static bodies, an implantable neural probe may be treated as a simple cantilevered beam, where the beam is fixed on one end, while a downward force is placed on the other end, causing a deflection [20]. The magnitude of the deflection is inversely proportional to the stiffness of the probe, with greater deflections associated with lower stiffness. Changes in the physical dimensions and/or the mechanical properties of the probe modulate its overall stiffness. The same is true for implantable devices. Devices with lower stiffness values, or greater flexibility, can be created by modifying the cross-sectional area (CSA) and/or by using softer constituent materials.

However, 'stiffness' (or 'flexibility') is often used synonymously to describe the softness or modulus of the implantable device or device substrate, even though stiffness must consider the contributions of device dimensions. For example, while polymer-based devices may be comprised of inherently soft materials, whether or not the device is highly flexible depends on more than just their material makeup. Instead, stiffness (k_b) assessments can be made based on calculations incorporating device dimensions to determine relative flexibility as compared to commercially available and other novel devices. The novelty of this study is the recognition that histological outcomes across material and geometric properties may be correlated to a single consolidated variable, k_b, as opposed to relating changes in histological outcomes to a single aspect of device design.

Here, we re-evaluated a number of studies reporting details on device design and the histological outcomes following implantation in rodent brain. The analysis draws upon studies utilizing a variety of devices fabricated from a wide range of materials and dimensions, yielding a range of stiffness values. Through quantitative analysis of previously published immunohistological images, we demonstrate that the severity of the immune response is highly correlated with device stiffness. This is a function of both elastic modulus and size, in contrast to correlations considering only modulus or cross-sectional dimensions independently.

2. Materials and Methods

2.1. Stiffness Calculations

Table 1 lists the studies and devices used in the meta-analysis. All devices were treated as simplified cantilevered beams (Figure 1) in order to solve for bending stiffness, k_b, as a function of area moment of inertia, I, device length, L, and Young's modulus, E, (Equation (1) [20]).

Device tip geometries and shank asymmetries were neglected for the sake of simplicity. It is important to note that many single shank devices do exhibit tapered geometries meaning that cross-sectional area, and area moment of inertia, are not necessarily uniform along the length of the device. However, preliminary computational modeling suggests that using average width values does not have a significant effect on stiffness calculations. Specifically, use of a simplified symmetric model resulted in a 12% difference in maximum tip deflection in the cantilevered device bending simulation, when compared to the original tapered geometries (Figure 2). It is important to mention, however, that the tapering angle used in this simulation was relatively high when compared to those reported. Therefore, this represents a 'worst-case scenario' for difference in tip deflection.

Table 1. Devices from studies used in meta-analysis.

Author, Year	Material	Modulus	CSA (μm^2)	Calculated Stiffness k_b (N/m)	Time Implanted	Stain Analyzed
Mercanzini et al., 2008 [21]	Polyimide	2.5 GPa	4200	0.00024	1 week	GFAP
Harris et al., 2011 [13]	Nanocomposite (poly(vinylacetate) and cellulose)	12 MPa	51,200	0.49	4 weeks	NeuN and GFAP
Biran et al., 2005 [11]	Silicon	179 GPa	3000	1.12	4 weeks	NeuN and GFAP
Knaack et al., 2016 [22]	Silicon	179 GPa	1875	0.15	4 weeks	NeuN and GFAP
Lee et al., 2017 [23]	OSTE soft (thiol-ene-epoxy)	6 MPa	5600	0.00016	4 weeks	NeuN and GFAP
Lewitus et al., 2014 [24]	Agarose with carbon nanotubes	Agarose-85 MPa	8220	0.02	4 weeks	GFAP
Kozai et al., 2012 [25]	Carbon fiber	234 GPa	38	0.01	2 weeks	NeuN and GFAP
Thelin et al., 2011 [26]	Stainless steel microwire (50 μm and 200 μm diameter)	200 GPa	50 μm: 1963 200 μm: 31416	50 μm: 32 200 μm: 8080	12 weeks	NeuN and GFAP
Lind et al., 2010 [27]	Bundled tungsten microwires in gelatin	Tungsten-411 GPa	70,686	7940	6 weeks	GFAP

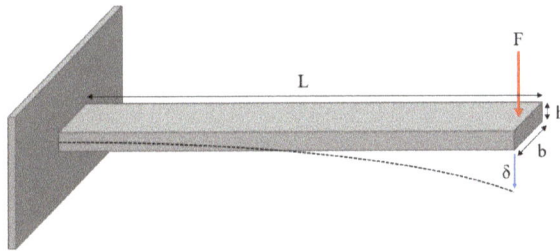

Figure 1. Diagram of a cantilevered beam. The beam is fixed on one end while a force on the opposite end produces a displacement, δ. Dimensions depicted are beam length, L, beam width, b, and beam thickness, h.

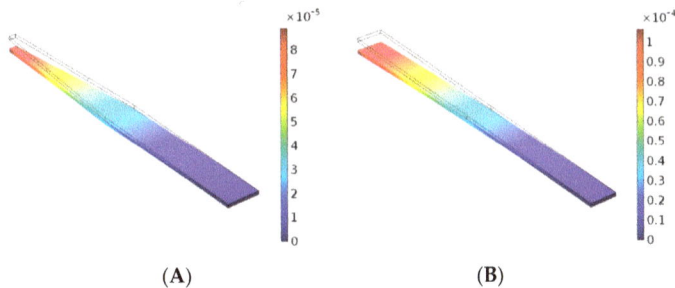

Figure 2. Computer simulated bend tests. Cantilever bend tests were used to determine the percent difference between device geometries with tapered and symmetrical shanks. In this case, shank (**A**) featured a width of 290 μm and tapered to 65 μm starting halfway down the shank. Shank (**B**) featured a width of 234 μm, calculated based on the weighted average of width down the length of shank (**A**). Both shanks were 30 μm thick and 3 mm long. Colored scale bars indicate deflection in meters.

Bending simulations were performed in COMSOL Multiphysics® v. 5.2. (COMSOL AB, Stockholm, Sweden) and the setup mirrored the cantilever-style bend test depicted in Figure 1. Further evaluation using Linear Buckling Analysis in COMSOL revealed only an 8% difference in critical buckling force between either geometries, indicating they are mechanically similar. Therefore, representative stiffness values (Equation (1) [20]) were calculated using average values of device width along the length of the shank. For devices with polymer coatings, stiffness was assumed to be dominated by the stiffest constituent material, and calculated accordingly. Most devices did not exhibit tapering as severe as the simulation presented above; rather, this was to illustrate the worst-case scenario. As such, most of the devices exhibit less than an 8 or 12% difference in critical buckling force and maximum tip deflection, respectively. All devices were treated as having either rectangular cross sections with height, h, and width, b, or circular cross sections with diameter, d, affecting the way in which moment of inertia of the cross-sectional area was calculated (Equations (2) and (3) [20]). Length was taken to be the overall length of the device shank, unless the implantation depth was otherwise stated in the study.

$$k_b = \frac{3EI}{L^3} \tag{1}$$

$$I_{rectangle} = \frac{bh^3}{12} \tag{2}$$

$$I_{circle} = \frac{\pi d^4}{64} \tag{3}$$

2.2. Image Analysis

The immune response for each study was quantified by analysis of fluorescent immunohistochemical images, from staining with several cell markers commonly associated with the immune response. For the purposes of this analysis, we focused on stains for neurons and astrocytes, specifically neuronal nuclei (NeuN) and glial fibrillary acidic protein (GFAP), a protein expressed in astrocytes.

Images were analyzed using Fiji [28], an open source image processing software based on ImageJ [29] (NIH). A custom macro was created to select the perimeter of the device within the image, and subsequently create concentric bands in 50 μm increments, while calculating the area in each band. For GFAP analysis, we computed the average intensity of GFAP immunofluorescence within each concentric band surrounding the probe (Figure 3a). For NeuN analysis, neurons were manually counted within each band using Fiji's Cell Counter plugin to quantify neuronal density (Figure 3b). Both GFAP intensity and neuronal density were normalized by dividing each band by the value in a band at least 200–250 μm from the device perimeter. This was done to ensure normalization with respect to tissue expected to be relatively unaffected by the implant. If healthy tissue samples were provided by the study, values were normalized with respect to areas from those samples.

While several of these studies reported their own analyses of fluorescent images, we chose not to include these quantifications in this meta-analysis. This was done in order to ensure that all NeuN density and GFAP intensity values were measured and normalized consistently across all studies, for accurate comparison. However, it is important to note that studies often feature figures that best illustrate the point of the study, i.e., fluorescent images that exemplify a reduced immune response. Therefore, our results likely reflect a conservative estimate of correlations between immune markers and device parameters.

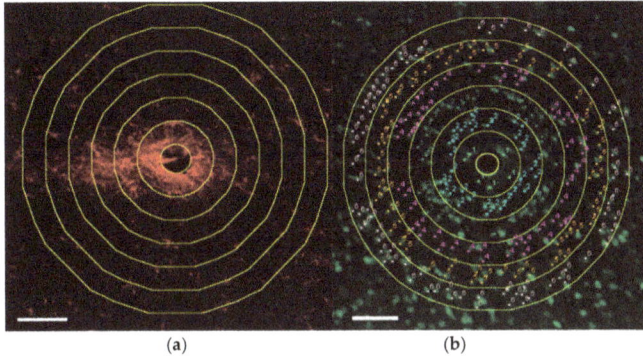

(a)   (b)

Figure 3. Example image analysis on a stainless steel microwire. Scale bar 100 μm. (**a**) glial fibrillary acidic protein (GFAP) intensity and (**b**) neuronal density quantification in 50 μm concentric bands. Adapted from Thelin et al., 2011 [26]. Scale bar = 100 μm.

2.3. Statistical Analysis

To examine the possible relationships between material properties, dimensions, and device flexibility with both neuronal density and GFAP intensity, a Spearman rank correlation coefficient was calculated for each data set using functions available in MATLAB R2017a (MathWorks, Natick, MA, USA). Spearman correlation is a nonparametric test which assesses the monotonic relationship between ranked datasets. Good correlation is indicated by ρ values closest to 1 or 1 for positive and negative correlations respectively, with a high correlation being between 0.70 to 1.00 (or -0.70 to -1.0) [30]. A *p*-value less than 0.05 was taken as indicative of a significant correlation.

3. Results

Calculated stiffness levels varied over six orders of magnitude ranging from 8×10^3 to 1.6×10^{-4} N/m. Statistical analysis across multiple studies showed a high positive correlation ($\rho = 0.89$, $p < 0.05$) between device stiffness and normalized GFAP intensity, within a 50-μm band of the device perimeter, indicating that gliosis is more severe when using a stiffer implant (Figure 4).

Additionally, there was a high negative correlation ($\rho = -0.92$, $p < 0.05$) between device stiffness and normalized NeuN density in the same area, indicating that neuronal loss is increased when using a stiffer implant.

Device modulus and cross-sectional area did not exhibit significant correlation values within the same band, for either GFAP intensity or NeuN density, suggesting that the dependence on stiffness is a contributing factor in the severity of the immune response (Table 2). However, results also suggest that this trend is only relevant within the first 50 μm around the device. Outside of the first 50 μm band, neither GFAP intensity nor neuronal density show good, significant correlation with device stiffness, with the exception of GFAP intensity in the 100–150 μm band, therefore these data was not shown.

Table 2. Spearman's rho correlation results for 0–50 μm band.

			Stiffness	Modulus	CSA
Spearman's rho	GFAP Intensity	Correlation Coefficient	0.89 *	0.62	0.42
		Significance (two-tailed)	0.001	0.06	0.23
		N	10	10	10
	Neuronal Density	Correlation Coefficient	−0.92 *	−0.09	−0.5
		Significance (two-tailed)	0.01	0.85	0.27
		N	7	7	7

*: $p < 0.05$.

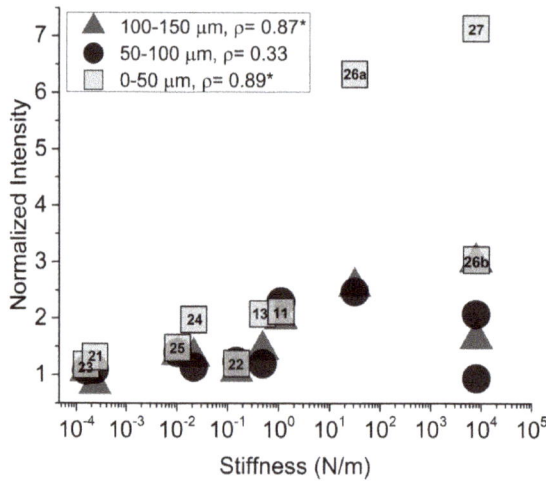

Figure 4. GFAP intensity analysis from GFAP-stained fluorescent images. Normalized intensity as a function of device stiffness three concentric 50 μm bands from device perimeter. * $p < 0.05$. Numbers indicate reference from Table 1. References are only included for 0–50 μm data, but all points aligned vertically are from the same reference. 26a and 26b reference the 50 μm and 200 μm stainless steel devices, respectively.

4. Discussion

Our meta-analysis across multiple studies indicated that the tissue response triggered during implantation may be most closely correlated with stiffness of an implanted device, as opposed to material moduli or geometric properties independently. Devices featured in this study exhibit stiffness values ranging from 10^{-4} to 10^3 N/m. For reference, a commercially available Michigan-style silicon probe might exhibit a stiffness around 10^2 N/m. Devices with a lower calculated bending stiffness exhibited decreased amounts of gliosis and neuronal death around the perimeter of the implant when compared with stiffer devices. These results were found to be significant within the first 50 μm of the device boundary, which is of critical importance in the context of functional neural recordings. Typically, neurons must be within 50 μm of the device electrodes in order to resolve single unit recordings at appropriate signal to noise ratios [31], and a severe immune response within this range would limit the device capabilities. Previously published studies have also reported on immune response with respect to 50 μm bands as important landmarks for histological outcomes [13,23]. Improved histological outcomes with respect to both GFAP intensity and NeuN density appeared to level off when a device reached the 10^{-1} to 10^{-2} N/m stiffness range (Figures 4 and 5) indicating that this could serve as a threshold for optimal device stiffness. This stiffness could be achieved with a commercially available Michigan-style probe by reducing the thickness from 50 μm to 10 μm while maintaining an average width of 125 μm and an implantation length of 2 mm. Stiffness of tapered devices may be more accurately calculated using cantilevered setups or computational models.

Overall, high correlation between device stiffness and the severity of the immune response may be a representation of how well these devices are able to move with the brain. Cross-sectional area or elastic modulus alone do not provide a full picture: a soft object may be so large that it is stiff and cannot flex with the brain. Conversely, a small device made from a material with a high elastic modulus may face the same issue. It has been well documented that the brain experiences significant micromotion due to breathing and vascular pulsation [32]. It is likely that decreased stiffness allows these devices to move with the brain, and therefore put less strain on the surrounding tissue, perhaps leading to a less significant tissue response.

In general, these findings support approaches to changing either the material properties, or physical dimensions of devices, to reduce the severity of the tissue response. Ideally, devices featuring both soft materials and small dimensions would offer improved tissue response, but in the absence of an insertion aid, mechanical considerations must also inform the minimal stiffness required to successfully penetrate the brain. This specific limitation explains a lack of histological studies in the literature performed, using highly soft and flexible devices which would provide additional insight into the relationship between flexibility and tissue response. Additionally, very stiff devices made from high modulus materials are prone to brittle fracture, which places limits on the minimum achievable dimensions during fabrication. Furthermore, ultra-small devices have limited available surface area for electrode sites on device structures, limiting the creation of high-density probes.

The results of this meta-analysis should however encourage further exploration of materials for devices which can be fabricated in a way that limits overall stiffness (k_b). This can be done through a reduction of material modulus (E) or a cross-sectional moment of inertia (I), with the goal of better matching stiffness to that of brain tissue, and subsequently improving chronic integration with surrounding tissue. Additionally, the possibility remains that the immune response may be a result of cells responding to stress concentrations due to material mismatch, as opposed to stiffness of the device itself. This hypothesis could be tested directly using an approach in which probe geometries are kept constant while varying material stiffness, or similarly, maintaining stiffness but using varied cross-sectional geometries.

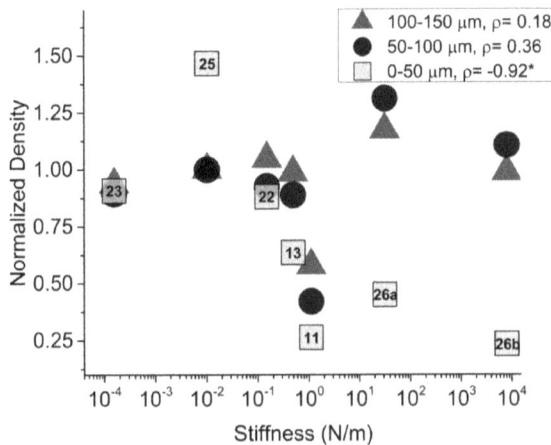

Figure 5. Neuronal density analysis from neuronal nuclei (NeuN)-stained fluorescent images. Normalized neuronal density as a function of device stiffness three concentric 50 μm bands from device perimeter. * $p < 0.05$. Numbers indicate reference from Table 1. References are only included for 0–50 μm data, but all points aligned vertically are from the same reference. 26a and 26b reference the 50 and 200 μm stainless steel devices, respectively.

5. Conclusions

Intracortical device stiffness may influence the severity of the chronic immune response, more than size or material properties of the device independently. Our novel results, which draw upon findings from multiple studies, indicate that device stiffness is especially important in close proximity to the device perimeter, which may profoundly affect the ability of devices to record from nearby neurons.

Author Contributions: Conceptualization, J.J.P. and A.M.S.; Methodology, A.M.S., B.J.B., and J.J.P.; Software, B.J.B. and A.M.S.; Validation, A.M.S.; Formal Analysis, A.M.S.; Investigation, A.M.S., C.K., and A.A.; Resources, J.J.P.; Data Curation, A.M.S.; C.K., and A.A.; Writing—Original Draft Preparation, A.M.S.; Writing—Review & Editing, A.M.S., B.J.B., S.F.C., V.D.V., and J.J.P.; Visualization, A.M.S. and B.J.B.; Supervision, J.J.P.; Project Administration, J.J.P.; Funding Acquisition, J.J.P.

Funding: This work was supported by the Office of the Assistant Secretary of Defense for Health Affairs through the Peer Reviewed Medical Research Program [grant No. W81XWH-15-1-0607]. Opinions, interpretations, conclusions and recommendations are those of the authors and are not necessarily endorsed by the Department of Defense. Additional support was provided by Defense Advanced Research Projects Agency (DARPA) BTO [grant No. HR0011-15-2-0017]; and the Eugene McDermott Graduate Fellowship Program, Richardson, TX [grant No. 201606] at University of Texas at Dallas.

Conflicts of Interest: The authors declare no conflicts of interest. The funders had no role in the design of the study; in the collection, analyses, or interpretation of data; in the writing of the manuscript, and in the decision to publish the results.

References

1. White, N.H.; Black, N.H. Spinal cord injury facts and figures at a glance. *Natl. Spinal Cord Inj. Stat. Cent.* **2017**, *35*, 197–198. [CrossRef]
2. Ziegler-Graham, K.; MacKenzie, E.J.; Ephraim, P.L.; Travison, T.G.; Brookmeyer, R. Estimating the prevalence of limb loss in the United States: 2005 to 2050. *Arch. Phys. Med. Rehabilit.* **2008**, *89*, 422–429. [CrossRef] [PubMed]
3. Tsu, A.P.; Burish, M.J.; GodLove, J.; Ganguly, K. Cortical neuroprosthetics from a clinical perspective. *Neurobiol. Dis.* **2015**, *83*, 154–160. [CrossRef] [PubMed]
4. Jorfi, M.; Skousen, J.L.; Weder, C.; Capadona, J.R. Progress towards biocompatible intracortical microelectrodes for neural interfacing applications. *J. Neural Eng.* **2015**, *12*, 011001. [CrossRef] [PubMed]
5. Hochberg, L.R.; Bacher, D.; Jarosiewicz, B.; Masse, N.Y.; Simeral, J.D.; Vogel, J.; Haddadin, S.; Liu, J.; Cash, S.S.; van der Smagt, P.; et al. Reach and grasp by people with tetraplegia using a neurally controlled robotic arm. *Nature* **2012**, *485*, 372–375. [CrossRef] [PubMed]
6. Pancrazio, J.J.; Peckham, P.H. Neuroprosthetic devices: How far are we from recovering movement in paralyzed patients? *Expert Rev. Neurother.* **2009**, *9*, 427–430. [CrossRef] [PubMed]
7. Chestek, C.A.; Gilja, V.; Nuyujukian, P.; Foster, J.D.; Fan, J.M.; Kaufman, M.T.; Churchland, M.M.; Rivera-alvidrez, Z.; Cunningham, J.P.; Ryu, S.I.; et al. Long-term stability of neural prosthetic control signals from silicon cortical arrays in rhesus macaque motor cortex. *J. Neural Eng.* **2011**, *8*, 045005. [CrossRef] [PubMed]
8. Barrese, J.C.; Rao, N.; Paroo, K.; Triebwasser, C.; Vargas-Irwin, C.; Franquemont, L.; Donoghue, J.P. Failure mode analysis of silicon-based intracortical microelectrode arrays in non-human primates. *J. Neural Eng.* **2013**, *10*, 066014. [CrossRef] [PubMed]
9. Ward, M.P.; Rajdev, P.; Ellison, C.; Irazoqui, P.P. Toward a comparison of microelectrodes for acute and chronic recordings. *Brain Res.* **2009**, *1282*, 183–200. [CrossRef] [PubMed]
10. Polikov, V.S.; Tresco, P.A.; Reichert, W.M. Response of brain tissue to chronically implanted neural electrodes. *J. Neurosci. Methods* **2005**, *148*, 1–18. [CrossRef] [PubMed]
11. Biran, R.; Martin, D.C.; Tresco, P.A. Neuronal cell loss accompanies the brain tissue response to chronically implanted silicon microelectrode arrays. *Exp. Neurol.* **2005**, *195*, 115–126. [CrossRef] [PubMed]
12. Andrei, A.; Welkenhuysen, M.; Nuttin, B.; Eberle, W. A response surface model predicting the in vivo insertion behavior of micromachined neural implants. *J. Neural Eng.* **2011**, *9*, 016005. [CrossRef] [PubMed]
13. Harris, J.P.; Capadona, J.R.; Miller, R.H.; Healy, B.C.; Shanmuganathan, K.; Rowan, S.J.; Weder, C.; Tyler, D.J. Mechanically adaptive intracortical implants improve the proximity of neuronal cell bodies. *J. Neural Eng.* **2011**, *8*, 066011. [CrossRef] [PubMed]
14. Moshayedi, P.; Ng, G.; Kwok, J.C.F.; Yeo, G.S.H.; Bryant, C.E.; Fawcett, J.W.; Franze, K.; Guck, J. The relationship between glial cell mechanosensitivity and foreign body reactions in the central nervous system. *Biomaterials* **2014**, *35*, 3919–3925. [CrossRef] [PubMed]
15. Sridharan, A.; Nguyen, J.K.; Capadona, J.R.; Muthuswamy, J. Compliant intracortical implants reduce strains and strain rates in brain tissue in vivo. *J. Neural Eng.* **2015**, *12*, 036002. [CrossRef] [PubMed]

16. Pancrazio, J.J.; Deku, F.; Ghazavi, A.; Stiller, A.M.; Rihani, R.; Frewin, C.L.; Varner, V.D.; Gardner, T.J.; Cogan, S.F. Thinking small: Progress on microscale neurostimulation technology. *Neuromodulation* **2017**, *20*, 745–752. [CrossRef] [PubMed]

17. Deku, F.; Cohen, Y.; Joshi-Imre, A.; Kanneganti, A.; Gardner, T.J.; Cogan, S.F. Amorphous silicon carbide ultramicroelectrode arrays for neural stimulation and recording. *J. Neural Eng.* **2018**, *15*. [CrossRef] [PubMed]

18. Simon, D.M.; Charkhkar, H.; John, C., St.; Rajendran, S.; Kang, T.; Reit, R.; Arreaga-Salas, D.; McHail, D.G.; Knaack, G.L.; Sloan, A.; et al. Design and demonstration of an intracortical probe technology with tunable modulus. *J. Biomed. Mater. Res. Part A* **2017**, *105*, 159–168. [CrossRef] [PubMed]

19. Weltman, A.; Yoo, J.; Meng, E. Flexible, penetrating brain probes enabled by advances in polymer microfabrication. *Micromachines* **2016**, *7*, 180. [CrossRef]

20. Hibbeler, R.C. *Mechanics of Materials*, 10th ed.; Pearson: London, UK, 2016; ISBN 0134319656.

21. Mercanzini, A.; Cheung, K.; Buhl, D.L.; Boers, M.; Maillard, A.; Colin, P.; Bensadoun, J.C.; Bertsch, A.; Renaud, P. Demonstration of cortical recording using novel flexible polymer neural probes. *Sens. Actuators A Phys.* **2008**, *143*, 90–96. [CrossRef]

22. Knaack, G.L.; McHail, D.G.; Borda, G.; Koo, B.; Peixoto, N.; Cogan, S.F.; Dumas, T.C.; Pancrazio, J.J. In vivo characterization of amorphous silicon carbide as a biomaterial for chronic neural interfaces. *Front. Neurosci.* **2016**, *10*, 301. [CrossRef] [PubMed]

23. Lee, H.C.; Ejserholm, F.; Gaire, J.; Currlin, S.; Schouenborg, J.; Wallman, L.; Bengtsson, M.; Park, K.; Otto, K.J. Histological evaluation of flexible neural implants; Flexibility limit for reducing the tissue response? *J. Neural Eng.* **2017**, *14*, 036026. [CrossRef] [PubMed]

24. Lewitus, D.Y.; Smith, K.L.; Landers, J.; Neimark, A.V.; Koh, J. Bioactive agarose carbon-nanotube composites are capable of manipulating brain-implant interface. *J. Appl. Polym. Sci.* **2014**, *131*, 317–323. [CrossRef] [PubMed]

25. Yoshida Kozai, T.D.; Langhals, N.B.; Patel, P.R.; Deng, X.; Zhang, H.; Smith, K.L.; Lahann, J.; Kotov, N.A.; Kipke, D.R. Ultrasmall implantable composite microelectrodes with bioactive surfaces for chronic neural interfaces. *Nat. Mater.* **2012**, *11*, 1065–1073. [CrossRef] [PubMed]

26. Thelin, J.; Jörntell, H.; Psouni, E.; Garwicz, M.; Schouenborg, J.; Danielsen, N.; Linsmeier, C.E. Implant size and fixation mode strongly influence tissue reactions in the CNS. *PLoS ONE* **2011**, *6*, e16267. [CrossRef] [PubMed]

27. Lind, G.; Linsmeier, C.E.; Thelin, J.; Schouenborg, J. Gelatine-embedded electrodes—A novel biocompatible vehicle allowing implantation of highly flexible microelectrodes. *J. Neural Eng.* **2010**, *7*. [CrossRef] [PubMed]

28. Schindelin, J.; Arganda-Carreras, I.; Frise, E.; Kaynig, V.; Longair, M.; Pietzsch, T.; Preibisch, S.; Rueden, C.; Saalfeld, S.; Schmid, B.; et al. Fiji: An open-source platform for biological-image analysis. *Nat. Methods* **2012**, *9*, 676–682. [CrossRef] [PubMed]

29. Schneider, C.A.; Rasband, W.S.; Eliceiri, K.W. NIH Image to ImageJ: 25 years of image analysis. *Nat. Methods* **2012**, *9*, 671–675. [CrossRef] [PubMed]

30. Mukaka, M.M. Statistics corner: A guide to appropriate use of correlation coefficient in medical research. *Malawi Med. J.* **2012**, *24*, 69–71. [CrossRef] [PubMed]

31. Buzsáki, G. Large-scale recording of neuronal ensembles. *Nat. Neurosci.* **2004**, *7*, 446–451. [CrossRef] [PubMed]

32. Gilletti, A.; Muthuswamy, J. Brain micromotion around implants in the rodent somatosensory cortex. *J. Neural Eng.* **2006**, *3*, 189–195. [CrossRef] [PubMed]

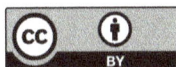

micromachines

MDPI

Article

A Mechanically-Adaptive Polymer Nanocomposite-Based Intracortical Probe and Package for Chronic Neural Recording

Allison Hess-Dunning [1,2,*] and Dustin J. Tyler [1,2,3]

[1] Rehabilitation Research and Development, Louis Stokes Cleveland VA Medical Center, Cleveland, OH 44106, USA
[2] Advanced Platform Technology Center, Cleveland, OH 44106, USA
[3] Department of Biomedical Engineering, Case Western Reserve University, Cleveland, OH 44106, USA; dustin.tyler@case.edu
* Correspondence: ahess@aptcenter.org; Tel.: +1-216-368-8541

Received: 14 September 2018; Accepted: 2 November 2018; Published: 8 November 2018

Abstract: Mechanical, materials, and biological causes of intracortical probe failure have hampered their utility in basic science and clinical applications. By anticipating causes of failure, we can design a system that will prevent the known causes of failure. The neural probe design was centered around a bio-inspired, mechanically-softening polymer nanocomposite. The polymer nanocomposite was functionalized with recording microelectrodes using a microfabrication process designed for chemical and thermal process compatibility. A custom package based upon a ribbon cable, printed circuit board, and a 3D-printed housing was designed to enable connection to external electronics. Probes were implanted into the primary motor cortex of Sprague-Dawley rats for 16 weeks, during which regular recording and electrochemical impedance spectroscopy measurement sessions took place. The implanted mechanically-softening probes had stable electrochemical impedance spectra across the 16 weeks and single units were recorded out to 16 weeks. The demonstration of chronic neural recording with the mechanically-softening probe suggests that probe architecture, custom package, and general design strategy are appropriate for long-term studies in rodents.

Keywords: neural probe; intracortical; microelectrodes; bio-inspired; polymer nanocomposite; cellulose nanocrystals; photolithography; Parylene C

1. Introduction

Intracortical neural interfaces enable both fundamental neuroscience advances and engineering strategies to restore motor, sensory, and cognitive functions to individuals who have suffered neurological injury or disease. Though electrical interfaces have dominated the field [1], recent advances in neural interfacing technologies also include single- and bi-directional chemical [2–4], ultrasound [5], and optical interfaces [6] for interrogating or modulating neural function. Intracortical brain-machine interfaces (BMIs) rely upon the detection of extracellular neural electrical activity in the tens-of-microvolts range using microelectrodes implanted several millimeters into the cortex. Mechanical, materials, and biological failures all contribute to the poor long-term stability and functionality of intracortical neural interfaces that continue to limit long-term, chronic studies and applications [7–9]. The harsh physiological environment, combined with the need to make a connection to external systems for control or recording, requires a system-level engineering design to maintain a stable interface with a microscale device requiring sensitive measurements. The probes, leads, and connectors can fail due to sudden applied forces or fatigue-related damage [9]. Electrode and insulating materials can degrade due to the harsh physiological environment, and may be accelerated by reactive oxygen species that accumulate as a result of an inflammatory tissue response to the implant [10–12]. Chronic inflammation also results in glial encapsulation, and further may be responsible for neuronal degradation near the implant [13–15]. Intracortical implant design should aim to: (1) maintain a high neuronal density at the biotic-abiotic interface, and (2) minimize chronic inflammation. Though these issues have primarily impacted intracortical probes for electrical recording, they extend to any intracortical interface and modality of interfacing, as well as to other implanted devices such as for deep brain stimulation. Therefore, engineering a reliable intracortical interface system will be impactful across a variety of applications requiring a device implanted into the cortex.

Solutions to poor long-term intracortical interface reliability largely focus on addressing the biological tissue response through geometric or materials design of neural probes [16–20]. Relative micromotion arising from constant, repetitive displacements in tissue due to respiration and vascular pulsations produce strain on tissue surrounding the implant due to mechanical mismatch at the implant-tissue interface for high modulus implants. The differential strain on tissue is considered to be a primary contributor to glial scar formation [21,22], which is further supported by in vitro studies reporting that components of astroglial scarring proliferate in response to mechanical strain [23] and high modulus substrates [24], while neurite outgrowth and extension is stimulated on low-modulus substrates with mechanical properties approaching brain tissue ($E_{brain} \sim 10$ kPa) [25]. Intracortical implants based on a lower modulus material reduce the differential strain on tissue during micromotion [26,27], which may also reduce the problematic neuroinflammatory response. The correlation between mechanics and the neural tissue response has led to the development of soft intracortical probes based on polymers with established microfabrication processes, such as polyimide [20,28,29], parylene [30–33], and SU-8 [34–37] polymer-based intracortical probes with much lower Young's moduli ($E_{polymer} \sim 2$–4 GPa) than standard silicon-based devices ($E_{Si} \sim 160$ GPa) or tungsten microwire ($E_W \sim 411$ GPa) arrays [8,38,39], thereby alleviating implant-tissue mechanical mismatch. However, mechanically-flexible, polymer-based neural probes may buckle during implantation. In some cases, probe width or thickness of polymer-based probes may be relatively large to ensure that the critical buckling force is greater than the insertion force [37,40,41]. Several strategies have also been developed to provide enhancement of temporary stiffness, including removeable rigid shuttles to guide the probe into place and dissolvable coatings [28,33,42]. Alternatively, the effective length of the probe can be shortened to increase the critical buckling strength by partial reinforcement of the probe shank with polyethylene glycol (PEG) [43] or with the use of an insertion guide [44]. Regardless of the insertion strategy, these commercially-available polymers retain a six order-of-magnitude mechanical mismatch with brain tissue after insertion. An ideal implant for improving integration with tissue and reducing strain would have a lower modulus that more closely matches brain tissue, and can be scaled to multi-shank arrays without requiring complex removable support structures.

The biological mechanism underlying the mechanical stiffness modulation of the sea cucumber dermis inspired the development of a polymer nanocomposite with a modulus that can be controlled by temperature and degree of saturation [45–47]. A soft poly(vinyl acetate) (PVAc) matrix polymer with a percolated network of high-aspect-ratio cellulose nanocrystals (CNC) harvested from tunicate mantles form the nanocomposite (Figure 1). The polymer nanocomposite (PVAc-CNC) has a high Young's modulus ($E \sim 4$–5 GPa) when dry due to the reinforcing effects of a percolating CNC network through the material. When swollen with water, the CNC network disengages, thus "turning off" the reinforcing effect. Bulk PVAc-CNC films swell 70% by weight [48], which is anisotropically distributed with a 3% increase in the lateral dimensions of water-saturated films and a 24% increase in film thickness [49]. The water-swollen matrix polymer is also plasticized, reducing the glass transition temperature (T_g) to ~20° C. The CNC disengagement and T_g reduction effects combine to yield a dramatic reduction in modulus to $E \sim 10$ MPa [40,50,51]. For intracortical neural interfaces, this single material is both sufficiently rigid for needle-like insertion into tissue without buckling, while also offering softening after insertion to reduce mechanical mismatch with surrounding tissue [40]. This material reduces strain on tissue and neuroinflammation compared to standard, rigid (E ~ 160 GPa) silicon-based implants [22,26,52].

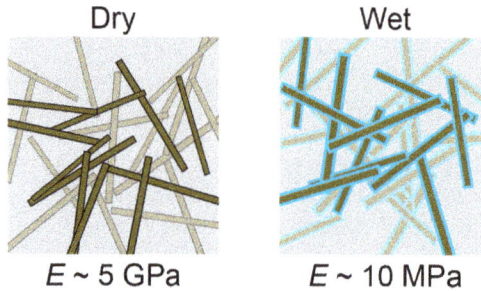

Figure 1. Schematic demonstrating the sea cucumber dermis-inspired PVAc-CNC softening mechanism. In the dry state (**left**), cellulose nanocrystals joined by hydrogen bonds form a reinforcing network throughout the nanocomposite. When saturated with water (**right**), the inter-nanocrystal hydrogen bonds are displaced with water molecule-nanocrystal bonds, leading to an overall reduction in storage modulus.

PVAc-CNC has a much wider mechanical range than other mechanically-softening polymers used for neural interface applications [18,41,53]. In its stiff state, PVAc-CNC has a modulus approximately seven times higher than the thiol-ene-based shape memory polymer [53]. In its mechanically-compliant state, PVAc-CNC has a modulus approximately four times lower than the shape memory polymer [53]. The higher stiff-state modulus for PVAc-CNC allows for a probe with a smaller cross-sectional area that will still penetrate through the pia and into the cortex without buckling. As a result of a smaller required cross-sectional area and a lower compliant-state modulus, the bending stiffness of PVAc-CNC implants can have a bending stiffness less than 5% of the bending stiffness of a shape memory polymer neural interface with the same length. However, PVAc-CNC has more extensive fabrication process limitations compared to the shape memory polymer [53,54]. Specifically, PVAc-CNC is incompatible with wet chemicals and with temperatures exceeding 100 °C [49,55]. Exposure to acids and bases will interfere with the surface properties of the cellulose nanocrystals, exposure to organic solvents will dissolve the PVAc matrix, and temperatures exceeding 100 °C will cause CNC degradation [56]. Further, PVAc-CNC is dependent upon water absorption to soften and therefore: (1) cannot serve as an insulating moisture barrier for thin-film metal traces and electrodes, and (2) cannot be completely coated with an insulating moisture barrier film.

Intracortical interfaces based upon PVAc-CNC require processes for forming a neural probe geometry and functionalizing the material with microelectrodes for recording, as well as a robust packaging system for making connection to external electronics. A complete system must consider the biological system, material properties, and forces to which the system is subjected during and after the insertion procedure. The design and method of packaging microscale neural interfaces are critical, yet often neglected, components of the implant system. For the mechanically-softening PVAc-CNC, the package must include a compatible method for making electrical connection between a rigid commercial connector and the mechanically-softening probe. The electrical interconnections between the probe and the connector must be insulated from the physiological environment and should avoid mechanical failure modalities. The connector itself must be protected to prevent mechanical breakage or removal. Finally, the entire headcap must be anchored securely to the skull for successful chronic studies. We previously reported on the fabrication and benchtop studies of an early-stage PVAc-CNC neural probe [49,51,55]. These studies demonstrated the feasibility of using PVAc-CNC as a mechanical substrate for microfabricated neural interfaces, that the thin-film metal and insulation layers do not contribute significantly to the mechanical behavior of the device, and that the device architecture remains stable through 60 days of soaking under physiological conditions [49,51,55].

Advancing PVAc-CNC neural interfaces to use in chronic studies required the refinement of the fabrication processes to include multiple microelectrodes along the shank, as well as a packaging scheme compatible with PVAc-CNC and the demands of chronic implantation. Here, we report on the progress we have made toward advancing PVAc-CNC neural interfaces to chronic implant studies.

2. Materials and Methods

2.1. Design and Overview

Our goal was to produce a planar microelectrode array with up to 8 recording sites on the PVAc-CNC polymer nanocomposite structural material. Planar microelectrode arrays allow for simultaneously measuring from multiple depths within the cortex [57]. The PVAc-CNC neural probe has a five-layer architecture comprising a PVAc-CNC structural substrate layer, a Parylene C barrier layer, Au electrodes and interconnections with a Ti adhesion layer, and a Parylene C capping layer. Additionally, probe length, width, and thickness must be chosen such that the critical buckling force, as determined by Euler's buckling formula, is greater than the force required to insert the probe [40]. The probe must be able to withstand an insertion force of 10 mN, based upon a typical insertion force of 5 mN [40] and a safety factor of 2. For a 40 μm-thick PVAc-CNC probe with a length of 3 mm, the probe width must be at least 140 μm.

2.2. Materials

2.2.1. PVAc-CNC

The polyvinyl acetate-cellulose nanocrystal polymer nanocomposite serves as the structural material for the neural probe. The methods for synthesizing PVAc-CNC have been described in detail elsewhere [45,46,48,58]. Briefly, poly(vinyl acetate) was dissolved in dimethylformamide (DMF). Cellulose nanocrystals were dispersed in DMF in a second beaker. The two solutions were mixed, then cast into a Teflon dish before drying under vacuum at 65 °C for 7 days [48]. The dry PVAc-CNC films were then pressed to a thickness of 30–60 μm at a temperature of 90 °C and a pressure of 3000 psi [59].

2.2.2. Parylene C

Parylene C serves as an insulating moisture barrier for the interconnection traces between the recording sites and connection contacts. Parylene is an FDA Class VI material and is a good moisture barrier with a 24-h water absorption of 0.06% and 0.14 g-mil/100 in^2 for 24 h at 37C, 90%RH moisture vapor transmission [60]. The Parylene C used in this application was vapor deposited with a Specialty Coating Systems Labcoter$^®$ 2 Parylene Deposition System (Specialty Coating Systems, Inc., Indianapolis, IN, USA).

2.2.3. Au/Ti

Sputter-deposited, thin-film Au was chosen for the microelectrode recording sites, connector contacts, and interconnecting traces due to its biocompatibility, inertness, and low residual stress.

2.3. Fabrication

The PVAc-CNC neural probe fabrication process averts PVAc-CNC exposure to wet chemicals or temperatures exceeding 100 °C. Exposure to acids and bases will interfere with the surface properties of the cellulose nanocrystals, exposure to organic solvents will dissolve the PVAc, and temperatures exceeding 100 °C will cause CNC degradation [56]. The microfabrication steps are illustrated in Figure 2a–j. First, a freestanding PVAc-CNC film was prepared by solution-casting and melt-pressing [48]. A silicon wafer provided a rigid support for the PVAc-CNC film during the fabrication process. The PVAc-CNC film was adhered to a silicon wafer by heating the assembly to

75 °C on a hotplate and pressing the film onto the silicon wafer (Figure 2a). It was important to avoid air bubbles between the wafer and the PVAc-CNC film. Next, a 2 μm-thick Parylene C barrier layer was vapor-deposited onto the PVAc-CNC film and silicon wafer (Figure 2b). This layer provided a moisture barrier necessary for protecting the PVAc-CNC film during wet chemical processing steps. Additionally, this layer was required to insulate the thin-film Ti/Au features from the electrolytic fluid absorbed by PVAc-CNC in vivo [49,55]. Next, a 20 nm-thick Ti adhesion layer and a 250 nm-thick Au conductive layer were sputter-deposited on the parylene film (Figure 2c). The Ti/Au films were patterned by photolithography using an iodine-based Au etchant (Gold Etch Type TFA, Transene Company, Inc., Danvers, MA, USA) and a buffered oxide etchant (Buffered Oxide Etchant 7:1 with Surfactant, Transene Company, Inc., Danvers, MA, USA), followed by removal of the photoresist with acetone and isopropanol (Figure 2d,e). A second 2 μm-thick parylene layer was then vapor-deposited to provide a capping layer to insulate conductive interconnect traces (Figure 2f). Openings in the Parylene C at the recording sites and connector contacts, as well as the outer geometry of the Parylene C layers were etched using reactive ion etching (RIE) with O_2 and CF_4 through a photoresist mask (Figure 2g). The outer probe geometry was then defined by laser-micromachining with a picosecond laser (Oxford Lasers, Didcot, UK) (Figure 2h). The excess material between probes was peeled from the handle wafer (Figure 2i). Finally, the completed probes were removed from the wafer with the aid of a razor blade (Figure 2j).

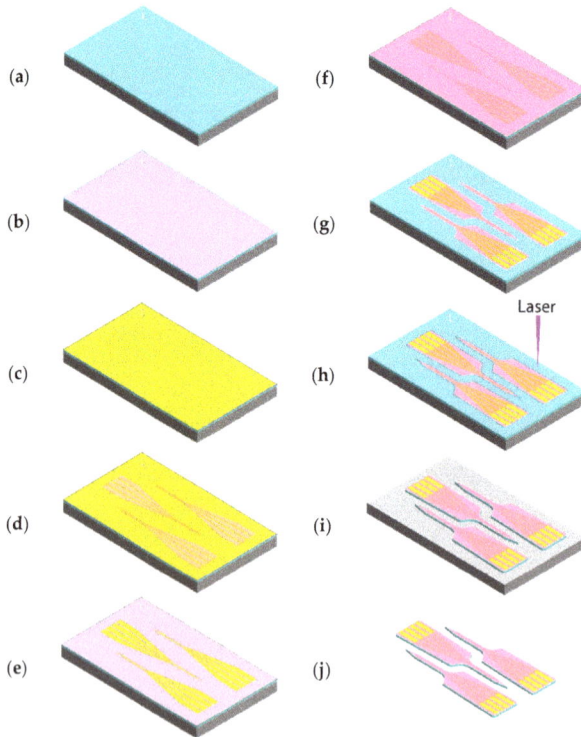

Figure 2. Microfabrication process for PVAc-CNC intracortical probes. (**a**) PVAc-CNC film mounted to bare Si probe; (**b**) Parylene C deposition; (**c**) Ti/Au deposition; (**d**) Photoresist spin-coating and patterning; (**e**) Wet etching of Ti/Au films; (**f**) Second Parylene C deposition; (**g**) Parylene C patterned using oxygen plasma; (**h**) Laser micromachining the PVAc-CNC substrate; (**i**) Remove excess PVAc-CNC in field region; (**j**) Release probes.

2.4. Packaging

The packaging scheme was designed to be modular such that the components could be tested at various levels of assembly and could be modified for compatibility with alternate applications. Probes were directly attached to polyimide-based ribbon cables (Pyralux, DuPont, Wilmington, DE, USA) designed to interface with a Hirose FH-19 Flexible circuit board connector (Hirose Electric Group, Shinagawa, Tokyo, Japan). Both the flexible circuit connector and an Omnetics Nano Strip connector (Omnetics Connector Corporation, Minneapolis, MN, USA) were mounted to a printed circuit board (Figure 3a), providing a means to connect to external electronics for neural recording and for impedance measurements. A 3D-printed housing was custom-designed and fabricated to hold the PCB, connectors, and ribbon cable (Figure 3b).

The ribbon cables were fabricated by etching the Pyralux copper cladding with a sodium persulfate solution through a laser-printed toner etch mask. The toner was then removed from the surface of the copper using acetone. The copper traces were insulated with an acrylic spray through a shadow mask, then the ribbon cable was cut out by laser micromachining. Probes were attached to the flexible ribbon cable using a cyanoacrylic adhesive. Electrical connection between the copper ribbon cable pads and the gold probe pads was made with conductive epoxy (MG Chemicals 8331S, MC Chemicals, Surrey, British Columbia, Canada). To insulate the electrical connections, a 2-part epoxy was applied using a needle to the exposed conductive epoxy and contact pads on both the probe and ribbon cable. The ribbon cables were inserted into the flexible circuit connector on the PCB, then the assembly was pushed into the 3D-printed housing. The PCB slides into one section of the housing, while a separate section holds the ribbon cable to ensure that the probe shank was normal to the housing. The components were secured with insulating epoxy.

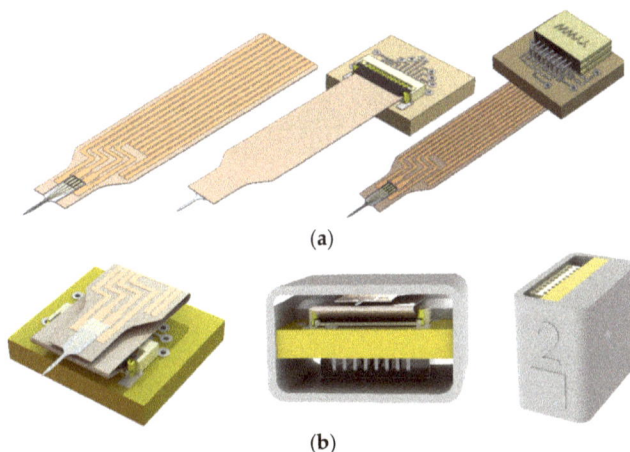

(a)

(b)

Figure 3. Packaging scheme for PVAc-CNC intracortical probes. (**a**) The probes are attached to a polyimide-based ribbon cable with patterned Cu traces. The ribbon cable is designed for insertion into a flexible circuit connector mounted on a printed circuit board with an Omnetics connector for interfacing with external electronics; (**b**) The ribbon cable/PCB/connector assembly is inserted into a custom-designed, 3D-printed housing to protect the components.

2.5. Benchtop Impedance Measurements

Fully-packaged PVAc-CNC probes were immersed in phosphate buffered saline in a heated water bath at 37 °C, then the impedance spectra of recording sites were measured over 48 days. An EZStat Pro potentiostat (NuVant Systems Inc., Crown Point, IN, USA) was used to measure the impedance versus a platinum reference wire between 10 Hz and 10 kHz, with 25 points per decade. The impedance magnitude at a frequency of 1 kHz was used to compare frequency over time.

2.6. Chronic In Vivo Experiments

2.6.1. Surgical Procedure

Three male Sprague-Dawley rats (225–250 g) were implanted with a single PVAc-CNC neural probe in the primary motor cortex, which was then left in place for 16 weeks. The PVAc-CNC probes were sterilized using ethylene oxide. All procedures and animal care practices were approved by and performed in accordance with the Case Western Reserve University Institutional Animal Care and Use Committee. The surgical procedures followed standard protocols [52,61,62]. Briefly, the rats were initially anesthetized by a mixture of ketamine (80 mg/kg) and xylazine (10 mg/kg) administered intraperitoneally (IP). After preparing the animal's head by shaving and cleaning, a one-inch incision was made down the midline; then the surrounding tissue was retracted to expose the skull. An opening approximately 3 mm in diameter was drilled into the skull in the left hemisphere approximately 3 mm lateral to the midline and 2 mm anterior to bregma. The dura was deflected using a dura pick to expose the pia. Three stainless steel screws (#2-56) were implanted in the skull, and the ground and reference wires were attached to the base of two of the screws, then secured in place with silver print. The probe was brought within 2 mm of the brain surface for positioning while ensuring that the shank remained dry. Once in place, the probe was rapidly lowered using a manual micromanipulator at a rate of approximately 0.5 mm·s^{-1} to a final depth of approximately 2 mm. After the PVAc-CNC probe and housing were set in place, silicone elastomer (Kwik-Sil, World Precision Instruments) was applied to seal the craniotomy. The connector housing was secured in place with dental acrylic anchored by the screws. Finally, the skin on the scalp was closed around the housing with 1–2 sutures.

2.6.2. Neural Recording and EIS Measurements

Eleven neural recording sessions took place during the 16-week implant duration. Each recording session lasted for approximately 10 min and involved cleaning and drying the housing and Omnetics connector, connecting a pre-amplifier and cable, then allowing the rat to freely move within a clean cage. Neural potentials were recorded with a 16-channel Tucker David Technologies (TDT) Pentusa Z5 system (Tucker-Davis Technologies, Alachua, FL, USA), using a sampling rate of 24.4 kHz. EIS measurements were made with the rat under isoflurane anesthesia using an amplitude of 10 mV between 1 Hz and 10 kHz with 10 frequencies per decade.

2.6.3. Neural Recording Data Analysis

Data from each trial was processed by a MATLAB (R2013, MathWorks, Natick, MA, USA) analysis program based on code from the Kipke Lab [63,64]. Signals were separated into local field potential (LFP) (0.1–140 Hz) and neural spike (300–5000 Hz) components in MATLAB. For spike analysis, a negative threshold at 3.5 times the standard deviation of the signal was set to identify candidate samples. Any sample crossing the threshold was considered for further processing. The samples were considered within a 2.4 ms window, and the minimum potential was chosen to be the center of the spike snippet window at 1.2 ms. A principal component analysis (PCA) was performed on a voltage amplitude matrix ($N_{spikes} \times 100$ timepoints) corresponding to the collection of spike snippet windows to cluster the spikes. Neural units were identified by choosing the clusters with more than 20 spikes in a cluster. A mean spike waveform was created from the spikes in the cluster, and the peak-to-peak voltage of the mean waveform determined the peak-to-peak signal voltage. The peak-to-peak noise voltage of each channel and block was determined by first removing the spike snippets windows from the signal and determining the standard deviation of the remaining signal. The peak-to-peak noise voltage was then defined as 3 times the standard deviation of the remaining noise signal.

3. Results and Discussion

3.1. Device Fabrication

Multi-electrode arrays with between 4 and 8 individually-addressable microelectrode recording sites were fabricated on the PVAc-CNC polymer nanocomposite, as shown in Figure 4. Thin-film metal feature sizes down to 7 μm were resolved on the Parylene C-coated PVAc-CNC surface. The solution-cast and compressed PVAc-CNC films have surface height variations of up to 4 μm over a 100 μm lateral distance, yielding a much larger surface roughness than a standard silicon wafer with sub-nanometer surface roughness. The minimum resolvable feature size is therefore limited by the roughness and uniformity of the PVAc-CNC surface, and can be decreased further by refining PVAc-CNC film manufacturing processes. An important aspect of our refined fabrication process is the use of a picosecond UV micromachining laser with alignment capability to pattern the PVAc-CNC probe outer geometry after the photolithography steps, instead of as one of the first fabrication steps. This allowed for photolithography steps on a much more planar surface, thus improving yield and minimum feature size. In the 4-electrode design shown in Figure 4A,B, the parylene capping layer covers the entire front-side of the probe. To maximize the benefits of the PVAc-CNC material properties, the Parylene C footprint was minimized in the 8-electrode design shown in Figure 4C,D. This change in geometry was made possible with improved precision in photolithography, etching, and PVAc-CNC patterning. These improvements also facilitated a reduction in interconnect trace width from 15 μm to 7 μm without sacrificing yield. This microfabrication process is scalable and can be used for multiple shanks or to increase the number of recording sites per shank.

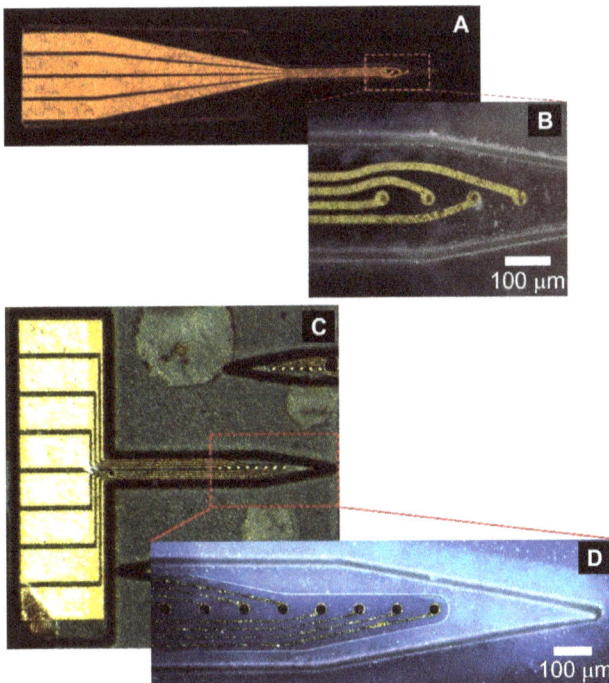

Figure 4. PVAc-CNC neural probes: (**A**) 4-channel probe overview; (**B**) Close-up of 15 μm-diameter Au microelectrode sites on 4-electrode probe; (**C**) 8-channel probe overview; (**D**) Close-up of 30 μm-diameter Au microelectrode sites on 8-electrode probe.

Device yield was largely dependent upon the elimination of air from between the PVAc-CNC film and the underlying silicon handle wafer. Unlike spin-cast or vapor-deposited polymers, PVAc-CNC begins as a free-standing film. Air trapped between the wafer and PVAc-CNC film can expand during microfabrication steps that occur under vacuum, particularly during sputter deposition when the nanocomposite softens with an increase in temperature. Additionally, the in-line design of the 4-channel design had fewer mechanical failures during release from the wafer than the wide connector contact pad layout with the sharp transition to the shank featured in the 8-contact design.

3.2. Probe Packaging

We considered materials and process compatibility, modularity, and robustness when designing and developing a package for the PVAc-CNC probes. In our packaging scheme, the probe, reference, and ground wires were attached to a polyimide-based Pyralux ribbon cable with copper traces running from the probe to an end designed to interface with a flexible circuit connector. Electrical connection between the Au contact pads on the probe and the Cu contact pads on the ribbon cable was made with Ag-based conductive epoxy. The contact resistance between the Au contact pads on the probe and the Cu contact pads on the ribbon cable was less than 5 Ω, which is negligible compared to the overall trace resistance and electrode-electrolyte interface impedance. The ribbon cable provides a modular approach to making electrical connection to the probe, thus allowing for testing before assembling the complete package. Further, electrical connection via a ribbon cable lends itself to design flexibility, as the ribbon cable length can be increased to reduce tethering forces, and the configuration can be modified to enable more bending and stretching without putting undue stress on the ribbon cable traces. In our in vivo studies, the ribbon cable was folded and inserted into the 3D printed housing (Figures 3 and 5). The ribbon cable connected to a printed circuit board via a flexible circuit connector (Hirose FH-12-10SH). The neural recording system was then connected via cable to an Omnetics Nanostrip connector also mounted on the PCB. The completed assembly is shown in Figure 5. The housing made it possible to grip the housing for insertion purposes and protect the circuit board and all connections while implanted. The package can be easily scaled up to accommodate more recording contacts.

The labor-intensive process required to package the PVAc-CNC probes presents several risks for failure of a mechanically-brittle probe. To reduce these risks and improve yield of packaged probes, PVAc-CNC probes are packaged while the shanks are slightly moist and are therefore less brittle. Future designs will include a monolithically-integrated ribbon cable that will reduce the level of skill required to make a connection between the PVAc-CNC and connectors to external electronics.

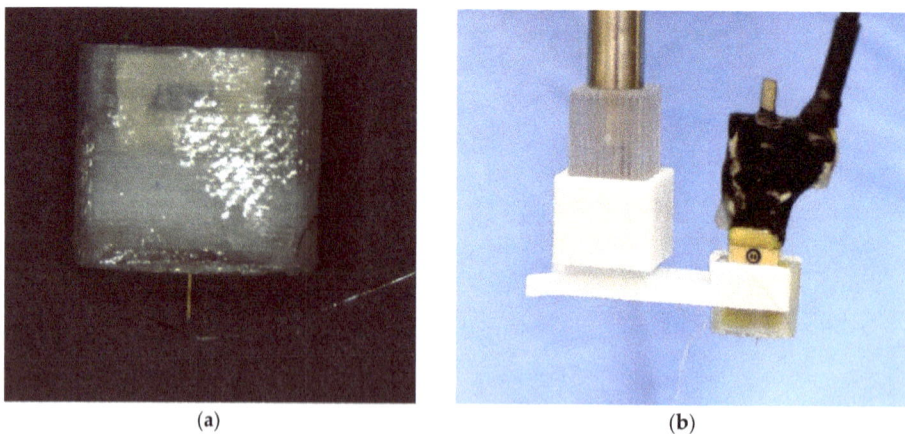

(a)   (b)

Figure 5. *Cont.*

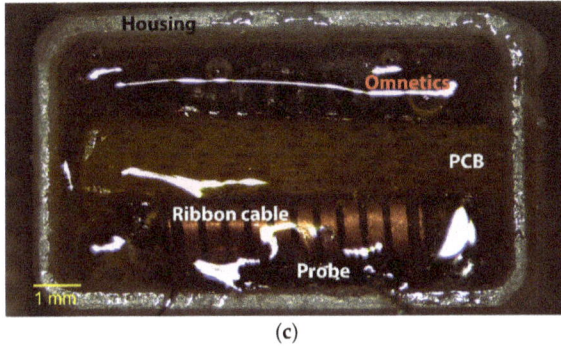

(c)

Figure 5. Packaged PVAc-CNC neural probes: (**a**) Front-view of probe in connector housing; (**b**) Assembly held with a custom clip for insertion; (**c**) Underside view of probe in connector housing, which shows the ribbon cable folded into the connector housing.

3.3. Benchtop Characterization

EIS results for the 50 μm-diameter PVAc-CNC microelectrode sites in PBS indicated impedance magnitude values between 55.1 and 190.7 kΩ at a frequency of 1 kHz. EIS results from a typical recording site are shown in Figure 6a. The average impedance magnitude at a frequency of 1 kHz of six channels across two devices measured over 48 days is shown in Figure 6b. The electrode-electrolyte interface properties are typical for 50 μm-diameter Au microelectrodes and remained relatively stable throughout the soak test. These results indicated that the microelectrodes remained intact and the Parylene C served as a moisture barrier for the soak test duration. Based on this data, we determined that these probes were sufficiently robust for preliminary in vivo investigations for chronic recording and electrochemical impedance spectroscopy measurements.

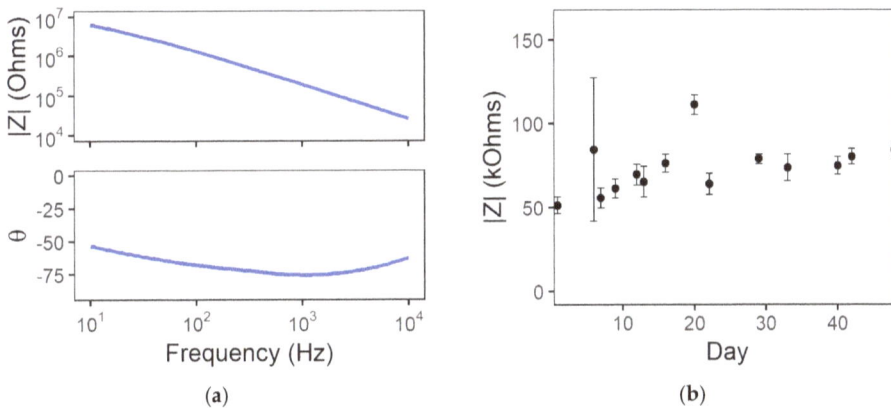

(a)   (b)

Figure 6. Representative results from PVAc-CNC soak testing with 50 μm-diameter microelectrodes: (**a**) Impedance spectra at 1 h after immersion in PBS; (**b**) Impedance magnitude at a 1 kHz frequency over time.

3.4. Chronic Implant Experiments

3.4.1. Surgery/Insertion

Using the custom, 3D-printed clip to hold the probe housing, the probes were inserted into the cortex cleanly and securely. The insertion needed to be performed within a few seconds due to the rapid softening of the PVAc-CNC material [40,49,50]. The headcaps remained firmly in place for the 16-week duration of the experiment.

PVAc-CNC swelling is primarily a concern only during the insertion process because swelling corresponds to a reduction in material stiffness. Further, damage during implantation can be minimized by completing the insertion process before the probe is able to swell appreciably. Though an increase in implant size has generally correlated with an increase in glial scarring and a decrease local neuronal density [65,66], a decrease in mechanical modulus [26,52,67] and material density [68] of the structural material can improve the tissue response and neuronal density. PVAc-CNC swelling is anisotropic, favoring the through-thickness dimension by 8-fold. The minimal swelling across the film prevents probe curling or bending, even though one surface of the film is constrained by the parylene films, electrodes, and interconnects. Though additional study is required to understand the effects of PVAc-CNC swelling on recording quality, we speculate that through-thickness swelling may have a positive effect on neural recording quality by reducing the distance between recording electrode sites and active neurons after deployment.

3.4.2. Electrochemical Impedance Spectroscopy

EIS results, averaged across functional channels, measured across the duration of the implant time period, are shown in Figure 7. At 1 kHz, the impedance magnitude initially ranges from 0.32 to 1.28 MΩ, which increases to a range of 0.82–1.31 MΩ on the final day. The smaller area of the implanted microelectrodes sites (15 μm-diameter) compared to the microelectrode sites on the soak-tested devices (50 μm-diameter) (Figure 6) resulted in a higher electrochemical impedance. These valued scaled as expected with $1/r^2$ [69]. Further, these are typical impedance values for gold microelectrodes of a similar area [70]. Overall, there is no clear trend in impedance magnitude over the 16 weeks, and the spectra are quite stable across the duration. This stability indicates that the electrode contacts, insulating barrier and capping layers, and the surrounding tissue properties remained quite stable for the duration of the implant duration.

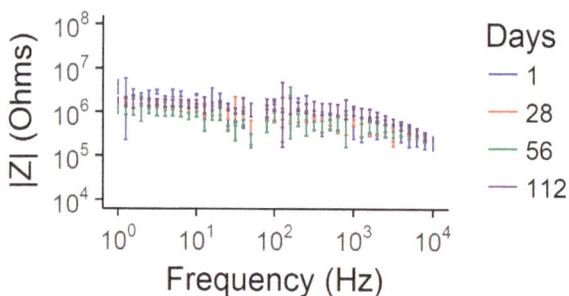

Figure 7. Comparison of impedance magnitude spectra from EIS over the 16-week implant period.

3.4.3. Chronic Neural Recording

Neural activity with a signal-to-noise ratio between 2.6 and 4.3 was recorded using the PVAc-CNC neural probes during the 16-week implant duration (Figure 8B). Average unit waveforms from pile-plots of 50 isolated spike snippets recorded at 1-week (Figure 8A, top) and 16-week (Figure 8A, bottom) timepoints indicate that the PVAc-CNC probes are sufficiently robust in terms of probe architecture and packaging to be able to record isolated units at a 16-week timepoint. The mean signal-to-noise ratio (SNR) for isolated units from each recording session with the same probe is shown in Figure 8B. The SNR was relatively stable, especially beyond the 30-day timepoint. There were two recording sessions during which no action potentials were recorded. With the exception of these two recording sessions, isolated units were recorded on at least one channel for each recording session. For some sessions, units were recorded on two or three channels. High-pass filtered (>300 Hz) voltage traces recorded from adjacent channels at the 16-week timepoint are shown in Figure 8C. Each trace contains unique features and spikes, indicating that crosstalk between traces is minimal, even at the 16-week timepoint. These results are the first demonstration of neural recording using the PVAc-CNC material, and therefore offers encouraging results for the chronic functional use of the mechanically-softening polymer nanocomposite.

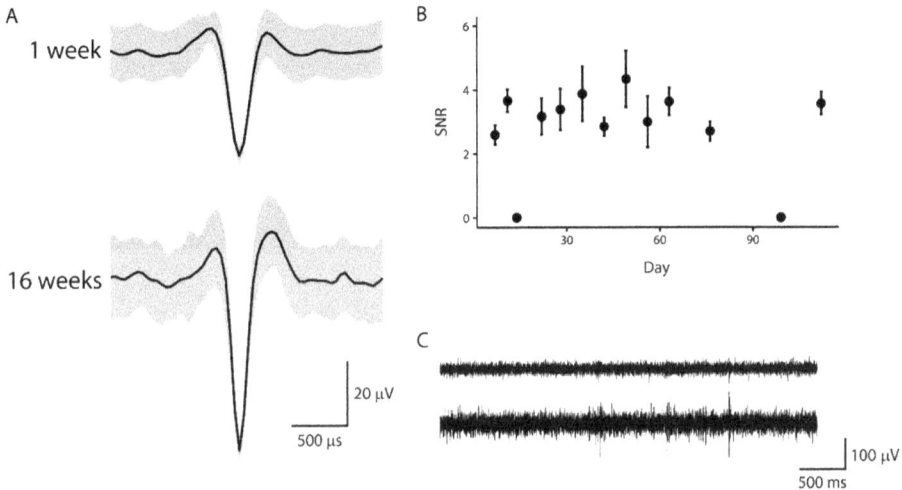

Figure 8. Demonstration of neural recording with PVAc-CNC neural probes. (**A**) Average waveform from 50 isolated and clustered spike snippets at the1-week timepoint (top) and 16-week timepoint (bottom); (**B**) Mean SNR +/− s.e. for isolated units detected for each recording session during the 16-week implant period; (**C**) High-pass (>300 Hz) filtered traces for two adjacent microelectrodes at the 16-week timepoint.

4. Conclusions

We developed a neural probe system based on a mechanically-adaptive polymer nanocomposite using a microfabrication process flow designed for compatibility with the chemical and thermal sensitivities of PVAc-CNC. Importantly, the polymer nanocomposite was designed specifically for biocompatibility and biological integration as an implant material, which contrasts strongly with the focus on processability for silicon- and mechanically-static polymer-based neural implants. PVAc-CNC is a sufficiently rigid material in its dry state to penetrate the cortex before dramatically softening and reducing mechanical mismatch at the interface. To overcome the incompatibility of PVAc-CNC with standard microfabrication processes, the process flow used to develop PVAc-CNC neural probes was reliant upon laser micromachining and the use of a conformal Parylene C coating that protects PVAc-CNC from exposure to wet chemicals during processing and insulates thin-film traces from electrolytic fluid absorbed by PVAc-CNC while implanted. A custom, robust package was also designed to interface the microscale polymer nanocomposite-based probes with external electronics and maintain the ability to connect to external electronics for at least 16 weeks. For the first time, we have demonstrated that the PVAc-CNC probes remain electrically functional and stable for an extended duration and are capable of recording electrical neural activity for at least 16 weeks.

Author Contributions: Conceptualization, D.J.T. and A.H.-D.; Methodology, D.J.T. and A.H.-D.; Validation, A.H.-D.; Formal Analysis, A.H.-D.; Investigation, D.J.T. and A.H.-D.; Resources, D.J.T. and A.H.-D.; Data Curation, D.J.T. and A.H.-D.; Writing-Original Draft Preparation, A.H.-D.; Writing-Review & Editing, D.J.T. and A.H.-D.; Supervision, D.J.T.; Project Administration, D.J.T.; Funding Acquisition, D.J.T. and A.H.-D.

Funding: This research was funded by grant number R21-NS053798 from the National Institute of Neurological Disorders and Stroke, the Advanced Platform Technology Center of the Rehabilitation Research and Development Service of the United States (U.S.) Department of Veterans Affairs (Center #C3819C, A6791C, 1I50RX001871) and Career Development Awards #IK1RX000959 (CDA-1, AHD) and #IK2RX001841 (CDA-2, AHD) from the U.S. Department of Veterans Affairs Rehabilitation Research and Development Service. The contents do not represent the views of the U.S. Department of Veterans Affairs or the United States Government.

Acknowledgments: The authors would like to acknowledge Stuart Rowan and Yefei Zhang for preparing and providing the polymer nanocomposite materials, Jeffrey Capadona and Evon Ereifej for their assistance and training for the implant surgeries, and Christian Zorman for the use of equipment and space in his laboratory.

Conflicts of Interest: The authors declare no conflict of interest.

References

1. Flesher, S.N.; Collinger, J.L.; Foldes, S.T.; Weiss, J.M.; Downey, J.E.; Tyler-Kabara, E.C.; Bensmaia, S.J.; Schwartz, A.B.; Boninger, M.L.; Gaunt, R.A. Intracortical microstimulation of human somatosensory cortex. *Sci. Transl. Med.* **2016**. [CrossRef] [PubMed]
2. Ferreira, N.R.; Ledo, A.; Laranjinha, J.; Gerhardt, G.A.; Barbosa, R.M. Simultaneous measurements of ascorbate and glutamate in vivo in the rat brain using carbon fiber nanocomposite sensors and microbiosensor arrays. *Bioelectrochemistry* **2018**, *121*, 142–150. [CrossRef] [PubMed]
3. Clark, J.J.; Sandberg, S.G.; Wanat, M.J.; Gan, J.O.; Horne, E.A.; Hart, A.S.; Akers, C.A.; Parker, J.G.; Willuhn, I.; Martinez, V.; et al. Chronic microsensors for longitudinal, subsecond dopamine detection in behaving animals. *Nat. Methods* **2010**, *7*, 126–129. [CrossRef] [PubMed]
4. Sim, J.Y.; Haney, M.P.; Park, S., II; McCall, J.G.; Jeong, J.-W. Microfluidic neural probes: In vivo tools for advancing neuroscience. *Lab Chip* **2017**, *17*, 1406–1435. [CrossRef] [PubMed]
5. Seo, D.; Carmena, J.M.; Rabaey, J.M.; Maharbiz, M.M.; Alon, E. Model validation of untethered, ultrasonic neural dust motes for cortical recording. *J. Neurosci. Methods* **2015**, *244*, 114–122. [CrossRef] [PubMed]
6. Aravanis, A.M.; Wang, L.P.; Zhang, F.; Meltzer, L.A.; Mogri, M.Z.; Schneider, M.B.; Deisseroth, K. An optical neural interface: In vivo control of rodent motor cortex with integrated fiberoptic and optogenetic technology. *J. Neural Eng.* **2007**, *4*, S143. [CrossRef] [PubMed]
7. Ward, M.P.; Rajdev, P.; Ellison, C.; Irazoqui, P.P. Toward a comparison of microelectrodes for acute and chronic recordings. *Brain Res.* **2009**, *1282*, 183–200. [CrossRef] [PubMed]
8. Prasad, A.; Xue, Q.-S.S.; Sankar, V.; Nishida, T.; Shaw, G.; Streit, W.J.; Sanchez, J.C. Comprehensive characterization and failure modes of tungsten microwire arrays in chronic neural implants. *J. Neural Eng.* **2012**, *9*, 56015. [CrossRef] [PubMed]
9. Kozai, T.D.Y.; Catt, K.; Li, X.; Gugel, Z.V.; Olafsson, V.T.; Vazquez, A.L.; Cui, X.T. Mechanical failure modes of chronically implanted planar silicon-based neural probes for laminar recording. *Biomaterials* **2015**, *37*, 25–39. [CrossRef] [PubMed]
10. Potter-Baker, K.A.; Capadona, J.R. Reducing the "Stress": Antioxidative Therapeutic and Material Approaches May Prevent Intracortical Microelectrode Failure. *ACS Macro Lett.* **2015**, *4*, 275–279. [CrossRef]
11. Potter-Baker, K.A.; Stewart, W.G.; Tomaszewski, W.H.; Wong, C.T.; Meador, W.D.; Ziats, N.P.; Capadona, J.R. Implications of chronic daily anti-oxidant administration on the inflammatory response to intracortical microelectrodes. *J. Neural Eng.* **2015**, *12*, 046002. [CrossRef] [PubMed]
12. Takmakov, P.; Ruda, K.; Scott Phillips, K.; Isayeva, I.S.; Krauthamer, V.; Welle, C.G. Rapid evaluation of the durability of cortical neural implants using accelerated aging with reactive oxygen species. *J. Neural Eng.* **2015**, *12*, 026003. [CrossRef] [PubMed]
13. Polikov, V.S.; Tresco, P.A.; Reichert, W.M. Response of brain tissue to chronically implanted neural electrodes. *J. Neurosci. Methods* **2005**, *148*, 1–18. [CrossRef] [PubMed]
14. Biran, R.; Martin, D.C.; Tresco, P.A. Neuronal cell loss accompanies the brain tissue response to chronically implanted silicon microelectrode arrays. *Exp. Neurol.* **2005**, *195*, 115–126. [CrossRef] [PubMed]
15. Woolley, A.J.; Desai, H.A.; Otto, K.J. Chronic intracortical microelectrode arrays induce non-uniform, depth-related tissue responses. *J. Neural Eng.* **2013**, *10*, 026007. [CrossRef] [PubMed]
16. Seymour, J.P.; Kipke, D.R. Neural probe design for reduced tissue encapsulation in CNS. *Biomaterials* **2007**, *28*, 3594–3607. [CrossRef] [PubMed]

17. Kozai, T.D.Y.; Langhals, N.B.; Patel, P.R.; Deng, X.; Zhang, H.; Smith, K.L.; Lahann, J.; Kotov, N.A.; Kipke, D.R. Ultrasmall implantable composite microelectrodes with bioactive surfaces for chronic neural interfaces. *Nat. Mater.* **2012**, *11*, 1065–1073. [CrossRef] [PubMed]

18. Ware, T.; Simon, D.; Arreaga-Salas, D.E.; Reeder, J.; Rennaker, R.; Keefer, E.W.; Voit, W. Fabrication of Responsive, Softening Neural Interfaces. *Adv. Funct. Mater.* **2012**, *22*, 3470–3479. [CrossRef]

19. Takeuchi, S.; Ziegler, D.; Yoshida, Y.; Mabuchi, K.; Suzuki, T. Parylene flexible neural probes integrated with microfluidic channels. *Lab Chip* **2005**, *5*, 519–523. [CrossRef] [PubMed]

20. Rousche, P.J.; Pellinen, D.S.; Pivin, D.P., Jr.; Williams, J.C.; Vetter, R.J.; Kirke, D.R.; Member, S.; Pivin, D.P.; Kipke, D.R.; Williams, J.C.; et al. Flexible polyimide-based intracortical electrode arrays with bioactive capability. *IEEE Trans. Biomed. Eng.* **2001**, *48*, 361–371. [CrossRef] [PubMed]

21. Gilletti, A.; Muthuswamy, J. Brain micromotion around implants in the rodent somatosensory cortex. *J. Neural Eng.* **2006**, *3*, 189. [CrossRef] [PubMed]

22. Sridharan, A.; Nguyen, J.K.; Capadona, J.R.; Muthuswamy, J. Compliant intracortical implants reduce strains and strain rates in brain tissue in vivo. *J. Neural Eng.* **2015**, *12*, 036002. [CrossRef] [PubMed]

23. Spencer, K.C.; Sy, J.C.; Falcón-Banchs, R.; Cima, M.J. A three dimensional in vitro glial scar model to investigate the local strain effects from micromotion around neural implants. *Lab Chip* **2017**, *17*, 795–804. [CrossRef] [PubMed]

24. Moshayedi, P.; Ng, G.; Kwok, J.C.F.; Yeo, G.S.H.; Bryant, C.E.; Fawcett, J.W.; Franze, K.; Guck, J. The relationship between glial cell mechanosensitivity and foreign body reactions in the central nervous system. *Biomaterials* **2014**, *35*, 3919–3925. [CrossRef] [PubMed]

25. Khoshakhlagh, P.; Moore, M.J. Photoreactive interpenetrating network of hyaluronic acid and Puramatrix as a selectively tunable scaffold for neurite growth. *Acta Biomater.* **2015**, *16*, 23–34. [CrossRef] [PubMed]

26. Nguyen, J.K.; Park, D.J.; Skousen, J.L.; Hess-Dunning, A.E.; Tyler, D.J.; Rowan, S.J.; Weder, C.; Capadona, J.R. Mechanically-compliant intracortical implants reduce the neuroinflammatory response. *J. Neural Eng.* **2014**, *11*, 056014. [CrossRef] [PubMed]

27. Subbaroyan, J.; Martin, D.C.; Kipke, D.R. A finite-element model of the mechanical effects of implantable microelectrodes in the cerebral cortex. *J. Neural Eng.* **2005**, *2*, 103. [CrossRef] [PubMed]

28. Xiang, Z.; Yen, S.-C.; Xue, N.; Sun, T.; Tsang, W.M.; Zhang, S.; Liao, L.-D.; Thakor, N.V.; Lee, C. Ultra-thin flexible polyimide neural probe embedded in a dissolvable maltose-coated microneedle. *J. Micromech. Microeng.* **2014**, *24*, 065015. [CrossRef]

29. Fomani, A.A.; Mansour, R.R. Fabrication and characterization of the flexible neural microprobes with improved structural design. *Sens. Actuators A Phys.* **2011**, *168*, 233–241. [CrossRef]

30. Sohal, H.S.; Jackson, A.; Jackson, R.; Clowry, G.J.; Vassilevski, K.; O'Neill, A.; Baker, S.N. The sinusoidal probe: A new approach to improve electrode longevity. *Front. Neuroeng.* **2014**, *7*, 10. [CrossRef] [PubMed]

31. Hara, S.A.; Kim, B.J.; Kuo, J.T.W.; Lee, C.D.; Meng, E.; Pikov, V. Long-term stability of intracortical recordings using perforated and arrayed Parylene sheath electrodes. *J. Neural Eng.* **2016**, *13*, 066020. [CrossRef] [PubMed]

32. Lecomte, A.; Castagnola, V.; Descamps, E.; Dahan, L.; Blatché, M.C.; Leclerc, E.; Bergaud, C. Silk and PEG as means to stiffen parylene probes for insertion in the brain: A comparison. *J. Micromech. Microeng.* **2015**, *25*, 125003. [CrossRef]

33. Wu, F.; Tien, L.W.; Chen, F.; Berke, J.D.; Kaplan, D.L.; Yoon, E. Silk-backed structural optimization of high-density flexible intracortical neural probes. *J. Microelectromech. Syst.* **2015**, *24*, 62–69. [CrossRef]

34. Altuna, A.; Gabriel, G.; Menéndez de la Prida, L.; Tijero, M.; Guimerá, A.; Berganzo, J.; Salido, R.; Villa, R.; Fernández, L.J. SU-8-based microneedles for in vitro neural applications. *J. Micromech. Microeng.* **2010**, *20*, 064014. [CrossRef]

35. Tijero, M.; Gabriel, G.; Caro, J.; Altuna, A.; Hernández, R.; Villa, R.; Berganzo, J.; Blanco, F.J.; Salido, R.; Fernández, L.J. SU-8 microprobe with microelectrodes for monitoring electrical impedance in living tissues. *Biosens. Bioelectron.* **2009**, *24*, 2410–2416. [CrossRef] [PubMed]

36. Luan, L.; Wei, X.; Zhao, Z.; Siegel, J.J.; Potnis, O.; Tuppen, C.A.; Lin, S.; Kazmi, S.; Fowler, R.A.; Holloway, S.; et al. Ultraflexible nanoelectronic probes form reliable, glial scar–free neural integration. *Sci. Adv.* **2017**, *3*, e1601966. [CrossRef] [PubMed]

37. Altuna, A.; Berganzo, J.; Fernández, L.J. Polymer SU-8-Based Microprobes for Neural Recording and Drug Delivery. *Front. Mater.* **2015**, *2*, 47. [CrossRef]

38. Rousche, P.J.; Normann, R.A. Chronic recording capability of the Utah Intracortical Electrode Array in cat sensory cortex. *J. Neurosci. Methods* **1998**, *82*, 1–15. [CrossRef]
39. Hoogerwerf, A.C.; Wise, K.D. A three-dimensional microelectrode array for chronic neural recording. *IEEE Trans. Biomed. Eng.* **1994**, *41*, 1136–1146. [CrossRef] [PubMed]
40. Harris, J.P.; Hess, A.E.; Rowan, S.J.; Weder, C.; Zorman, C.A.; Tyler, D.J.; Capadona, J.R. In vivo deployment of mechanically adaptive nanocomposites for intracortical microelectrodes. *J. Neural Eng.* **2011**, *8*, 46010. [CrossRef] [PubMed]
41. Ware, T.; Simon, D.; Liu, C.; Musa, T.; Vasudevan, S.; Sloan, A.; Keefer, E.W.; Rennaker, R.L.; Voit, W. Thiol-ene/acrylate substrates for softening intracortical electrodes. *J. Biomed. Mater. Res. Part B* **2014**, *102*, 1–11. [CrossRef] [PubMed]
42. Lo, M.; Wang, S.; Singh, S.; Damodaran, V.B.; Kaplan, H.M.; Kohn, J.; Shreiber, D.I.; Zahn, J.D. Coating flexible probes with an ultra fast degrading polymer to aid in tissue insertion. *Biomed. Microdevices* **2015**, *17*, 34. [CrossRef] [PubMed]
43. Xu, H.; Hirschberg, A.W.; Scholten, K.; Berger, T.W.; Song, D.; Meng, E. Acute in vivo testing of a conformal polymer microelectrode array for multi-region hippocampal recordings. *J. Neural Eng.* **2018**, *15*. [CrossRef] [PubMed]
44. Shoffstall, A.J.; Srinivasan, S.; Willis, M.; Stiller, A.M.; Ecker, M.; Voit, W.E.; Pancrazio, J.J.; Capadona, J.R. A Mosquito Inspired Strategy to Implant Microprobes into the Brain. *Sci. Rep.* **2018**, *8*, 122. [CrossRef] [PubMed]
45. Capadona, J.R.; Shanmuganathan, K.; Tyler, D.J.; Rowan, S.J.; Weder, C. Stimuli-Responsive Polymer Nanocomposites Inspired by the Sea Cucumber Dermis. *Science* **2008**, *319*, 1370–1374. [CrossRef] [PubMed]
46. Shanmuganathan, K.; Capadona, J.R.; Rowan, S.J.; Weder, C. Bio-inspired mechanically-adaptive nanocomposites derived from cotton cellulose whiskers. *J. Mater. Chem.* **2010**, *20*, 180. [CrossRef]
47. Capadona, J.R.; Tyler, D.J.; Zorman, C.A.; Rowan, S.J.; Weder, C. Mechanically adaptive nanocomposites for neural interfacing. *MRS Bull.* **2012**, *37*, 581–589. [CrossRef]
48. Shanmuganathan, K.; Capadona, J.R.; Rowan, S.J.; Weder, C. Biomimetic mechanically adaptive nanocomposites. *Prog. Polym. Sci.* **2010**, *35*, 212–222. [CrossRef]
49. Hess, A.E.; Capadona, J.R.; Shanmuganathan, K.; Hsu, L.; Rowan, S.J.; Weder, C.; Tyler, D.J.; Zorman, C.A. Development of a stimuli-responsive polymer nanocomposite toward biologically optimized, MEMS-based neural probes. *J. Micromech. Microeng.* **2011**, *21*, 54009. [CrossRef]
50. Hess, A.E.; Potter, K.A.; Tyler, D.J.; Zorman, C.A.; Capadona, J.R. Environmentally-controlled microtensile testing of mechanically-adaptive polymer nanocomposites for ex vivo characterization. *J. Vis. Exp.* **2013**, e50078. [CrossRef] [PubMed]
51. Hess-Dunning, A.E.; Tyler, D.J.; Harris, J.P.; Capadona, J.R.; Weder, C.; Rowan, S.J.; Zorman, C.A. Microscale Characterization of a Mechanically Adaptive Polymer Nanocomposite with Cotton-Derived Cellulose Nanocrystals for Implantable BioMEMS. *J. Microelectromech. Syst.* **2014**, *23*, 774–784. [CrossRef]
52. Harris, J.P.; Capadona, J.R.; Miller, R.H.; Healy, B.C.; Shanmuganathan, K.; Rowan, S.J.; Weder, C.; Tyler, D.J. Mechanically adaptive intracortical implants improve the proximity of neuronal cell bodies. *J. Neural Eng.* **2011**, *8*, 066011. [CrossRef] [PubMed]
53. Arreaga-Salas, D.E.; Avendaño-Bolívar, A.; Simon, D.; Reit, R.; Garcia-Sandoval, A.; Rennaker, R.L.; Voit, W. Integration of High-Charge-Injection-Capacity Electrodes onto Polymer Softening Neural Interfaces. *ACS Appl. Mater. Interfaces* **2015**, *7*, 26614–26623. [CrossRef] [PubMed]
54. Simon, D.; Ware, T.; Marcotte, R.; Lund, B.R.; Smith, D.W.; Di Prima, M.; Rennaker, R.L.; Voit, W. A comparison of polymer substrates for photolithographic processing of flexible bioelectronics. *Biomed. Microdevices* **2013**, *15*, 925–939. [CrossRef] [PubMed]
55. Hess, A.E.; Zorman, C.A. Fabrication and Characterization of MEMS-Based Structures from a Bio-Inspired, Chemo-Responsive Polymer Nanocomposite. *MRS Proc.* **2011**, *1299*. [CrossRef]
56. Lu, P.; Hsieh, Y.-L. Preparation and properties of cellulose nanocrystals: Rods, spheres, and network. *Carbohydr. Polym.* **2010**, *82*, 329–336. [CrossRef]
57. Drake, K.L.; Wise, K.D.; Farraye, J.; Anderson, D.J.; BeMent, S.L. Performance of planar multisite microprobes in recording extracellular single-unit intracortical activity. *IEEE Trans. Biomed. Eng.* **1988**, *35*, 719–732. [CrossRef] [PubMed]

58. Dagnon, K.L.; Shanmuganathan, K.; Weder, C.; Rowan, S.J. Water-Triggered Modulus Changes of Cellulose Nanofiber Nanocomposites with Hydrophobic Polymer Matrices. *Macromolecules* **2012**, *45*, 4707–4715. [CrossRef]

59. Shanmuganathan, K.; Capadona, J.R.; Rowan, S.J.; Weder, C. Stimuli-responsive mechanically adaptive polymer nanocomposites. *ACS Appl. Mater. Interfaces* **2010**, *2*, 165–174. [CrossRef] [PubMed]

60. V&P Scientific, Inc. Parylene C Data Sheet. Available online: http://www.vp-scientific.com/parylene_properties.htm (accessed on 15 August 2018).

61. Hermann, J.K.; Ravikumar, M.; Shoffstall, A.J.; Ereifej, E.S.; Kovach, K.M.; Chang, J.; Soffer, A.; Wong, C.; Srivastava, V.; Smith, P.; et al. Inhibition of the cluster of differentiation 14 innate immunity pathway with IAXO-101 improves chronic microelectrode performance. *J. Neural Eng.* **2018**, *15*, 025002. [CrossRef] [PubMed]

62. Goss-Varley, M.; Dona, K.R.; McMahon, J.A.; Shoffstall, A.J.; Ereifej, E.S.; Lindner, S.C.; Capadona, J.R. Microelectrode implantation in motor cortex causes fine motor deficit: Implications on potential considerations to Brain Computer Interfacing and Human Augmentation. *Sci. Rep.* **2017**, *7*, 15254. [CrossRef] [PubMed]

63. Ludwig, K.A.; Uram, J.D.; Yang, J.; Martin, D.C.; Kipke, D.R. Chronic neural recordings using silicon microelectrode arrays electrochemically deposited with a poly(3,4-ethylenedioxythiophene) (PEDOT) film. *J. Neural Eng.* **2006**, *3*, 59–70. [CrossRef] [PubMed]

64. Ludwig, K.A.; Miriani, R.M.; Langhals, N.B.; Joseph, M.D.; Anderson, D.J.; Kipke, D.R. Using a common average reference to improve cortical neuron recordings from microelectrode arrays. *J. Neurophysiol.* **2009**, *101*, 1679–1689. [CrossRef] [PubMed]

65. Spencer, K.C.; Sy, J.C.; Ramadi, K.B.; Graybiel, A.M.; Langer, R.; Cima, M.J. Characterization of Mechanically Matched Hydrogel Coatings to Improve the Biocompatibility of Neural Implants. *Sci. Rep.* **2017**, *7*, 1952. [CrossRef] [PubMed]

66. Thelin, J.; Jörntell, H.; Psouni, E.; Garwicz, M.; Schouenborg, J.; Danielsen, N.; Linsmeier, C.E. Implant Size and Fixation Mode Strongly Influence Tissue Reactions in the CNS. *PLoS ONE* **2011**, *6*, e16267. [CrossRef] [PubMed]

67. Lee, H.C.; Ejserholm, F.; Gaire, J.; Currlin, S.; Schouenborg, J.; Wallman, L.; Bengtsson, M.; Park, K.; Otto, K.J. Histological evaluation of flexible neural implants; flexibility limit for reducing the tissue response? *J. Neural Eng.* **2017**, *14*, 036026. [CrossRef] [PubMed]

68. Lind, G.; Linsmeier, C.E.; Schouenborg, J. The density difference between tissue and neural probes is a key factor for glial scarring. *Sci. Rep.* **2013**, *3*, 2942. [CrossRef] [PubMed]

69. Ahuja, A.K.; Behrend, M.R.; Whalen, J.J.; Humayun, M.S.; Weiland, J.D. The Dependence of Spectral Impedance on Disc Microelectrode Radius. *IEEE Trans. Biomed. Eng.* **2008**, *55*, 1457–1460. [CrossRef] [PubMed]

70. Cui, X.; Martin, D.C. Fuzzy gold electrodes for lowering impedance and improving adhesion with electrodeposited conducting polymer films. *Sens. Actuators A Phys.* **2003**, *103*, 384–394. [CrossRef]

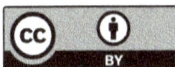

Article

Amorphous Silicon Carbide Platform for Next Generation Penetrating Neural Interface Designs

Felix Deku [1,*], Christopher L. Frewin [1], Allison Stiller [1], Yarden Cohen [2], Saher Aqeel [1], Alexandra Joshi-Imre [1], Bryan Black [1], Timothy J. Gardner [2], Joseph J. Pancrazio [1] and Stuart F. Cogan [1]

[1] Department of Bioengineering, University of Texas at Dallas, Richardson, TX 75080, USA; christopher.frewin@utdallas.edu (C.L.F.); axs169031@utdallas.edu (A.S.); saher.aqeel@utdallas.edu (S.A.); alexandra.joshi-imre@utdallas.edu (A.J.-I.); bjb140530@utdallas.edu (B.B.); joseph.pancrazio@utdallas.edu (J.J.P.); stuart.cogan@utdallas.edu (S.F.C.)
[2] Department of Biology and Biomedical Engineering, Boston University, Boston, MA 02215, USA; yardenc@bu.edu (Y.C.); timothyg@bu.edu (T.J.G.)
*   Correspondence: felix.deku@utdallas.edu; Tel.: +1-469-667-0634

Received: 31 July 2018; Accepted: 17 September 2018; Published: 20 September 2018

Abstract: Microelectrode arrays that consistently and reliably record and stimulate neural activity under conditions of chronic implantation have so far eluded the neural interface community due to failures attributed to both biotic and abiotic mechanisms. Arrays with transverse dimensions of 10 μm or below are thought to minimize the inflammatory response; however, the reduction of implant thickness also decreases buckling thresholds for materials with low Young's modulus. While these issues have been overcome using stiffer, thicker materials as transport shuttles during implantation, the acute damage from the use of shuttles may generate many other biotic complications. Amorphous silicon carbide (a-SiC) provides excellent electrical insulation and a large Young's modulus, allowing the fabrication of ultrasmall arrays with increased resistance to buckling. Prototype a-SiC intracortical implants were fabricated containing 8 - 16 single shanks which had critical thicknesses of either 4 μm or 6 μm. The 6 μm thick a-SiC shanks could penetrate rat cortex without an insertion aid. Single unit recordings from SIROF-coated arrays implanted without any structural support are presented. This work demonstrates that a-SiC can provide an excellent mechanical platform for devices that penetrate cortical tissue while maintaining a critical thickness less than 10 μm.

Keywords: amorphous silicon carbide; neural stimulation and recording; insertion force; microelectrodes; neural interfaces

1. Introduction

Penetrating microelectrode arrays (MEAs) that stimulate or record neural activity usually consist of a base substrate material which may be an insulator or conductor. Typical conducting substrates include silicon [1], tungsten, iridium wire [2,3], and carbon fiber [4–7], which provide the backbone and structural stiffness necessary to penetrate neural tissue. For the Utah array, silicon is doped to provide conductivity [8], and is usually insulated so that current conduction is restricted to the doped silicon. A common polymeric coating used to isolate the conducting substrate from the surrounding electrolyte is Parylene C. It is also common practice to use thin-film dielectric materials, such as low pressure chemical vapor deposited (LPCVD) SiO_2, to encapsulate polycrystalline silicon traces [9]. In most cases another dielectric material, such as Si_3N_4, is deposited over the SiO_2 to control the intrinsic compressive stress in the SiO_2 [10,11] or to create a multilayer passivation stack of PECVD $SiO_2/Si_3N_4/SiO_2$ over the conducting trace [12]. The silicon - based microelectrodes, however, have been shown to deteriorate when chronically implanted [13–15]. Failure modes associated with silicon - based MEA degradation were recently described following array implantation in non-human primates [14].

Recent studies have shown that flexible neural interfaces may provide an alternative to traditional silicon-based implants and have the potential to greatly improve the chronic longevity of the implanted microelectrodes [2,16]. Polymers such as polyimide [17,18], Parylene-C [19,20], SU-8 [21], polydimethylsiloxane (PDMS) [22], and shape memory polymers [23,24] have been investigated as substrates for neural stimulation and recording microelectrodes. Their low Young's modulus reduces the mechanical mismatch between neural tissue and the implanted device. Thin-film metal conducting traces such as gold or platinum are used between layers of the polymer substrate connecting electrode sites and bond pads. The insulating layers effectively sandwich the conducting traces. Electrode sites are then created by removing or etching the top layer through a precise and controlled microfabrication process.

Implantation of some penetrating polymer-based MEAs have been aided by a delivery vehicle [5,25–28] or temporary support structure [5,29–31] to minimize buckling during insertion by increasing the critical buckling load [32]. To penetrate neural tissue without the assistance of support structures, a minimum cross-sectional dimension of the shank (the part that penetrates the neural tissue) is typically greater than 20 µm [18,21,33]. Unfortunately, this cross-sectional dimension may still be higher than that required to ameliorate the foreign body reaction, noting that the prevailing thought has been that the minimum geometric dimension requirement, at least in one dimension, should be under 10 µm [34]. We recently described the development of multielectrode arrays based on PECVD amorphous silicon carbide (a-SiC) [35]. Amorphous SiC was chosen because it exhibits robust chemical inertness [36], high electronic and ionic resistivity [37], biocompatibility [37–40], and is amenable to thin-film fabrication processes [35]. Crystalline SiC has also been used as a material in the fabrication of MEAs and, because it is a wide bandgap semiconductor that can be doped for electronic conductivity, it may be used for conductive traces or as a low-impedance electrode, as well as an insulator [41–45]. The 16 channel MEAs were developed with two a-SiC layers sandwiching a thin-film Au conducting trace. Each shank was 10 µm wide and 2 mm long and had a shank cross-sectional area below 45 µm². The greatly reduced shank cross-sectional dimensions may promote compliance with neural tissue when implanted [46]. The electrode sites were opened at the distal tips by removing the top a-SiC layer and were coated with sputtered iridium oxide films (SIROF) or titanium nitride (TiN) to reduce electrode impedance [35].

Here, we evaluate different approaches of reducing the critical buckling load of a-SiC MEAs having individual shank cross-sectional area below 45 µm², and demonstrate insertion of multiple a-SiC MEA shanks into rat cortex. Acute extracellular neural recording from the a-SiC MEAs following array insertion is also presented.

2. Materials and Methods

2.1. Thin Film Deposition and Array Fabrication

Plasma enhanced chemical vapor deposited a-SiC films using the Plasmatherm Unaxis 790 series deposition system are used as substrates for MEA development. The a-SiC films are deposited at 1000 mTorr, 350 °C, and 0.27 W/cm² using a SiH_4:CH_4 gas ratio of 1:3. A 2 µm or 4 µm thick a-SiC film forms the bottom layer of the MEA. The bottom a-SiC layer is followed by the deposition of approximately 350 nm thick patterned gold layer that forms the interconnecting traces. A thin (<50 nm) film of titanium is deposited as an adhesion layer between the a-SiC and gold on both surfaces of the metal to form a trilayer metal structure of Ti/Au/Ti. A second 2 µm a-SiC layer was deposited over the metal traces and bottom a-SiC layer to produce either a 4 µm or 6 µm thick a-SiC superstructure. The details of the fabrication have been reported previously [35]. Briefly, a 1 µm polyimide (HD Microsystems PI 2610) release layer is spin-coated on to a 100 mm silicon wafer and cured at 350 °C under N_2 for 1 h. The bottom a-SiC layer is deposited on the polyimide followed by a bilayer photolithography process, using LOR5A (Microchem Inc., Westborough, MA, USA) and Shipley S1813 (Microposit, Marlborough, MA, USA) photoresists, to define the metallization pattern. The metal was sputtered or evaporated, and the sample soaked in EBR-PG (Microchem Inc. Westborough, MA, USA) to complete the lift-off process. The second a-SiC layer was then deposited over the metallization and the bottom a-SiC the complete the thin-film stack. The 350 °C deposition temperature of the second a-SiC results in an increase in tensile stress of the metallization by about 400 MPa, for either the evaporated or sputtered trilayers. For the overall device, the effect of the increase in metal tensile stress is a reduction in the overall device stress from about 100 MPa compressive to near-neutral (<20 MPa compressive), recognizing that the overall stress in the device is dependent on the thickness and processing of the individual layers. Another photolithography process, using a positive photoresist, was used to define the electrode sites, bond pads and shape of the individual devices on the wafer. The devices were then formed by reactive ion etching of the exposed a-SiC in SF_6 plasma using an inductively coupled plasma (ICP) etcher. After the etching process, the remaining resist was stripped and the wafer with the a-SiC MEAs are soaked in deionized water until the arrays release. An example of a 16-channel MEA fabricated by the process described is shown in Figure 1. The device is intended for intracortical studies with only the 2-mm long distal shanks penetrating the cortex. Photolithographic patterning provides a means of creating a variety of array geometries including straight and curved shanks (Figure 2).

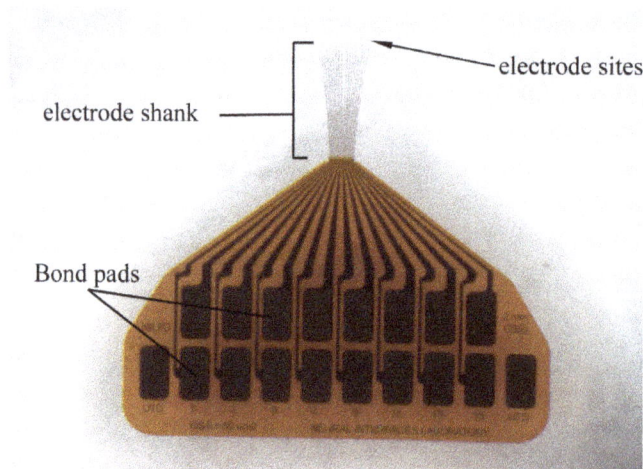

Figure 1. Example of the 16-channel a-SiC microelectrode array (MEA) showing bond pads at the proximal end, 2 mm long electrode shanks, and electrode sites located at the distal tips.

2.2. Buckling and Insertion Mechanics

Force measurements were made using a 20 g S-Beam load cell (Futek Advanced Sensor Technology, Inc., Irvine, CA, USA) mounted to a pneumatically controlled micro-positioner (Model 2650 Micropositioner, Kopf Instruments, Tujunga, CA, USA) which has predefined speed settings ranging from 1 μ/s to 4 mm/s. The micromanipulator is hydraulically driven and thus the motion is continuous. The steps in the forcetime curves are due to the sampling frequency of the recording equipment used to measure the load cell output. The sample probe was mounted on a screw which was directly threaded into the bottom of the load cell so that compression forces could be measured as the MEA was inserted into the brain tissue. Before implantation, the probe was lowered until it was directly above the surface of the brain. The load cell was then tared, and the probe inserted 2 mm into the brain at a constant rate of 50 μm/s. For the measurements of buckling forces on glass substrates, the load cell was tared with a slight compressive stress on the tip and then retracted from the surface.

This procedure results in an initial tensile deflection in the force-time curve immediately prior to the probe tip striking the glass surface.

2.3. Surgery and a-SiC Implantation

All surgical procedures were performed under the approval of the University of Texas at Dallas Institutional Animal Care and Use Committee (IACUC). Long Evans rats were deeply anaesthetized with 5% isoflurane vapor and administered an intraperitoneal KXA cohort consisting of ketamine (65 mg/kg), xylazine (13.33 mg/kg), and acepromazine (1.5 mg/kg) cocktail. The anesthesia was maintained at 0.5 to 1.5% throughout the remainder of the procedure. A 1 to 2 mm square craniotomy was centered 2.5 mm rostral and 2.5 mm lateral to bregma, and bone debris was carefully removed using sterile phosphate buffered solution (PBS). The dura was reflected using a dura pick and the surface of the brain was kept moist with sterile PBS. The Omnetics 18 pin male connector attached to the a-SiC cortical implant was placed within a NeuroNexus IST implantation tool (NeuroNexus, Ann Arbor, MI, USA) and loaded onto a Kopf Model 2650 hydraulic micropositioner (David Kopf Instruments, Tujunga, CA, USA). The implant was inserted to a depth of 1.5 to 2 mm from the cortical surface at an insertion rate of 50 μm/s at a location at the center of the craniotomy, deviating only enough to avoid large surface vasculature. The dura was sealed using Kwik Cast silicone elastomer (World Precision Instruments, Saratosa, FL, USA), followed by a layer of GLUture Octyl/Butyl cyanoacrylate glue (World Precision Instruments, Sarasota, FL, USA). A protective head cap was constructed using two-part dental cement (Stoelting Co., Wood Dale IL, USA) which served to secure and support the implant as well as protect the surgical site. The scalp wound was sutured, and the animal was administered an intramuscular injection of Cefazolin (5 mg/Kg), a subcutaneous injection of sustained release Buprenorphine (0.15 mg/Kg), and 2 mL of 0.9% saline. The rat was individually housed following implantation. Clavamox was administered orally and buprenorphine was administered every 72 h for one week.

2.4. In Vivo Recording and Analysis

Following construction and curing of the surgical head cap, recordings for a period of 10 min were collected using an OmniPlex Neural Acquisition System (Plexon Inc., Dallas, TX, USA) connected to the a-SiC array via Omnetics connector and a 16-channel digital headstage. Wideband signals (0.1–7000 Hz) were recorded simultaneously from all 16 electrodes at 40 kHz sampling frequency and later filtered offline using a 4-pole Butterworth high pass filter (250 Hz). A -4σ threshold based on RMS noise calculations was applied to filtered continuous data to identify potential waveforms (or spikes). Single units were identified manually based on 2D principal component clustering using Plexon's Offline Sorter software (Plexon, Dallas, TX, USA). Sorted units which were not comprised of at least 100 individual spikes or which exhibited greater than 0.5% spike refractory period violations were excluded from analysis. Signal-to-noise ratios (SNR) were calculated by dividing the mean peak-to-peak amplitude of each unit by the adjusted RMS noise of the associated channel, which excluded values greater or less than $\pm4\sigma$ of the filtered continuous signal.

3. Results and Discussions

The 16-channel a-SiC MEAs were generally designed to mate with the 16-channel Omnetics connectors (A79040-001, Omnetics, Minneapolis, MN, USA). Gold bonding pads located at the proximal end of the MEA superstructure, 750×500 μm dimensions and pitch of 635 μm ensured that the 16 a-SiC channels mated well with the connector. A solder reflow process using an indium-tin eutectic solder paste consisting of 52% In to 48% Sn (IND.1E, Indium Corporation, Clinton, NY, USA) was used to bond the pads on the connector to the gold bond pads on the MEA.

To characterize the functionality of the a-SiC platform, MEAs consisting of 16 penetrating shanks with one electrode per shank were fabricated (Figure 1). Each shank was 4 or 6 μm thick, 2–4 mm long, and 7–10 μm wide with 25 μm intershank separation. The shanks were designed with a straight outline and with 'arrow head' tip geometry. The shanks are sometimes intrinsically curved with the expectation that such geometry will direct the deployment of the shanks to a larger volume of brain tissue when implanted.

Figure 2 shows shank arrangements of the as-fabricated 16 channel a-SiC penetrating MEAs with (a) straight shanks of identical length and (b) intrinsically curve shanks. Tip profiles are shown in (c). Metal traces are 2 μm wide and run centrally along the length of the shank. The electrode sites are located at the distal tip and are constrained in size and shape by the width of the shanks, such that the 50 μm² electrode sites were 2 μm wide and 25 μm long.

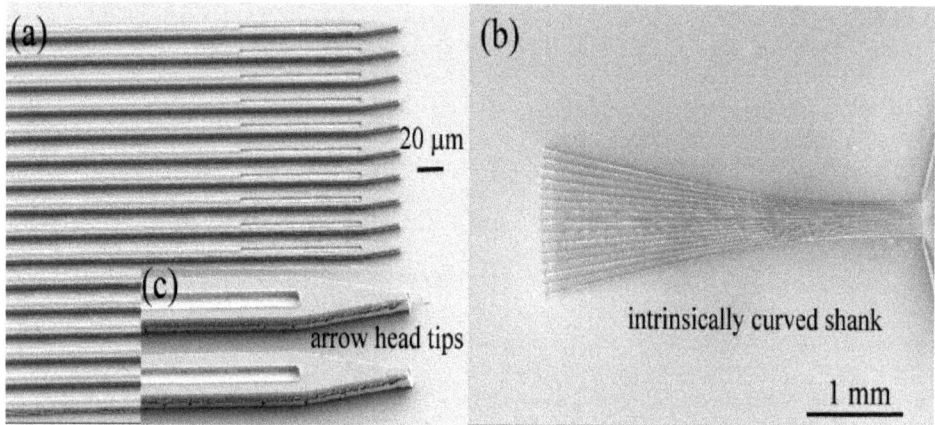

Figure 2. Scanning electron micrographs of as-fabricated 16 channel a-SiC intracortical ultramicroelectrode arrays with straight shanks of identical length (**a**) or intrinsically curve shanks (**b**). Tip profile and electrode site opening are shown in (**c**).

3.1. Insertion of Ultrathin Shanks into Cortex

3.1.1. PEG-Stabilized Shanks

While shanks with very small cross-sectional area offer the promise of reduced FBR, insertion of individual shanks into the neural tissue is challenging. Coating the shanks with polyethylene glycol (PEG) that temporarily stiffens the shanks while leaving a small portion of the tips exposed [5] is an approach previously shown to successfully aid insertion. The PEG coating increases the buckling threshold of the shanks and allows the arrays to be implanted. Using this method, we have inserted 4 μm thick versions of the a-SiC arrays into rat brain.

An example of an array coated with PEG (MW 2000, Alfa Aesar, Tewksbury, MA, USA) prior to implantation is shown in Figure 3. Prior to PEG coating, the assembled a-SC array is placed on a mineral oiled aluminum surface. A single flake of PEG is placed on the proximal end of the separated shanks. The PEG is then melted onto the shanks with a soldering gun. As shown in Figure 3, the PEG coating was only used to strengthen the shanks towards the base of the MEA leaving the tips free to individually penetrate the brain. An insertion rate of 50 μm/s was used to insert the shanks so that, as the array is slowly advanced into the brain, the PEG coating dissolves on the surface of the brain without itself penetrating the tissue, preserving the sub 10-μm dimensions of the shanks that are inserted into the brain. Based on visual observation with a surgical microscope, the shanks appear to penetrate the parenchyma of the brain without dimpling the cortex.

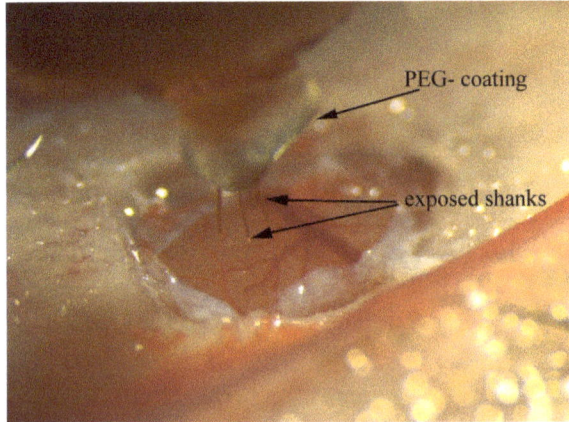

Figure 3. Insertion of a PEG-stabilized a-SiC MEA into rat motor cortex. The PEG temporarily provides mechanical support to the 4 µm thick a-SiC shanks prior to insertion. An insertion rate of 50 µm/s ensures that the PEG completely dissolves as the array is advanced into the brain.

3.1.2. Bundled Shanks

Another successful approach introduced by Guitchounts et al. when working with carbon fiber ultramicroelectrodes was to draw the fibers into a bundle allowing the individual fibers to provide mechanical support to each other during array insertion [4]. This approach also increases the overall cross-sectional area of the bundled fibers and increases the buckling threshold for insertion. Since the fibers on the bundled array are held together by weak Van der Waals forces, they separate upon insertion and spread out into the brain following the path of least resistance defined by the mechanical heterogeneity of the brain [4]. The 4 µm thick a-SiC arrays were successfully inserted using this approach, however unlike carbon fibers, we observed that the shanks of the a-SiC MEA twisted together or intertwined when drawn out of water. The tangled shanks prevented the individual shanks from separating and splaying when implanted. Further work is needed to find an appropriate surface treatment that would aid shank separation. Figure 4a shows a bundled a-SiC array formed when the shanks are drawn out of water. Figure 4b shows the tip geometry of the bundle and Figure 4c shows a bundled 8-channel a-SiC array prior to rat cortical implantation.

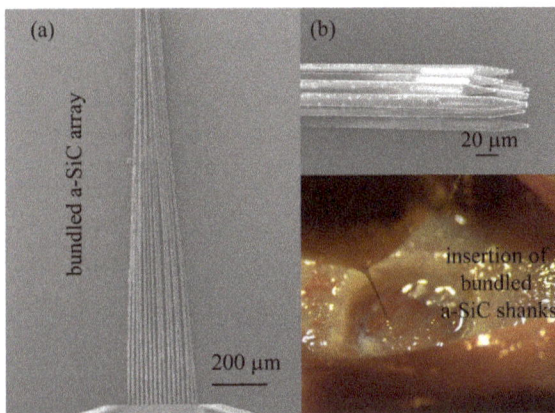

Figure 4. Bundles of 16-channel a-SiC MEA when drawn out of water (**a**) showing tip geometry (**b**). Insertion of a bundled 8-channel a-SiC array into rat cortex (**c**).

3.1.3. Reduction of Effective Shank Length

Another factor that influences the critical buckling load is the effective length of the shanks. The effective length of a beam or a shank corresponds to the distance between the points of inflection in the buckled mode. The buckling threshold increases with decreasing effective length of the shank. Patel et al. [5], while working with carbon fibers, developed silicon support structures that enabled the insertion of 0.5 mm long carbon fibers to deeper structures within rat brain. For the carbon fibers, this was the minimum length that could be inserted into the brain without buckling [5]. The advantage of the a-SiC technology over the carbon fiber approach is that structures that will reduce the effective length of the shanks can be designed as part of the MEA geometry. The a-SiC thin film technology allows in situ designs in the a-SiC without the need for additional support structures and micro-assembly. As a result, shorter ultrathin a-SiC array shanks can be developed for insertion into deeper structures within the brain.

We designed and developed webbed a-SiC arrays as shown in Figure 5b with an effective shank length below 1 mm for an overall insertion depth of 2 mm (including the hinged part). The individual shanks are fused in pairs by a-SiC film interconnects as the shanks approach the base of the MEA 5d while maintaining the ultrathin geometries at the distal end 5a. Electrode sites are located at the distal end 5c. Amorphous SiC MEAs with ultrathin shank geometries (4 μm thick × 10 μm wide) have been successfully implanted when the shanks are webbed. This a-SiC lateral interconnect strategy increases the width of the shank towards the base and may induce lateral stresses in tissue and potentially induce host immune response. We are yet to evaluate the chronic response to these arrays. Since the electrode sites are located on shanks that maintain the critical dimension of 10 μm or less, it is expected that the host immune response, at least around the electrode sites, will be minimized.

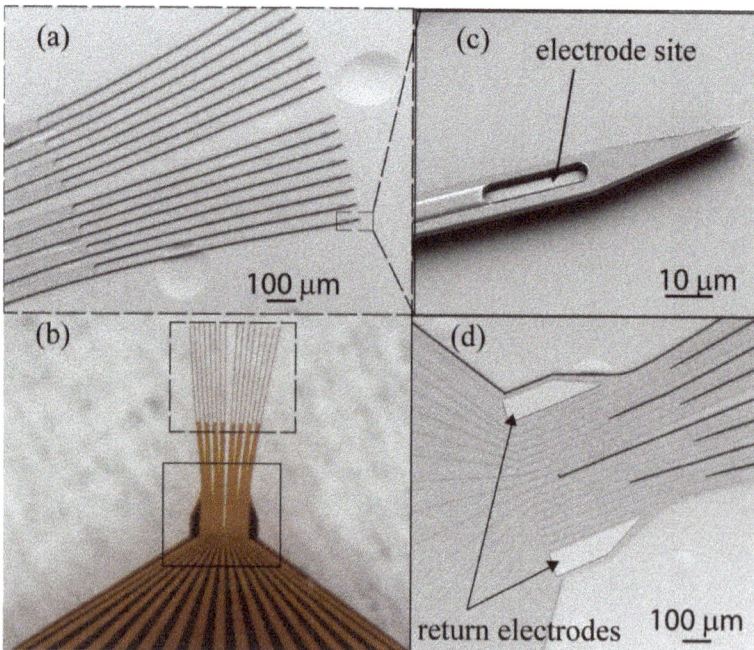

Figure 5. Webbed a-SiC MEA with an effective shank length of 1 mm and a monopolar stimulation current return electrode as part of the MEA structure.

3.1.4. Insertion of Individual Shanks

A trade-off between flexibility and stiffness is required when developing compliant microelectrode arrays for cortical application [32]. Insertion of ultrathin flexible microelectrodes into neural tissue usually fails during implantation. The flexural rigidity (a product of the Young's modulus of the material and moments of inertia of the cross-section) of the shank is related to the critical buckling load by Equation (1) where P_{cr} is the critical buckling load, E is the Young's modulus, I is the moment of inertia of cross-section, l is the length, and K is the column effective length factor (one fixed end, one pinned end = 0.7). A Young's modulus of 300 GPa was used for numerical calculations and simulation purposes. The Young's modulus of a-SiC films depends on deposition conditions and values between 150 and 321 GPa have been reported in the literature [47–49].

$$P_{cr} = \frac{\pi^2 EI}{(Kl)^2} \tag{1}$$

The critical buckling load is the maximum axial load a shank can experience that will not cause lateral deflections. For a microelectrode shank to successfully penetrate the pia mater of a rat brain it is generally expected that its critical buckling load to be larger than tissue insertion force estimated to be approximately 0.5 to 2 mN [50–54]. Since the moment of inertia of the cross-section, which influences critical buckling load, depends greatly on the thickness of the shank, COMSOL Multiphysics v. 5.2 (COMSOL AB, Stockholm, Sweden) finite element modeling was used to predict the critical buckling load of a 2 mm long shank when the a-SiC thickness is increased from 4 μm to 6 μm.

Force values during a buckling test with a single shank dummy a-SiC probe with a 6 μm thick and 7 μm wide cross-section are shown in Figure 6a. The probe was lowered against a glass surface at a speed of 50 μm/s. No sliding of the probe tip on the glass surface was observed. The lowering was paused when buckling was observed visually, as shown by the plateau at 0.69 mN in Figure 6a. Since the visually observed buckling occurs well-beyond the first deflection of the probe, the 0.69 mN overestimates the buckling force that would be calculated from Equation (1), which is ~0.2 mN for the probe in Figure 6. The recorded buckling force of 0.69 mN should also be adjusted for the nonzero compressive force on the tip when the load cell is tared, which is approximately 0.15 mN. The combined total force of 0.84 mN is notably larger than the COMSOL modeling prediction of 0.17 mN, which is likely due to the uncertainty in the visual assessment of buckling onset and changing boundary conditions as the probe inserts into the brain. The visually observed deflection profile (Figure 6b) was generally in agreement with predictions from the modeling (Figure 6c). Penetration forces are highly dependent on the tip geometry of the implanted device, with larger devices generally exhibiting greater implantation forces. Sridharan et al. [55] measured penetration forces greater than 1 mN using nanocomposite-based devices and observed significant dimpling upon implantation. Welkenhuysen et al. [56] demonstrated penetration forces greater than 0.6 mN using silicon devices, again with significant dimpling.

A preliminary investigation of the forces involved in inserting a single a-SiC shank into rat cortex was conducted. The force-time curve during implantation of a single shank with a 6 × 7 μm² cross-section at 50 μm/s is shown in Figure 7. From the curve, the point of penetration of the probe corresponds to an insertion force of 0.35 mN. Dimpling of the cortex was not evident. The maximum length of a 6 × 7 μm probe that can be inserted into brain without buckling is 1.4 mm based on Equation (1), using an insertion force of 0.35 mN, an a-SiC modulus of 300 GPa, and K = 0.7, corresponding to boundary conditions at which the probe is pinned at the probe-brain interface and fixed at the proximal end. The calculated length likely underestimates that actual length that can be inserted without buckling. As the sharp tips of the probe penetrate the brain, the boundary condition at the probe-brain interface changes to a less challenging fixed condition and the effective length of the shank also decreases slightly. Forces due to brain micromotion (inset) after the probe was implanted to the full 2 mm depth show that the indwelling shank experience an extremely low tissue force which relaxed at a rate of ~2.2 μN/s. We have successfully implanted a single shank and multiple colinear shanks with thickness of 6 μm into a 0.6% agarose gel phantom and into rat brain at an insertion rate of 50 μm/s. To prevent the a-SiC arrays from forming bundles, a minimum intershank distance of 100 μm was found necessary for the 7–10 μm wide shanks investigated. The data in Figure 7 represent the results of a single measurement only and additional studies are required to more fully quantify the forces involved in insertion of these devices into cortex, particularly with respect to the effects of tip geometry, shank cross-sectional dimensions, and shank length.

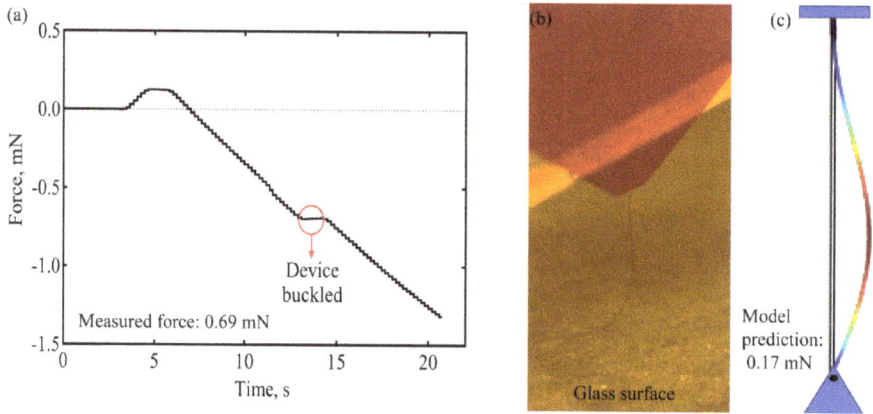

Figure 6. Buckling test. Force measured when a single shank a-SiC probe is lowered against a glass surface (**a**). An image of the buckled state of a 2 mm long shank (**b**) and a COMSOL prediction of the buckled state (**c**).

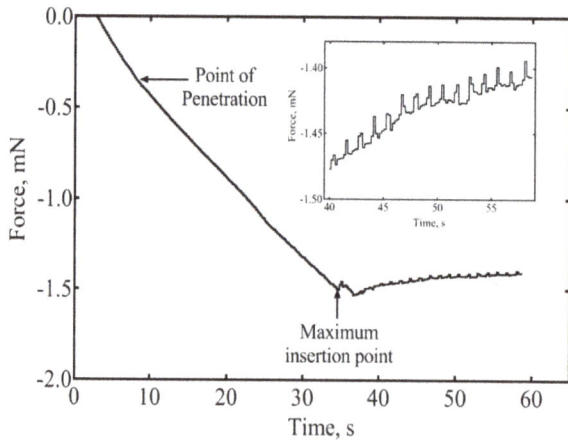

Figure 7. A representative example of the insertion force recorded during the insertion of a 6 μm × 7 μm a-SiC shank into rat cortex. An insertion force of 0.35 mN was recorded at the point of insertion. Inset shows forces experienced by the indwelling shank at 2 mm insertion depth.

3.2. Neural Recording

To determine whether 6 μm a-SiC and SIROF MEAs could be used for in vivo single-unit extracellular recordings, we performed 10-min electrophysiological recordings immediately following implantation. Figure 8a shows three representative filtered continuous recordings from a single a-SiC array. Extracellular spikes were well-resolved and sorted based on characteristic waveform shape and 2D PC-space clustering into single units (Figure 8b). We observed distinguishable single units on between 25 and 75% of electrode sites, with the total number of units ranging from 4 to 16. These units had mean peak-to-peak amplitudes ranging from 118.5 to 287.7 µV, with a mean amplitude of 179.4 ± 18.4 µV and SNR of 24.1 ± 2.2. Table 1 contains RMS noise, mean amplitude, and SNR values for all three implanted arrays as well as cumulative means. These data suggest that 6 µm a-SiC MEAs are stiff enough to penetrate the cortex without compromising their mechanical/electrical stability and their ability to record single-unit activity.

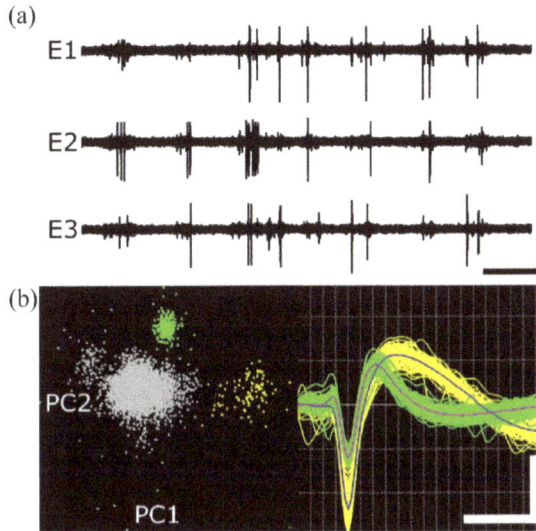

Figure 8. Acute extracellular action potentials recorded using 6 µm a-SiC MEAs. (**a**) Filtered continuous data traces from three representative electrodes on Array 1. Vertical and horizontal scale bar represents 125 µV and 1.75 s, respectively. (**b**) Left—Representative 2D principal component space indicating clear separation from the noise (central gray cluster). Right—Associated single units, indicating characteristic extracellular waveform shape. Vertical and horizontal scale bar represents 175 µV and 0.6 ms, respectively.

Table 1. Active electrode yield (AEY) percentage, total number of units, mean peak-to-peak amplitude, RMS noise, and SNR per array, and cumulative values across all arrays.

Array #	AEY (%)	# of Units	Mean Vpp (µV)	RMS Noise (µV)	SNR
Array 1	75	16	179.0 ± 19.8	10.2 ± 1.8	25.6 ± 2.9
Array 2	25	4	287.7 ± 64.4	8.8 ± 0.2	30.8 ± 6.8
Array 3	31.3	7	118.5 ± 12.2	7.8 ± 0.4	16.7 ± 1.7
Cumulative	43.75%	27	179.4 ± 18.4	8.9 ± 0.6	24.1 ± 2.2

4. Conclusions

The a-SiC platform allows a wide design space to create next generation ultrathin neural interfaces. To reduce overall impedance associated with small electrodes of small geometric surface area, electrode sites could also be coated with common low impedance coating materials, such as TiN or SIROF which decrease the impedance by 2 orders of magnitude over a range of frequencies [35]. For MEAs developed with an overall a-SiC thickness of 4 µm, we have described various techniques which increase the critical buckling force of the individual shanks and enable penetration of the shanks without buckling. These methods include the addition of a temporary stiffening structure, bundling the individual shanks, or through in situ designs which reduced the effective length of the shanks while allowing for targeted depth penetration. With just the addition of a minimal amount of a-SiC material to a thickness of 6 μm, individual single shanks or colinear 2 mm long a-SiC fibers were successfully implanted into rat cortex without buckling. We have also demonstrated the ability to record neural signals using 6 μm thick a-SiC MEAs acutely in rat motor cortex. Our results also indicated that SIROF-coated sites showed high amplitude and high SNR of the recorded neural signals.

Author Contributions: Conceptualization, F.D., J.J.P., and S.F.C.; Funding acquisition, T.J.G. and S.F.C.; Investigation, F.D., Y.C., and A.J.-I.; Methodology, F.D., C.L.F., A.S., S.A., and B.B.; Supervision, J.J.P. and S.F.C.; Writing—original draft, F.D. and C.L.F.; Writing—review & editing, A.S., Y.C., S.A., A.J.-I., B.B., T.J.G., J.J.P., and S.F.C.

Funding: This research was funded by the National Institute of Health under grant number U01NS090454.

Acknowledgments: The University of Texas at Dallas Natural Sciences and Engineering Research Laboratory cleanroom staffers Gordon Pollock and Ronald Scott Riekena are acknowledged for their support in the maintenance of the PECVD tool.

Conflicts of Interest: The authors declare no conflicts of interest. The funders had no role in the design of the study; in the collection, analyses, or interpretation of data; in the writing of the manuscript, and in the decision to publish the results.

References

1. Jun, J.J.; Steinmetz, N.A.; Siegle, J.H.; Denman, D.J.; Bauza, M.; Barbarits, B.; Lee, A.K.; Anastassiou, C.A.; Andrei, A.; Aydın, Ç.; et al. Fully integrated silicon probes for high-density recording of neural activity. *Nature* **2017**, *551*, 232–236. [CrossRef] [PubMed]
2. Freire, M.A.M.; Morya, E.; Faber, J.; Santos, J.R.; Guimaraes, J.S.; Lemos, N.A.M.; Sameshima, K.; Pereira, A.; Ribeiro, S.; Nicolelis, M.A.L. Comprehensive Analysis of Tissue Preservation and Recording Quality from Chronic Multielectrode Implants. *PLoS ONE* **2011**, *6*, e27554. [CrossRef] [PubMed]
3. McCreery, D.B.; Yuen, T.G.H.; Agnew, W.F.; Bullara, L.A. Stimulation with chronically implanted microelectrodes in the cochlear nucleus of the cat: Histologic and physiologic effects. *Hear. Res.* **1992**, *62*, 42–56. [CrossRef]
4. Guitchounts, G.; Markowitz, J.E.; Liberti, W.A.; Gardner, T.J. A carbon-fiber electrode array for long-term neural recording. *J. Neural Eng.* **2013**, *10*, 046016. [CrossRef] [PubMed]
5. Patel, P.R.; Na, K.; Zhang, H.; Kozai, T.D.Y.; Kotov, N.A.; Yoon, E.; Chestek, C.A. Insertion of linear 8.4 μm diameter 16 channel carbon fiber electrode arrays for single unit recordings. *J. Neural Eng.* **2015**, *12*, 046009. [CrossRef] [PubMed]
6. Deku, F.; Joshi-Imre, A.; Mertiri, A.; Gardner, T.J.; Cogan, S.F. Electrodeposited Iridium Oxide on Carbon Fiber Ultramicroelectrodes for Neural Recording and Stimulation. *J. Electrochem. Soc.* **2018**, *165*, D375–D380. [CrossRef]
7. Gillis, W.F.; Lissandrello, C.A.; Shen, J.; Pearre, B.W.; Mertiri, A.; Deku, F.; Cogan, S.; Holinski, B.J.; Chew, D.J.; White, A.E.; et al. Carbon fiber on polyimide ultra-microelectrodes. *J. Neural Eng.* **2018**, *15*, 016010. [CrossRef] [PubMed]
8. Seto, J.Y.W. The electrical properties of polycrystalline silicon films. *J. Appl. Phys.* **1975**, *46*, 5247–5254. [CrossRef]
9. Batey, J.; Tierney, E. Low-temperature deposition of high-quality silicon dioxide by plasma-enhanced chemical vapor deposition. *J. Appl. Phys.* **1986**, *60*. [CrossRef]
10. Yang, T.-C.; Saraswat, K.C. Effect of physical stress on the degradation of thin SiO/sub 2/ films under electrical stress. *IEEE Trans. Electron. Devices* **2000**, *47*, 746–755. [CrossRef]
11. Sheikholeslami, A.; Parhami, F.; Puchner, H.; Selberherr, S. Planarization of Silicon Dioxide and Silicon Nitride Passivation Layers. *J. Phys. Conf. Ser.* **2007**, *61*, 1051–1055. [CrossRef]
12. Hetke, J.F.; Lund, J.L.; Najafi, K.; Wise, K.D.; Anderson, D.J. Silicon Ribbon Cables for Chronically Implantable Microelectrode Arrays. *IEEE Trans. Biomed. Eng.* **1994**, *41*, 314–321. [CrossRef] [PubMed]
13. Barrese, J.C.; Aceros, J.; Donoghue, J.P. Scanning electron microscopy of chronically implanted intracortical microelectrode arrays in non-human primates. *J. Neural Eng.* **2016**, *13*, 026003. [CrossRef] [PubMed]

14. Barrese, J.C.; Rao, N.; Paroo, K.; Triebwasser, C.; Vargas-Irwin, C.; Franquemont, L.; Donoghue, J.P. Failure mode analysis of silicon-based intracortical microelectrode arrays in non-human primates. *J. Neural Eng.* **2013**, *10*, 066014. [CrossRef] [PubMed]

15. Kane, S.R.; Cogan, S.F.; Ehrlich, J.; Plante, T.D.; McCreery, D.B.; Troyk, P.R. Electrical performance of penetrating microelectrodes chronically implanted in cat cortex. *IEEE Trans. Biomed. Eng.* **2013**, *60*, 2153–2160. [CrossRef] [PubMed]

16. Hassler, C.; Boretius, T.; Stieglitz, T. Polymers for neural implants. *J. Polym. Sci. Part B Polym. Phys.* **2011**, *49*, 18–33. [CrossRef]

17. Metz, S.; Bertsch, A.; Bertrand, D.; Renaud, P. Flexible polyimide probes with microelectrodes and embedded microfluidic channels for simultaneous drug delivery and multi-channel monitoring of bioelectric activity. *Biosens. Bioelectron.* **2004**, *19*, 1309–1318. [CrossRef] [PubMed]

18. Rousche, P.J.; Pellinen, D.S.; Pivin, D.P.; Williams, J.C.; Vetter, R.J.; Kipke, D.R. Flexible polyimide-based intracortical electrode arrays with bioactive capability. *IEEE Trans. Biomed. Eng.* **2001**, *48*, 361–371. [CrossRef] [PubMed]

19. Kim, B.J.; Kuo, J.T.W.; Hara, S.A.; Lee, C.D.; Yu, L.; Gutierrez, C.A.; Hoang, T.Q.; Pikov, V.; Meng, E. 3D Parylene sheath neural probe for chronic recordings. *J. Neural Eng.* **2013**, *10*, 045002. [CrossRef] [PubMed]

20. Takeuchi, S.; Ziegler, D.; Yoshida, Y.; Mabuchi, K.; Suzuki, T. Parylene flexible neural probes integrated with microfluidic channels. *Lab Chip* **2005**, *5*, 519. [CrossRef] [PubMed]

21. Altuna, A.; Bellistri, E.; Cid, E.; Aivar, P.; Gal, B.; Berganzo, J.; Gabriel, G.; Guimerà, A.; Villa, R.; Fernández, L.J.; et al. SU-8 based microprobes for simultaneous neural depth recording and drug delivery in the brain. *Lab Chip* **2013**, *13*, 1422. [CrossRef] [PubMed]

22. Liang, G.; DeWeerth, S.P. PDMS-based conformable microelectrode arrays with selectable novel 3-D microelectrode geometries for surface stimulation and recording. *Conf. Proc. IEEE Eng. Med. Biol. Soc.* **2009**, *2009*, 1623–1626. [CrossRef]

23. Ware, T.; Simon, D.; Rennaker, R.L.; Voit, W. Smart Polymers for Neural Interfaces. *Polym. Rev.* **2013**, *53*, 108–129. [CrossRef]

24. Simon, D.M.; Charkhkar, H.; St. John, C.; Rajendran, S.; Kang, T.; Reit, R.; Arreaga-Salas, D.; McHail, D.G.; Knaack, G.L.; Sloan, A.; et al. Design and demonstration of an intracortical probe technology with tunable modulus. *J. Biomed. Mater. Res. Part A* **2017**, *105*, 159–168. [CrossRef] [PubMed]

25. Wei, X.; Luan, L.; Zhao, Z.; Li, X.; Zhu, H.; Potnis, O.; Xie, C. Nanofabricated Ultraflexible Electrode Arrays for High-Density Intracortical Recording. *Adv. Sci.* **2018**, *5*, 1700625. [CrossRef] [PubMed]

26. Gopalakrishnaiah, S.K.; Joseph, K.; Hofmann, U.G. Microfluidic drive for flexible brain implants. *Curr. Dir. Biomed. Eng.* **2017**, *3*, 675–678. [CrossRef]

27. Kozai, T.D.Y.; Kipke, D.R. Insertion shuttle with carboxyl terminated self-assembled monolayer coatings for implanting flexible polymer neural probes in the brain. *J. Neurosci. Methods* **2009**, *184*, 199–205. [CrossRef] [PubMed]

28. Shoffstall, A.J.; Srinivasan, S.; Willis, M.; Stiller, A.M.; Ecker, M.; Voit, W.E.; Pancrazio, J.J.; Capadona, J.R. A Mosquito Inspired Strategy to Implant Microprobes into the Brain. *Sci. Rep.* **2018**, *8*, 122. [CrossRef] [PubMed]

29. Lo, M.; Wang, S.; Singh, S.; Damodaran, V.B.; Kaplan, H.M.; Kohn, J.; Shreiber, D.I.; Zahn, J.D. Coating flexible probes with an ultra fast degrading polymer to aid in tissue insertion. *Biomed. Microdevices* **2015**, *17*, 34. [CrossRef] [PubMed]

30. Lewitus, D.; Smith, K.L.; Shain, W.; Kohn, J. Ultrafast resorbing polymers for use as carriers for cortical neural probes. *Acta Biomater.* **2011**, *7*, 2483–2491. [CrossRef] [PubMed]

31. Lind, G.; Linsmeier, C.E.; Thelin, J.; Schouenborg, J. Gelatine-embedded electrodes—A novel biocompatible vehicle allowing implantation of highly flexible microelectrodes. *J. Neural Eng.* **2010**, *7*, 046005. [CrossRef] [PubMed]

32. Lecomte, A.; Descamps, E.; Bergaud, C. A review on mechanical considerations for chronically-implanted neural probes. *J. Neural Eng.* **2018**, *15*, 031001. [CrossRef] [PubMed]

33. Sohal, H.S.; Clowry, G.J.; Jackson, A.; O'Neill, A.; Baker, S.N. Mechanical Flexibility Reduces the Foreign Body Response to Long-Term Implanted Microelectrodes in Rabbit Cortex. *PLoS ONE* **2016**, *11*, e0165606. [CrossRef] [PubMed]

34. Seymour, J.P.; Kipke, D.R. Neural probe design for reduced tissue encapsulation in CNS. *Biomaterials* **2007**, *28*, 3594–3607. [CrossRef] [PubMed]

35. Deku, F.; Cohen, Y.; Joshi-Imre, A.; Kanneganti, A.; Gardner, T.J.; Cogan, S.F. Amorphous silicon carbide ultramicroelectrode arrays for neural stimulation and recording. *J. Neural Eng.* **2018**, *15*, 016007. [CrossRef] [PubMed]

36. Azevedo, R.G.; Zhang, J.; Jones, D.G.; Myers, D.R.; Jog, A.V.; Jamshidi, B.; Wijesundara, M.B.J.; Maboudian, R.; Pisano, A.P. Silicon carbide coated MEMS strain sensor for harsh environment applications. Proceeding of the 2007 IEEE 20th International Conference on Micro Electro Mechanical Systems (MEMS), Hyogo, Japan, 21–25 January 2007; IEEE: Piscataway, NJ, USA, 2007; pp. 643–646.

37. Cogan, S.F.; Edell, D.J.; Guzelian, A.A.; Liu, Y.P.; Edell, R. Plasma-enhanced chemical vapor deposited silicon carbide as an implantable dielectric coating. *J. Biomed. Mater. Res. A* **2003**, *67*, 856–867. [CrossRef] [PubMed]

38. Knaack, G.L.; Charkhkar, H.; Cogan, S.F.; Pancrazio, J.J. Amorphous Silicon Carbide for Neural Interface Applications. *Silicon Carbide Biotechnol.* **2016**, 249–260. [CrossRef]

39. Knaack, G.L.; McHail, D.G.; Borda, G.; Koo, B.S.; Peixoto, N.; Cogan, S.F.; Dumas, T.C.; Pancrazio, J.J. In vivo Characterization of Amorphous Silicon Carbide as a Biomaterial for Chronic Neural Interfaces. *Front. Neurosci.* **2016**, *10*, 301. [CrossRef] [PubMed]

40. Iliescu, C.; Chen, B.; Poenar, D.P.; Lee, Y.Y. PECVD amorphous silicon carbide membranes for cell culturing. *Sensors Actuators, B Chem.* **2008**, *129*, 404–411. [CrossRef]

41. Frewin, C.L.; Locke, C.; Saddow, S.E.; Weeber, E.J. Single-crystal cubic silicon carbide: An in vivo biocompatible semiconductor for brain machine interface devices. Proceeding of the 2011 Annual International Conference of the IEEE Engineering in Medicine and Biology Society, Boston, MA, USA, 30 August–3 September 2011; IEEE: Piscataway, NJ, USA, 2011; pp. 2957–2960.

42. Oliveros, A.; Guiseppi-Elie, A.; Saddow, S.E. Silicon carbide: a versatile material for biosensor applications. *Biomed. Microdevices* **2013**, *15*, 353–368. [CrossRef] [PubMed]

43. Diaz-Botia, C.A.; Luna, L.E.; Chamanzar, M.; Carraro, C.; Sabes, P.N.; Maboudian, R.; Maharbiz, M.M. Fabrication of all-silicon carbide neural interfaces. Proceeding of the 2017 8th International IEEE/EMBS Conference on Neural Engineering (NER), Shanghai, China, 25–28 May 2017; IEEE: Piscataway, NJ, USA, 2017; pp. 170–173.

44. Bernardin, E.; Frewin, C.; Everly, R.; Ul Hassan, J.; Saddow, S.; Bernardin, E.K.; Frewin, C.L.; Everly, R.; Ul Hassan, J.; Saddow, S.E. Demonstration of a Robust All-Silicon-Carbide Intracortical Neural Interface. *Micromachines* **2018**, *9*, 412. [CrossRef]

45. Frewin, C.L.; Bernardin, E.E.; Deku, F.; Everly, R.; Hassan, J.; Pancrazio, J.J.; Saddow, S.E. Silicon Carbide as a Robust Neural Interface. *ECS Trans.* **2016**, *75*, 39–45. [CrossRef]

46. Pancrazio, J.J.; Deku, F.; Ghazavi, A.; Stiller, A.M.; Rihani, R.; Frewin, C.L.; Varner, V.D.; Gardner, T.J.; Cogan, S.F. Thinking Small: Progress on Microscale Neurostimulation Technology. *Neuromodulation Technol. Neural Interface* **2017**, *20*, 745–752. [CrossRef] [PubMed]

47. El Khakani, M.A.; Chaker, M.; Jean, A.; Boily, S.; Kieffer, J.C.; O'Hern, M.E.; Ravet, M.F.; Rousseaux, F. Hardness and Young's modulus of amorphous a-SiC thin films determined by nanoindentation and bulge tests. *J. Mater. Res.* **1994**, *9*, 96–103. [CrossRef]

48. Cros, B.; Gat, E.; Saurel, J. Characterization of the elastic properties of amorphous silicon carbide thin films by acoustic microscopy. *J. Non. Cryst. Solids* **1997**, *209*, 273–282. [CrossRef]

49. Xue, K.; Niu, L.-S.; Shi, H.-J. Mechanical Properties of Amorphous Silicon Carbide. *Silicon Carbide IntechOpen* **2011**. [CrossRef]

50. Jensen, W.; Yoshida, K.; Hofmann, U.G. In-vivo implant mechanics of flexible, silicon-based ACREO microelectrode arrays in rat cerebral cortex. *IEEE Trans. Biomed. Eng.* **2006**, *53*, 934–940. [CrossRef] [PubMed]

51. Wester, B.A.; Lee, R.H.; LaPlaca, M.C. Development and characterization of in vivo flexible electrodes compatible with large tissue displacements. *J. Neural Eng.* **2009**, *6*, 024002. [CrossRef] [PubMed]

52. Howard, M.A.; Abkes, B.A.; Ollendieck, M.C.; Noh, M.D.; Ritter, C.; Gillies, G.T. Measurement of the force required to move a neurosurgical probe through in vivo human brain tissue. *IEEE Trans. Biomed. Eng.* **1999**, *46*, 891–894. [CrossRef] [PubMed]

53. Molloy, J.A.; Ritter, R.C.; Grady, M.S.; Howard, M.A.; Quate, E.G.; Gillies, G.T. Experimental determination of the force required for insertion of a thermoseed into deep brain tissues. *Ann. Biomed. Eng.* **1990**, *18*, 299–313. [CrossRef] [PubMed]
54. Tian, C.X.; He, J. Monitoring Insertion Force and Electrode Impedance during Implantation of Microwire Electrodes. Proceeding of the 2005 IEEE Engineering in Medicine and Biology 27th Annual Conference, Shanghai, China, 17–18 January 2006; IEEE: Piscataway, NJ, USA, 2006; pp. 7333–7336.
55. Sridharan, A.; Nguyen, J.K.; Capadona, J.R.; Muthuswamy, J. Compliant intracortical implants reduce strains and strain rates in brain tissue in vivo. *J. Neural Eng.* **2015**, *12*, 036002. [CrossRef] [PubMed]
56. Welkenhuysen, M.; Andrei, A.; Ameye, L.; Eberle, W.; Nuttin, B. Effect of Insertion Speed on Tissue Response and Insertion Mechanics of a Chronically Implanted Silicon-Based Neural Probe. *IEEE Trans. Biomed. Eng.* **2011**, *58*, 3250–3259. [CrossRef] [PubMed]

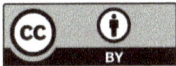

micromachines

MDPI

Article

Chronic Intracortical Recording and Electrochemical Stability of Thiol-ene/Acrylate Shape Memory Polymer Electrode Arrays

Allison M. Stiller [1,*], Joshua Usoro [1], Christopher L. Frewin [1], Vindhya R. Danda [1,2],
Melanie Ecker [3], Alexandra Joshi-Imre [1], Kate C. Musselman [1], Walter Voit [2,3], Romil Modi [2],
Joseph J. Pancrazio [1] and Bryan J. Black [1]

[1] Department of Bioengineering, The University of Texas at Dallas, Richardson, TX 75080, USA;
    Joshua.usoro@utdallas.edu (J.U.); Christopher.frewin@utdallas.edu (C.L.F.);
    vxd160030@utdallas.edu (V.R.D.); Alexandra.Joshi-imre@utdallas.edu (A.J.-I.);
    kate.musselman@utdallas.edu (K.C.M.); joseph.pancrazio@utdallas.edu (J.J.P.);
    bjb140530@utdallas.edu (B.J.B.)
[2] Qualia, Inc., Dallas, TX 75252, USA; walter.voit@utdallas.edu (W.V.); romil@qualiamedical.com (R.M.)
[3] Department of Materials Science and Engineering, The University of Texas at Dallas, Richardson, TX 75080,
    USA; Melanie.ecker@utdallas.edu
* Correspondence: Allison.stiller@utdallas.edu; Tel.: +1-972-883-2138

Received: 18 August 2018; Accepted: 27 September 2018; Published: 29 September 2018

Abstract: Current intracortical probe technology is limited in clinical implementation due to the short functional lifetime of implanted devices. Devices often fail several months to years post-implantation, likely due to the chronic immune response characterized by glial scarring and neuronal dieback. It has been demonstrated that this neuroinflammatory response is influenced by the mechanical mismatch between stiff devices and the soft brain tissue, spurring interest in the use of softer polymer materials for probe encapsulation. Here, we demonstrate stable recordings and electrochemical properties obtained from fully encapsulated shape memory polymer (SMP) intracortical electrodes implanted in the rat motor cortex for 13 weeks. SMPs are a class of material that exhibit modulus changes when exposed to specific conditions. The formulation used in these devices softens by an order of magnitude after implantation compared to its dry, room-temperature modulus of ~2 GPa.

Keywords: intracortical implant; microelectrodes; softening; immunohistochemistry; immune response; neural interface; shape memory polymer

1. Introduction

Successful clinical application of brain-machine interfaces (BMIs) requires stable, chronic, selective recordings from task-associated neural networks. Noninvasive techniques for the acquisition of neural signals include electroencephalography and electrocorticography [1–3]; however, these methods cannot achieve high-density, single-unit resolution, and are therefore limited as high information content BMI systems [4–6]. Multichannel intracortical microelectrode arrays (MEAs) are able to record single units and local field potentials from adjacent neural tissue within the brain. While several styles of intracortical MEAs are commercially available, they are limited in clinical implementation due to a relatively short functional lifetime, only recording distinguishable units in non-human primates for an average of 1-6 years post-implantation [7–10].

While there are various factors that contribute to MEA failure, findings suggest that the tissue response may be one component that contributes to the premature loss of stable neural recordings [11–14]. The chronic foreign body response stems from the recruitment of activated support cells to the injury site, initiating signaling cascades that result in upregulated local production of inflammatory and neurotoxic cytokines [14,15]. This leads to the accumulation of glial cells around the implant (i.e., encapsulation) concurrent with local neuronal death [11,15–18], both of which are obstacles for reliable signal acquisition.

State-of-the-art, commercially available devices are fabricated using very stiff (high elastic modulus) materials, such as silicon or tungsten (50–400 GPa). Current research suggests that this mechanical mismatch between the low modulus of the brain (~1–10 kPa) and the high modulus of the device may play a major role in aggravating the chronic immune response [17,19,20]. This effect is exacerbated by constant micromotion of the brain around the implant [21], which results in the development of strain fields in tissue adjacent to the probe [22,23]. Several groups have demonstrated that softer implants may mitigate the tissue response over time when compared to stiffer counterparts [24,25]. However, these materials are often too soft to provide appropriate mechanical support for successful penetration into the brain tissue without the aid of insertion guides [26,27]. Conversely, stiffer devices are brittle and prone to fracture, making them difficult to handle in a clinical setting.

Shape memory polymers (SMPs) are a class of materials that undergo dramatic programmed mechanical deformations or modulus changes when exposed to external stimuli such as light, electric currents, or heat [28–30]. Recently, softening thiol-ene/acrylate-based SMPs, which exhibit changes in modulus when transitioning from ambient to physiological conditions, have been investigated for their use as substrate and encapsulation materials for neural interfaces [31,32]. Specifically, this type of SMP can maintain a high modulus and mechanical stability necessary for the implantation of a thin device, but softens by an order of magnitude within only a few minutes [33]. However, to date, no published study has evaluated the chronic recording and electrochemical performance of fully encapsulated thiol-ene/acrylate-based SMP MEAs in vivo. To address this issue, we have implanted 15-channel Michigan-style SMP devices in the motor cortex of five rats and conducted electrophysiological recordings as well as electrochemical impedance spectroscopy (EIS) and cyclic voltammetry (CV) over a 13-week period. Additionally, we have performed immunohistochemistry (IHC) to evaluate tissue response. Our results demonstrate that these SMP devices consistently recorded units for 13 weeks and induced a minimal immune response in the surrounding tissue.

2. Materials and Methods

2.1. Shape Memory Polymer Devices

All experiments were carried out using IC-5-16E devices (Figure 1) provided by Qualia, Inc. (Dallas, TX, USA). Devices featured 15 electrode sites coated with sputtered iridium oxide film (SIROF) with an electrode area of 180 μm^2. Parylene C encapsulated the thin metal traces to ensure proper electrical insulation. Shanks were 5 mm long, 290 μm wide at the base, and 35 $\pm$ 5 μm thick, with an asymmetric geometry that tapered toward the device tip. The SMP formulation used in these devices softens by an order of magnitude from its dry room-temperature modulus of ~2 GPa to ~300 MPa after implantation. This transition occurs within a few minutes of implantation.

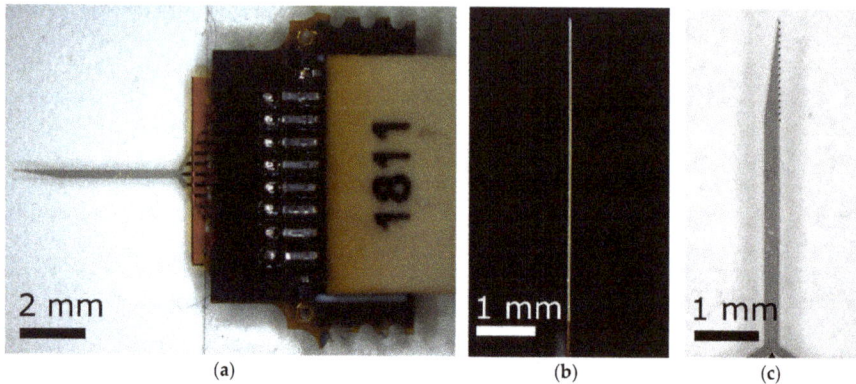

Figure 1. Optical images of shape memory polymer (SMP) probes. (**a**) Device with Omnetics connector, (**b**) side view demonstrating a straight shank prior to implantation, (**c**) tip with sputtered iridium oxide film (SIROF)-coated electrodes.

2.2. Surgical Implantation

All animal handling, housing, and surgical procedures were approved by the University of Texas Institutional Animal Care and Use Committee. Long Evans rats (n = 5, Charles River), weighing 300–450 g, were implanted with functional SMP devices. Devices underwent brief electrochemical impedance testing before implantation to ensure all electrode sites were below 1 MΩ at 1 kHz frequency. Animals were anesthetized by an intraperitoneal (IP) injection of KXA cocktail consisting of ketamine (65 mg/kg), xylazine (13.33 mg/kg) and acepromazine (1.5 mg/kg) followed by an intramuscular injection of atropine sulfate (0.05 mg/kg) to counteract the cardiovascular depression induced by KXA. After reaching a deep anesthesia plane, confirmed by tail and toe pinches, the scalp was shaved using small hair clippers. Ophthalmic ointment was applied to the animal's eyes to mitigate drying and post-operative irritation. The anesthetic plane was supplemented and maintained using 1–2% isoflurane mixed with 100% oxygen for the duration of the surgery.

Three alternating rounds of 10% iodine solution and 70% ethanol, ending with ethanol, were used to sterilize and clean the point of incision on the scalp. Dexamethasone was then administered subcutaneously between the shoulders (2 mg/kg), followed by subcutaneous injection of 0.4 mL 0.5% lidocaine at the incision cite. A surgical blade was used to make a midline incision down the scalp and the surrounding skin and muscle were retracted with hemostatic forceps. All loose tissue and debris was removed from the skull surface using sterile cotton swabs, and the skull was roughened using the surgical blade to promote binding of the head cap post-surgery.

A surgical drill was used to create a 1–2 mm^2 craniotomy centered in the right motor cortex, approximately 2.5 mm rostral and 2.5 mm lateral from bregma. Three anchoring screws were positioned approximately 1 cm from the perimeter of the insertion site. The dura was resected and the device was implanted at 1000 µm/s to a depth of 1.5–2 mm using a pneumatically controlled micropositioner (Kopf Instruments, Tujunga, CA, USA). No significant curvature or bending of the device was observed prior to or during implantation. Collagen-based dural grafts (Biodesign Dural Graft, Cook Medical, Bloomington, IN, USA) were placed around the implanted device to act as a dura replacement, and then set in place with Gluture topical adhesive (World Precision Instruments, Sarasota, FL, USA). We applied dental cement around the device and all three anchoring screws to construct a protective head cap, promoting chronic mechanical stability. Before being removed from the isoflurane, the animal was given 0.15 mg/kg of sustained release buprenorphine SR LAB (ZooPharm, Windsor, CO, USA) and 5 mg/kg of cefazolin antibiotic along with subcutaneous sterile saline to prevent dehydration. All animals received follow-up analgesic injections of buprenorphine SR 72 h following surgery. None of the animals showed signs of post-operative complications including chronic bleeding, signs of infection, or skin ulcers.

2.3. Electrophysiological Recordings and Single-Unit Analysis

Electrophysiological recordings were carried out on lightly anesthetized animals (0.5–1.5% isoflurane) immediately following surgical implantation and once per week for 13 weeks afterward. Spontaneous wideband recordings (0.1–7000 Hz) were collected using 15-channel Michigan style SMP arrays (IC-5-16E, Qualia, Inc.) and an Omniplex acquisition system (Plexon, Inc., Dallas, TX, USA) from all 15 recording sites simultaneously at 40,000 Hz for 10 min. Wideband data were processed using a four-pole Butterworth high pass filter with a cutoff frequency of 250 Hz. Individual waveforms (spikes) were identified by filtered continuous data crossing a threshold of -4σ, based on the root mean square (RMS) of the filtered continuous signal. Single units were manually identified from collections of spikes using 2D principal component space, but were excluded from further analysis if they did not contain at least 100 individual spikes, or if >3% of spikes violated a 1.5-ms minimum refractory period. The signal to noise ratio (SNR) was calculated by dividing the mean peak-to-peak voltage of each unit (Vpp) by the RMS noise of its associated channel. The RMS noise was calculated as the RMS of the filtered continuous signal after removing all samples exceeding the 4σ threshold.

2.4. EIS and CV Measurements

EIS and CV measurements were carried out on all electrodes each week immediately following in vivo electrophysiological recordings. The Plexon headstage was removed and replaced with a pre-wired 18 pin dual strip Nano-D female connector (NSD-18-WD-18.0-C-GS, Omnetics Connector Corporation, Minneapolis, MN, USA) attached to multiplexor inputs of a model 604E Series Electrochemical Analyzer/Workstation (CH Instruments Inc., Austin, TX, USA). EIS was performed using a 10 mV RMS sinusoidal signal (Vrms), starting at a frequency of 100 kHz and decreasing to 1 Hz, recording current 12 times per decade of frequency. The impedance magnitude at each frequency was calculated by the CH instruments software. CV evaluations were performed by applying a negative potential ramp starting at the open circuit potential (vs. 316 stainless steel) with no external direct current bias applied. The potential was reduced to -0.6 V and then cycled at 50 mV/s for two complete cycles between -0.6 V and 0.8 V while recording current every 10 ms. A second CV measurement was performed under the same conditions, but at a sweep rate of 50,000 mV/s.

Electrochemistry results were process in MATLAB to extract the values of real impedance (Ω) directly from the EIS recordings at the physiological frequencies of 0.01, 1, and 10 kHz. MATLAB scripts also determined cathodal charge storage capacity (CSCc), a measure of the total cathodal charge available per unit of geometric area, from the CV cathodal current between the limits of -0.6 to 0.8 V.

2.5. Immunohistochemistry

2.5.1. Tissue Preparation

Rats were administered a 200 mg/kg IP injection of sodium pentobarbital. After confirming unconsciousness through tail and toe pinches, the rats were transcardially perfused with room-temperature phosphate buffered saline (PBS) followed by room-temperature 4% paraformaldehyde (PFA) solution. The brain was removed such that the device was kept intact with the connector and surrounding skull. The brain was stored in PFA at 4 °C overnight, then transferred to PBS with sodium azide and stored at 4 °C until sectioning.

Prior to sectioning, brains were submerged in a 4% (m/V) agarose solution for stability. Vibratome sections (Leica VT 1000 S, Leica Biosystems Inc., Buffalo Grove, IL, USA) were collected from the surface of the brain to a 2 mm depth (200 µm slices) and then stored in PBS with 0.1% (*w*/*v*) sodium azide (Alfa Aesar, Tewksbury, MA, USA) at 4 °C until staining.

2.5.2. Antibody Staining

Brain slices were blocked in 4% (*v*/*v*) normal goat serum (Abcam Inc., Cambridge, UK) with 0.3% (*v*/*v*) Triton X-100 (Sigma-Aldrich, Saint Louis, MO, USA) in 1× PBS with 0.1% sodium azide (Alfa Aesar) for one hour. Slices were then incubated overnight with primary antibodies targeting neuronal nuclei (NeuN), astrocytes (GFAP), and activated microglia/macrophages (CD68) (Table 1) at 4 °C in a buffer solution containing only 0.1% (*v*/*v*) Triton X-100.

Table 1. Primary antibodies.

Primary	Vendor	ID#	Dilution	Labeling
NeuN	Sigma-Aldrich	ABN91	1:500	Neuronal nuclei
GFAP	Millipore-Sigma	AB5541	1:500	Astrocytes
CD68	Fisher Scientific	MS397P0	1:1000	Activated microglia/macrophages

The following day, slices were washed and incubated for one hour in blocking solution with secondary antibodies, goat anti-rabbit IgG (TRITC), goat anti-mouse IgG (Alexa Fluor 488), goat anti-chicken IgY (Alexa Fluor 647), at 1:1000 dilution, and DAPI (0.6 µM) (Abcam Inc.). Slices were subsequently washed and mounted on glass slides with Fluoromount aqueous mounting medium (Sigma-Aldrich).

2.5.3. IHC Imaging

Stained tissue slices were imaged using an inverted confocal microscope (Nikon Ti eclipse + A1R, Tokyo, Japan) controlled by Nikon Instruments Software package (version AR 4.40.00). Briefly, z-stack images were collected at 1024 × 1024 transverse resolution and 5 µm per axial slice using a 20× Ph2 objective. Fluorescence signal-to-noise was increased by enabling 2× pixel averaging and bleed-over between emission lines was reduced by collecting each emission line in series. All microscope hardware and software settings were conserved between individual image collections and imaging sessions. Following acquisition, z-stack images were collapsed to single maximum intensity projection image.

2.5.4. IHC Quantification

Astrogliosis (GFAP intensity) and neuronal density were quantified as described in [34]. Briefly, images were imported into Fiji [35], and open source imaging software based on ImageJ [36]. Using a custom macro, GFAP intensities and NeuN+ nuclei per area were calculated within at least eight concentric bands of 50 µm thickness generated from a user-defined implant site. All reported values were normalized to measurements from the band located 350–400 µm from the device edge.

2.6. Statistical Analysis

Statistical analysis and graphing were carried out in OriginPro 2017 (Origin Lab, Northampton, MA, USA). In all cases, statistical significance of increasing/decreasing differences ($p < 0.05$) was determined by carrying out analysis of variance (ANOVA) tests on residuals. In the case of both EIS and CV measurements, a single-tiered Grubb's test was applied at a 0.05 significance level to exclude aberrant statistical outliers.

3. Results

3.1. Chronic Single Unit Recordings

To evaluate the chronic recording performance of thiol-ene/acrylate-based SMP devices, we implanted 15-channel Michigan-style single shank electrode arrays in the motor cortex of five Long Evans rats and collected spontaneous wide-band 10-min recordings for 13 weeks post-implantation (Figure 2). Immediately following implantation, we observed that $18.3 \pm 6.9\%$ (mean $\pm$ SEM, $n = 60$)

of electrode sites across all devices exhibited distinguishable single units (termed "Active electrode yield %") (Figure 3b). At this time, the mean peak-to-peak voltage of sorted waveforms (Figure 3a) was 66.8 ± 3.1 µV, $n = 75$, resulting in an excellent mean signal-to-noise ratio (SNR) of 9.80 ± 0.47 (Figure 3c). One week post-implantation, the active electrode yield increased to 41.3 ± 12.7%. While, there was no significant change in active electrode yield or SNR over the remaining 13-week period, the total number of recorded units (Figure 2d) increased slightly ($R^2 = 0.02$, $p = 0.02$). Overall, these data suggest that our SMP electrodes were stable with regard to their recording capabilities.

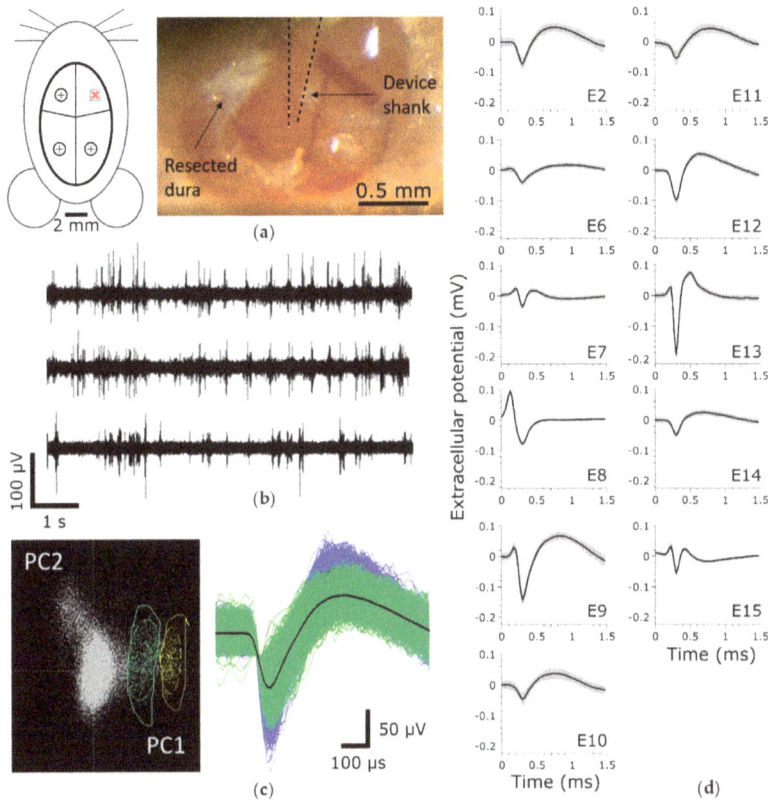

Figure 2. Neural data acquisition and waveform analysis. (**a**) Implantation schematic denoting the implantation site (red "x") and stabilizing screws, (**b**) filtered continuous data from three representative electrodes on a single array, (**c**) representation of single-unit sorting principals (left) and representative multi-unit activity from a single recording electrode (right), (**d**) single units recorded on a single array during a single recording session, ordered from array tip (E2) to base (E15).

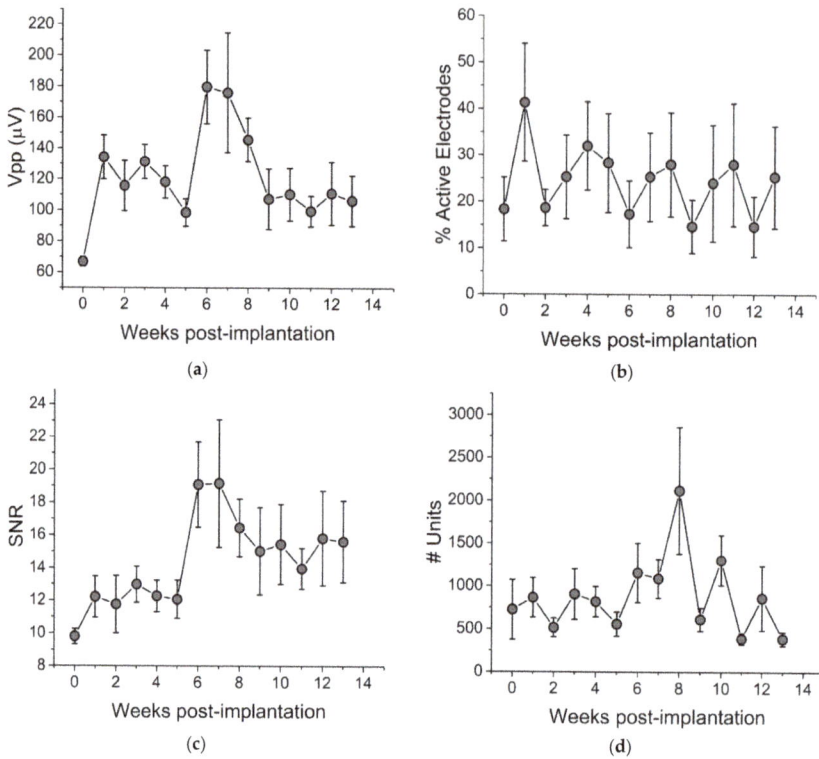

Figure 3. Chronic recording stability. (**a**) peak-to-peak voltage (Vpp), (**b**) active electrode yield %, (**c**) signal-to-noise ratio (SNR), and (**d**) number of units. Each time point reflects n = 75 electrodes, except weeks 0 and 5, which reflect n = 60 electrodes. Linear regression analysis indicates no change in Vpp, active electrode yield %, or SNR, while number of units increased slightly (R^2 = 0.016, p = 0.02). Week 0 represents data taken on the day of implantation. Data are shown as mean $\pm$ SEM.

3.2. Chronic In Vivo Electrochemistry

To evaluate the electrochemical stability of the SMP devices over time, we performed EIS and CV measurements on each array across all electrode sites for 13 weeks post-implantation. EIS and CV data are also presented for week 0 data points indicating pre-implantation measurements taken in room temperature PBS. Figure 4a shows representative traces for mean EIS for a single device prior to implantation (in vitro), immediately following implantation, and at five, nine, and 13 weeks following implantation. To evaluate the stability over a frequency relevant to extracellular spikes, the mean 1 kHz impedance across all devices is plotted in Figure 4b over the 13-week time period.

All electrodes exhibited a significant increase in impedance magnitude one week post-implantation (1.23 ± 0.07 MΩ) versus in vitro measurements (0.62 ± 0.09 MΩ), similar to observations made in [37]. Impedance magnitudes remained largely consistent at this value across the first seven weeks of the study, and then decreased slightly during the remaining six weeks. This decrease did not show any correlation with the mean active electrode yield, however, suggesting that although there may have been degradation of the insulating material, this degradation did not hinder the devices' ability to resolve and record single unit activity.

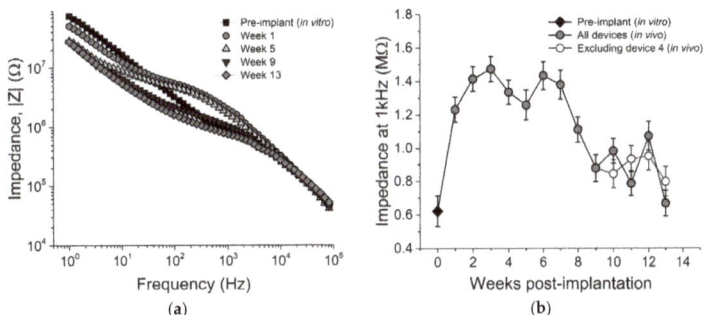

Figure 4. Electrochemical impedance spectroscopy. (**a**) Impedance across 1–10 kHz frequency range for a representative electrode at five time points and (**b**) impedance magnitude at 1 kHz across all electrodes on all devices. Impedance was initially low (~600 kΩ) upon testing before implantation, but increased following implantation. From week 1 until week 13, impedance magnitude decreased over time. Pre-implantation data are from $n = 45$ electrodes. All other time point reflect $n = 75$ electrodes, except weeks 0 and 5, which reflect $n = 60$ electrodes.

Figure 5a–d shows representative CV traces for a single electrode at two different sweep rates (50 and 50,000 mV/s) at selected time points, as well as mean CSC_C for both sweep rates across all devices and time points. Faster sweep rates are indicative of conductive pathways that are near the tip of the device, while slower sweep rates allow access to conductive pathways proximal to the tip.

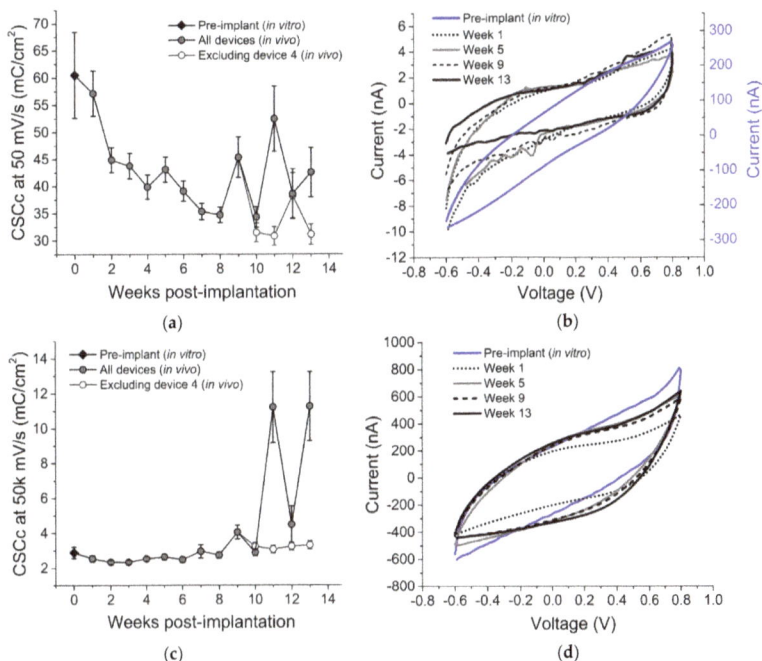

Figure 5. Cyclic voltammetry (CV) results. (**a,c**) slow (50 mV/s) and fast (50 k mV/s) CV over 13 weeks, (**b,d**) slow and fast CV curves across five time points on a representative electrode.

We observed an increase over time in CSC_C at 50,000 mV/s, ($R^2 = 0.07$, $p < 0.001$) likely indicating increased access to conductive paths that could be due to cracks or separation between the insulating and conductive layers near the tip. CSC_C at 50 mV/s decreased within the first two weeks post-implantation as compared to in vitro measurements, and continued to decrease until week 8, suggesting a possible loss of the SIROF coating. After week 10, however, the CSC_C increased. This change was attributable to values recorded from a single device (device 4), as demonstrated in Figure 5a,c, and also supported by EIS results (Figure 4b). Nevertheless, the majority of the devices exhibited stable electrochemistry over time, as also supported by the stable neural recordings.

3.3. Histology

To evaluate the induced FBR related to chronic implantation of softening SMP devices, we performed histology targeting neuronal cell bodies (NeuN), astrocytes (GFAP), and activated microglia/macrophages (CD68). Figure 6a shows representative fluorescence images for each marker with respect to increasing depth along the shank of the device.

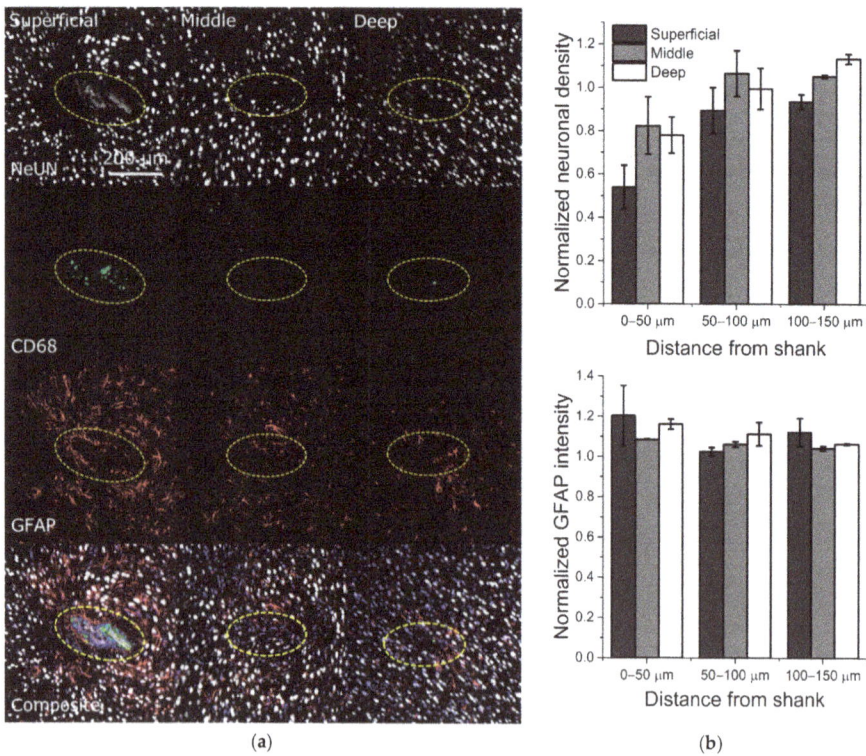

(a) (b)

Figure 6. Immunohistochemistry for SMP implant after 13 weeks in vivo. (**a**) Columns represent tissue collected at superficial, middle, and deep slices in relation to the surface of the motor cortex. Rows represent neuronal nuclei (NeUN) (gray, top), activated microglia/macrophages (CD68) (green), astrocytes (GFAP) (red), and Composite (bottom) images. Scale bar represents 200 µm in the transverse plane across all images. Yellow ellipses indicate probe location. (**b**) Quantification of NeuN and GFAP for $n = 2$ animals at varying slice depths (one slice per region) with respect to the shank location in the brain.

While Figure 6 demonstrates promising histological outcomes, these results are preliminary and require a more comprehensive analysis comparing SMP with standard silicon devices to make statistical claims. The most severe apparent immune response was observed at the base of the shank, represented by "superficial" slices, within the first 50 μm of the device perimeter (Figure 6b). However, this effect tapered off along the length of the probe, represented by "middle" and "deep" slices. Additionally, consistent with previous studies reporting histological outcomes, we observed slight astrogliosis in areas with neuronal dieback, again with the most severe response near the base of the shank but tapered off toward the tip. This is in contrast to previous reports of significant neuroinflammatory response within 100 μm of the device when using silicon-based arrays [15]. Additionally, there were few or no apparent activated microglia around the device at "middle" and "deep" slices. It is important to note that the microelectrode sites on this device are located near the end of the device shank, and therefore best represented by the "middle" and "deep" slices. Therefore, it appears that the neuroinflammatory response was modest proximal to the microelectrode site locations.

4. Discussion

Significant efforts have been directed toward developing penetrating intracortical MEAs that mitigate the FBR. Prior work has made use of three general strategies or combinations thereof: (1) decreasing MEAs dimensions [38,39], (2) utilizing soft or softening materials for MEAs [24,25], and (3) coating MEAs with biomimetic gels, proteins, or growth factors to depress the foreign body response or facilitate local regeneration [40,41]. While these approaches have all yielded varying levels of success in terms of histological response, the chronic recording reliability of penetrating intracortical MEAs remains a significant challenge. Here, for the first time, we have demonstrated stable chronic recordings from a fully encapsulated softening SMP-based electrode array implanted in the motor cortex of rats. Importantly, we observed no significant decrease in active electrode yield over a 13-week indwelling period. Additionally, we performed electrochemical measurements to evaluate the electrical stability of these arrays. While we initially observed an increase in 1 kHz impedance magnitude, most likely associated with acute inflammation, the impedance approached its pre-implantation values over time, suggesting a resolution of the acute immune response over the first eight weeks in vivo [42]. This is further supported by the limited FBR we observed following device explantation. Cathodal charge storage capacity was also found to be largely consistent over the indwelling period. However, in the case of one electrode array, the CSC increased dramatically over the final three weeks of implantation (approximately 2 orders of magnitude). Concurrently, this electrode array exhibited reduced impedances. This was most likely due to trace or wire bundle breakage.

Table 2 summarizes previous studies using state-of-the-art single-shank silicon- and SMP-based electrode arrays. While there are important differences in all these studies in terms of N number, study duration, implantation site, single-unit sorting criteria, and electrode material/deposition, our results (top row) compare well in terms of terminal AEY% with the current state of the art (25 ± 11% versus 10–59%). Additionally, there have been significant prior efforts to leverage soft or softening polymers as either an insulator or a structural material for intracortical MEAs. Luan et al. demonstrated chronic recording capability with a comparable active electrode yield (20–25%), and also exhibited minimal tissue response [43]. However, due to their extreme flexibility, they required an insertion guide, which may not be practical for applications using multi-shank structures. This highlights one of the inherent advantages of softening over soft material approaches. Other groups have investigated Parylene C [44,45] and polyimide [46], but have not achieved chronic recordings up to or longer than one month. Others have investigated softening polymers [24,25], but face significant challenges in fabricating functional devices due to water absorption during softening.

Table 2. Planar single-shank electrode array comparison. Active electrode yield (AEY) percentage represents spontaneous single-unit activity unless otherwise indicated.

Ref	Model (R/M), Implant Site	N, Study Duration	AEY%	Substrate, Electrode Material
-	R, MC	N = 5, 13 weeks	25 ± 11%	SMP, SIROF
[32]	R, MC	N = 2, 11 weeks	* 37 ± 13%	SMP, PEDOT:PSS
[47]	R, MC	N = 8, 6 weeks	59% (Ir, SNR > 2)	Si, Ir or PEDOT
[37]	R, MC	N = 5, 12 weeks	33 and 39%	Si, Au or PEDOT:TFB
[7]	R, MC	N = 4, 4 weeks	* 27%	Si, Ir
[48]	M, VC	N = 4, 27 weeks	* 10% (spontaneous)	Si, Ir

* Represents approximate or recalculated values in the case that AEY was not reported. (R/M)—Rat or Mouse model. MC—motor cortex, VC—visual cortex.

The feasibility of SMP-based recording MEAs has been demonstrated in both rat auditory [31] and motor cortex [32]. The work presented here takes full advantage of SMP as an encapsulation material. Whereas previous studies have assessed devices that are SMP on one side and Parylene C on the other, the devices used here are completely sandwiched between layers of both Parylene C and SMP. In this way, we show that SMP is viable for use as a substrate material for neural device encapsulation, along with a thin layer of Parylene C necessary for electrical isolation. Additionally, SEM images collected post-explantation (Figure 7) reveal no evident signs of encapsulation failure or cracking.

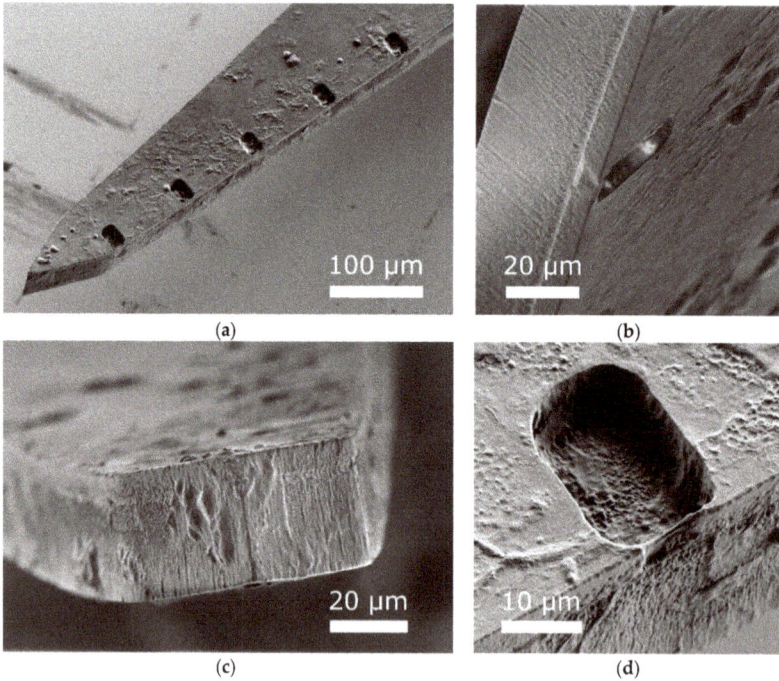

Figure 7. SEM post-explantation. (a) Explanted array showing some, but limited, biofouling, (b) interface between SMP layers at an electrode site, indicating no apparent layer separation, (c) interface between SMP layers at the tip of the array, (d) representative electrode site, showing no apparent signs of SIROF delamination.

Future studies focused on the design and development of SMP-based MEAs should take advantage of both geometrical and chemical considerations. For example, recently developed SMP formulations may extend the dynamic softening range of SMP devices [48]. Additionally, one inherent disadvantage of thiol-ene/acrylate polymers based on ester linkages is that they may exhibit degradation due to hydrolysis. The development of hydrolytically stable SMP formulations may provide a more chronically useful substrate. Nevertheless, for experiments over the time course of 13 weeks in vivo, the present SMP formulation appears sufficient to realize functional devices.

5. Conclusions

Here we demonstrated stable neural recordings and electrochemistry using IC-5-16E devices fully encapsulated with SMP. Devices consistently recorded single units for 13 weeks in the rat motor cortex and preliminary histology demonstrated only a modest tissue response in the tissue adjacent to the insertion site. Our results establish a valuable baseline for the evaluation of other softening probe technologies including devices comprised of SMPs capable of increased softening after implantation.

Author Contributions: Conceptualization, A.M.S., B.J.B. and J.J.P.; Methodology, A.M.S., B.J.B., J.U. and C.L.F.; Software, A.M.S., B.J.B. and C.L.F.; Validation, A.M.S. and B.J.B.; Formal Analysis, A.M.S., J.U. and B.J.B.; Investigation, A.M.S., B.J.B., J.U. and C.L.F.; Resources, J.J.P.; Data Curation, A.M.S., J.U., C.L.F., K.C.M. and A.J.-M. and B.J.B.; Writing—Original Draft Preparation, A.M.S., J.U. and B.J.B.; Writing—Review & Editing, A.M.S., B.J.B., M.E., W.V., R.M., V.R.D., C.L.F. and J.J.P.; Visualization, A.M.S. and B.J.B.; Supervision, B.J.B. and J.J.P.; Project Administration, A.M.S., B.J.B. and J.J.P.; Funding Acquisition, J.J.P.

Funding: This work was supported by the Office of the Assistant Secretary of Defense for Health Affairs through the Peer-Reviewed Medical Research Program (grant number W81XWH-15-1-0607). Opinions, interpretations, conclusions, and recommendations are those of the authors and are not necessarily endorsed by the Department of Defense. Additional support was provided by the Eugene McDermott Graduate Fellowship Program, Richardson, TX (grant number 201606) at the University of Texas at Dallas.

Conflicts of Interest: Qualia Labs, Inc. provided the intracortical electrodes used in this study. W.V. is the president of Qualia Labs, Inc. R.M. and V.D. are paid employees of Qualia Labs, Inc. W.V., R.M., and V.D. had no role in the design of the study; in the collection, analysis, or interpretation of the data; or in the decision to publish the results. The senior author of this work (B.B.) serves as an unpaid advisor to Qualia Labs, Inc.

References

1. Kübler, A.; Kotchoubey, B.; Kaiser, J.; Wolpaw, J.R.; Birbaumer, N. Brain-computer communication: Unlocking the locked in. *Psychol. Bull.* **2001**, *127*, 358–375. [CrossRef] [PubMed]

2. Obermaier, B.; Müller, G.R.; Pfurtscheller, G. "Virtual keyboard" controlled by spontaneous EEG activity. *IEEE Trans. Neural Syst. Rehabil. Eng.* **2003**, *11*, 422–426. [CrossRef] [PubMed]

3. Pailla, T.; Jiang, W.; Dichter, B.; Chang, E.F.; Gilja, V. ECoG data analyses to inform closed-loop BCI experiments for speech-based prosthetic applications. In Proceedings of the 38th Annual International Conference of the IEEE Engineering in Medicine and Biology Society (EMBC), Orlando, FL, USA, 16–20 August 2016; pp. 5713–5716.

4. Birbaumer, N. Brain-computer-interface research: Coming of age. *Clin. Neurophysiol.* **2006**, *117*, 479–483. [CrossRef] [PubMed]

5. Lebedev, M.A.; Nicolelis, M.A. Brain-machine interfaces: Past, present and future. *Trends Neurosci.* **2006**, *29*, 536–546. [CrossRef] [PubMed]

6. Kipke, D.R.; Shain, W.; Buzsaki, G.; Fetz, E.; Henderson, J.M.; Hetke, J.F.; Schalk, G. Advanced neurotechnologies for chronic neural interfaces: New horizons and clinical opportunities. *J. Neurosci.* **2008**, *28*, 11830–11838. [CrossRef] [PubMed]

7. Ward, M.P.; Rajdev, P.; Ellison, C.; Irazoqui, P.P. Toward a comparison of microelectrodes for acute and chronic recordings. *Brain Res.* **2009**, *1282*, 183–200. [CrossRef] [PubMed]

8. Barrese, J.C.; Rao, N.; Paroo, K.; Triebwasser, C.; Vargas-Irwin, C.; Franquemont, L.; Donoghue, J.P. Failure mode analysis of silicon-based intracortical microelectrode arrays in non-human primates. *J. Neural Eng.* **2013**, *10*, 066014. [CrossRef] [PubMed]

9. Barrese, J.C.; Aceros, J.; Donoghue, J.P. Scanning electron microscopy of chronically implanted intracortical microelectrode arrays in non-human primates. *J. Neural Eng.* **2016**, *13*, 026003. [CrossRef] [PubMed]

10. Suner, S.; Fellows, M.R.; Vargas-Irwin, C.; Nakata, G.K.; Donoghue, J.P. Reliability of signals from a chronically implanted, silicon-based electrode array in non-human primate primary motor cortex. *IEEE Trans. Neural Syst. Rehabil. Eng.* **2005**, *13*, 524–541. [CrossRef] [PubMed]

11. Polikov, V.S.; Tresco, P.A.; Reichert, W.M. Response of brain tissue to chronically implanted neural electrodes. *J. Neurosci. Methods* **2005**, *148*, 1–18. [CrossRef] [PubMed]
12. Seymour, J.P.; Kipke, D.R. Neural probe design for reduced tissue encapsulation in CNS. *Biomaterials* **2007**, *28*, 3594–3607. [CrossRef] [PubMed]
13. Leach, J.; Achyuta, A.K.H.; Murthy, S.K. Bridging the divide between neuroprosthetic design, tissue engineering and neurobiology. *Front. Neuroeng.* **2010**, *2*, 1–19. [CrossRef] [PubMed]
14. Karumbaiah, L.; Saxena, T.; Carlson, D.; Patil, K.; Patkar, R.; Gaupp, E.A.; Betancur, M.; Stanley, G.B.; Carin, L.; Bellamkonda, R.V. Relationship between intracortical electrode design and chronic recording function. *Biomaterials* **2013**, *34*, 8061–8074. [CrossRef] [PubMed]
15. Biran, R.; Martin, D.C.; Tresco, P.A. Neuronal cell loss accompanies the brain tissue response to chronically implanted silicon microelectrode arrays. *Exp. Neurol.* **2005**, *195*, 115–126. [CrossRef] [PubMed]
16. McConnell, G.C.; Rees, H.D.; Levey, A.I.; Gutekunst, C.-A.; Gross, R.E.; Bellamkonda, R.V. Implanted neural electrodes cause chronic, local inflammation that is correlated with local neurodegeneration. *J. Neural Eng.* **2009**, *6*, 056003. [CrossRef] [PubMed]
17. Moshayedi, P.; Ng, G.; Kwok, J.C.; Yeo, G.S.; Bryant, C.E.; Fawcett, J.W.; Franze, K.; Guck, J. The relationship between glial cell mechanosensitivity and foreign body reactions in the central nervous system. *Biomaterials* **2014**, *35*, 3919–3925. [CrossRef] [PubMed]
18. Nolta, N.F.; Christensen, M.B.; Crane, P.D.; Skousen, J.L.; Tresco, P.A. BBB leakage, astrogliosis, and tissue loss correlate with silicon microelectrode array recording performance. *Biomaterials* **2015**, *53*, 753–762. [CrossRef] [PubMed]
19. Andrei, A.; Welkenhuysen, M.; Nuttin, B.; Eberle, W. A response surface model predicting the in vivo insertion behavior of micromachined neural implants. *J. Neural Eng.* **2011**, *9*, 016005. [CrossRef] [PubMed]
20. Karumbaiah, L.; Norman, S.E.; Rajan, N.B.; Anand, S.; Saxena, T.; Betancur, M.; Patkar, R.; Bellamkonda, R.V. The upregulation of specific interleukin (IL) receptor antagonists and paradoxical enhancement of neuronal apoptosis due to electrode induced strain and brain micromotion. *Biomaterials* **2012**, *33*, 5983–5996. [CrossRef] [PubMed]
21. Gilletti, A.; Muthuswamy, J. Brain micromotion around implants in the rodent somatosensory cortex. *J. Neural Eng.* **2006**, *3*, 189–195. [CrossRef] [PubMed]
22. Sridharan, A.; Nguyen, J.K.; Capadona, J.R.; Muthuswamy, J. Compliant intracortical implants reduce strains and strain rates in brain tissue in vivo. *J. Neural Eng.* **2015**, *12*, 036002. [CrossRef] [PubMed]
23. Subbaroyan, J.; Martin, D.C.; Kipke, D.R. A finite-element model of the mechanical effects of implantable microelectrodes in the cerebral cortex. *J. Neural Eng.* **2005**, *2*, 103–113. [CrossRef] [PubMed]
24. Harris, J.P.; Capadona, J.R.; Miller, R.H.; Healy, B.C.; Shanmuganathan, K.; Rowan, S.J.; Weder, C.; Tyler, D.J. Mechanically adaptive intracortical implants improve the proximity of neuronal cell bodies. *J. Neural Eng.* **2011**, *8*, 066011. [CrossRef] [PubMed]
25. Lee, H.C.; Ejserholm, F.; Gaire, J.; Currlin, S.; Schouenborg, J.; Wallman, L.; Bengtsson, M.; Park, K.; Otto, K.J. Histological evaluation of flexible neural implants; Flexibility limit for reducing the tissue response? *J. Neural Eng.* **2017**, *14*, 036026. [CrossRef] [PubMed]
26. Shoffstall, A.J.; Srinivasan, S.; Willis, M.; Stiller, A.M.; Ecker, M.; Voit, W.E.; Pancrazio, J.J.; Capadona, J.R. A mosquito inspired strategy to implant microprobes into the brain. *Sci. Rep.* **2018**, *8*, 1–10. [CrossRef] [PubMed]
27. Lo, M.C.; Wang, S.; Singh, S.; Damodaran, V.B.; Kaplan, H.M.; Kohn, J.; Shreiber, D.I.; Zahn, J.D. Coating flexible probes with an ultra fast degrading polymer to aid in tissue insertion. *Biomed. Microdevices* **2015**, *17*. [CrossRef] [PubMed]
28. Mather, P.T.; Luo, X.; Rousseau, I.A. Shape memory polymer research. *Annu. Rev. Mater. Res.* **2009**, *39*, 445–471. [CrossRef]
29. Wang, K.; Strandman, S.; Zhu, X.X. A mini review: Shape memory polymers for biomedical applications. *Front. Chem. Sci. Eng.* **2017**, *11*, 143–153. [CrossRef]
30. Leng, J.; Lan, X.; Liu, Y.; Du, S. Shape-memory polymers and their composites: Stimulus methods and applications. *Prog. Mater. Sci.* **2011**, *56*, 1077–1135. [CrossRef]
31. Ware, T.; Simon, D.; Liu, C.; Musa, T.; Vasudevan, S.; Sloan, A.; Keefer, E.W.; Ii, R.L.R.; Voit, W. Thiol-ene/acrylate substrates for softening intracortical electrodes. *Appl. Biomater.* **2013**, *102*, 1–11.

32. Simon, D.M.; Charkhkar, H.; St. John, C.; Rajendran, S.; Kang, T.; Reit, R.; Arreaga-Salas, D.; McHail, D.G.; Knaack, G.L.; Sloan, A.; et al. Design and demonstration of an intracortical probe technology with tunable modulus. *J. Biomed. Mater. Res. Part A* **2017**, *105*, 159–168. [CrossRef] [PubMed]

33. Do, D.-H.; Ecker, M.; Voit, W.E. Characterization of a thiol-ene/acrylate-based polymer for neuroprosthetic implants. *ACS Omega* **2017**, *2*, 4604–4611. [CrossRef] [PubMed]

34. Stiller, A.; Black, B.; Kung, C.; Ashok, A.; Cogan, S.; Varner, V.; Pancrazio, J. A meta-analysis of intracortical device stiffness and its correlation with histological outcomes. *Micromachines* **2018**, *9*, 443. [CrossRef]

35. Schindelin, J.; Arganda-Carreras, I.; Frise, E.; Kaynig, V.; Longair, M.; Pietzsch, T.; Preibisch, S.; Rueden, C.; Saalfeld, S.; Schmid, B.; et al. Fiji: An open-source platform for biological-image analysis. *Nat. Methods* **2012**, *9*, 676–682. [CrossRef] [PubMed]

36. Schneider, C.A.; Rasband, W.S.; Eliceiri, K.W. NIH Image to ImageJ: 25 years of image analysis. *Nat. Methods* **2012**, *9*, 671–675. [CrossRef] [PubMed]

37. Charkhkar, H.; Knaack, G.L.; Mchail, D.G.; Mandal, H.S.; Peixoto, N.; Rubinson, J.F.; Dumas, T.C.; Pancrazio, J.J. Chronic intracortical neural recordings using microelectrode arrays coated with PEDOT-TFB. *Acta Biomater.* **2016**, *32*, 57–67. [CrossRef] [PubMed]

38. Pancrazio, J.J.; Deku, F.; Ghazavi, A.; Stiller, A.M.; Rihani, R.; Frewin, C.L.; Varner, V.D.; Gardner, T.J.; Cogan, S.F. Thinking small: Progress on microscale neurostimulation technology. *Neuromodul. Technol. Neural Interfaces* **2017**, *20*, 745–752. [CrossRef] [PubMed]

39. Deku, F.; Cohen, Y.; Joshi-Imre, A.; Kanneganti, A.; Gardner, T.J.; Cogan, S.F. Amorphous silicon carbide ultramicroelectrode arrays for neural stimulation and recording. *J. Neural Eng.* **2018**, *15*, 016007. [CrossRef] [PubMed]

40. Lewitus, D.Y.; Smith, K.L.; Landers, J.; Neimark, A.V.; Koh, J. Bioactive agarose carbon-nanotube composites are capable of manipulating brain-implant interface. *J. Appl. Polym. Sci.* **2014**, *131*. [CrossRef] [PubMed]

41. Spencer, K.C.; Sy, J.C.; Ramadi, K.B.; Graybiel, A.M.; Langer, R.; Cima, M.J. Characterization of mechanically matched hydrogel coatings to improve the biocompatibility of neural implants. *Sci. Rep.* **2017**, *7*, 1–16.

42. Cody, P.A.; Eles, J.R.; Lagenaur, C.F.; Kozai, T.D.Y.; Cui, X.T. Unique electrophysiological and impedance signatures between encapsulation types: An analysis of biological Utah array failure and benefit of a biomimetic coating in a rat model. *Biomaterials* **2018**, *161*, 117–128. [CrossRef] [PubMed]

43. Luan, L.; Wei, X.; Zhao, Z.; Siegel, J.J.; Potnis, O.; Tuppen, C.A.; Lin, S.; Kazmi, S.; Fowler, R.A.; Holloway, S.; et al. Ultraflexible nanoelectronic probes form reliable, glial scar–free neural integration. *Sci. Adv.* **2017**, *3*, e1601966. [CrossRef] [PubMed]

44. Takeuchi, S.; Ziegler, D.; Yoshida, Y.; Mabuchi, K.; Suzuki, T. Parylene flexible neural probes integrated with microfluidic channels. *Lab Chip* **2005**, *5*, 519–523. [CrossRef] [PubMed]

45. Xu, H.; Weltman, A.; Scholten, K.; Meng, E.; Berger, T.W.; Song, D. Chronic multi-region recording from the rat hippocampus in vivo with a flexible Parylene-based multi-electrode array. In Proceedings of the 39th Annual International Conference of the IEEE Engineering in Medicine and Biology Society (EMBC), Seogwipo, Korea, 11–15 July 2017; pp. 1716–1719.

46. Mercanzini, A.; Cheung, K.; Buhl, D.L.; Boers, M.; Maillard, A.; Colin, P.; Bensadoun, J.C.; Bertsch, A.; Renaud, P. Demonstration of cortical recording using novel flexible polymer neural probes. *Sens. Actuators A Phys.* **2008**, *143*, 90–96. [CrossRef]

47. Ludwig, K.A.; Uram, J.D.; Yang, J.; Martin, D.C.; Kipke, D.R. Chronic neural recordings using silicon microelectrode arrays electrochemically deposited with a poly (3,4-ethylenedioxythiophene)(PEDOT) film. *J. Neural Eng.* **2006**, *3*, 59–70. [CrossRef] [PubMed]

48. Kozai, T.D.Y.; Du, Z.; Gugel, Z.V.; Smith, M.A.; Chase, S.M.; Bodily, L.M.; Caparosa, E.M.; Friedlander, R.M.; Cui, X.T. Comprehensive chronic laminar single-unit, multi-unit, and local field potential recording performance with planar single shank electrode arrays. *J. Neurosci. Methods* **2015**, *242*, 15–40. [CrossRef] [PubMed]

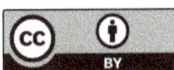

micromachines

MDPI

Article

Characterization of the Neuroinflammatory Response to Thiol-ene Shape Memory Polymer Coated Intracortical Microelectrodes

Andrew J. Shoffstall [1,2], Melanie Ecker [2,3], Vindhya Danda [3,4,5,6], Alexandra Joshi-Imre [4], Allison Stiller [5], Marina Yu [1,2], Jennifer E. Paiz [1,2], Elizabeth Mancuso [1,2], Hillary W. Bedell [1], Walter E. Voit [3,4,5,6], Joseph J. Pancrazio [5] and Jeffrey R. Capadona [1,2,*]

[1] Department of Biomedical Engineering, Case Western Reserve University, Cleveland, OH, USA; andrew.shoffstall@case.edu (A.J.S.); mhy7@case.edu (M.Y.); jep141@case.edu (J.E.P.); mancuso.33@buckeyemail.osu.edu (E.M.); hillary.bedell1@gmail.com (H.W.B.)
[2] Advanced Platform Technology Center, Rehabilitation Research and Development, Louis Stokes Cleveland Department of Veteran Affairs Medical Center, Cleveland, OH, USA
[3] Department of Materials Science and Engineering, The University of Texas at Dallas, Richardson, TX, USA; melanie.ecker@utdallas.edu (M.E.); vxd160030@utdallas.edu (V.D.); walter.voit@utdallas.edu (W.E.V.)
[4] Center for Engineering Innovation, The University of Texas at Dallas, Richardson, TX, USA; alexandra.joshi-imre@utdallas.edu
[5] Department of Bioengineering, The University of Texas at Dallas, Richardson, TX, USA; axs169031@utdallas.edu (A.S.); joseph.pancrazio@utdallas.edu (J.J.P.)
[6] Department of Mechanical Engineering, The University of Texas at Dallas, Richardson, TX, USA
* Correspondence: jrc35@case.edu; Tel.: +1-(216)-368-5486

Received: 31 July 2018; Accepted: 18 September 2018; Published: 24 September 2018

Abstract: Thiol-ene based shape memory polymers (SMPs) have been developed for use as intracortical microelectrode substrates. The unique chemistry provides precise control over the mechanical and thermal glass-transition properties. As a result, SMP substrates are stiff at room temperature, allowing for insertion into the brain without buckling and subsequently soften in response to body temperatures, reducing the mechanical mismatch between device and tissue. Since the surface chemistry of the materials can contribute significantly to the ultimate biocompatibility, as a first step in the characterization of our SMPs, we sought to isolate the biological response to the implanted material surface without regards to the softening mechanics. To accomplish this, we tightly controlled for bulk stiffness by comparing bare silicon 'dummy' devices to thickness-matched silicon devices dip-coated with SMP. The neuroinflammatory response was evaluated after devices were implanted in the rat cortex for 2 or 16 weeks. We observed no differences in the markers tested at either time point, except that astrocytic scarring was significantly reduced for the dip-coated implants at 16 weeks. The surface properties of non-softening thiol-ene SMP substrates appeared to be equally-tolerated and just as suitable as silicon for neural implant substrates for applications such as intracortical microelectrodes, laying the groundwork for future softer devices to improve upon the prototype device performance presented here.

Keywords: intracortical; microelectrodes; shape-memory-polymer; electrophysiology

1. Introduction

Intracortical microelectrodes are used for electrophysiology recordings from the brain in a number of applications across both basic neuroscience and rehabilitation [1–4]. The specific needs of the given application dictate how long the microelectrode must endure, what type of signal is required (e.g., single units versus local field potential), and the design of the electrode required for reaching the targeted location [5–9]. Unfortunately, the currently available implantable microelectrode arrays do not demonstrate long-term robustness, as evidenced by a gradual decline in the signal-to-noise ratio and ultimately a diminishing percentage of contacts that are able to record spiking behavior [10–13]. Therefore, there are many types of intracortical microelectrodes under development [3,4].

The failure mechanisms of recording microelectrodes are multifaceted and include a number of interrelated processes involving mechanical, material, and biological pathways [14–18]. Among these interrelated processes, the neuroinflammatory response is thought to play a central role in microelectrode failure. Prolonged neuroinflammation can cause a build-up of oxidative species that can promote neurodegeneration while also initiating the degradation of implanted materials, resulting in a positive feedback cycle [19,20]. Numerous materials-based and therapeutic strategies have the potential to intervene in several of the failure modes by combining mechanical strategies, bioactive coatings, and/or drug-eluting substrates [21].

To reduce the tissue response and combat chronic neurodegeneration around implanted intracortical microelectrodes, the neural engineering field has been increasingly moving toward smaller, softer materials and electrode designs [21–23]. Using soft polymer substrates, like polyimides [24–26] or Parylene-C [27], compliant devices appear to reduce the appearance of chronic inflammation in end-point histology [28–30]. Ultra-small concepts have also proven to work well for reaching superficial cortical targets of the brain [28,31–33]. However, such devices may not be compatible with implantation strategies for more difficult to access structures of the brain.

Thiol-ene and thiol-ene/acrylate shape memory polymers (SMPs) comprise a new class of substrate under development for neural interfaces [34,35]. Thiol-ene/acrylate acts as a versatile material that is stiff at room temperature and softens after implantation in response to body temperatures and fluid exposure. The softening effect can be as large as a transition from 1 GPa to 18 MPa [35]. The combination of thiol, alkene and acrylate monomers modulates the rubbery modulus and allows for the adjustment of the glass transition temperature via a composition ratio (i.e., relative concentrations of multivalent monomers from all three groups) [36–38]. Sterilization methods have been optimized [39], allowing for the first demonstration of acute recordings signals from the primary auditory cortex of rats [40]. While thiol-ene-based SMPs appear to be promising, thus far, there have not been robust analyses of the neuroinflammatory response elicited by their long-term implantation in the cortex.

The objective of the current study was to quantify the neuroinflammatory response to implanted SMP materials. Here, we chose to first compare our SMP to a bare silicon substrate similar to those used in commercially available planar microelectrodes. The goal was to first understand the biological response to the thiol-ene material itself, without the confounding variable of stiffness (and resulting differential tissue strains). To that end, the SMP material was dip-coated onto a silicon surface and compared to a size-matched bare silicon substrate. As a result, the bulk flexibility of the microelectrode was held consistent, while only the tissue-exposed surface varied. Given the similar size and stiffness, we hypothesized that stiff silicon microelectrodes dip-coated with a shape memory polymer would elicit a similar or reduced neuroinflammatory response compared to size-matched bare silicon microelectrodes after implantation into the rat cortex.

2. Materials and Methods

2.1. Study Design

Male Sprague Dawley rats (200–250 g, $n = 11$ per group) were implanted with either stiff silicon microelectrode probes dip-coated with shape memory polymer or size-matched bare silicon microelectrode probes. As performed previously by our group and others, microelectrode probes were implanted bilaterally (one in each hemisphere) and treated as independent of one another [41,42]. After implantation, animals were housed for 2 or 16 weeks, spanning the periods of initial and late-onset neurodegeneration [43,44]. Immunohistochemistry markers tested included neuronal density (NeuN), activated microglia (CD68), blood-brain barrier permeability (Immunoglobulin G (IgG)), and reactive astrocytes (glial fibrillary acidic protein (GFAP)) [20,43,45–49].

2.2. Device Fabrication and Sterilization

Silicon 'dummy' probe devices, substrates without a recording functionality, were fabricated by a photolithographic process using a deep-reactive ion etching procedure as described below. In detail, silicon shanks of the desired thickness were fabricated from the appropriate SOI (silicon on insulator) wafer. These SOI wafers contained a device silicon layer and a buried oxide layer of 2 µm on top of 400 µm silicon handle layer. A hard mask of 2 µm thermal oxide was grown on these SOI wafers using a Tystar Diffusion/Oxidation Furnace. The wafers were then patterned using standard lithography techniques to yield the desired probe pattern. The thermal oxide hard mask and the device silicon layer were etched using CHF_3/Ar plasma and a Bosch sequence (SF_6/Ar and C_4F_8 plasmas) using a Plasma-Therm deep silicon etcher respectively. The buried oxide layer was used as the etch stop layer for the device silicon etch. The wafers were then soaked in solvent to remove the photoresist residues and in diluted 10:1 hydrofluoric acid overnight to lift-off the silicon shanks before they were triple rinsed in distilled water. The silicon shanks were further singulated from each other by breaking the tab that connects them using very fine metal tweezers under a microscope. The use of two different thickness of silicon wafers allowed us to generate devices that were either 30 µm or 14 µm thick (25 µm prior to etching). The latter devices were then modified with a dip-coating process to add a thiol-ene shape memory polymer to generate a nearly equivalent ~30 µm thick SMP dip-coated device (Figure 1).

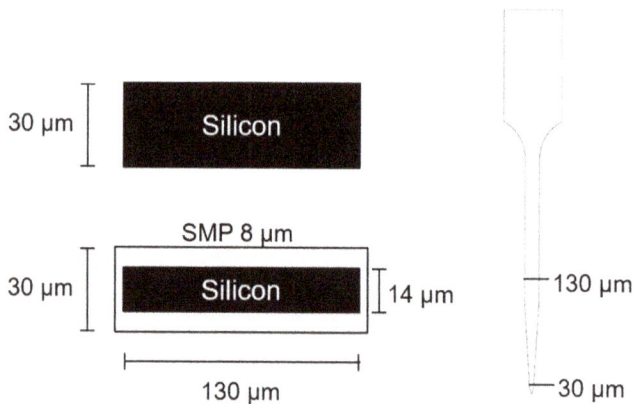

Figure 1. Probe design schematic. Cross-sectional dimensions of the silicon (**top**) and dip-coated (**bottom**) devices and view of the profile from the side (right). Here, 30 µm thick silicon wafers were used to fabricate the bare silicon probes whereas a 14 µm thick silicon wafer (after etching) was used to produce the dip-coating substrate so that the overall device thickness resulted as ~30 µm for both device types. Due to the photomasks used, the widths of the etched silicon devices were held constant so that the bare silicon probes were 130 µm in width and after coating, the dip-coated probes were slightly larger, ~135 µm, in width. The actual coating thickness varied slightly along the length of the probe as shown in Supplementary Figure S1.

SMP pre-polymer solution was prepared as described previously [39]. The material is characterized by a glass transition temperature (T_g) of 45 °C in the dry state, and a T_g of 30 °C after being soaked in phosphate buffered saline (PBS) at 37 °C for at least 30 min. The storage modulus E' of the materials decreases from 1.7 GPa (dry) to 20 MPa (wet) due to plasticization effects. The monomer ratios were 50 mol% 1,3,5-Triallyl-1,3,5-triazine-2,4,6(1H,3H,5H)-trione (TATATO), 45 mol% trimethylolpropane tris(3-mercaptopropionate) (TMTMP), and 5 mol%

Tris[2-mercaptopropionyloxy)ethyl] isocyanurate (TMICN). All monomers were mixed with 0.1 wt% of photoinitiator 2,2-dimethoxy-2-phenylacetophenone (DMPA) before they were used for dip coating.

The silicon shanks were individually mounted on ethylene oxide indicator tape for handling purposes. To enhance the SMP adhesion, bare silicon shanks were subjected to a surface treatment prior to the dip-coating which included a roughening step via O_2/Ar plasma in a March reactive ion etching (RIE) system for 16 min at 200 mT/50 W followed by SF_6 plasma treatments at 120 mT/100 W for 5 min in a Technics RIE system on both sides. The surface-treated silicon shanks were then held with tweezers and dipped manually at an average speed of 7–13 mm·s^{-1} (assessed by videotaping) into the pre-polymer solution. The viscosity (h) of the thiol-ene pre-polymer solution was 0.18 ± 0.1 Pa·s (TA discovery HR3 rheometer (TA Instruments, New Castle, DE, USA), sweep from 1 to 1000 s^{-1}). The SMP solution was prepared immediately before dip-coating. The coated pre-polymer was cured on all sides using a 365 nm handheld UV gun for about 30 s. The probes were inspected under an optical microscope to ensure the shank was coated successfully (i.e., showing full polymer coverage and no beads). Only sufficiently coated probes were selected and fully cured for 1 h in a cross-linking chamber (UVP CL-1000 (UVP, LLC, Upland, CA, USA) with five overhead bulbs) followed by an overnight post-cure at 120 °C under vacuum. To verify the thickness of the SMP layer and to ensure evenly coated surfaces, the fully cured samples were investigated using scanning electron microscope (SEM) (Zeiss Supra 40 and Zeiss EVO LS 15 Scanning Electron Microscopes, Zeiss, Inc., Oberkochen, Germany). SEM parameters included: EHT (accelerating voltage) between 0.5 kV and 5.0 kV and various magnifications. Individual parameters are displayed at the bottoms of the SEM images. The contact angle of water for the SMP material was ~70° while the silicon had a contact angle of ~40°.

Devices were sterilized using ethylene oxide (EtO) as previously described [39]. Briefly, the devices were loaded into a liner bag along with gas indicator tape and a glass ampoule containing 18 g of liquid EtO before it was sealed using Velcro wrap and placed into the ethylene oxide sterilizer (AN 74i, Anprolene, Andersen Sterilizers Inc., Haw River, NC, USA). The sterilization cycle at atmospheric pressure lasted for 24 h followed by a 2 h purge/aeration. To remove any residual EtO from the samples, they were subjected to an addition degassing for 72 h at 37 °C under vacuum. To validate the effectiveness of this sterilization method, we have previously performed residual endotoxin testing on pre- and post-sterilization materials as well as a host of mechanical testing (e.g., dynamic mechanical analysis (DMA)) to ensure that the mechanical properties were not adversely impacted in the described process [39].

2.3. Device Implantation

All procedures were reviewed and approved by the Louis Stokes Cleveland Department of Veterans Affairs Institutional Animal Care and Use Committee. Sprague Dawley rats were anesthetized (3–5%) and kept under anesthesia (1–3%) using an isoflurane vaporizer to maintain a surgical plane of anesthesia. Once anesthetized, eye lubricant was applied and the fur on the scalp was shaved and cleaned. Prior to surgery, the rats received 16 mg/kg cefazolin and 1 mg/kg meloxicam subcutaneously as a prophylactic antibiotic and analgesic, respectively. Additionally, a single dose of 0.2 mL of 0.25% bupivacaine (local anesthetic) was administered subcutaneously at the incision site. The surgical site was cleaned in triplicate with betadine followed by isopropyl alcohol scrubs. Surgery was performed under an operating microscope. Craniotomies were performed carefully with a combination of intermittent pausing and saline application, to prevent overheating from drilling [50]. A sterile ruler and forceps were used to mark the area to be drilled, 2 mm lateral to midline, 3 mm posterior to bregma (corresponding to a region of the sensory cortex). Removal of the final thinned bone flap was performed with ultrafine rongeurs to prevent incidental mechanical damage to the brain from the drill tip. After careful reflection of the dura, microelectrodes were implanted ~2 mm deep by hand using micro-forceps, avoiding superficially visible vasculature. Kwik-Cast was applied to cover the craniotomy and allowed to cure, followed by application of cold-cure dental acrylic to build up a stable cement base around the implant. Given the low profile of the dummy probe implants (e.g., as compared to functional recording microelectrodes that require an exposed head-stage), the skin was sutured together and treated with a non-prescription triple-antibiotic cream. A post-operative analgesic was provided for 2 days following implantation (1 mg/kg meloxicam q.d.) and post-operative prophylactic antibiotics were provided for 1 day following implantation (16 mg/kg cefazolin, b.i.d.). There were no complications with post-operative infection or observations of overtly unmanaged pain from the procedure.

2.4. Tissue Extraction and Preparation

At the pre-determined end points (2 or 16 weeks), animals were perfused transcardially under deep anesthesia to prepare the tissue for histological processing. After achieving a deep plane of anesthesia, using a ketamine/xylazine cocktail (80 mg/kg and 10 mg/kg respectively), rat aortas were cannulated with a gavage needle via an incision in the left ventricle and connected to a perfusion pump. Phosphate buffered saline (1×) was perfused until the fluid exiting the excised vena cava/right atrium appeared clear. Tissue was then fixed by perfusion with ~200 mL of 4% w/v paraformaldehyde solution. The tissue was post-fixed in 4% w/v paraformaldehyde solution overnight. After careful extraction, brains were subsequently cryoprotected with a gradient of sucrose (with 0.1% sodium azide) from 10 % to 30% w/v and frozen in OCT (Opjmal Cu ng. Temperature) blocks and stored at −80 °C until sectioning. Tissue sections, 20 μm thick, were generated on a cryostat and were collected on Fisherbrand 'Superfrost Plus' glass slides.

2.5. Quantification of Immunohistochemistry

Immunohistochemistry was performed as previously described for neuronal density (NeuN), activated microglia (CD68), blood-brain barrier permeability (IgG), and astrocytes (GFAP) [45,51]. To account for the known variation of the histological response along the depth of the implant, horizontal (transverse) slices were collected and compared at an array of locations spanning randomized depths of 500–1500 microns. Stained slides were imaged using a 10× objective on an AxioObserver Z1 (Zeiss, Inc.) and AxioCam MRm (Zeiss Inc.). All images except those stained for NeuN were analyzed using SECOND (version 030918, MathWorks, Inc., Natick, MA, USA), a custom MATLAB program developed to analyze fluorescent intensity profiles around the electrode [52]. In summary, the void in the tissue left by the explanted microelectrode was manually defined by tracing each image on-screen. The area defined by this tracing was collected and used to tabulate the explanted hole size. Fluorescent intensity was then tabulated by the program in expanding concentric contours around the microelectrode-tissue interface edge. To quantify neuron populations around the implant site, the number of neurons in each ring was manually counted to obtain the number of neurons per area for each radial distance [19,43]. In each case a normalized metric was generated, where the average intensity for a given concentric bin was divided by a concentric bin far enough away from the microelectrode implant that the neuroinflammatory response was minimal: 600–650 μm for intensity-based measures (IgG, GFAP, CD68), and 250–300 μm for count-based measures (NeuN).

Statistics were calculated in Minitab 18 (State College, PA, USA). The continuous outcome measures, including neuronal density, captured at endpoint histology were evaluated to compare inter-group differences for individual distance buckets (i.e., 0–50 μm, 50–100 μm,) using two-sample t-tests, with a significance at level $p < 0.05$. Intensity-based histological measures (GFAP, CD68, IgG) were analyzed using previously established quantification methods [43,46], wherein the fluorescent intensity was plotted as a function of distance from the electrode surface and the statistical outcome was the area-under-the-curve, corresponding to the level of overall tissue response for a given stain. Similarly, inter-group differences for individual distance buckets were calculated by two-sample t-tests, with a significance at level $p < 0.05$.

2.6. Characterization

2.6.1. Dip-Coating Silicon 'Dummy' Microelectrodes with Thiol-ene Polymer

Dummy microelectrodes were successfully dip-coated with a thiol-ene polymer (Figure 2). Multiple parameters appeared to influence the coating thickness and ability to form a uniform layer, especially the surface of the silicon shanks and the rate of removal from the polymer solution. If the silicon shanks were unmodified, the SMP did not adhere well to the surface (Figure 2A). However, after applying a surface treatment to the bare silicon shanks (O_2/Ar and SF_6 plasma), the shanks could be uniformly coated with SMP (Figure 2B). The viscosity of the pre-polymer solution, $h = 0.18 \pm 0.1$ Pa·s, was set by the previously defined composition of monomers. A change in the composition would result in a change of thermomechanical properties and was therefore not desired. Another way to change the viscosity of the solution would be by the addition of solvent. However, the addition of solvent would alter the curing kinetics and cross-link density and thus the thermomechanical properties as well. Therefore, only the removal speed could be varied to alter the surface coating. An average speed of 7 to 13 mm·s^{-1} of manual dip-coating turned out to result in sufficient coatings (Figure 2B). In some cases, more dominant at lower speeds, beading of the coating was visible along the microelectrode shank (Figure 2C). Only probes which showed full coating and no visible beads were used for the in vivo study.

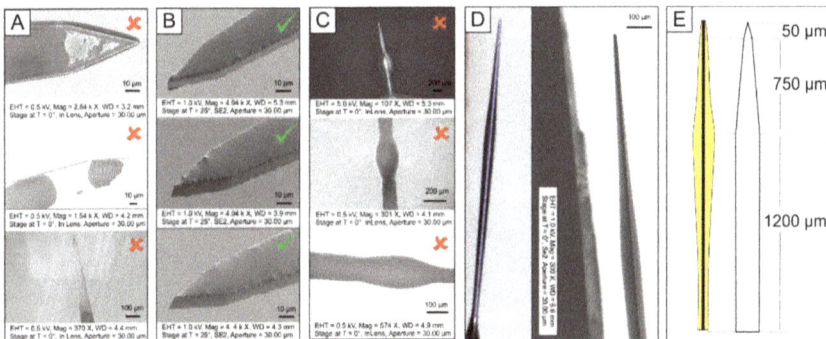

Figure 2. Characterization of silicon 'dummy' microelectrode with thiol-ene polymer. Dip coating of 25 μm thick microelectrodes with a uniform layer of shape memory polymer (SMP) to generate approximately 30 μm thick coated devices; (**A**) the polymer detached before surface modification of silicon probes, (**B**) nicely coated the silicon shanks after surface modification. (**C**) In some cases, the coating would form 'beads' due to slow removal. Checkmarks and crosses indicate whether probes were used for in vivo studies or not. (**D**) Optical and scanning electron microscope (SEM) images in the side view to assess the thickness of the coating, and (**E**) schematic drawing of coating thickness with respect to the shank geometry.

Dip coating quality and uniformity were approximated using optical microscopy and SEM on several representative devices. We found that the coating profile was consistent across various probes. The thickness of the coating, however, had no uniform thickness throughout the length of the shanks (Figure 2D). The tip of the probes had a very thin layer of polymer (less than 1 μm), whereas the rest of the probe had a layer thickness of about 10 to 30 μm on the top and bottom, respectively. The thickest coating was consistently found at the part of the probes where the shank started to narrow down about 850 μm distance from the tip (Figure 2E). This can be explained by the dipping process. The pre-polymer solution was flowing down the probes due to gravity before they were cured and accumulated at the abovementioned part of the probe due to an abrupt change of geometrical surface area. After the surface modification of the bare silicon shank, which included reactive ion etching, the thickness of the shanks was reduced from 25 μm to 14 μm. The averaged thickness of the SMP coating across the surface was approximately 8 μm on either side, which adds up to an overall probe thickness of about 30 μm. Even if the coating had no consistent thickness throughout the probe, the overall probe volume, and with that the averaged footprint of the implanted part of the dip-coated probes, was still similar to that of bare silicon probes.

2.6.2. Durability of Dip Coated Probes

The thiol-ene formulation used here was stable under physiological conditions for up to 13 months without any signs of hydrolytic degradation (paper under review). In order to directly test the dip-coating stability after in vivo implantation, explanted polymer coated silicon probes were investigated after 2 weeks (Figure 3A,B) and 16 weeks of dwelling in the rat cortex (Figure 3C,D). The coating of the probes was investigated before and after aging by means of SEM imaging. It was found that the coating was stable and did not show any signs of degradation over the course of implantation. The coating looked intact after being implanted into rat cortex for 2 weeks and 16 weeks, as demonstrated by the representative SEM images in Figure 3. In order to further assess the durability of the SMP coating and its adhesion to the silicon shanks, the dip-coated probes were further tested in vitro under accelerated aging conditions. The dip-coated probes were mounted onto the cap of a glass jar and were immersed into phosphate buffered saline (PBS) at 57 °C for a minimum of 84 h. While the surfaces of the probes became rougher, they remained visibly intact under SEM imaging (Supplementary Figure S2).

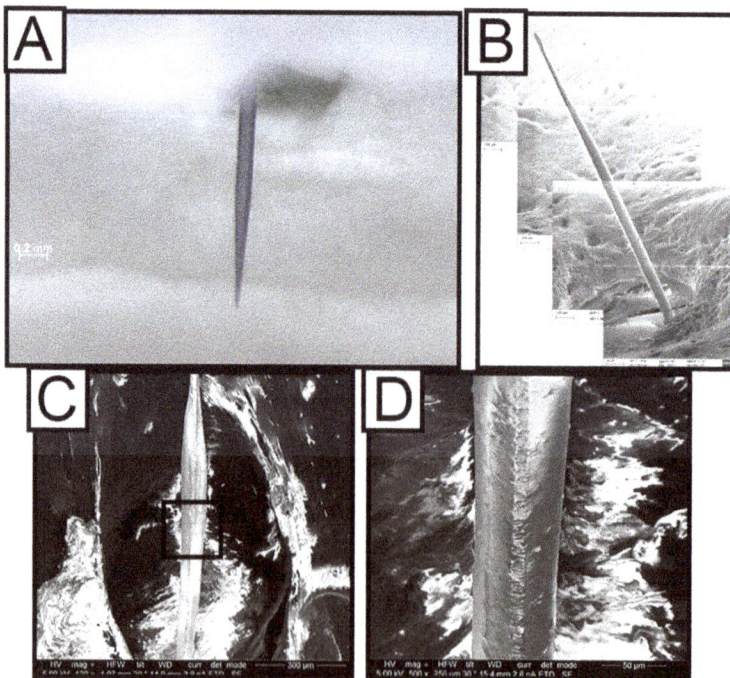

Figure 3. Ex vivo Characterization of coating stability. Dip-coated probes inside the skull with all tissue removed captured using optical microscopy (**A**) and SEM (**B**) showing that the SMP coating of the silicon shanks is still intact after two weeks. (**C**) Side-view SEM image of a dip-coated probe, explanted after 16 weeks in the rat cortex, showing the SMP coating intact. Black rectangle inset is blown up further in (**D**).

2.6.3. Tissue Void from Device Explantation

To verify that the cross-sectional area was held consistent between the two types of implants, we quantified the remnant hole in the tissue after device explantation. As expected, the hole sizes were similar to, but slightly larger than, the cross-sectional area of the actual probe devices ($\sim$3900 μm^2, Figure 4A,B). The difference in the hole to device size could be due to a thin layer of tissue remaining adhered to the microelectrode, or any slicing (edge) artifact. Interestingly, the remnant tissue hole size variability appeared to be higher at 2 weeks compared to 16 weeks and may have resulted from a looser, more immature scar or increased edema at that time.

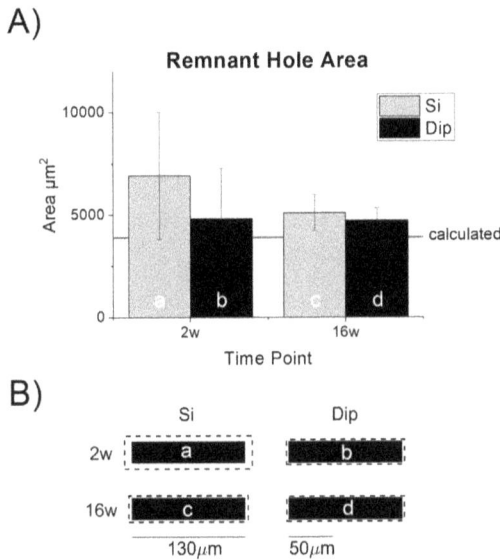

Figure 4. Characterization of the remnant tissue hole after explantation and 'dummy' probe device dimensions. (**A**) Remnant hole size after probe extraction was consistent (no statistically significant differences) across both implant types. The hole was slightly larger than the theoretical cross-sectional area denoted by the horizontal line; n = 9 (Si-2w), 10 (Si-16w), 10 (dip-2w), 10 (Dip-16w). (**B**) Mean explanted hole size (dashed line) drawn in relative scale to the actual device dimensions. The letters correspond with the matching bar in the chart shown in (**A**). The 130 μm scale bar is shown to provide context for the microelectrode dummy probe width. The 50 μm scale bar provides context for the analysis of bucket widths for the histological analysis. Tissue responses can extend several hundred microns away from the tissue-device interface.

As described above, the size of the dip-coated probe devices was controlled by applying a $\sim$8 μm thick layer of SMP to a bare silicon device with 14 μm thickness to achieve an approximately 30 μm overall thickness (Figure 1). Compared to the actual device sizes, the increased hole diameters appeared to be marginal (Figure 4B). In the largest group, two-week silicon implants ('2w-Si'), the equivalent mean increase in radius was calculated to be $\sim$16 microns (Figure 4B).

3. Results

3.1. Endpoint Histological Analysis

3.1.1. Astrocyte Response

Astrocytes, a glial cell, play a number of important roles in the brain, including contributing to the blood-brain barrier [16,53]. They react to injury and foreign implanted materials in the brain by changing morphology, migrating toward the implant, and expressing or upregulating the expression of a host of proteins, including glial fibrillary acidic protein (GFAP) [18,54].

While there were no significant differences between silicon and SMP dip-coated devices at 2 weeks (Figure 5A), there was a significantly lower response for dip-coated implants at 16 weeks compared to the bare silicon control. Specifically, the statistically significant differences were in the concentric ranges 50–100 μm and 100–150 μm from the hole remaining after device extraction (Figure 5B).

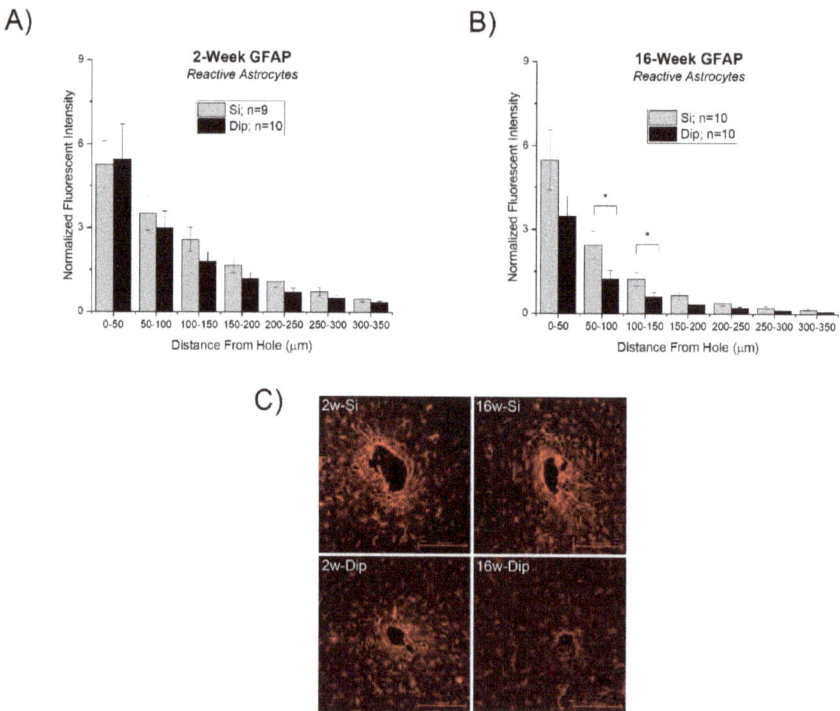

Figure 5. Astrocytic response to silicon vs. SMP dip-coated implants. (**A**) Astrocytic scarring at 2 weeks and (**B**) 16 weeks. There were significant differences between the silicon and dip-coated glial fibrillary acidic protein (GFAP) response at 16 weeks, specifically at bucketed distances 50–100 μm and 100–150 μm from the hole. There were no differences between the groups at 2 weeks or any other regions from the hole at 16 weeks post-implantation. (**C**) Representative images of the GFAP staining results with 200 μm scale bars in the bottom right-hand corner.

3.1.2. Activation of Microglia and Macrophages and Blood-Brain Barrier Permeability

CD68 is a marker of activated microglia and macrophages and has been associated with heightened neuroinflammatory responses to implanted foreign materials in the brain [55–58]. IgG is a blood immunoglobulin protein not normally found in the brain and is therefore commonly used as a marker for blood-brain barrier permeability [59]. All the stains followed a typical decay profile with the largest expression at the explant hole edge, returning to a baseline response within a few hundred microns. While overall there was a trend of a reduced response in both CD68 (Figure 6A,B) and IgG (Figure 6C,D), there were no statistically significant differences between any of the silicon and SMP dip-coated implants for either stain at each time point.

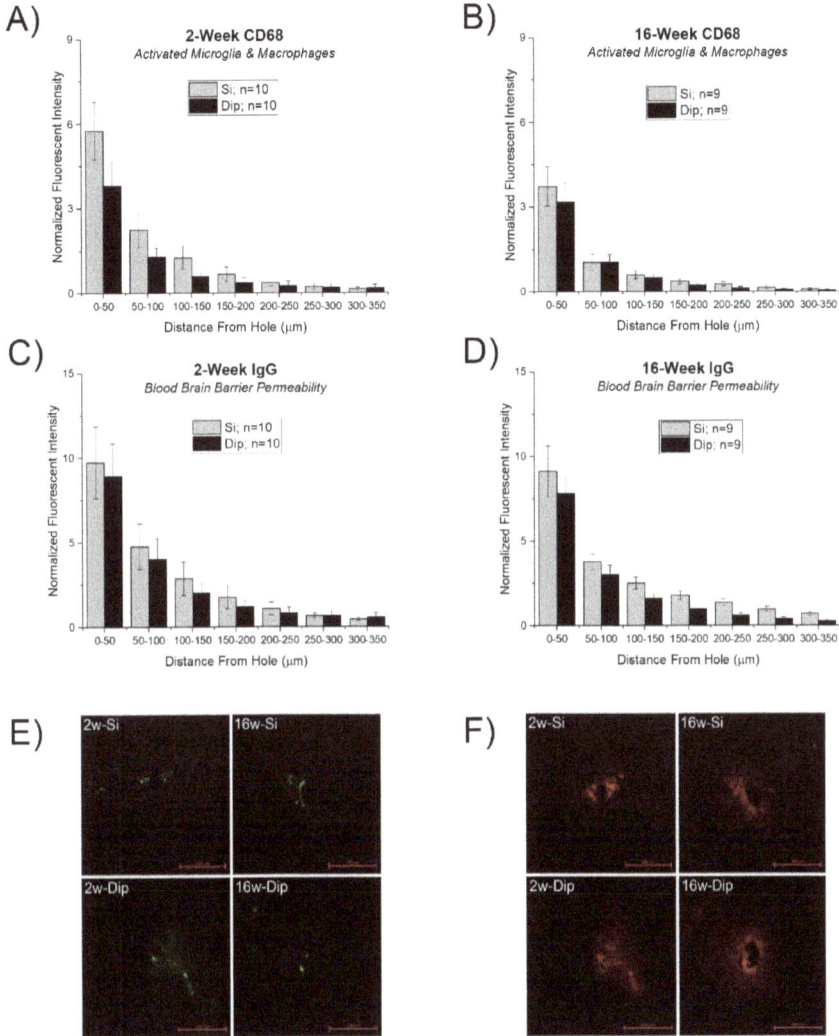

Figure 6. Microglia and BBB response to silicon vs. SMP dip-coated implants. Activated macrophages and microglia (CD68) at (**A**) 2 weeks and (**B**) 16 weeks. Blood-brain barrier (BBB) permeability marked by immunoglobulin G (IgG) staining at (**C**) 2 weeks and (**D**) 16 weeks after microelectrode implantation. There were no differences in either stain between each probe type for either time point tested. (**E,F**) Representative images of the CD68 (**E**) and IgG (**F**) staining results with 200 μm scale bars in the bottom right-hand corner.

3.1.3. Neuronal Density

Insertion surgery and the subsequent neuroinflammatory response is thought to contribute to neuronal loss near the microelectrode interface [60]. In our studies, a decrease in neuronal density near the explanted microelectrode site was observed both at 2 weeks and 16 weeks for both probe types (Figure 7). For both probe types, neuronal densities returned to background levels by 200–250 μm at 2 weeks post-implantation and by 50–100 μm at 16 weeks post-implantation. There were no statistically significant differences between the silicon and dip-coated implants.

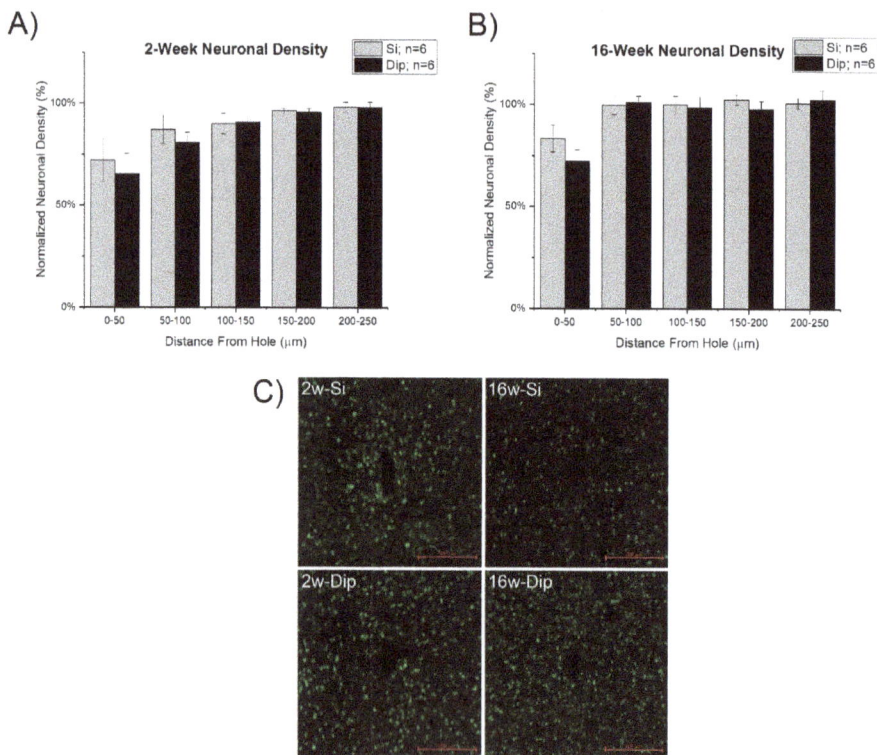

Figure 7. Neuronal density (NeuN staining) at (**A**) 2 weeks and (**B**) 16 weeks after microelectrode implantation. There were no significant differences between either material group, silicon vs dip-coated, at the two time points tested. (**C**) Representative images of the NeuN staining results with 200 μm scale bars in the bottom right-hand corner.

4. Discussion

Thiol-ene and thiol-ene/acrylate shape memory polymers (SMP) are under development for use as an implanted microelectrode substrate [35]. The materials are advantageous owing to their unique and highly tunable chemistry, the potential for reproducible manufacturing, and ability to soften after implantation in the brain [40]. We have previously demonstrated that intracortical probes that reduce their modulus after implantation into the brain significantly reduce the resulting neuroinflammatory response [45,61–63], likely due to the reduction in tissue strain and micro-motion [64]. We have also shown that the protein, cellular, and tissue responses to synthetic materials are highly correlated to the surface chemistry [65–69]. Therefore, in order to disentangle the potential differential effects on the biological response from both the new material chemistry and the unique mechanics, in this study, we first sought to hold the bulk mechanics as constant as possible while only varying the surface exposed to the brain tissue after implantation. By dip-coating SMP onto the surface of silicon probe devices, we were able to compare the biological response to implanted thiol-ene polymer materials without regards to their bulk stiffness or flexibility.

The only marker with statistically significant results was in the astrocytic response after 16 weeks of implantation, where the dip-coated silicon devices exhibited a significantly lower response than the bare silicon control devices at distances of 50–150 μm from the implant surface (Figure 5B). We found no statistically significant differences between the two implanted probes with regards to microglia and macrophage activation, blood-brain barrier permeability, or neuronal density. While the surface mechanics of the dip-coating layer may have played a minor role, we have shown before that the overall flexibility of the devices is driven by the underlying silicon [62]. Several studies have investigated the effects of substrate stiffness (modulus) on the astrocytic response, both in vitro [70,71] and in vivo [70,72], showing an enhanced response around stiff materials (~10 kPa) compared to softer materials (~100 Pa). While consistent with our overall observations of a decrease in activated astrocytes proximal to the implant, it is important to note that the modulus of the SMP coating here was at least twice as stiff as the "stiffer" substrates in each of the mentioned studies, with "soft" substrates often an order(s) of magnitude softer than the SMP reported here.

As the neuroinflammatory events surrounding the implanted microelectrode are constantly changing with respect to glial cell density, biochemical environment, neuron viability, and blood-brain barrier leakage [13,73,74], it is important to consider several time points. Here, we chose 2 weeks and 16 weeks, as they correspond with both early-onset and late-stage neurodegeneration [43]. Upon implantation, microelectrodes immediately disrupt brain tissue and neurovasculature, initiating a multi-phasic inflammatory response [3,43]. The acute response plateaus within the first few weeks of implantation and inflammation thereafter is driven in a chronic state by various mechanisms, including the fibrotic glial scar formation, microglial and macrophage activation, free radical oxidation and chronic dysfunction of the blood-brain barrier [43,49,75,76].

In the current study, the astrocytic response was observed to be greater for the non-coated silicon at the 16 week time point but not the 2 week time point. Since GFAP expression was only greater at the later-stage time point, our results suggest that the main differences appear after the normal wound-healing response has subsided. The overall magnitude of the response to the silicon implants at 16 weeks was similar to that of the silicon and dip-coated material at 2 weeks. Therefore, the increased astrocyte response for silicon versus the dip-coated at 16 weeks appears as a prolonged state of activation phase (or inability to 'de-activate') rather than the increased initial magnitude of astrocyte activation. Furthermore, differences were not observed in any of the other markers, including microglial/macrophage activation, blood-brain barrier permeability, or neuronal density, suggesting that the different response may be uniquely centered around astrocytes (at least of the markers tested). Increased astrocytic scarring has been associated with negatively impacting signal quality, either through directly increasing tissue impedance, or through physical separation and increased distance between the microelectrode contacts and viable neurons [77]. Results demonstrating that the SMP material exhibits a reduction in GFAP expression at 16 weeks are promising and deserve further exploration in future recording studies.

The SMP polymer formulation used here demonstrated a slightly higher contact angle (more hydrophobic) compared to bare silicon. We have previously demonstrated that slight changes in contact angle measurements can have profound impacts on the nature of protein adsorption and the resulting cell adhesion [68]. Upon initial observation, the higher contact angle (more hydrophobic) SMP material would have been thought to lend itself to a greater adsorption of proteins that promote the development of the glial scar. On the contrary, we found less GFAP expression for the SMP group compared to bare silicon at 16 weeks. It is possible that the dip-coated surface may preferentially attract a different composition or conformation of adsorbed proteins that does not react with astrocytes as strongly. Similar results have been demonstrated with other coating approaches to microelectrode substrates.

By comparison, Lee found that coating planar silicon microelectrodes with polyethylene glycol (PEG) previously demonstrated no effect on the foreign body response [41]. Considering that PEG is highly hydrophilic, this is somewhat contradictory to the expected results. However, as noted by the authors of the paper, it is unlikely the PEG coatings remained intact over the course of the entire 4 week study. Considering the work reported by Lee, and our current study together, it is unclear if a high degree of hydrophobicity alone is enough to influence the long-term foreign body response.

Future studies will investigate the recording performance and neuroinflammatory response to probes made entirely from the SMP materials. Preliminary experiments with dummy (non-functional) SMP probes have suggested that stereotactic insertion of the SMP microelectrodes will be challenging. Due to their thin and flexible nature, many of the fabricated SMP devices have a curved surface that prevents their successful insertion using stereotactic methods. The probes bend, deflect, or buckle at a relatively high frequency. Since the current study was planned to be compared to a study of microelectrodes made completely of the SMP material, all implantations were performed by-hand to allow for cross-comparability between the experimental conditions. However, it is likely that the error injected into the study is minimal compared to other experimental confounds. We have previously compared the neuroinflammatory response of microelectrodes implanted by either stereotactic or by-hand method and found the variability of the histological responses to be negligible compared the larger subject-to-subject variability inherent with both methods (Supplementary Figure S3). While the magnitude of the impact may be debated, the discrepancy must be noted as a known limitation of the present study.

In conclusion, thiol-ene and thiol-ene/acrylate shape memory polymers are currently under development for a wide range of neural implant applications, including intracortical microelectrodes, spinal cord stimulators, sciatic-tibial-sural 'Y' electrodes, longitudinal intrafascicular electrodes, and self-coiling nerve cuff electrodes [22,35,40,78–80]. Here, our initial study sought to investigate the foreign body response to the material in absence of its mechanical softening properties so that as many extra and potentially confounding variables as possible could be eliminated. From the results of the current study, we can conclude that the thiol-ene polymer material performs similar to, or better than, bare silicon in terms of the biological markers tested over 16 weeks of implantation in the rat cortex. It is well documented that silicon-based microelectrodes, such as the controls used here, are not a long-term solution for intracortical microelectrodes. Therefore, the fact that our thiol-ene shape memory polymer merely performs as well is not overly inspiring. However, the anticipated advantage of the thiol-ene shape memory polymer system is in the mechanical softening, which was not exploited here. Therefore, at worst, our SMP is adequate as an intracortical microelectrode substrate. Additional studies are required to test how the mechanics (dynamically softening after implantation) will affect the neuroinflammatory response.

Supplementary Materials: The following are available online at http://www.mdpi.com/2072-666X/9/10/486/s1, Figure S1: SEM measurement of dip-coating thickness along the length of the probe, Figure S2: Accelerated aging representative SEM, Figure S3: Comparing neuronal density around stereotactically and hand inserted Michigan-style microelectrodes 16 weeks post implantation.

Author Contributions: Conceptualization W.E.V., J.J.P., J.R.C.; methodology A.J.S., M.E., V.D.; software A.J.S.; validation M.E., V.D., A.S.; formal analysis A.J.S., M.E., V.D., M.Y., J.E.P., E.M.; investigation A.J.S., M.E., V.D., H.W.B., A.S.; resources W.E.V., J.J.P., J.R.C.; data curation A.J.S., M.Y., J.E.P., E.M.; writing—original draft preparation A.J.S., M.E., A.J.-I., V.D., H.W.B.; writing—review and editing A.J.S., M.E., V.D., W.E.V., J.J.P., J.R.C.; visualization A.J.S.; supervision W.E.V., J.J.P., J.R.C.; project administration W.E.V., J.J.P., J.R.C.; funding acquisition W.E.V., J.J.P., A.J.S., J.R.C.

Funding: This work was supported in part by the Office of the Assistant Secretary of Defense for Health Affairs through the Peer Reviewed Medical Research Program under Award No. W81XWH-15-1-0607 (Pancrazio) and W81XWH-15-1-0608 (Capadona) in part by Merit Review Awards #B1495-R and #B2611 (Capadona), Presidential Early Career Award for Scientist and Engineers (PECASE, Capadona), and a Career Development Award-1 #1IK1RX002492-01A2 (Shoffstall) from the United States (US) Department of Veterans Affairs Rehabilitation Research and Development Service, and by the National Institute of Health, National Institute of Neurological Disorders and Stroke, (Grant # 1R01NS082404-Q3 01A1). None of the funding sources aided in collection, analysis and interpretation of the data, in writing of the manuscript, or in the decision to submit the manuscript for publication. The contents do not represent the views of the U.S. Department of Defense, the U.S. Department of Veterans Affairs or the United States Government.

Acknowledgments: We would like to acknowledge the following individuals for their contribution to the image process and surgical assistance: Suraj Srinivasan, Mitchell Willis, Dhariyat Menendez, Carmen Toth, Rachel Welscott, Noel Jeansonne.

Conflicts of Interest: The authors declare no conflicts of interest.

References

1. Pancrazio, J.J.; Peckham, P.H. Neuroprosthetic devices: How far are we from recovering movement in paralyzed patients? *Expert Rev. Neurother.* **2009**, *9*, 427–430. [CrossRef] [PubMed]
2. Ajiboye, A.B.; Willett, F.R.; Young, D.R.; Memberg, W.D.; Murphy, B.A.; Miller, J.P.; Walter, B.L.; Sweet, J.A.; Hoyen, H.A.; Keith, M.W.; et al. Restoration of reaching and grasping movements through brain-controlled muscle stimulation in a person with tetraplegia: A proof-of-concept demonstration. *Lancet* **2017**, *389*, 1821–1830. [CrossRef]
3. Jorfi, M.; Skousen, J.L.; Weder, C.; Capadona, J.R. Progress towards biocompatible intracortical microelectrodes for neural interfacing applications. *J. Neural Eng.* **2015**, *12*, 011001. [CrossRef] [PubMed]
4. Seymour, J.P.; Wu, F.; Wise, K.D.; Yoon, E. State-of-the-art MEMS and microsystem tools for brain research. *Microsyst. Nanoeng.* **2017**, *3*, 16066. [CrossRef]
5. Teleńczuk, B.; Dehghani, N.; Le Van Quyen, M.; Cash, S.S.; Halgren, E.; Hatsopoulos, N.G.; Destexhe, A. Local field potentials primarily reflect inhibitory neuron activity in human and monkey cortex. *Sci. Rep.* **2017**, *7*, 40211. [CrossRef] [PubMed]
6. Turner, D.A.; Patil, P.G.; Nicolelis, M.A.L. Conceptual and technical approaches to human neural ensemble recordings. In *Methods for Neural Ensemble Recordings*, 2nd ed.; Nicolelis, M.A.L., Ed.; CRC Press/Taylor & Francis: Boca Raton, FL, USA, 2008.
7. Perel, S.; Sadtler, P.T.; Oby, E.R.; Ryu, S.I.; Tyler-Kabara, E.C.; Batista, A.P.; Chase, S.M. Single-unit activity, threshold crossings, and local field potentials in motor cortex differentially encode reach kinematics. *J. Neurophysiol.* **2015**, *114*, 1500–1512. [CrossRef] [PubMed]
8. Sendhilnathan, N.; Basu, D.; Murthy, A. Simultaneous analysis of the LFP and spiking activity reveals essential components of a visuomotor transformation in the frontal eye field. *Proc. Natl. Acad. Sci. USA* **2017**, *114*, 6370–6375. [CrossRef] [PubMed]
9. Sharma, G.; Annetta, N.; Friedenberg, D.; Blanco, T.; Vasconcelos, D.; Shaikhouni, A.; Rezai, A.R.; Bouton, C. Time stability and coherence analysis of multiunit, single-unit and local field potential neuronal signals in chronically implanted brain electrodes. *Bioelectron. Med.* **2015**, *2*, 63–71.
10. Rennaker, R.L.; Miller, J.; Tang, H.; Wilson, D.A. Minocycline increases quality and longevity of chronic neural recordings. *J. Neural Eng.* **2007**, *4*, L1–L5. [CrossRef] [PubMed]
11. Williams, J.C.; Rennaker, R.L.; Kipke, D.R. Long-term neural recording characteristics of wire microelectrode arrays implanted in cerebral cortex. *Brain Res.* **1999**, *4*, 303–313. [CrossRef]
12. Tresco, P.A.; Winslow, B.D. The challenge of integrating devices into the central nervous system. *Crit. Rev. Biomed. Eng.* **2011**, *39*, 29–44. [CrossRef] [PubMed]
13. McConnell, G.C.; Rees, H.D.; Levey, A.I.; Gutekunst, C.-A.; Gross, R.E.; Bellamkonda, R.V. Implanted neural electrodes cause chronic, local inflammation that is correlated with local neurodegeneration. *J. Neural Eng.* **2009**, *6*, 056003. [CrossRef] [PubMed]
14. Kozai, T.D.Y.; Catt, K.; Li, X.; Gugel, Z.V.; Olafsson, V.T.; Vazquez, A.L.; Cui, X.T. Mechanical failure modes of chronically implanted planar silicon-based neural probes for laminar recording. *Biomaterials* **2015**, *37*, 25–39. [CrossRef] [PubMed]
15. Shoffstall, A.; Capadona, J.R. Prospects for a robust cortical recording interface. In *Neuromodulation*, 2nd ed.; Krames, E.S., Peckham, P.H., Rezai, A.R., Eds.; Academic Press: Cambridge, MA, USA, 2018; pp. 393–413.
16. Michelson, N.J.; Vazquez, A.L.; Eles, J.R.; Salatino, J.W.; Purcell, E.K.; Williams, J.J.; Cui, X.T.; Kozai, T.D.Y. Multi-scale, multi-modal analysis uncovers complex relationship at the brain tissue-implant neural interface: New emphasis on the biological interface. *J. Neural Eng.* **2018**, *15*, 033001. [CrossRef] [PubMed]

17. Miranda, R.A.; Casebeer, W.D.; Hein, A.M.; Judy, J.W.; Krotkov, E.P.; Laabs, T.L.; Manzo, J.E.; Pankratz, K.G.; Pratt, G.A.; Sanchez, J.C.; et al. Darpa-funded efforts in the development of novel brain–computer interface technologies. *J. Neurosci. Methods* **2015**, *244*, 52–67. [CrossRef] [PubMed]

18. Cody, P.A.; Eles, J.R.; Lagenaur, C.F.; Kozai, T.D.Y.; Cui, X.T. Unique electrophysiological and impedance signatures between encapsulation types: An analysis of biological utah array failure and benefit of a biomimetic coating in a rat model. *Biomaterials* **2018**, *161*, 117–128. [CrossRef] [PubMed]

19. Potter-Baker, K.A.; Nguyen, J.K.; Kovach, K.M.; Gitomer, M.M.; Srail, T.W.; Stewart, W.G.; Skousen, J.L.; Capadona, J.R. Development of superoxide dismutase mimetic surfaces to reduce accumulation of reactive oxygen species surrounding intracortical microelectrodes. *J. Mater. Chem. B* **2014**, *2*, 2248–2258. [CrossRef] [PubMed]

20. Potter-Baker, K.A.; Stewart, W.G.; Tomaszewski, W.H.; Wong, C.T.; Meador, W.D.; Ziats, N.P.; Capadona, J.R. Implications of chronic daily anti-oxidant administration on the inflammatory response to intracortical microelectrodes. *J. Neural Eng.* **2015**, *12*, 046002. [CrossRef] [PubMed]

21. Wellman, S.M.; Eles, J.R.; Ludwig, K.A.; Seymour, J.P.; Michelson, N.J.; McFadden, W.E.; Vazquez, A.L.; Kozai, T.D.Y. A materials roadmap to functional neural interface design. *Adv. Funct. Mater.* **2018**, *28*. [CrossRef] [PubMed]

22. Ware, T.; Simon, D.; Arreaga-Salas David, E.; Reeder, J.; Rennaker, R.; Keefer Edward, W.; Voit, W. Fabrication of responsive, softening neural interfaces. *Adv. Funct. Mater.* **2012**, *22*, 3470–3479. [CrossRef]

23. Pancrazio, J.J.; Deku, F.; Ghazavi, A.; Stiller, A.M.; Rihani, R.; Frewin, C.L.; Varner, V.D.; Gardner, T.J.; Cogan, S.F. Thinking small: Progress on microscale neurostimulation technology. *Neuromodulation* **2017**, *20*, 745–752. [CrossRef] [PubMed]

24. Mercanzini, A.; Cheung, K.; Buhl, D.L.; Boers, M.; Maillard, A.; Colin, P.; Bensadoun, J.-C.; Bertsch, A.; Renaud, P. Demonstration of cortical recording using novel flexible polymer neural probes. *Sens. Actuators A Phys.* **2008**, *143*, 90–96. [CrossRef]

25. Cheung, K.C.; Renaud, P.; Tanila, H.; Djupsund, K. Flexible polyimide microelectrode array for in vivo recordings and current source density analysis. *Biosens. Bioelectron.* **2007**, *22*, 1783–1790. [CrossRef] [PubMed]

26. Metz, S.; Bertsch, A.; Bertrand, D.; Renaud, P. Flexible polyimide probes with microelectrodes and embedded microfluidic channels for simultaneous drug delivery and multi-channel monitoring of bioelectric activity. *Biosens. Bioelectron.* **2004**, *19*, 1309–1318. [CrossRef] [PubMed]

27. Takeuchi, S.; Ziegler, D.; Yoshida, Y.; Mabuchi, K.; Suzuki, T. Parylene flexible neural probes integrated with microfluidic channels. *Lab Chip* **2005**, *5*, 519–523. [CrossRef] [PubMed]

28. Luan, L.; Wei, X.; Zhao, Z.; Siegel, J.J.; Potnis, O.; Tuppen, C.A.; Lin, S.; Kazmi, S.; Fowler, R.A.; Holloway, S.; et al. Ultraflexible nanoelectronic probes form reliable, glial scar-free neural integration. *Sci. Adv.* **2017**, *3*, e1601966. [CrossRef] [PubMed]

29. Liu, J.; Fu, T.-M.; Cheng, Z.; Hong, G.; Zhou, T.; Jin, L.; Duvvuri, M.; Jiang, Z.; Kruskal, P.; Xie, C.; et al. Syringe-injectable electronics. *Nat. Nanotechnol.* **2015**, *10*, 629. [CrossRef] [PubMed]

30. Sohal, H.S.; Jackson, A.; Jackson, R.; Clowry, G.J.; Vassilevski, K.; O'Neill, A.; Baker, S.N. The sinusoidal probe: A new approach to improve electrode longevity. *Front. Neuroeng.* **2014**, *7*, 10. [CrossRef] [PubMed]

31. Kozai, T.D.; Gugel, Z.; Li, X.; Gilgunn, P.J.; Khilwani, R.; Ozdoganlar, O.B.; Fedder, G.K.; Weber, D.J.; Cui, X.T. Chronic tissue response to carboxymethyl cellulose based dissolvable insertion needle for ultra-small neural probes. *Biomaterials* **2014**, *35*, 9255–9268. [CrossRef] [PubMed]

32. McCallum, G.A.; Sui, X.; Qiu, C.; Marmerstein, J.; Zheng, Y.; Eggers, T.E.; Hu, C.; Dai, L.; Durand, D.M. Chronic interfacing with the autonomic nervous system using carbon nanotube (cnt) yarn electrodes. *Sci. Rep.* **2017**, *7*, 11723. [CrossRef] [PubMed]

33. Patel, P.R.; Zhang, H.; Robbins, M.T.; Nofar, J.B.; Marshall, S.P.; Kobylarek, M.J.; Kozai, T.D.; Kotov, N.A.; Chestek, C.A. Chronic in vivo stability assessment of carbon fiber microelectrode arrays. *J. Neural Eng.* **2016**, *13*, 066002. [CrossRef] [PubMed]

34. Reit, R.; Zamorano, D.; Parker, S.; Simon, D.; Lund, B.; Voit, W.; Ware, T.H. Hydrolytically stable thiol-ene networks for flexible bioelectronics. *ACS Appl. Mater. Interfaces* **2015**, *7*, 28673–28681. [CrossRef] [PubMed]

35. Ware, T.; Simon, D.; Liu, C.; Musa, T.; Vasudevan, S.; Sloan, A.; Keefer, E.W.; Rennaker, R.L., 2nd; Voit, W. Thiol-ene/acrylate substrates for softening intracortical electrodes. *J. Biomed. Mater. Res. B Appl. Biomater.* **2014**, *102*, 1–11. [CrossRef] [PubMed]

36. Senyurt, A.F.; Wei, H.; Hoyle, C.E.; Piland, S.G.; Gould, T.E. Ternary thiol−ene/acrylate photopolymers: Effect of acrylate structure on mechanical properties. *Macromolecules* **2007**, *40*, 4901–4909. [CrossRef]

37. Wei, H.; Senyurt Askim, F.; Jönsson, S.; Hoyle Charles, E. Photopolymerization of ternary thiol–ene/acrylate systems: Film and network properties. *J. Polym. Sci. Part A: Polym. Chem.* **2007**, *45*, 822–829. [CrossRef]

38. Do, D.-H.; Ecker, M.; Voit, W.E. Characterization of a thiol-ene/acrylate-based polymer for neuroprosthetic implants. *ACS Omega* **2017**, *2*, 4604–4611. [CrossRef] [PubMed]

39. Ecker, M.; Danda, V.; Shoffstall Andrew, J.; Mahmood Samsuddin, F.; Joshi-Imre, A.; Frewin Christopher, L.; Ware Taylor, H.; Capadona Jeffrey, R.; Pancrazio Joseph, J.; Voit Walter, E. Sterilization of thiol-ene/acrylate based shape memory polymers for biomedical applications. *Macromol. Mater. Eng.* **2016**, *302*, 1600331. [CrossRef]

40. Simon, D.M.; Charkhkar, H.; St. John, C.; Rajendran, S.; Kang, T.; Reit, R.; Arreaga-Salas, D.; McHail Daniel, G.; Knaack Gretchen, L.; Sloan, A.; et al. Design and demonstration of an intracortical probe technology with tunable modulus. *J. Biomed. Mater. Res. Part A* **2016**, *105*, 159–168. [CrossRef] [PubMed]

41. Lee, H.C.; Gaire, J.; Currlin, S.W.; McDermott, M.D.; Park, K.; Otto, K.J. Foreign body response to intracortical microelectrodes is not altered with dip-coating of polyethylene glycol (peg). *Front. Neurosci.* **2017**, *11*, 513. [CrossRef] [PubMed]

42. Lind, G.; Gallentoft, L.; Danielsen, N.; Schouenborg, J.; Pettersson, L.M. Multiple implants do not aggravate the tissue reaction in rat brain. *PLoS ONE* **2012**, *7*, e47509. [CrossRef] [PubMed]

43. Potter, K.A.; Buck, A.C.; Self, W.K.; Capadona, J.R. Stab injury and device implantation within the brain results in inversely multiphasic neuroinflammatory and neurodegenerative responses. *J. Neural Eng.* **2012**, *9*, 046020. [CrossRef] [PubMed]

44. McConnell, G.C. *Chronic Inflammation Surrounding Intra-Cortical Electrodes Is Correlated with a Local Neurodegenerative State*; Georgia Institute of Technology: Atlanta, GA, USA, 2008.

45. Harris, J.P.; Capadona, J.R.; Miller, R.H.; Healy, B.C.; Shanmuganathan, K.; Rowan, S.J.; Weder, C.; Tyler, D.J. Mechanically adaptive intracortical implants improve the proximity of neuronal cell bodies. *J. Neural Eng.* **2011**, *8*, 066011. [CrossRef] [PubMed]

46. Potter, K.A.; Simon, J.S.; Velagapudi, B.; Capadona, J.R. Reduction of autofluorescence at the microelectrode-cortical tissue interface improves antibody detection. *J. Neurosci. Methods* **2012**, *203*, 96–105. [CrossRef] [PubMed]

47. Potter, K.A.; Buck, A.C.; Self, W.K.; Callanan, M.E.; Sunil, S.; Capadona, J.R. The effect of resveratrol on neurodegeneration and blood brain barrier stability surrounding intracortical microelectrodes. *Biomaterials* **2013**, *34*, 7001–7015. [CrossRef] [PubMed]

48. Potter, K.A.; Jorfi, M.; Householder, K.T.; Foster, E.J.; Weder, C.; Capadona, J.R. Curcumin-releasing mechanically-adaptive intracortical implants improve the proximal neuronal density and blood-brain barrier stability. *Acta Biomater.* **2014**, *10*, 2209–2222. [CrossRef] [PubMed]

49. Potter-Baker, K.A.; Ravikumar, M.; Burke, A.A.; Meador, W.D.; Householder, K.T.; Buck, A.C.; Sunil, S.; Stewart, W.G.; Anna, J.P.; Tomaszewski, W.H.; et al. A comparison of neuroinflammation to implanted microelectrodes in rat and mouse models. *Biomaterials* **2014**, *34*, 5637–5646. [CrossRef] [PubMed]

50. Shoffstall, A.J.; Paiz, J.E.; Miller, D.M.; Rial, G.M.; Willis, M.T.; Menendez, D.M.; Hostler, S.R.; Capadona, J.R. Potential for thermal damage to the blood-brain barrier during craniotomy: Implications for intracortical recording microelectrodes. *J. Neural Eng.* **2018**, *15*, 034001. [CrossRef] [PubMed]

51. Potter, K.; Gui, B.; Capadona, J.R. Biomimicry at the cell-material interface. In *Biomimetics—Innovation Thru Mimicking natures Inventions*; Bar-Cohen, Y., Ed.; CRC Press: Boca Raton, FL, USA, 2011; Volume 2, pp. 95–129.

52. Hermann, J.K.; Ravikumar, M.; Shoffstall, A.J.; Ereifej, E.S.; Kovach, K.M.; Chang, J.; Soffer, A.; Wong, C.; Srivastava, V.; Smith, P.; et al. Inhibition of the cluster of differentiation 14 innate immunity pathway with iaxo-101 improves chronic microelectrode performance. *J. Neural Eng.* **2018**, *15*, 025002. [CrossRef] [PubMed]

53. Abbott, N.J. Astrocyte–endothelial interactions and blood–brain barrier permeability. *J. Anat.* **2002**, *200*, 629–638. [CrossRef] [PubMed]

54. Cavanagh, J.B. The proliferation of astrocytes around a needle wound in the rat brain. *J. Anat.* **1970**, *106*, 471–487. [PubMed]

55. Woolley, A.J.; Desai, H.A.; Otto, K.J. Chronic intracortical microelectrode arrays induce non-uniform, depth-related tissue responses. *J. Neural Eng.* **2013**, *10*, 026007. [CrossRef] [PubMed]

56. Hanisch, U.-K. Microglia as a source and target of cytokines. *Glia* **2002**, *40*, 140–155. [CrossRef] [PubMed]
57. Bedell, H.W.; Hermann, J.K.; Ravikumar, M.; Lin, S.; Rein, A.; Li, X.; Molinich, E.; Smith, P.D.; Selkirk, S.M.; Miller, R.H.; et al. Targeting cd14 on blood derived cells improves intracortical microelectrode performance. *Biomaterials* **2018**, *163*, 163–173. [CrossRef] [PubMed]
58. Graeber, M.B.; Streit, W.J.; Kiefer, R.; Schoen, S.W.; Kreutzberg, G.W. New expression of myelomonocytic antigens by microglia and perivascular cells following lethal motor neuron injury. *J. Neuroimmunol.* **1990**, *27*, 121–132. [CrossRef]
59. Aihara, N.; Tanno, H.; Hall, J.J.; Pitts Lawrence, H.; Noble, L.J. Immunocytochemical localization of immunoglobulins in the rat brain: Relationship to the blood-brain barrier. *J. Comp. Neurol.* **1994**, *342*, 481–496. [CrossRef] [PubMed]
60. Biran, R.; Martin, D.C.; Tresco, P.A. Neuronal cell loss accompanies the brain tissue response to chronically implanted silicon microelectrode arrays. *Exp. Neurol.* **2005**, *195*, 115–126. [CrossRef] [PubMed]
61. Nguyen, J.K.; Jorfi, M.; Buchanan, K.L.; Park, D.J.; Foster, E.J.; Tyler, D.J.; Rowan, S.J.; Weder, C.; Capadona, J.R. Influence of resveratrol release on the tissue response to mechanically adaptive cortical implants. *Acta Biomater.* **2016**, *29*, 81–93. [CrossRef] [PubMed]
62. Nguyen, J.K.; Park, D.J.; Skousen, J.L.; Hess-Dunning, A.E.; Tyler, D.J.; Rowan, S.J.; Weder, C.; Capadona, J.R. Mechanically-compliant intracortical implants reduce the neuroinflammatory response. *J. Neural Eng.* **2014**, *11*, 056014. [CrossRef] [PubMed]
63. Capadona, J.R.; Tyler, D.J.; Zorman, C.A.; Rowan, S.J.; Weder, C. Mechanically adaptive nanocomposites for neural interfacing. *MRS Bull.* **2012**, *37*, 581–589. [CrossRef]
64. Sridharan, A.; Nguyen, J.K.; Capadona, J.R.; Muthuswamy, J. Compliant intracortical implants reduce strains and strain rates in brain tissue in vivo. *J. Neural Eng.* **2015**, *12*, 036002. [CrossRef] [PubMed]
65. Raynor, J.E.; Capadona, J.R.; Collard, D.M.; Petrie, T.A.; Garcia, A.J. Polymer brushes and self-assembled monolayers: Versatile platforms to control cell adhesion to biomaterials (review). *Biointerphases* **2009**, *4*, FA3–FA16. [CrossRef] [PubMed]
66. Petrie, T.A.; Capadona, J.R.; Reyes, C.D.; Garcia, A.J. Integrin specificity and enhanced cellular activities associated with surfaces presenting a recombinant fibronectin fragment compared to rgd supports. *Biomaterials* **2006**, *27*, 5459–5470. [CrossRef] [PubMed]
67. Capadona, J.R.; Petrie, T.A.; Fears, K.P.; Latour, R.A.; Collard, D.M.; García, A.J. Surface-nucleated assembly of fibrillar extracellular matrices. *Adv. Mater.* **2005**, *17*, 2604–2608. [CrossRef]
68. Capadona, J.R.; Collard, D.M.; García, A.J. Fibronectin adsorption and cell adhesion to mixed monolayers of tri(ethylene glycol)- and methyl-terminated alkanethiols. *Langmuir* **2003**, *19*, 1847–1852. [CrossRef]
69. Kovach, K.M.; Capadona, J.R.; Gupta, A.S.; Potkay, J.A. The effects of peg-based surface modification of pdms microchannels on long-term hemocompatibility. *J. Biomed. Mater. Res. A* **2014**, *102*, 4195–4205. [PubMed]
70. Moshayedi, P.; Ng, G.; Kwok, J.C.F.; Yeo, G.S.H.; Bryant, C.E.; Fawcett, J.W.; Franze, K.; Guck, J. The relationship between glial cell mechanosensitivity and foreign body reactions in the central nervous system. *Biomaterials* **2014**, *35*, 3919–3925. [CrossRef] [PubMed]
71. Wilson, C.L.; Hayward, S.L.; Kidambi, S. Astrogliosis in a dish: Substrate stiffness induces astrogliosis in primary rat astrocytes. *RSC Adv.* **2016**, *6*, 34447. [CrossRef]
72. Spencer, K.C.; Sy, J.C.; Ramadi, K.B.; Graybiel, A.M.; Langer, R.; Cima, M.J. Characterization of mechanically matched hydrogel coatings to improve the biocompatibility of neural implants. *Sci. Rep.* **2017**, *7*, 1952. [CrossRef] [PubMed]
73. McConnell, G.C.; Butera, R.J.; Bellamkonda, R.V. Bioimpedance modeling to monitor astrocytic response to chronically implanted electrodes. *J. Neural Eng.* **2009**, *6*, 055005. [CrossRef] [PubMed]
74. He, W.; Bellamkonda, R.V. A molecular perspective on understanding and modulating the performance of chronic central nervous system (CNS) recording electrodes. In *Indwelling Neural Implants: Strategies for Contending with the In Vivo Environment*; Reichert, W.M., Ed.; CRC Press: Boca Raton, FL, USA, 2008.
75. Skousen, J.L.; Bridge, M.J.; Tresco, P.A. A strategy to passively reduce neuroinflammation surrounding devices implanted chronically in brain tissue by manipulating device surface permeability. *Biomaterials* **2015**, *36*, 33–43. [CrossRef] [PubMed]
76. Nguyen, D.; Cho, N.; Satkunendrarajah, K.; Austin, J.W.; Wang, J.; Fehlings, M.G. Immunoglobulin g (IgG) attenuates neuroinflammation and improves neurobehavioral recovery after cervical spinal cord injury. *J. Neuroinflamm.* **2012**, *9*, 224. [CrossRef] [PubMed]

77. Douglas, M.; Stuart, C.; Sheryl, K.; Victor, P. Correlations between histology and neuronal activity recorded by microelectrodes implanted chronically in the cerebral cortex. *J. Neural Eng.* **2016**, *13*, 036012.

78. Ware, T.; Simon, D.; Hearon, K.; Liu, C.; Shah, S.; Reeder, J.; Khodaparast, N.; Kilgard, M.P.; Maitland, D.J.; Rennaker, R.L., 2nd; et al. Three-dimensional flexible electronics enabled by shape memory polymer substrates for responsive neural interfaces. *Macromol. Mater. Eng.* **2012**, *297*, 1193–1202. [CrossRef] [PubMed]

79. Ware, T.; Simon, D.; Hearon, K.; Kang, T.H.; Maitland, D.J.; Voit, W. Thiol-click chemistries for responsive neural interfaces. *Macromol. Biosci.* **2013**, *13*, 1640–1647. [CrossRef] [PubMed]

80. Garcia-Sandoval, A.; Pal, A.; Mishra, A.M.; Sherman, S.; Parikh, A.R.; Joshi-Imre, A.; Arreaga-Salas, D.; Gutierrez-Heredia, G.; Duran-Martinez, A.C.; Nathan, J.; et al. Chronic softening spinal cord stimulation arrays. *J. Neural Eng.* **2018**, *15*, 045002. [CrossRef] [PubMed]

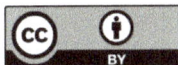

micromachines

MDPI

Article

Liquid Crystal Elastomer-Based Microelectrode Array for In Vitro Neuronal Recordings

Rashed T. Rihani [†], Hyun Kim [†], Bryan J. Black, Rahul Atmaramani, Mohand O. Saed, Joseph J. Pancrazio and Taylor H. Ware *

Department of Bioengineering, University of Texas at Dallas, Richardson, TX 75080, USA;
Rashed.Rihani@utdallas.edu (R.T.R.); kimhyun@utdallas.edu (H.K.); bjb140530@utdallas.edu (B.J.B.);
rxa162330@utdallas.edu (R.A.); Mohand.Saed@utdallas.edu (M.O.S.); Joseph.Pancrazio@utdallas.edu (J.J.P.)
* Correspondence: taylor.ware@utdallas.edu; Tel.: +1-972-883-4937
† These authors contributed equally to this work.

Received: 31 July 2018; Accepted: 16 August 2018; Published: 20 August 2018

Abstract: Polymer-based biomedical electronics provide a tunable platform to interact with nervous tissue both in vitro and in vivo. Ultimately, the ability to control functional properties of neural interfaces may provide important advantages to study the nervous system or to restore function in patients with neurodegenerative disorders. Liquid crystal elastomers (LCEs) are a class of smart materials that reversibly change shape when exposed to a variety of stimuli. Our interest in LCEs is based on leveraging this shape change to deploy electrode sites beyond the tissue regions exhibiting inflammation associated with chronic implantation. As a first step, we demonstrate that LCEs are cellular compatible materials that can be used as substrates for fabricating microelectrode arrays (MEAs) capable of recording single unit activity in vitro. Extracts from LCEs are non-cytotoxic (>70% normalized percent viability), as determined in accordance to ISO protocol 10993-5 using fibroblasts and primary murine cortical neurons. LCEs are also not functionally neurotoxic as determined by exposing cortical neurons cultured on conventional microelectrode arrays to LCE extract for 48 h. Microelectrode arrays fabricated on LCEs are stable, as determined by electrochemical impedance spectroscopy. Examination of the impedance and phase at 1 kHz, a frequency associated with single unit recording, showed results well within range of electrophysiological recordings over 30 days of monitoring in phosphate-buffered saline (PBS). Moreover, the LCE arrays are shown to support viable cortical neuronal cultures over 27 days in vitro and to enable recording of prominent extracellular biopotentials comparable to those achieved with conventional commercially-available microelectrode arrays.

Keywords: microelectrode array; liquid crystal elastomer; neuronal recordings

1. Introduction

Neural interfaces allow for communication with nervous tissue both in vitro and in vivo. In vitro neural interfaces, such as planar microelectrode arrays (MEAs), allow for characterization of cultured neural networks, which is effective in a variety of in vitro model applications such as neuropharmacological applications and cell compartmentalization [1–3]. The use of polymers for in vitro neural interfaces has proven advantageous and gained traction over the past years [3–6]. This includes the fabrication of mechanically flexible planar MEAs to reduce the tissue-interface mechanical mismatch [7] or using polymer actuators to allow for advanced interface control in the case of cell compartmentalization [8]. In vivo neural interfaces, such as implantable microelectrode arrays, offer a means of functional restoration in patients who suffer paralysis, strokes, limb loss, or neurodegenerative disease [9]. However, the reliability of such neural interfaces is compromised, in part, by the body's own foreign body response (FBR), leading to localized astrogliosis and fibrotic encapsulation of the device [10]. These factors may lead to accelerated mechanical/electrical device failure and/or loss of neurons at the site of implantation [11,12]. While conventional implantable microelectrode arrays are comprised of inherently stiff materials, flexible polymer substrates have gained interest for their potential in mitigating the mechanical mismatch at the tissue–device interface and reduce FBR-induced encapsulation [13,14].

Biostable and biocompatible polymer packaging may provide important advantages over traditional ceramic devices including mechanical flexibility and compatibility with tissue. These polymer-based hybrid devices consist of a metallic electrode array and a polymeric package [15]. It is critical that the chosen polymer also form a sufficient barrier to insulate the electronics from the moist physiological environment [16]. Various types of polymers—such as polyimide [17], Parylene [18], shape memory polymers [19], and liquid crystal polymer (LCP) [15,20]—have been tested as compliant, insulating materials in neural interfaces. Particularly, LCPs have gained significant attention as a promising substrate material for long-term implantable neural interfaces due to its low moisture absorption, which is equivalent to that of polytetrafluoroethylene (PTFE) and glass (<0.04%) [21,22]. This absorption is significantly lower than those of other polymers such as polyimide (~2.8%), Parylene-C (0.06–0.6%) and silicone elastomers (~1%) [20]. Certain classes of LCPs may offer additional functionality beyond serving as a robust barrier, including by enabling deployable neural interfaces.

Most polymer-based bioelectronic devices are planar in nature, as photolithography is used to fabricate the devices. Three-dimensional and reconfigurable bioelectronic systems may enable devices that dynamically adapt to external physiological environments [23]. To go beyond the capability of current static devices, we aim to integrate shape-changing materials and microelectronic devices into a single dynamic reconfigurable system. LCEs [24–26], a subclass of LCPs, contain light crosslinking density and tunable transition temperatures which allows for a reversible shape change in response to a stimulus such as heat [27,28], light [29,30], or solvent [31,32]. This approach potentially enables the controlled deployment of small recording or stimulation electrode sites to regions beyond that of the FBR-induced tissue encapsulation zone surrounding an implanted shank (50–100 µm) [33–37]. Recently several publications have suggested that some compositions of LCEs may be cytocompatible [38–40]. However, there have been no prior studies evaluating cytotoxicity, neurotoxicity, or manufacturability of LCE as a functional electrode array package. Notably, the performance of LCEs as barriers to the physiological environment has not been evaluated. Here, we apply International Organization for Standards (ISO) protocol 10993-5 to evaluate the cytotoxicity of LCEs using both NCTC clone 929 fibroblasts and primary murine cortical neurons. Additionally, we evaluate the functional neurotoxicity of LCE materials in vitro using primary neuronal networks cultured on commercially available planar microelectrode arrays. Finally, we report the fabrication and characterization of functional planar MEAs using LCEs as an insulating package material.

2. Materials and Methods

2.1. Fabrication of LCE MEAs

Figure 1a,b depict the fabrication of the MEA and a schematic of the layers that comprise the MEA. To fabricate MEAs, microscope glass slides (75 mm × 51 mm × 1.2 mm, Electron Microscopy Sciences, Hatfield, PA, USA) were serially cleaned with acetone, isopropanol, and deionized water and subsequently dried with nitrogen (Figure 1). Then, 5 nm of chromium and 400 nm of gold were serially deposited via e-beam evaporation (Temescal BJD-1800, Ferrotec Corporation, Livermore, CA, USA). The deposition rate in this process was set to 2–3 Å/s. After coating of the Cr/Au to the glass slides, a positive photoresist (Shipley S1805, Dow Chemical, Midland, MI, USA) was spun at 2000 rpm with an acceleration of 3000 rpm/s for 60 s and soft baked at 85 °C for 12 min. The photoresist was exposed to 75 mJ/cm^2 of UV light using a Karl Suss MA6 Mask Aligner (SÜSS MicroTec, Garching, Germany). Photoresist development was performed in Micropost MF-319 (Dow Chemical, Midland, MI, USA) for 60 s. Etching of the Au was performed using gold etchant (Transene Company, Midland, MI,

USA) for approximately 60 s. Etching of the Cr was performed using chrome etchant (KMG Electronic Chemicals, Pueblo, CO, USA) for approximately 10 s. The remaining photoresist was removed by a flood exposure of 150 mJ/cm^2 UV light and subsequent development in MF-319.

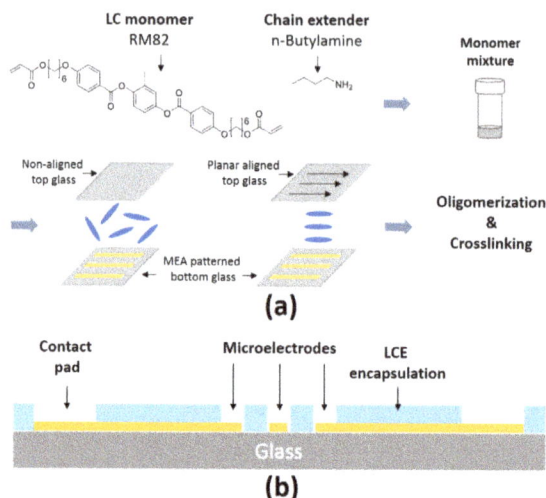

Figure 1. Chemistry of LCE and MEA fabrication: (**a**) Molecular structure of monomers used to synthesize the LCE and device fabrication procedure; (**b**) Cross-sectional schematic of LCE MEA devices.

To encapsulate MEAs with LCEs, a previously described chemistry was used [27,31]. The liquid crystal monomer, 1,4-bis-[4-(6-acryloyloxyhexyloxy)-benzoyloxy]-2-methylbenzene (RM82), was purchased from Wilshire Chemicals (Princeton, NJ, USA). The chain extender molecule, n-butylamine, was purchased from Sigma Aldrich (St. Louis, MO, USA). The photoinitiator, Irgacure I-369, was donated by BASF (Ludwigshafen, Germany). The photoalignable dye, brilliant yellow, was purchased from Sigma Aldrich. To prepare the top side glass slide, a solution of Brilliant yellow (1 wt. %) in dimethylformamide (DMF, Fisher Scientific, Pittsburgh, PA, USA) was prepared and filtered through a 0.45 μm filter (Whatman, Maidstone, UK). Clean glass slides were treated with oxygen plasma for 1 min at 100 mTorr pressure and 50 mW power (Sirius T2, Trion Technology, Tempe, AZ, USA). The brilliant yellow solution was then spin-coated onto the cleaned slides at 750 rpm with an acceleration of 1500 rpm/s for 10 s and 1500 rpm with an acceleration of 1500 rpm/s for 30 s. A previously described photoalignment procedure was adopted [41]. Dye-coated glass slides were exposed to broadband, linearly polarized light at an intensity of 10 mW/cm^2 (Vivitek D912HD, Vivitek, Fremont, CA, USA). A pair of glass substrates, one with the patterned electrodes and one coated with the dye (uniaxial alignment or non-aligned) were spaced 25 μm apart using a spacer (Precision Brand, Downers Grove, IL, USA) along the edges. This mold was filled with a monomer mixture of an equimolar amount RM82 and n-butylamine mixed with 1.5 wt. % of photoinitiator I-369. The monomer mixtures were filled by capillary force and kept for 15 h at 65 °C for oligomerization. Then, oligomerized samples were crosslinked with 250 mW/cm^2 intensity of 365 nm UV light (OmniCure® LX400+, Lumen Dynamics, Mississauga, ON, Canada) for 5 min. After crosslinking, the top-side glass slide was removed yielding an electrode array covered with a layer of LCE. The optical images of LCE MEA devices were observed by a polarized optical microscope (POM) (Olympus BX51, Olympus Corporation, Tokyo, Japan).

To finalize fabrication of LCE MEA devices, the fully insulated MEAs were coated by 800 nm silicon nitride at 150 °C using Plasma Enhanced Chemical Vapor Deposition Unaxis 790 PECVD (Mykrolis Corporation, Billerica, MA, USA). Then hexamethyldisilazane (HMDS, Sigma Aldrich, St. Louis, MO, USA) was vapor-deposited onto the silicon nitride to serve as an adhesion layer for photoresist. A positive photoresist (Shipley S1813, Dow Chemical, Midland, MI, USA) was spun at 500 rpm for 10 s with an acceleration of 100 rpm/s and 2000 rpm for 60 s with an acceleration of 3000 rpm/s and soft baked at 85 °C for 12 min. The photoresist was exposed to 150 mJ/cm^2 of UV light using a Karl Suss MA6 Mask Aligner. The silicon nitride was patterned using dry etching by 120 mTorr pressure and 100 mW power with SF$_6$ (Sirius T2, Trion Technology, Tempe, AZ, USA). Next, the encapsulated LCE layer was patterned via dry etching by 220 mTorr pressure and 200 mW power with oxygen plasma. The remaining hard mask was removed with a 60 s rinse of hydrofluoric acid (1:10) (HF) treatment. Lastly, a polycarbonate ring (0.6 cm height, 2.0 cm inner diameter, and 2.2 cm outer diameter) was attached to the surface of the LCE MEA devices with a silicone adhesive (MED1-4213, Nu-Sil, USA) as described in a previous study [5].

2.2. Electrochemical Characterization of LCE MEAs

All devices were sterilized by exposure to ethylene oxide prior to testing. Electrochemical impedance spectroscopy (EIS) measurements were carried out on eight randomly selected electrodes from LCE microelectrode arrays for 30 consecutive days in PBS at 37 °C. For impedance measurements, the experimental setup consisted of a three-electrode configuration (working, ground, reference), wherein the external MEA pads were used to deliver a sinusoidal 20 mV signal, and impedance was measured by a CH 604E potentiostat (CH Instruments, Austin, TX, USA) between 10 Hz and 100 kHz. Between measurements, MEAs were housed in a cell culture incubator at 37 °C and 95% humidity between measurements. Fresh PBS was replaced prior to each measurement to account for any evaporation and subsequent osmolarity changes. The sample size of four MEAs decreased to three MEAs starting on day 24 due to inadvertent manual damage to one of the MEAs.

2.3. In Vitro Cytotoxicity Testing

All handling, housing, and surgical procedures of the mice were approved by the University of Texas Institutional Animal Care and Use Committee. Cytotoxicity assays were carried out as previously described [42] and in accordance with the ISO protocol "10993-5: Biological evaluation of medical devices" using both NTC 929 fibroblasts (ATCC, Manassas, VA, USA) and embryonic day 15 (E15) mouse-derived cortical neurons. Briefly, 50 and 100% concentration LCE extract was evaluated against Tygon-F-4040-lubricant tubing extract (positive control) and cell medium (negative control) [42]. In accordance with the ISO protocol, materials were said to 'pass' if normalized cell viability percentages exceeded 70% following 24-h incubation with material extracts.

Cortices were surgically dissected from E18 mouse embryos, dissociated, and cultured as previously described [4,5]. Prior to seeding, 24 well polystyrene plates (Greiner Bio-One, Kremsminster, Austria) were treated with 50 µg/mL poly-d-lysine (PDL) (Sigma-Aldrich, Saint Louis, MO, USA) and 20 µg/mL laminin to facilitate cell adhesion. Cells were seeded at a density of 100,000 cells/well and incubated at 37 °C, 10% CO$_2$, and 95% humidity in proliferation medium (Dulbecco's Modified Eagle Medium, GlutaMAX, B-27, ascorbic acid, and 10% horse serum). Serum was reduced to 0% over the span of 5 days to avoid over-proliferation and ganglionation of supporting cells. Fibroblasts were sub-cultured prior to seeding in a 24 well polystyrene plate. Cells were incubated at 37 °C, 10% CO$_2$, and 95% humidity in complete medium (Dulbecco's Modified Eagle Medium and 10% horse serum). Material extracts were made by soaking strips of LCE (3 cm^2/mL) in normal cell medium (Dulbecco's Modified Eagle Medium) at 37 °C, 10% CO$_2$, and 95% humidity for 24 h. When cells formed a semi-confluent layer, cell medium was exchanged for 50% or 100% material extract concentrations. Cells were incubated in extract for 24 h prior to using a LIVE/DEAD cytotoxicity kit for mammalian cells according to manufacturer's protocol (Thermo Fisher, L3324, Waltham, MA, USA). Briefly, cells were stained with 2 µM Calcein-AM and 4 µM Ethidium homodimer for live and dead cells, respectively. Images were collected using a 10× objective on an inverted microscope (Nikon Ti eclipse, Nikon, Tokyo, Japan). Cell counts were carried out using a boutique ImageJ (NIH, Bethesda, MD, USA) macro, which applied a 2.0 Gaussian blur before locating local intensity maxima. Cells that were stained with both dyes were marked as "dual-stained" and were regarded as part of the dead cell count based on a MATLAB code.

2.4. In Vitro Functional Neurotoxicity Testing

Functional neurotoxicity assays were carried out as previously described [42]. Briefly, primary cortical neurons were seeded on 48 well Axion well plates (Axion Biosystems, Atlanta, GA, USA) after treating wells with 50 µg/mL PDL and 20 µg/mL laminin. On DIV 23, baseline spontaneous extracellular activity was recorded using Axion's Maestro recording system (Axion, Atlanta, GA, USA). Immediately following baseline recordings, cell medium was exchanged for LCE extract at concentrations of 50% or 100%. Spontaneous extracellular activity was recorded again on DIV 25. Spike and burst rates were determined using a custom MATLAB script. An active electrode was defined as an electrode exhibiting more than five spikes per minute. Inactive electrode sites recorded on DIV 23 were excluded from any further analysis. A burst was defined as at least five consecutive spikes with interspike intervals less than 100 ms [43].

2.5. In Vitro Neuronal Recordings and Pharmacology

Three polydomain and planar-aligned LCE MEAs were sterilized by ethylene oxide for 12 h, and then de-gassed at 37 °C for 48 h. LCE MEAs were treated as described in Section 2.3. Every other day, wide band extracellular potentials generated by cultured neurons were recorded for 5 min from 59 channels simultaneously at a 40 kHz sampling rate using an Omniplex data acquisition system (Plexon Inc., Dallas, TX, USA). Wideband data were band pass filtered (250–7000 Hz) and spikes were detected by voltage excursions exceeding a threshold set to 5.5σ based on RMS noise on a per electrode basis. Spikes were manually sorted using Plexon's offline sorter (Plexon Inc., Dallas, TX, USA). Additional data and statistical analyses were carried out using OriginPro software (Origin Labs, Farmington, ME, USA). Average spike rates were calculated using Neuroexplorer (NEX technologies, Reston, VA, USA). SNR was calculated as

$$\text{SNR} = \left(\frac{Signal}{RMS_{Noise}} \right), \tag{1}$$

where *Signal* and RMS_{Noise} are the mean peak-to-peak amplitude of the sorted unit and the RMS noise, respectively [43]. Active electrode yield percentage was calculated excluding electrodes with impedances over 5 MΩ that would not be capable of recording single units [5]. As a result, 8.2% of total electrodes were excluded.

2.6. Statistical and Data Analysis

All experiments were carried out in parallel using both polydomain and planar-aligned LCEs. This was done to determine if the alignment procedure itself affected any changes on the stability of the substrate. However, these groups are, in fact, chemically identical, and we observed no apparent differences between the groups in any of the results reported here. Therefore, these results derived from both polydomain and planar aligned have been pooled in the following sections.

All statistical analyses were carried out using OriginPro software (Origin Labs, Farmington, ME, USA). In the case of functional neurotoxicity tests, treatment groups were compared using a two-sample *t*-test. In the case of TTX treatments on LCE MEAs and electrochemical stability, a paired two-tailed *t*-test was applied. $p < 0.05$ was considered statistically significant in all cases.

3. Results

To investigate the use of LCEs as substrate materials for neural interfaces, we examine the cytotoxicity, functional neurotoxicity, and manufacturability of microelectrodes on LCEs. Here, we use ISO protocol 10993-5 to evaluate the cytotoxicity of LCEs using both fibroblasts and primary murine cortical neurons. Additionally, we evaluate the functional neurotoxicity of LCE materials in vitro using primary murine cortical neurons cultured on commercially available planar MEAs. Finally, we report the fabrication and characterization of functional planar MEAs using LCEs as an insulating layer.

3.1. In Vitro Cytotoxicity Testing

To determine whether LCEs induce cytotoxicity, live/dead assays were carried out in accordance to ISO protocol 10993-5 using both NTC fibroblasts and primary mouse-derived cortical neurons. Cells were stained with both live and dead markers after exposure to extract as seen in Figure 2a. The threshold for in vitro cytotoxicity is a normalized viability of greater than 70% after extract exposure. After 24 h of exposure to 50 or 100% LCE extracts, NTC fibroblasts exhibited normalized viability percentages of 99.7 ± 0.6 and 87.6 ± 4.9% (mean ± SEM, n = 5). On exposure to positive control material extract (Tygon tubing), NTC fibroblasts exhibited a significantly lower normalized viability percentage of 27.1% ± 4.3 (mean ± SEM, n = 5, $p < 0.0001$). The normalized viability of primary cortical neurons with exposure to 50 or 100% concentrations of LCE extracts was 91.0 ± 3.7 and 88.8 ± 3.6% (mean ± SEM, n = 5), respectively. In contrast, exposure to Tygon tubing (positive control) extract resulted in a statistically significant reduction in normalized viability percentage to 3.2% ± 1.6 (mean ± SEM, n = 5, $p < 0.0001$) (Figure 2b). While exposure to 100% LCE extracts caused a significant reduction in normalized viability percentage to both fibroblasts ($p = 0.04$) and cortical neurons ($p = 0.02$) when compared to the negative control, these values were well above the 70% threshold set by ISO standards, suggesting that the LCE material is not cytotoxic to either NTC fibroblasts or primary cortical neurons.

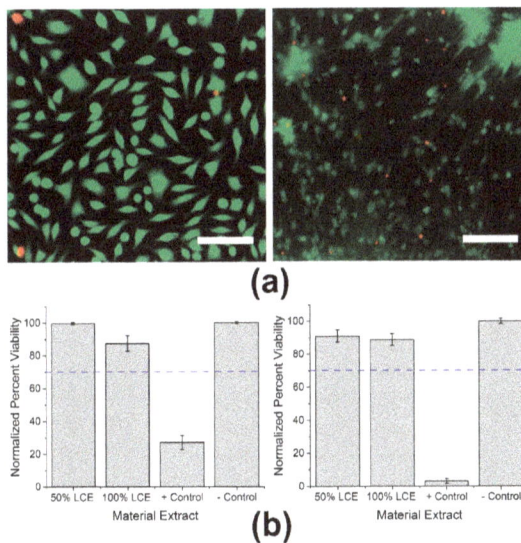

Figure 2. Cytotoxicity assays using both NCTC fibroblasts and primary cortical neurons: (**a**) Fluorescent images of NCTC fibroblasts (**left**) and primary murine-derived cortical neurons (**right**) stained with CaAM (green) for live cells and EthD-1 (red) for apoptotic cells. Scale bars represent 100 μm (**b**) Mean normalized fibroblast (**left**) and cortical neuron (**right**) viability percentages of LCE extract at 50% and 100% concentrations, positive control, and negative control. Blue dotted line at 70% represents the ISO threshold set for non-cytotoxic materials.

3.2. In Vitro Functional Neurotoxicity Testing

While it is paramount to maintain cell viability in the presence of LCE devices, it is equally important that LCE neural interfaces ultimately not affect neuronal network activity. To determine whether neuronal network activity is modulated in the presence of LCE material extracts, we measured mean firing rates and bursting rates in the presence and absence of 50% or 100% material extract treatments using cortical neurons cultured on commercially-available MEAs. After 21 days in culture, neuronal network activity reached a plateau with a mean spike rate of 2.72 ± 0.55 Hz (mean ± SEM) and a burst rate of 0.75 ± 0.11 Hz (mean ± SEM) (n = 19 wells). On DIV 23, a 10 minute baseline recording was taken, then medium was exchanged for LCE extract at 50% and 100% concentrations. Parallel experiments were performed with positive (Tygon extract) and negative control (cell medium) treatments. A second recording was taken to compare to baseline after 48 h of exposure. Exposure of primary cortical neurons to LCE extracts did not significantly change neuronal network parameters (Figure 3a). Normalized mean spike and burst rates after exposure to positive control extracts were significantly reduced to 0% ± 0 (mean ± SEM) (n = 4) ($p = 0.003$ for spike rate, $p = 0.008$ for burst rate). LCE extracts failed to significantly alter bursts ($p = 0.27$ at 50%, 0.31 at 100%) or spike rates ($p = 0.32$ at 50%, 0.46 at 100%) when compared to the negative control, suggesting functional biocompatibility (Figure 3b).

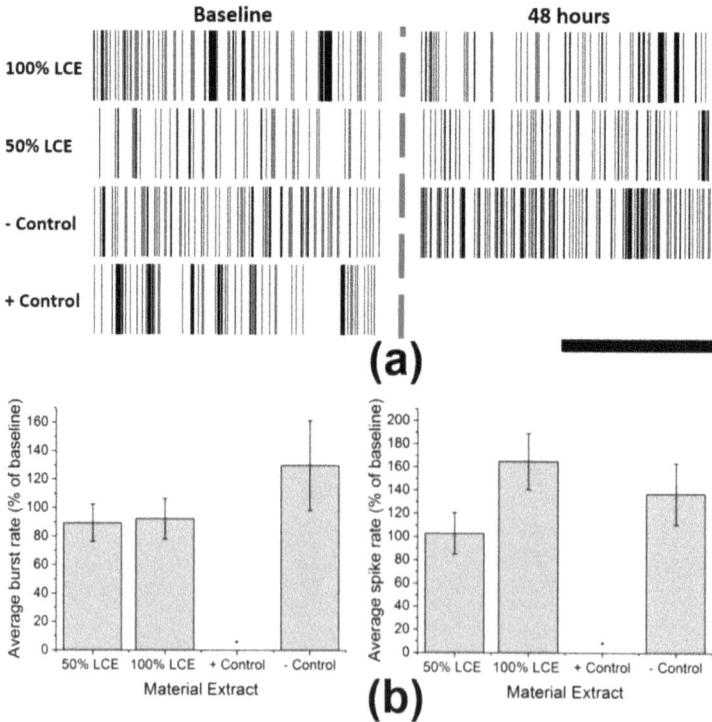

Figure 3. Functional neurotoxicity assays using primary cortical neurons: (**a**) Representative raster plots of spontaneous activity from single electrodes before (**left**) and after (**right**) each treatment. Scale bar represents 3 s. (**b**) Average Burst rate (**left**) and spike rate (**right**) of cortical neurons after 48 h exposure to LCE extract at 50% and 100% concentrations, positive control, and negative control.

3.3. Electrochemical Impedance Stability of MEAs

After evaluation of cytotoxicity and functional neurotoxicity, LCE MEAs (Figure 4a,b) were fabricated as described above. Initial impedances ranged from 248.7 kΩ to 627.1 kΩ at 1 kHz. To examine the electrochemical stability in LCE MEAs, MEAs were aged at 37 °C in PBS for 30 days. The initial recorded impedance magnitudes of electrode sites ranged from 248.7 kΩ to 627.1 kΩ at 1 kHz on day 0 and averaged 381.7 kΩ ± 22.3 (mean ± SEM, n = 32 electrodes, 8 each from 4 MEAs). The final recorded impedance magnitude at 1 kHz on day 30 was 120.3 kΩ ± 42.7 (mean ± SEM) (n = 24 electrodes, 8 from each MEA). While this change was statistically significant ($p < 0.05$), the decrease was relatively minor and was largely attributed to an initial decrease over days 0–4 followed by a prolonged period of apparent stability. The recorded phase on day 0 at 1 kHz was −53.9° ± 1.6 (mean ± SEM) (n = 32 electrodes, 8 from each MEA). The final recorded phase at 1 kHz on day 30 was −68.5° ± 0.6 (mean ± SEM) (n = 24 electrodes, 8 from each MEA). There was no significant trend found in the phase at 1 kHz over the span of 30 days ($p = 0.47$, ANOVA). Even though there is a significant change in the impedance magnitude at 1 kHz through the 30 days, the final recorded impedance at 1 kHz is still well within the range of impedances capable of recording physiological signals, suggesting that LCE MEAs are sufficiently electrochemically stable for neural interfaces [4,5,44].

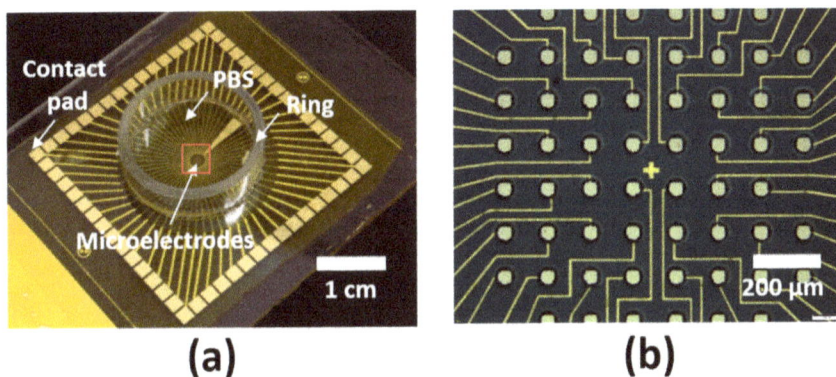

Figure 4. LCE encapsulated MEA devices: (**a**) Optical image of LCE encapsulated MEA device with polycarbonate ring attachment. Red square indicates microelectrode sites at the center of the device. (**b**) Reflection optical microscope image of the microelectrode site. 30 × 30 μm microelectrodes are exposed by 50 μm windows for recording of extracellular activity. Electrical traces are fully encapsulated with LCE.

3.4. In Vitro Neuronal Recordings and Pharmacology

To assess the neural recording capabilities of LCE MEAs, six MEAs were seeded with primary embryonic mouse-derived cortical neurons and recorded over the course of 27 days in vitro. Figure 5a shows that LCE MEAs supported cell adhesion as can be seen by the phase-dark cell bodies and minimal cell clumping on DIV 2 (Figure 5a). Five of the six arrays showed excellent adhesion and network activity and were selected for further analysis.

Using LCE MEAs, extracellular action potentials could be readily detected and sorted into collections of characteristic waveforms (single units, Figure 5b). By DIV 23, single units were detected on 56 ± 8% (mean ± SEM, n = 5) of electrode sites with a mean SNR of 8.9 ± 0.8 (mean ± SEM, n = 5). To confirm that the recorded spikes were biologically sourced, cortical cultures were exposed to 100 nM of TTX, a sodium channel blocker, on DIV 27. In the presence of TTX, mean spiking rates were significantly reduced from 2.8 ± 0.5 to 0.5 ± 0.2 Hz (mean ± SEM, n = 4) based on a paired *t*-test ($p = 0.03$), suggesting that recorded activity from MEAs was physiological (Figure 5c). Overall, mature cortical networks on DIV 23 exhibited a mean spiking rate of 2.7 ± 0.9 (mean $\pm$ SEM, n = 5), and mean bursting rate of 4.5 ± 1.5 (mean $\pm$ SEM, n = 5), suggesting development of synaptically-driven network activity. These values are all highly consistent with those reported in previous studies using commercial MEAs [4,42].

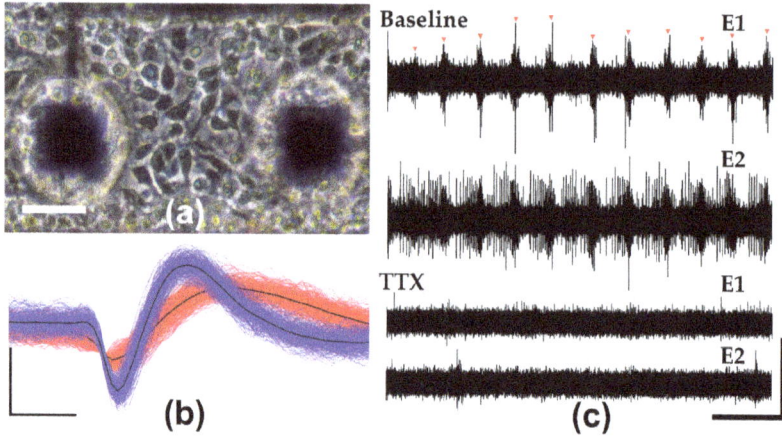

Figure 5. Neuronal Recordings and pharmacology on LCE MEAs: (**a**) Phase contrast image of cultured cortical neurons on LCE MEA DIV2. Scale bar represents 30 μm. (**b**) Representative extracellular waveforms recorded from LCE MEAs on DIV 21. Vertical and horizontal scale bars represent 40 μV and 280 μs. (**c**) Representative bandpass-filtered extracellular recordings from 2 representative electrodes on a single MEA (DIV 27) before and after application of TTX. Red arrowheads indicate network bursts. Vertical and horizontal scale bars represent 55 μV and 2 s.

4. Discussion

The goal of this study is to examine the cellular compatibility of LCE as a material to serve for novel neural interfaces and to demonstrate the manufacturability of the material for fabricating devices. LCEs are a class of smart materials that undergo reversible changes in shape on exposure to a variety of stimuli [33–37]. No previous study has evaluated the suitability of LCE as a substrate and/or insulating material for microelectrode arrays for neural interface applications. Here, we have demonstrated that material extract treatment assays, carried out in accordance with ISO protocol 10993-5, do not indicate significant cytotoxicity in cultures of either NTC fibroblasts or primary cortical neurons; material extract treatments do not significantly modulate primary cortical network activity; that LCE-encapsulated in vitro MEAs exhibit stable impedance measurements over 30 days at 37 °C; and that MEAs could be fabricated, sterilized, and used to record primary neuronal activity for 27 days in vitro. In total, these results suggest that LCE may be a viable substrate for designing and fabricating neural microelectrodes for in vitro and, potentially, in vivo applications. Such devices may provide new capabilities, including deployable microelectrodes.

Author Contributions: Conceptualization, R.T.R., H.K., J.J.P. and T.H.W.; Methodology, R.T.R. and H.K.; Software, R.T.R.; Validation, R.T.R. and H.K.; Formal Analysis, R.T.R.; Investigation, R.T.R., H.K., R.A. and M.O.S.; Resources, J.J.P. and T.H.W.; Data Curation, R.T.R.; Writing-Original Draft Preparation, R.T.R. and H.K.; Writing-Review & Editing, R.T.R., B.J.B., H.K., J.J.P. and T.H.W.; Visualization, R.T.R. and H.K.; Supervision, J.J.P., T.H.W. and B.J.B.; Project Administration, J.J.P. and T.H.W.; Funding Acquisition, J.J.P. and T.H.W.

Funding: This research was partially-funded by the National Science Foundation under grant No. 1711383 and by the University of Texas at Dallas.

Acknowledgments: The authors extend their appreciation to Hamid Charkhkar for providing custom MATLAB code.

Conflicts of Interest: The authors declare no conflict of interest. The funders had no role in the design of the study; in the collection, analyses, or interpretation of data; in the writing of the manuscript, and in the decision to publish the results.

References

1. Campenot, R.B.; Lund, K.; Mok, S.-A. Production of compartmented cultures of rat sympathetic neurons. *Nat. Protoc.* **2009**. [CrossRef] [PubMed]
2. Xiang, G.; Pan, L.; Huang, L.; Yu, Z.; Song, X.; Cheng, J.; Xing, W.; Zhou, Y. Microelectrode array-based system for neuropharmacological applications with cortical neurons cultured in vitro. *Biosens. Bioelectron.* **2007**. [CrossRef] [PubMed]
3. Kim, R.; Joo, S.; Jung, H.; Hong, N.; Nam, Y. Recent trends in microelectrode array technology for in vitro neural interface platform. *Biomed. Eng. Lett.* **2014**, *4*, 129–141. [CrossRef]
4. Charkhkar, H.; Arreaga-Salas, D.E.; Tran, T.; Hammack, A.; Voit, W.E.; Pancrazio, J.J.; Gnade, B.E. Novel disposable microelectrode array for cultured neuronal network recording exhibiting equivalent performance to commercially available arrays. *Sens. Actuators B Chem.* **2016**. [CrossRef]
5. Hammack, A.; Rihani, R.T.; Black, B.J.; Pancrazio, J.J.; Gnade, B.E. A patterned polystyrene-based microelectrode array for in vitro neuronal recordings. *Biomed. Microdevices* **2018**, *20*, 48. [CrossRef] [PubMed]
6. Wheeler, B.C.; Nam, Y. In Vitro Microelectrode Array Technology and Neural Recordings. *Crit. Rev. Biomed. Eng.* **2011**. [CrossRef]
7. Lacour, S.P.; Benmerah, S.; Tarte, E.; Fitzgerald, J.; Serra, J.; McMahon, S.; Fawcett, J.; Graudejus, O.; Yu, Z.; Morrison, B. Flexible and stretchable micro-electrodes for in vitro and in vivo neural interfaces. *Med. Biol. Eng. Comput.* **2010**, *48*, 945–954. [CrossRef] [PubMed]
8. Smela, E.; Jager, E.W.H.; Inganas, O.; Smela, E.; Inganäs, O. Microfabricating Conjugated Polymer Actuators. *Science* **2000**, *290*, 1540–1545. [CrossRef]
9. Hochberg, L.R.; Bacher, D.; Jarosiewicz, B.; Masse, N.Y.; Simeral, J.D.; Vogel, J.; Haddadin, S.; Liu, J.; Cash, S.S.; Van Der Smagt, P.; et al. Reach and grasp by people with tetraplegia using a neurally controlled robotic arm. *Nature* **2012**. [CrossRef] [PubMed]
10. Jorfi, M.; Skousen, J.L.; Weder, C.; Capadona, J.R. Progress towards biocompatible intracortical microelectrodes for neural interfacing applications. *J. Neural Eng.* **2015**. [CrossRef] [PubMed]
11. Biran, R.; Martin, D.C.; Tresco, P.A. Neuronal cell loss accompanies the brain tissue response to chronically implanted silicon microelectrode arrays. *Exp. Neurol.* **2005**. [CrossRef] [PubMed]
12. Leung, B.K.; Biran, R.; Underwood, C.J.; Tresco, P.A. Characterization of microglial attachment and cytokine release on biomaterials of differing surface chemistry. *Biomaterials* **2008**. [CrossRef] [PubMed]
13. Hassler, C.; Boretius, T.; Stieglitz, T. Polymers for neural implants. *J. Polym. Sci. Part B Polym. Phys.* **2011**, *49*, 18–33. [CrossRef]
14. Capadona, J.R.; Tyler, D.J.; Zorman, C.A.; Rowan, S.J.; Weder, C. Mechanically adaptive nanocomposites for neural interfacing. *MRS Bull.* **2012**. [CrossRef]
15. Jeong, J.; Bae, S.H.; Seo, J.; Chung, H.; Kim, S.J. Long-term evaluation of a liquid crystal polymer (LCP)-based retinal prosthesis. *J. Neural Eng.* **2016**, *13*. [CrossRef] [PubMed]
16. Teo, A.J.T.; Mishra, A.; Park, I.; Kim, Y.; Park, W.; Yoon, Y. Polymeric Biomaterials for Medical Implants and Devices. *ACS Biomater. Sci. Eng.* **2016**, *2*, 454–472. [CrossRef]
17. Kisban, S.; Herwik, S.; Seidl, K.; Rubehn, B.; Jezzini, A.; Umiltà, M.A.; Fogassi, L.; Stieglitz, T.; Paul, O.; Ruther, P. Microprobe Array with Low Impedance Electrodes and Highly Flexible Polyimide Cables for Acute Neural Recording. *IEEE Eng. Med. Biol. Soc.* **2007**, *3*, 175–178.
18. Pang, C.; Cham, J.G.; Nenadic, Z.; Musallam, S.; Tai, Y.; Burdick, J.W.; Andersen, R.A. A New Multi-Site Probe Array with Monolithically Integrated Parylene Flexible Cable for Neural Prostheses. *IEEE Eng. Med. Biol. Soc.* **2005**. [CrossRef]
19. Ware, T.; Simon, D.; Arreaga-salas, D.E.; Reeder, J.; Rennaker, R.; Keefer, E.W.; Voit, W. Fabrication of Responsive, Softening Neural Interfaces. *Adv. Funct. Mater.* **2012**, *22*, 3470–3479. [CrossRef]
20. Jeong, J.; Lee, S.W.; Min, K.S.; Shin, S.; Jun, S.B.; Kim, S.J. Liquid Crystal Polymer (LCP), an Attractive Substrate for Retinal Implant. *Sens. Mater.* **2012**, *24*, 189–203.

21. Chen, M.J.; Pham, A.H.; Member, S.; Evers, N.A.; Kapusta, C.; Iannotti, J.; Kornrumpf, W.; Maciel, J.J.; Karabudak, N. Design and Development of a Package Using LCP for RF/Microwave MEMS Switches. *IEEE Trans. Microw. Theory Tech.* **2006**, *54*, 4009–4015. [CrossRef]
22. Lee, S.W.; Min, K.S.; Jeong, J.; Kim, J.; Kim, S.J.; Member, S. Monolithic Encapsulation of Implantable Neuroprosthetic Devices Using Liquid Crystal Polymers. *IEEE Trans. Biomed. Eng.* **2011**, *58*, 2255–2263.
23. Zhu, J.; Dexheimer, M.; Cheng, H. Reconfigurable systems for multifunctional electronics. *NPJ Flex. Electron.* **2017**, *1*. [CrossRef]
24. White, T.J.; Broer, D.J. Programmable and adaptive mechanics with liquid crystal polymer networks and elastomers. *Nat. Mater.* **2015**, *14*, 1087–1098. [CrossRef] [PubMed]
25. Kularatne, R.S.; Kim, H.; Boothby, J.M.; Ware, T.H. Liquid crystal elastomer actuators: Synthesis, alignment, and applications. *J. Polym. Sci. Part B Polym. Phys.* **2017**, *55*, 395–411. [CrossRef]
26. Küpfer, J.; Finkelmann, H. Nematic liquid single crystal elastomers. *Die Makromol. Chem. Rapid Commun.* **1991**, *12*, 717–726. [CrossRef]
27. Ware, T.H.; McConney, M.E.; Wie, J.J.; Tondiglia, V.P.; White, T.J. Voxelated liquid crystal elastomers. *Science* **2015**, *347*, 982–984. [CrossRef] [PubMed]
28. Wermter, H.; Finkelmann, H. Liquid crystalline elastomers as artificial muscles. *E-Polymers* **2001**, *1*, 1–13. [CrossRef]
29. Gelebart, A.H.; Mulder, D.J.; Varga, M.; Konya, A.; Vantomme, G.; Meijer, E.W.; Selinger, L.B.R.; Broer, D.J. Making waves in a photoactive polymer film. *Nature* **2017**, *546*, 632–636. [CrossRef] [PubMed]
30. Yu, H.; Ikeda, T. Photocontrollable liquid-crystalline actuators. *Adv. Mater.* **2011**. [CrossRef] [PubMed]
31. Boothby, J.M.; Kim, H.; Ware, T.H. Shape changes in chemoresponsive liquid crystal elastomers. *Sens. Actuators B Chem.* **2017**, *240*, 511–518. [CrossRef]
32. De Haan, L.T.; Verjans, J.M.N.; Broer, D.J.; Bastiaansen, C.W.M.; Schenning, A.P.H.J. Humidity-responsive liquid crystalline polymer actuators with an asymmetry in the molecular trigger that bend, fold, and curl. *J. Am. Chem. Soc.* **2014**. [CrossRef] [PubMed]
33. Buzsáki, G. Large-scale recording of neuronal ensembles. *Nat. Neurosci.* **2004**, *7*, 446–451. [CrossRef] [PubMed]
34. Kozai, T.D.Y.; Gugel, Z.; Li, X.; Gilgunn, P.J.; Khilwani, R.; Ozdoganlar, O.B.; Fedder, G.K.; Weber, D.J.; Cui, X.T. Chronic tissue response to carboxymethyl cellulose based dissolvable insertion needle for ultra-small neural probes. *Biomaterials* **2014**. [CrossRef] [PubMed]
35. Luan, L.; Wei, X.; Zhao, Z.; Siegel, J.J.; Potnis, O.; Tuppen, C.A.; Lin, S.; Kazmi, S.; Fowler, R.A.; Holloway, S.; et al. Ultraflexible nanoelectronic probes form reliable, glial scar–free neural integration. *Sci. Adv.* **2017**. [CrossRef] [PubMed]
36. Patel, P.R.; Na, K.; Zhang, H.; Kozai, T.D.Y.; Kotov, N.A.; Yoon, E.; Chestek, C.A. Insertion of linear 8.4 μm diameter 16 channel carbon fiber electrode arrays for single unit recordings. *J. Neural Eng.* **2015**. [CrossRef] [PubMed]
37. Guitchounts, G.; Markowitz, J.E.; Liberti, W.A.; Gardner, T.J. A carbon-fiber electrode array for long-term neural recording. *J. Neural Eng.* **2013**. [CrossRef] [PubMed]
38. Yakacki, C.M.; Saed, M.; Nair, D.P.; Gong, T.; Reed, S.M.; Bowman, C.N. Tailorable and programmable liquid-crystalline elastomers using a two-stage thiol-acrylate reaction. *RSC Adv.* **2015**. [CrossRef]
39. Sharma, A.; Neshat, A.; Mahnen, C.J.; Nielsen, A.D.; Snyder, J.; Stankovich, T.L.; Daum, B.G.; Laspina, E.M.; Beltrano, G.; Gao, Y.; et al. Biocompatible, biodegradable and porous liquid crystal elastomer scaffolds for spatial cell cultures. *Macromol. Biosci.* **2015**. [CrossRef] [PubMed]
40. Martella, D.; Paoli, P.; Pioner, J.M.; Sacconi, L.; Coppini, R.; Santini, L.; Lulli, M.; Cerbai, E.; Wiersma, D.S.; Poggesi, C.; et al. Liquid Crystalline Networks toward Regenerative Medicine and Tissue Repair. *Small* **2017**. [CrossRef] [PubMed]
41. Boothby, J.M.; Ware, T.H. Dual-responsive, shape-switching bilayers enabled by liquid crystal elastomers. *Soft Matter* **2017**, *13*, 4349–4356. [CrossRef] [PubMed]
42. Charkhkar, H.; Frewin, C.; Nezafati, M.; Knaack, G.L.; Peixoto, N.; Saddow, S.E.; Pancrazio, J.J. Use of cortical neuronal networks for in vitro material biocompatibility testing. *Biosens. Bioelectron.* **2014**, *53*, 316–323. [CrossRef] [PubMed]

43. Black, B.J.; Atmaramani, R.; Pancrazio, J.J. Spontaneous and Evoked Activity from Murine Ventral Horn Cultures on Microelectrode Arrays. *Front. Cell. Neurosci.* **2017**. [CrossRef] [PubMed]
44. Spira, M.E.; Hai, A. Multi-electrode array technologies for neuroscience and cardiology. *Nat. Nanotechnol.* **2013**, *8*, 83–94. [CrossRef] [PubMed]

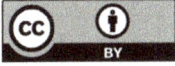

micromachines

Article

Dextran as a Resorbable Coating Material for Flexible Neural Probes

Dries Kil [1,*], Marta Bovet Carmona [2], Frederik Ceyssens [1], Marjolijn Deprez [3], Luigi Brancato [1], Bart Nuttin [3], Detlef Balschun [2] and Robert Puers [1]

[1]   ESAT-MICAS, KU Leuven, Kasteelpark Arenberg 10, 3001 Leuven, Belgium;
      fceyssen@esat.kuleuven.be (F.C.); luigi.brancato@esat.kuleuven.be (L.B.); puers@esat.kuleuven.be (R.P.)
[2]   Laboratory for Biological Psychology, Brain & Cognition, KU Leuven, Tiensestraat 102,
      3000 Leuven, Belgium; marta.bovetcarmona@kuleuven.be (M.B.C.); detlef.balschun@kuleuven.be (D.B.)
[3]   Experimental Neurosurgery and Neuroanatomy, UZ Herestraat 49 box 7003, 3000 Leuven, Belgium;
      marjolijn.deprez@kuleuven.be (M.D.); bart.nuttin@uzleuven.be (B.N.)
*   Correspondence: dries.kil@esat.kuleuven.be; Tel.: +32-16-327-985

Received: 13 November 2018; Accepted: 15 January 2019; Published: 17 January 2019

Abstract: In the quest for chronically reliable and bio-tolerable brain interfaces there has been a steady evolution towards the use of highly flexible, polymer-based electrode arrays. The reduced mechanical mismatch between implant and brain tissue has shown to reduce the evoked immune response, which in turn has a positive effect on signal stability and noise. Unfortunately, the low stiffness of the implants also has practical repercussions, making surgical insertion extremely difficult. In this work we explore the use of dextran as a coating material that temporarily stiffens the implant, preventing buckling during insertion. The mechanical properties of dextran coated neural probes are characterized, as well as the different parameters which influence the dissolution rate. Tuning parameters, such as coating thickness and molecular weight of the used dextran, allows customization of the stiffness and dissolution time to precisely match the user's needs. Finally, the immunological response to the coated electrodes was analyzed by performing a histological examination after four months of in vivo testing. The results indicated that a very limited amount of glial scar tissue was formed. Neurons have also infiltrated the area that was initially occupied by the dissolving dextran coating. There was no noticeable drop in neuron density around the site of implantation, confirming the suitability of the coating as a temporary aid during implantation of highly flexible polymer-based neural probes.

Keywords: dextran; neural probe; microfabrication; foreign body reaction; immunohistochemistry; polymer; chronic

1. Introduction

Ever since Italian physician Luigi Galvani discovered that nerves and muscles were electrically excitable (1791) neural electrodes have proven to be an essential tool in neuroscience research as well as emerging clinical applications [1]. An example of such a development is the field of neuroprosthetics, which is concerned with the development and implementation of devices that can replace a motor, sensor or cognitive modality that might have been lost as a result of an injury or a disease [2]. The most well-known example is the cochlear implant which consists of an external unit that collects sound waves, processes them and in turn transfers the signals to the auditory nerve through a microelectrode array, substituting the function of the ear drum and stapes [3].

Things get more complex when we try to use this concept to replace lost brain function as is the case for, e.g., motor prosthetics [4]. Although penetrating microelectrodes that are suitable for this kind of application have undergone great improvements regarding the high density recording and stimulation of neuronal tissue, even at single-cell resolution, their limited chronic reliability is still the major limitation blocking widespread applicability [5]. Earlier experiments have shown that electrode performance typically starts to decrease a few weeks after implantation due to a progressive inflammatory tissue response, also known as the Foreign Body Reaction (FBR) [6–8]. The FBR causes the number of active channels to decrease, and the quality of the recorded signal to drop over time as scar tissue is formed around the implant, eventually leading to sensing inaccuracies, instability and failure of the implant. The FBR is considered the main reason behind the deterioration of microelectrode systems. The dynamic progression of the response results in instability in the recording quality over time, eventually leading to failure [9–11].

The trend mentioned above is recognized quite often in old as well as recent literature. Researchers describe a steady increase in impedance over the first four to six weeks after implantation which can be attributed to the expanding glial scar [12]. This is confirmed by the noticeable decrease in quality of the electrical recordings over time, as well as the post-mortem immunohistochemical analysis of the brain tissue [13]. From this information, it is evident that most of the problems related to chronic reliability can be traced back to the electrode design and its material properties, especially during the acute phase of the FBR. When comparing the characteristics of traditional materials for electrode fabrication to those of brain tissue, we immediately notice a large difference in Young's modulus. Silicon and metals have moduli in the order of hundreds of GPa, while the stiffness of brain tissue is around 0.1 to 1.2 MPa [14]. After implantation, this mismatch will result in micromotions between the electrode and the tissue as the brain pulsates under influence of, e.g., blood flow, creating a constant source of irritation and thus a prolonged inflammatory reaction [5]. Several studies have examined the effect of implant stiffness on the surrounding brain tissue, providing evidence that using softer materials with a stiffness resembling that of the brain tissue reduces the aforementioned mismatch and attenuates the adverse foreign body reaction [15].

In general, it can be stated that the use of soft polymers increases the chronic reliability of penetrating microelectrodes. Practically however, this does come with some limitations. The most important one is the complexity of the surgical insertion of the probes, since many are too soft to penetrate the brain tissue without buckling, let alone puncture the dura. A frequently used solution is the use of an additional stiffening structure. Examples include stiff backbone layers [16], insertion shuttles [17] and biodegradable coatings [18]. These options however do come with some disadvantages. The stiff backbone layer is permanently attached to the implant and does not dissolve, limiting the flexibility of the device. Insertion shuttles on the other hand are quite bulky and temporarily increase the footprint of the implant, resulting in dimpling during insertion and additional, unnecessary damage to the neural tissue during implantation. The least invasive solution is to temporarily stiffen the implant using a bioresorbable coating, allowing the implant to regain its flexibility after the dissolution. Several types of bioresorbable materials have already been analyzed as potential candidates. Popular choices include silk fibroin [19], hydrogels, poly(lactic-co-glycolic acid) (PLGA), sucrose [20] and maltose [21]. Choosing the correct material for application is however no easy task, as each class of materials has its own (dis)advantages [22]. Sugar-based materials are typically characterized as materials with high Young's moduli (35 GPa) and a fast resorption time. This allows the coated probe to regain its flexibility almost immediately after implantation. There is, however, a practical disadvantage. The user only has one chance for implantation, as the coating immediately softens upon contact with the cerebrospinal fluid (CSF). In an attempt to counter this problem, we research the use of dextran as a temporary coating material. Apart from its use in medicine as an antithrombic or volume expander for hypovolaemia [23], dextran not only limits non-specific cell adhesion [24] but as it is a complex branched glucan, its dissolution rate and mechanical stiffness can be tuned by varying the chain length of the molecule. First, a thorough characterization of the proposed material is executed in which the dissolution rate and mechanical properties are determined. Based on this analysis, the buckling force of a coated electrode can be calculated and compared to the force needed to puncture several anatomical regions of the brain. Afterwards, the dextran coated polymer probes are subjected to an in vivo experiment in which their performance is evaluated based on their ability to puncture the brain as well as the severity of the evoked FBR.

2. Materials and Methods

2.1. Selection of Materials

As stated in the introduction, the use of soft polymer materials is critical for the development of reliable chronic neural probes. For this research, Parylene-C (Specialty Coating Systems) was chosen as the base material. Its dielectric properties, high strength under bending and biocompatibility make it an excellent candidate for our application. The flexibility of Parylene-C significantly increases the mechanical compliance between the device and the soft biological tissue surrounding it. The Young's modulus of Parylene-C also closely resembles that of brain tissue. A unique feature of parylene-C is that it can be coated using chemical vapor deposition (CVD) in vacuum, which enables a conformal coating. Additionally, Parylene-C received United States Pharmacopeia (USP) Class VI and International Organization for Standardization (ISO) 10993 compliance, making it a Food and Drug Administration (FDA) approved material for implantation.

Platinum was chosen as the material of choice for the conductors due to its biocompatibility and inertness in a biological environment and high charge injection limit.

Dextran (Sigma-Aldrich) was chosen as the coating material. Three types of dextran, with varying molecular weights, were analyzed: 40, 100, and 500 kDa.

2.2. Electrode Design and Fabrication

All experiments were performed using a Parylene-C shank electrode with a tapered profile (Figure 1.). The probe width ranged from 72 µm at the tip to 218 µm at the base. The length of the shank was 700 µm, allowing it to penetrate all layers of the rat cortex after implantation. The microelectrode was fabricated using a standard two-mask, three-layer microfabrication process that was executed on a standard 4 inch silicon carrier wafer with a thickness of 500 µm. The following workflow was applied, as partially described in an earlier publication [25]:

- The 4 inch silicon carrier wafers were thoroughly cleaned using piranha etchant (4 H_2SO_4:1 H_2O_2) to remove any organic contaminants. Afterwards, a HF-dip (2% HF) was performed followed by a rinsing cycle in DI water. The substrate was dried using purified nitrogen.
- A 400 nm thin layer of silicon oxide was grown on the substrate using a wet thermal oxidation process. The oxide served as a sacrificial layer which aids in the final release of the devices from the carrier wafer in a later step.
- A first insulation layer of Parylene-C was deposited, yielding a 7 µm thick layer.
- The 400 nm thick Pt conductors were deposited by sputter coating on a lithographically patterned photoresist bilayer (LOR10B/S1818). The lift-off process was completed by soaking the wafers in n-methyl-2-pyrrolidone (NMP) overnight at room temperature.
- A second layer of Parylene-C, with a thickness of 7 µm, was deposited using a similar process.
- The device shape was defined by reactive ion etching (RIE) of the Parylene-C using an aluminum hard mask. The device outline was lithographically patterned using a negative photoresist on top of which a 40 nm thick layer of aluminum was thermally evaporated. After a lift-off step in acetone, the wafers were ready for RIE. As platinum is not etched by the RIE plasma, it also functions as an etch stop, which opens up the electrode contacts and bond pads.
- The wafer was annealed at a temperature of 200 °C for 4 h (2 °C/min ramping rate) in a nitrogen atmosphere to relax any residual stress that was built up during the processing, as well as to prevent delamination [26].
- Finally, the wafer was soaked in a 1% HF solution that removed the Al hard mask and underetched the sacrificial silicon oxide layer. After 1 h of etching, the adhesion between the Parylene-C

electrode and the carrier wafer was reduced to such a level that the electrodes could be peeled off the carrier wafer using tweezers.

After completing the fabrication process the implants were stored in 70% ethanol for disinfection purposes.

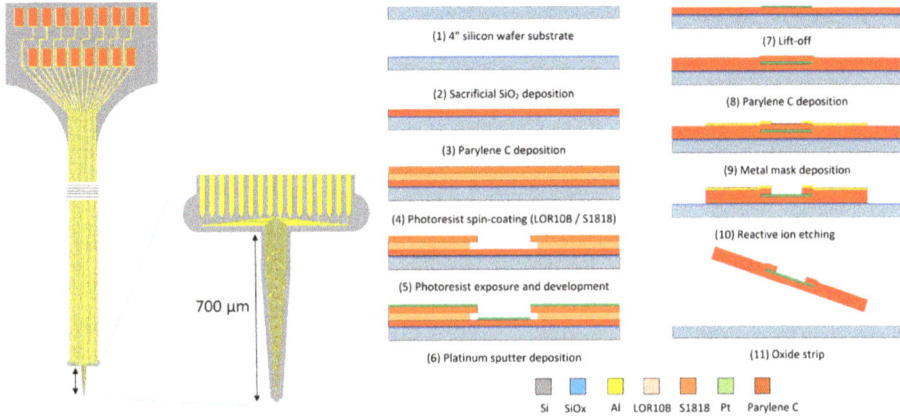

Figure 1. Electrode layout and microfabrication process.

To embed the electrode array, the neural probe was dipcoated in a highly viscous solution of molten dextran. Initially the dextran powder was dissolved in deionized water (50 wt %) before placement on a hotplate at 200 °C. After the evaporation of the water that was present in the solution, the dextran started to melt and take on a liquid state. The neural probe was fixed to a motorized z-stage and submerged in the solution. Afterwards, the probe was drawn from the solution, coating it with a layer of adhesive dextran, which immediately crystallized under influence of the lower room temperature.

The final film thickness was determined by the interplay between the entraining and draining forces acting on the film. This can be theoretically described by the Landau–Levich equation and the capillary regime equation which are a function of both the viscosity of the solution and the withdrawal speed of the probe. In order to characterize the aforementioned dipcoating process, an experiment was performed to determine the relationship between film thickness and withdrawal speed for dextran of different molecular weights (Figure 2). Six samples were tested for each combination of withdrawal speed and molecular weight. The plotted coating thickness consists of the combined thickness of dextran deposited on both sides of the shank.

As expected from the theoretical approximation, a higher molecular weight dextran (higher viscosity) resulted in a higher film thickness. For more information on the physical principles behind the dipcoating process, I refer to the review article by Rio and Boulogne [27].

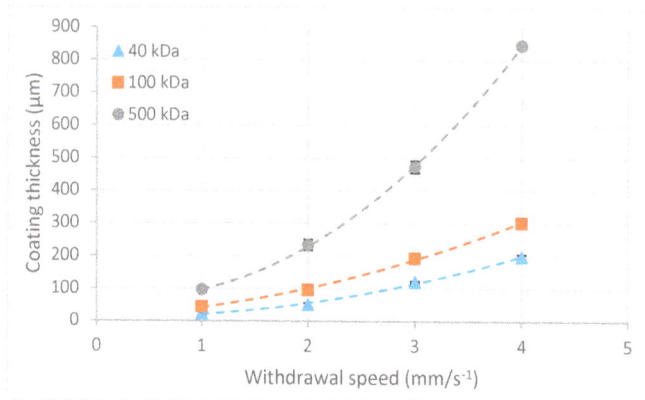

Figure 2. Coating thickness vs. withdrawal speed in function of molecular weight. The error bars represent the standard deviation ($n = 6$).

2.3. Micromechanical Characterization

In order to achieve successful surgical placement of neural probes, the main requirement is that the probes are mechanically robust enough to penetrate the brain. Ideally, the buckling force threshold of the neural probe must be higher than the penetration force needed for implantation. As in almost all cases, the thin polymer-based implants are too flexible for implantation and some sort of mechanical reinforcement is needed to temporarily increase the probe stiffness. Ideally, this mechanical augmentation is also temporary, allowing the electrode to regain its flexibility once it is implanted. Setting a fixed number on the amount of force needed to penetrate brain tissue is however very difficult, as the mechanical properties of brain tissue are highly dependent on a multitude of factors, such as the species of the subject animal, its age or the stiffness characteristics of the functional zone in the brain that is targeted. All of these tissue-specific variables are critical in determining the penetration force of neural probes for the application of interest [28].

For our intended application, which is a chronic implantation through the dura in the underlying sensorimotor cortex, we need to penetrate the stiffest part of the brain, the dura mater. The dura is the outermost meningeal covering of the brain and is made out of dense connective tissue. It has a Young's modulus that is several orders of magnitude higher than the cortex, cerebellum or the hippocampus. Many research groups prefer to remove the dura using sharp forceps to increase the ease of insertion of flexible neural probes. Performing a durotomy is however never without risk and should be avoided when trying to maximize the chronic reliability of the probe.

Based on earlier experiments reported in literature, we can make a rough estimation of the penetration force that is needed. A study by Jensen et al., which used silicon probes to penetrate rat cerebral cortex, concluded that penetration forces are in the range of 0.45 to 1.15 mN with an average of 0.775 mN [29]. Values in the range of 0.54 to 2.48 mN with a 1.25 mN average are reported by Sharp et al. in the case of individual stainless steel probes [30]. The small differences in penetration force ranges can be attributed to the difference in tip shape, as Sharp explored insertion of blunt implants, whereas Jensen focused on very sharp probe tips. Based on the information available in literature, we can make a safe estimation that individual tapered probes should be able to withstand a force of 1.5 mN to penetrate the rat cortex. This value can now be used as a design goal for the required buckling force threshold of neural probe.

By modeling penetrating neural probes as beams that are clamped at one end and pinned at the other, it is possible to make a mathematical estimation of the buckling force threshold of flexible probes. This simplification results in quite accurate results as the probes are fixed at their base since they are reversibly adhered to an insertion platform/stereotactic frame during implantation. They are considered pinned at the other end from the moment the tip contacts the dura. We can use Euler's formula to determine the critical load at which buckling occurs.

$$Pcr = \frac{(K \cdot pi^2 \cdot E \cdot I)}{L^2}, \tag{1}$$

$$I = \frac{1}{12} \cdot b \cdot h^3, \tag{2}$$

where Pcr = buckling force threshold, K = column effective length factor = 2.045, E = elasticity modulus, I = area moment of inertia, L = unsupported beam length, b = beam width, h = column thickness.

As an example, we can take a look at the critical load of our untreated Parylene-C shank electrode. The unsupported length of the electrode during implantation is 1 mm with a width of 190 μm and a thickness of 14 μm. The elasticity modulus of Parylene C is 2.8 GPa.

Theoretical analysis results in a buckling force threshold of 2.4 mN, indicating that the electrode is strong enough to withstand penetration in brain tissue without buckling. If we want to puncture the dura however, the electrode will need to be able to withstand a critical load of around 10 mN, which we would not be able to achieve with the electrode in its current form. This problem can be circumvented by fabricating a thicker electrode, but this will increase the stiffness of the implant and have an adverse effect on the 'mechanical match' of the electrode with the brain tissue, which is a critical requirement to improve long-term reliability of the implants. As stated earlier, the solution proposed in this paper is the use of a thin dextran coating that will temporarily stiffen the electrode.

To assess the level of mechanical reinforcement that can be obtained by a dextran coating, a set of micromechanical experiments was performed. Uncoated probes were taken as a reference.

The samples were fixed on a substrate with a known part of the shank extending over the edge. The floating part of the shank was displaced using a Femtotools FTA-M02 micromechanical testing system (Figures 3 and 4). Force measurements were taken during the displacement and the bending stiffness of the samples was calculated. The Young's modulus of the samples was approximated using the formula for bending of a beam under a point load:

$$E = \frac{k \cdot L^3}{3 \cdot I}. \tag{3}$$

With I the area moment of inertia:

$$I = \frac{b \cdot h^3}{12}. \tag{4}$$

In these formulas, L represents the distance between the hinging point and the contact point of the indenter tip, b is the measured width of the sample and h is the sample thickness. The stiffness of the coating is orders of magnitude higher than the stiffness of the uncoated implant, allowing us to simplify the implant to a solid dextran beam model during mechanical characterization.

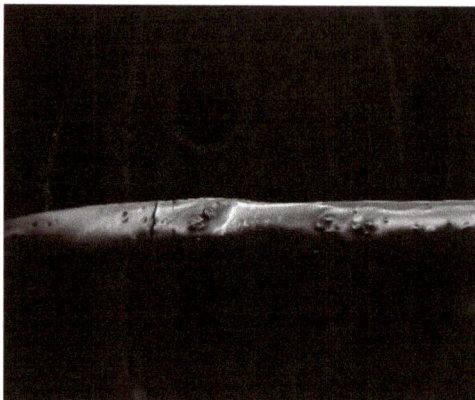

Figure 3. Electron micrograph of a dextran coated Parylene-C neural probe. A crack can be seen on the left-hand side of the probe which was formed after buckling. Reproduced with permission from [31]; published by IOPscience, 2017.

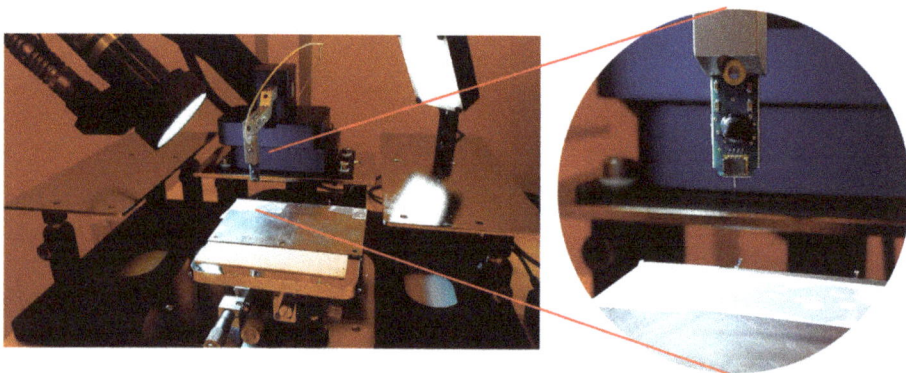

Figure 4. Test setup for measuring bending stiffness using the Femtotools FTA-M02 micromechanical testing system. Close-up shows the vertical indenter probe with integrated force sensor. Reproduced with permission from [31]; published by IOPscience, 2017.

2.4. Dissolution Rate

The dissolution rate of the coatings was determined in function of the molecular weight of the used dextran. Dextran slabs were prepared using a 1 cm × 1 cm × 1 cm mold, weighed and submerged in deionized water for a known amount of time. At regular time intervals, the samples were removed from the container, allowed to dry in an oven at slightly elevated temperature (40 °C), and weighed again. This provides an indication of the amount of dextran that dissolves over time. The dextran slabs were submerged while still in the mold to keep the surface area exposed to the dissolution rate constant in time, which results in a more accurate representation of the dissolution rate.

2.5. In Vivo Experiment

All experiments were performed in accordance with the Belgian and European laws, guidelines and policies for animal experimentation, housing and care (Belgian Royal Decree of 29 May and European Directive 2010/63/EU on the protection of animals used for scientific purposes of 20 October 2010). The animal experiments were performed on six male Wistar rats, weighing about 250 g on arrival. The animals were housed and maintained in standard cages under conventional laboratory conditions with ad libitum access to food and water and a 12 h light/12 h dark cycle. All experiments were conducted during the light phase of the animal's activity cycles.

2.5.1. Implantation Procedure

Prior to the surgical procedure the animals were anesthetized using an isoflurane/oxygen pump system (Iso-vet Surgivet at 3% isoflurane for induction and 1% to 2% for maintenance; O_2 1 L/min) after which they were placed in a stereotactic frame where constant isoflurane/oxygen was administered through a face mask. After removing the hair on the head, additional subcutaneous anesthetic (Xylocaine 2%, 1:200000 adrenaline, AstraZeneca) was applied. Then, the skin was opened and the skull was cleaned. Two holes were drilled, 4 mm distally from bregma, over the S1 sensorimotor cortex. First, the connector assembly was fixed on the skull together with a set of stainless steel screws that provide additional support. Afterwards, the electrode tip was inserted through the dura to a depth of roughly 700 μm and fixed in place using a drop of UV-cured dental cement (Tetric EvoFlow, Ivoclar Vivadent). Finally, the wound was sutured and pain relief was ensured for 24 h by administering 0.06 mg/kg of Vetergesic (Ecu phar). The implanted electrodes were temporarily stiffened using a 40 ± 7 μm thick dextran coating with a molecular weight of 40 kDa.

2.5.2. Perfusion

Four months after implantation the experiment was stopped. The animals were sacrificed by administering a lethal dose of pentobarbital. Afterwards, an intracardial perfusion was executed to fixate the brain tissue. First the animals were perfused with 250 mL of PBS followed by 200 mL of 4% PFA. After extraction of the brain, it was stored in 4% PFA for 24 h before rinsing and storing in a solution of 20% sucrose and 0.1% sodium aziide in preparation for histology. Prior to slicing, the tissue was embedded in a 4% agar gel. Coronal slices with a thickness of 80 μm were taken using a Leica VT1000S vibrotome (Leica Biosystems Inc., Buffalo Grove, IL, USA). It should be noted that due to the fixation of the tissue a small amount of shrinkage occurred, resulting a minor error during the subsequent analysis [32].

2.5.3. Histology

Before analysis the samples were stained for glial fibrillary acidic protein (GFAP) and neuronal nuclei (NeuN) which are standards for visualization of reactive astrocytes and neurons, respectively. The following procedure was performed:

- Overnight soak in blocking buffer (1% BSA, 0.1% Triton X100 in PBS) to reduce non-specific background staining
- Application of primary antibodies (1:100 MAB377 mouse anti-NeuN; 1:500 polyclonal rabbit anti-GFAP Z0334 in blocking buffer)
- Rinse in PBS (three times)
- 2 h incubation in blocking buffer
- Application of secondary antibodies (ALEXA fluor 488 (Abcam, Cambridge, UK) donkey anti-mouse IgG (H + L) and Cy3 Donkey Anti Rabbit IgG (H + L), 1:1000 in blocking buffer).
- Rinse in PBS (three times)

Subsequently, the samples were mounted on Superfrost microscope glasses using Sigma Fluoroshield. Imaging was done using a Leica TCS SP8 confocal microscope (Leica Microsystems, Wetzlar, Germany) using a 20× immersion objective (1024 × 1024 pixel imaging, 5% 488 nm laser power, 3% 552 nm laser power, Cy3 and ALEXA 488 filters and 950 and 830 amplifier gain, respectively). The analysis of the images was done using ImageJ image processing software. To quantify the amount of gliosis, the average thickness of the scar tissue was measured. Additionally, any change in neuronal density around the site of implantation was determined by counting neuronal cell bodies in concentric areas around the site of implantation.

3. Results

3.1. Micromechanical Characterization

In order to make an accurate comparison with the clamped beam model, which is proposed in Section 2.3., rectangular Parylene-C dummy probes were used for the micromechanical characterization. Measurements were performed on three groups (40, 100, and 500 kDa) of six samples each. The uncoated implants had an average thickness of 14 ± 1 μm and an average width of 500 ± 3 μm. The coated samples had an average thickness of 163 ± 21 μm and an average width of 641 ± 15 μm. By varying the withdrawal speed during dipcoating, we were able to achieve the same coating thickness for all dextran types. This allows us to easily detect any changes in mechanical properties that are related to the molecular weight of the used dextran. Micromechanical testing reveals an average bending stiffness of 0.029 ± 0.005 N·m^{-1} for the uncoated implants. Coating increased this average bending stiffness 360-fold to 10.5 ± 5.5 N·m^{-1}. The Young's modulus of all coated samples is measured to be only 0.6 ± 0.1 GPa, proving that the enhanced structural stiffness can be mainly attributed to the thickness of the coating and not to the molecular weight of the dextran. Based on the data gathered during the experiment, we can determine, by using Equations (1) and (2), that a dextran thickness of 37 μm is required to meet the critical load of 10 mN that is required for penetration of the dura mater.

3.2. Dextran Dissolution Rate

The results of the dissolution experiment are depicted in Figure 5. It is clearly visible that the higher the molecular weight of the dextran, the lower the weight loss over time becomes.

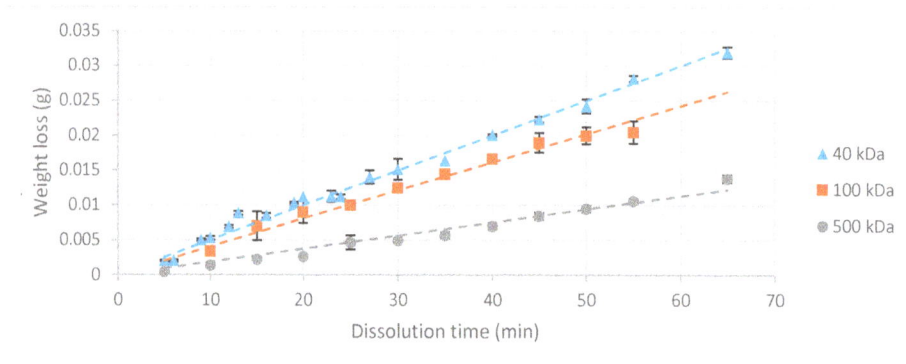

Figure 5. Weight loss in function of dissolution time ($n = 6$).

The aforementioned conclusions indicate a strong dependency between dissolution rate and molecular chain length that can be explained by the physical mechanism of sugar dissolution in water. When the sugar crystal comes into contact with water, the polar bonds of the water molecules form their own dipole-dipole bonds with the sugar molecules. These bonds are stronger than the intermolecular Vanderwaals forces which are present between the sugar molecules themselves, causing them to separate and bond to the water molecules. For molecules with high molecular weight (longer chain length) the formation of dipole-dipole interactions with the water molecules is more difficult. The surface area of the molecule exposed to the solute is relatively small compared to its size. This effect increases with the molecular weight, decreasing the dissolution rate. This allows tuning of the dissolution rate of dextran coatings by varying the molecular weight of the dextran. It is important to note that these three types of dextran can only be compared because the surface area exposed to the dissolution experiment was kept constant during the whole experiment. If the surface area is increased under constant volume, more dextran molecules would come into contact with the medium, increasing the rate at which the coating dissolves. This linear relationship was validated by an additional experiment in which the surface area exposed to the dissolution medium was varied by changing the dimensions of the dextran slabs (Figure 6).

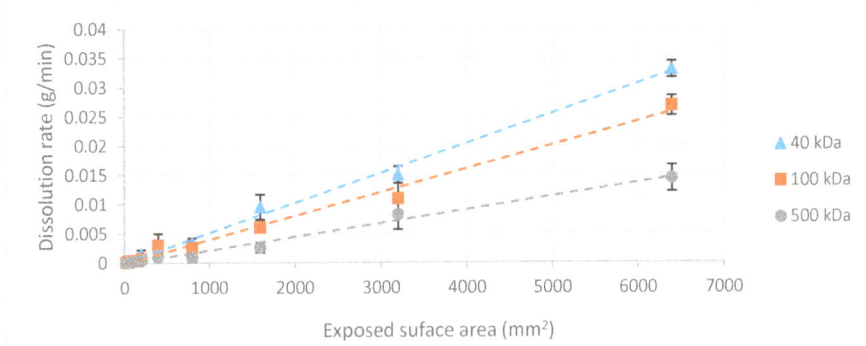

Figure 6. Dissolution rate in function of surface area exposed to the dissolution medium. The error bars represent the standard deviation (*n* = 3).

The dissolution mechanism can be considered as a 'layer-by-layer' process. The thickness of the coating has no influence on the dissolution rate. The total dissolution time is determined by the volume of the coating. As we now have information on all the factors influencing the dissolution time of a dextran coating, a formula can be presented, so that the dissolution time of an arbitrary dextran coating can be predicted. The density of the coating is dependent on the molecular weight of the dextran used and has already been published in earlier work [31].

Combining the results of the experiments, it is possible to create a formula that can be used by the reader to either determine the dissolution rate of a dextran coating with a known surface area to volume ratio or to determine the specifics of a coating with a desirable dissolution time.

$$\text{Dissolution time} = \frac{(\text{Surface area} * \text{coating thickness}) * \rho}{K(S, Mw)}, \tag{5}$$

$$\text{coating thickness} = \frac{(\text{Dissolution time} * K(S, Mw))}{\text{Surface area} * \rho}, \tag{6}$$

with *K(S, Mw)* being the dissolution rate in function of surface area and molecular weight of the used type of dextran.

This dissolution rate can be determined from Figure 5 in function of the surface area exposed to the dissolution medium and the molecular weight of the dextran. Using this formula, we now hold the tools to calculate the dissolution time of the probe we designed in the earlier sections The aforementioned layer-by-layer mechanism was verified by measuring the dissolution time of a known dextran coating and comparing it to its calculated value which was extracted from the "macro-model." A dextran coating with a thickness of 37 μm (MW = 40 kDa) resulted in a dissolution time of roughly 250 s. We have to take into account that this is the dissolution time when the sample is submerged in a large volume of water, meaning that the concentration gradient in the system can be considered to be maximal during the whole dissolution process.

3.3. Image Analysis

Analysis of the images shows the 'neuronless' zone in which the probe resided. The probe is no longer visible as it was removed from the brain during the brainectomy. This area has the same size as the cross section of the uncoated electrode, indicating that the active neurons have penetrated the area that was previously occupied by the dextran coating. As a reference, the outline of the coated electrode is visualized in Figure 7 by the dotted line. The implanted probe was coated with a ± 40 µm thick layer of dextran (40 kDa). The amount of gliosis was quantified using the GFAP stained slices (Figure 7b) and revealed an average thickness of 3.05 ± 0.73 µm. Counting of viable neurons in the vicinity of the implant showed that there was no significant decline in neuron density when approaching the implant. Figure 7 shows the average neuronal cell density at several distances from the site of implantation, normalized to the density in the outer concentric circle.

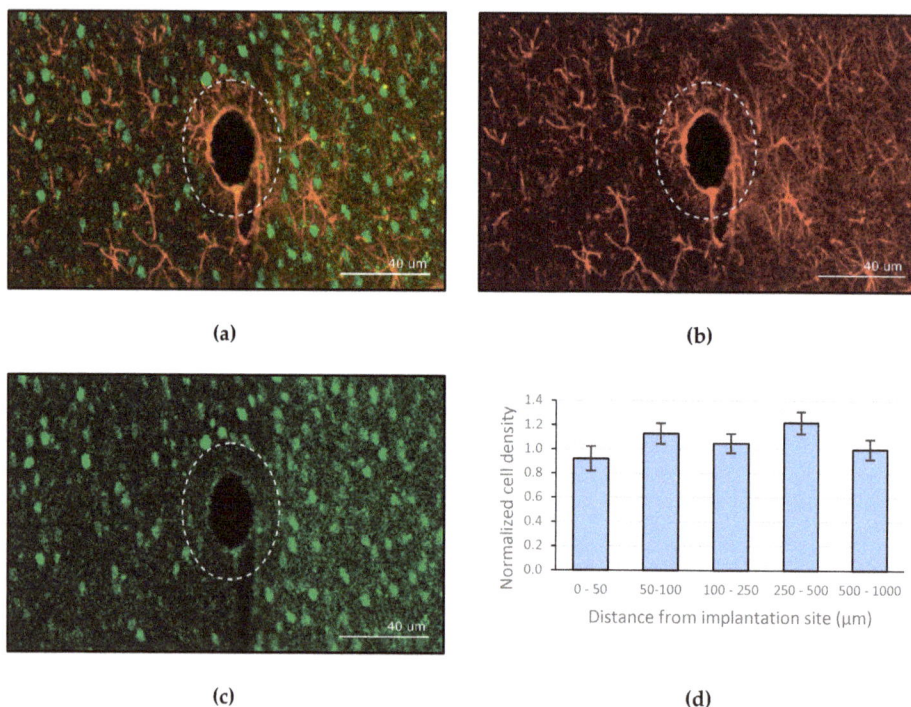

(a)

(b)

(c)

(d)

Figure 7. Confocal imaging of the brain slices (a) overlay of both the glial fibrillary acidic protein (GFAP) and neuronal nuclei (NeuN) stained channels. (b) GFAP channel. (c) NeuN channel. (d) Normalized neuronal density relative to site of implantation (the error bars represent the standard deviation, $n = 6$).

4. Discussion

The described experiments were executed to solve the practical problems that are associated with the use of highly flexible polymer-based neural probes. The goal we wanted to achieve was to find a coating material that could temporarily stiffen flexible probes, without evoking any additional effects concerning the FBR.

We started by going back to the origin of the problem, a simplified mechanical model was used to describe the buckling behavior of a bare Parylene-C electrode. Based on the results, it became evident that additional reinforcement is necessary if we aim to puncture the dura without buckling of the probe. In the quest to find a suitable material, dextran came forward as an ideal candidate as its chemical composition (polysaccharide) allowed tuning of different parameters. After performing a micromechanical experiment, we were able to deduce that a dextran coating of 37 µm increases the critical load of the assembly sufficiently to prevent buckling of the presented neural probe. Additionally, the dissolution rate of the coating can be controlled by varying the molecular weight and thickness of the used dextran. Practically, this means that a fast dissolution time allows the electrode to regain its highly flexible state after minutes, preventing micromotions in an early stage, and thus strongly limiting the chronic FBR and the associated glial scar formation. These hypotheses were analyzed by performing a long-term in vivo experiment. Not only did the results show that the glial sheath only had a thickness of roughly 3 μm, but also showed that the area initially taken up by the dextran coating was re-occupied with active neurons, which is most likely related to the quick dissolution of the coating. Moreover, there was no noticeable decrease in neuronal density in the vicinity of the implant.

With chronic applicability in mind, this may be a very important characteristic of the dextran coating. The functionality of neuroprosthetic devices depends on their capability to form electrical connections with nearby neuronal dendrites and axons, and the glial sheath prevents regrowing neuronal processes from contacting the implant. It is therefore important that this sheath is as thin as possible, as a smaller distance between the recording electrode and the neuron(s) of interest minimizes this electrically resistive barrier and has a positive effect on signal quality. Ideally, we would like to evolve to the use of ultra-thin polymer-based implants with thicknesses in the range of several micrometers or lower. Recent literature proved that such devices can be implanted, reliably, for up to a year without inducing the formation of any scar tissue [33–35]. Dextran would be a perfect temporary coating material for reliably implanting this type of neural probes.

Compared to the other available bioresorbable materials which are often used for the same application, dextran behaves quite well. The higher Young's modulus allows for a thinner coating, which leads to a smaller insertion footprint and dimpling effect. Especially, when the user aims to implant deep into the brain, a high Young's modulus coating is beneficial. Additionally, there are the practicalities related to the surgical implantation. Fast-resorbing polymers such as maltose only offer a single chance of implantation, as the coating softens immediately upon contact with the CSF [21]. This effect can be countered by dextran as it is available with chain lengths ranging from 3 to 2000 kDa. The disentanglement of large, high molecular weight, molecules from the particle surface and subsequent diffusion to the bulk solution takes a longer time, resulting in a slower dissolution rate.

In the literature, we can find several more examples of studies in which a resorbable biomaterial was used to temporarily stiffen flexible neural probes. An article by Lind et al. describes the use of a gelatin to embed thin, flexible microelectrodes [36]. In vivo experiments showed that the body was able to completely eliminate the gelatin, without forming a permanent scar. The neuronal cell density in the immediate vicinity of the implantation site was only slightly reduced, with viable neurons still remaining in the examined region of interest. The effect of the swelling of gelatin is however not described and might result in additional compressive stress on the surrounding cells. Lecomte et al. suggest the use of Polyethylene glycol (PEG) or silk as a coating material [37]. Despite its high Young's modulus, silk fibroin is not commercially available and tedious to process, making dextran a more interesting material. The alternative presented in the paper is the use of PEG, which dissolves within seconds after contact with cerebrospinal fluid, resulting in the practical problems that are mentioned before.

Overall, we can state that the conducted research proved that dextran is a practical and interesting coating material to stiffen flexible neural probes during the implantation phase. Future research will involve the use of dextran as a temporary coating material for an ultra-thin microelectrode array.

5. Conclusions

In this paper we presented and evaluated a novel coating method for flexible implants to improve the chronic reliability of neural probes, which is mainly afflicted by the FBR. By adjusting the probe stiffness to mimic that of brain tissue, this inflammatory reaction can be minimized, resulting in an increased lifetime. Using thin, flexible polymers as a base material solves this problem, but comes with its own limitations. To prevent buckling during surgical insertion the polymer probe needs to be stiffened temporarily. For this purpose, a thin dextran coating is applied which increases the critical load of the assembly. Additionally, the resulting stiffness and dissolution rate of the dextran coating can be tuned to the requirements of the user. All allegations were tested in a long-term in vivo experiment. After four months of electrode implantation only a small lesion remained, enveloped by scar tissue with an average thickness of 3 μm. Apart from a very small glial scar, no drop in neural density was observed, therefore proving that the presented technology allows successful implantation of highly flexible polymer-based neural probes without evoking a severe immune response.

Author Contributions: All experiments were conceived, designed and performed by D.K., F.C. and M.B.C. Fabrication of the microelectrode as well as the analysis of the collected data was performed by D.K. The original draft was written by D.K. All authors contributed to the critical review and editing of the manuscript.

Funding: The research leading to these results has received funding from the European Research Council under the European Union's Seventh Framework Programme (grant number FP7/2007-2013)/ERC grant agreement (grant number 340931), and the KU Leuven IDO program, project on electrical brain stimulation IDO/12/024, and FWO Research (grant numbers G0A5513N and G0D7516N), and the 2016 Research Grant of the European Society for Functional and Stereotactic Neurosurgery.

Acknowledgments: The authors would like to express their gratitude towards Karin Jonckers for the help with the histology and Erin Koos for granting access to the confocal microscope.

Conflicts of Interest: The authors declare no conflict of interest.

References

1. Galvani, L. De viribus eletricitatis in motu musculari commentarius. *Bon. Sci. Art. Inst. Acad. Comm.* **1791**, *7*, 363–418.
2. Krucoff, M.O.; Rahimpour, S.; Slutzky, M.W.; Edgerton, R.V.; Turner, D.A. Enhancing Nervous System Recovery through Neurobiologics, Neural Interface Training, and Neurorehabilitation. *Front. Neurosci.* **2016**, *10*, 584. [CrossRef] [PubMed]
3. Clark, G.M. The multi-channel cochlear implant: Multi-disciplinary development of electrical stimulation of the cochlea and the resulting clinical benefit. *Hear. Res.* **2015**, *322*, 4–13. [CrossRef]
4. Schwartz, A.B.; Cui, X.T.; Weber, D.J.; Moran, W. Brain-controlled interfaces: Movement restoration with neural prosthetics. *Neuron* **2006**, *52*, 205–220. [CrossRef] [PubMed]
5. Szarowski, D.H.; Anderse, M.D.; Retterer, S.; Spence, A.J.; Isaacson, M.; Craighead, H.G.; Shain, W. Brain responses to micro-machined silicon devices. *Brain Res.* **2003**, *983*, 23–35. [CrossRef]
6. Polikov, V.S.; Tresco, P.A.; Reichert, W.M. Response of brain tissue to chronically implanted neural electrodes. *J. Neurosci. Methods* **2005**, *148*, 1–18. [CrossRef] [PubMed]
7. Anderson, J.M.; Rodriguez, A.; Chang, D.T. Foreign body reaction to biomaterials. *Semin. Immunol.* **2008**, *20*, 86–100. [CrossRef]
8. Biran, R.; Martin, D.C.; Tresco, P.A. Neuronal cell loss accompanies the brain tissue response to chronicaly implanted silicon microelectrode arrays. *Exp. Neurol.* **2005**, *195*, 115–126. [CrossRef]
9. Rolfe, B.; Mooney, J.; Zhang, B.; Jahnke, S.; Le, S.J.; Chau, Y.Q.; Campbell, J. The fibrotic response to implanted biomaterials: Implications for tissue engineering. In *Regenerative Medicine and Tissue Engineering-Cells and Biomaterials*; InTech: London, UK, 2011.
10. Roitbak, T.; Sykova, E. Diffusion barriers evoked in the rat cortex by reactive astrogliosis. *Glia* **1999**, *28*, 40–48. [CrossRef]
11. McConnell, G.C.; Rees, H.D.; Levey, A.I.; Gutekunst, C.A.; Gross, R.E.; Bellamkonda, R.V. Implanted neural electrodes cause chronic, local inflammation that is correlated with local neurodegeneration. *J. Neural Eng.* **2009**, *6*, 056003. [CrossRef]
12. Turner, J.N.; Shain, W.; Szarowski, D.H.; Andersen, M.; Martins, S.; Isaacson, M.; Craighead, H. Cerebral astrocyte response to micromachined silicon implants. *Exp. Neurol.* **1999**, *156*, 33–49. [CrossRef] [PubMed]
13. Lago, N.; Ceballos, D.; Rodriguez, F.J.; Stieglitz, T.; Navarro, X. Long term assessment of axonal regeneration through polyimide regenerative electrodes to interface the peripheral nerve. *Biomaterials* **2005**, *26*, 2012–2031. [CrossRef] [PubMed]
14. Weltman, A.; Yoo, J.; Meng, E. Flexible, Penetrating Brain Probes Enabled by Advances in Polymer Microfabrication. *Micromachines* **2016**, *7*, 180. [CrossRef] [PubMed]

15. Sohal, H.S.; Clowry, G.J.; Jackson, A.; O'Neill, A.; Baker, S.N. Mechanical flexibility reduces the foreign body response to long-term implanted microelectrodes in rabbit cortex. *PLoS ONE* **2016**, *11*, e0165606. [CrossRef] [PubMed]

16. Lee, K.; He, J.; Singh, A.; Massia, S.; Ehteshami, G.; Kim, B.; Raupp, G. Polyimide-based intracortical neural implant with improved structural stiffness. *J. Micromech. Microeng.* **2004**, *14*, 32–37. [CrossRef]

17. Kozai, T.D.Y.; Kipke, D.R. Insertion shuttle with carboxyl terminated self-assembled monolayer coatings for implanting flexible polymer neural probes in the brain. *J. Neurosci. Methods* **2009**, *184*, 199–205. [CrossRef] [PubMed]

18. Li, W.; Rodger, D.C.; Pinto, A.; Meng, E.; Weiland, J.D.; Humayun, M.S.; Tai, Y.C. Parylene based integrated wireless single channel neurostimulator. *Sens. Actuators A* **2011**, *166*, 193–200. [CrossRef]

19. Tien, L.; Wu, F.; Tang-Schomer, M.D.; Yoon, E.; Omenetto, F.G.; Kaplan, D.L. Silk as a multifunctional biomaterial substrate for reduced glial scarring around brain-penetrating electrodes. *Adv. Funct. Mater.* **2013**, *23*, 3185–3193. [CrossRef]

20. Jeon, M.; Cho, J.; Kim, Y.K.; Jung, D.; Yoon, E.S.; Shin, S.; Cho, I.J. Partially flexible MEMS neural probe composed of polyimide and sucrose gel for reducing brain damage during and after implantation. *J. Micromech. Microeng.* **2014**, *24*, 025010. [CrossRef]

21. Xiang, Z.; Yen, S.C.; Xue, N.; Sun, T.; Tsang, W.M.; Zhang, S.; Liao, L.D.; Thakor, N.V.; Lee, C. Ultra-thin flexible polyimide neural probe embedded in a dissolvable maltose-coated microneedle. *J. Micromech. Microeng.* **2014**, *24*, 065015. [CrossRef]

22. Lecomte, A.; Descamps, E.; Bergaud, C. A review on mechanical considerations for chronically-implanted neural probes. *J. Neural Eng.* **2018**, *15*, 31001. [CrossRef] [PubMed]

23. Jones, C.; Payne, D.; Hayes, P.; Naylor, R.; Bell, P.; Thompson, M.; Goodall, A. The antithrobotic effect for dextran-40 is due to enhanced fibrinolysis in vivo. *J. Vasc. Surg.* **2008**, *48*, 715–722. [CrossRef] [PubMed]

24. Massia, S.P.; Stark, J.; Letbetter, D.S. Surface-immobilized dextran limits cell adhesion and spreading. *Biomaterials* **2000**, *21*, 2253–2261. [CrossRef]

25. Kil, D.; De Vloo, P.; Fierens, G.; Ceyssens, F.; Hunyadi, B.; Bertrand, A.; Nuttin, B.; Puers, R. A foldable electrode array for 3D recording of deep-seated abnormal brain cavities. *J. Neural Eng.* **2018**, *15*, 036029. [CrossRef] [PubMed]

26. Kim, H.-T.; Kim, C.-D.; Lee, S.-Y.; Sohn, Y.-S. Effects of Annealing Temperature on Parylene-C Films Formed by Chemical Vapor Condensation Method. *Mol. Cryst. Liquid Cryst.* **2015**, *618*, 139–145. [CrossRef]

27. Rio, E.; Boulogne, F. Withdrawing a solid from a bath: How much liquid is coated? *Adv. Colloid Interface Sci.* **2017**, *247*, 100–114. [CrossRef] [PubMed]

28. Elkin, B.S.; Ilankovan, A.; Morrison, B. Age-dependent regional mechanical properties of the rat hippocampus and cortex. *J. Biomech. Eng.* **2010**, *132*, 011010. [CrossRef]

29. Jensen, W.; Yoshida, K.; Hofmann, U.G. In vivo implant mechanics of flexible, silicon-based ACREO microelectrode arrays in rat cerebral cortex. *IEEE Trans. Biomed. Eng.* **2006**, *53*, 934–940. [CrossRef]

30. Sharp, A.; Ortage, A.M.; Restrepo, D.; Curran-Everett, D.; Gall, K. In vivo penetration mechanics and mechanical properties of mouse brain tissue at micrometer scales. *IEEE Trans. Biomed. Eng.* **2009**, *56*, 45–53. [CrossRef]

31. Kil, D.; Brancato, L.; Puers, R. Dextran as a fast resorbable and mechanically stiff coating for flexible neural probes. *J. Phys. Conf. Ser.* **2017**, *922*, 012016. [CrossRef]

32. Wehrl, H.F.; Bezrukov, I.; Wiehr, S.; Lehnhoff, M.; Fuchs, K.; Mannheim, J.G.; Quintanilla-Martinez, L.; Kohlhofer, U.; Kneilling, M.; Pichler, B.J.; et al. Assessment of murine brain tissue shrinkage caused by different histological fixatives using magnetic resonance and computed tomography imaging. *Histol. Histopathol.* **2015**, *30*, 601–613. [PubMed]

33. Zhou, T.; Hong, G.; Fu, T.M.; Yang, X.; Schuhmann, T.G.; Viveros, R.D.; Lieber, C.M. Syringe-injectable mesh electronics integrate seamlessly with minimal chronic immune response in the brain. *Proc. Natl. Acad. Sci. USA* **2017**, *114*, 5894–5899. [CrossRef] [PubMed]

34. Xie, C.; Liu, J.; Fu, T.M.; Dai, X.; Zhou, W.; Lieber, C.M. Three-dimensional macroporous nanoelectronic networks as minimally invasive brain probes. *Nat. Mater.* **2015**, *14*, 1286. [CrossRef] [PubMed]

35. Kozai, T.D.Y.; Gugel, Z.; Li, X.; Gilgunn, P.J.; Khilwani, R.; Ozdoganlar, O.B.; Fedder, G.K.; Weber, D.J.; Cui, X.T. Chronic tissue response to carboxymethyl cellulose based dissolvable insertion needle for ultra-small neural probes. *Biomaterials* **2014**, *35*, 9255–9268. [CrossRef] [PubMed]

36. Lind, G.; Linsmeier, C.E.; Thelin, J.; Schouenborg, J. Gelatine-embedded electrodes—A novel biocompatible vehicle allowing implantation of highly flexible microelectrodes. *J. Neural Eng.* **2010**, *7*, 046005. [CrossRef] [PubMed]
37. Lecomte, A.; Castagnola, V.; Descamps, E.; Dahan, L.; Blatché, M.C.; Dinis, T.M.; Leclerc, E.; Egles, C.; Bergaud, C. Silk and PEG as means to stiffen a parylene probe for insertion in the brain: Toward a double time-scale tool for local drug delivery. *J. Micromech. Microeng.* **2015**, *25*, 125003. [CrossRef]

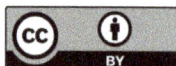

![micromachines]

MDPI

Article

Demonstration of a Robust All-Silicon-Carbide Intracortical Neural Interface

Evans K. Bernardin [1], Christopher L. Frewin [2], Richard Everly [3], Jawad Ul Hassan [4] and Stephen E. Saddow [5,*

[1] Department of Biomedical Engineering, University of South Florida, Tampa, FL 33620, USA; ebernardin@mail.usf.edu

[2] Department of Bioengineering, University of Texas at Dallas, Dallas, TX 75080, USA; Christopher.frewin@utdallas.edu

[3] Nanotechnology Research and Education Center @ USF, Tampa, FL 33617, USA; everly@usf.edu

[4] Department of Physics, Chemistry and Biology (IFM), Linköping University, SE-581 83 Linköping, Sweden; jawad.ul-hassan@liu.se

[5] Department of Electrical Engineering, University of South Florida, Tampa, FL 33620, USA

* Correspondence: saddow@ieee.org; Tel.: +1-813-974-4773

Received: 31 July 2018; Accepted: 12 August 2018; Published: 18 August 2018

Abstract: Intracortical neural interfaces (INI) have made impressive progress in recent years but still display questionable long-term reliability. Here, we report on the development and characterization of highly resilient monolithic silicon carbide (SiC) neural devices. SiC is a physically robust, biocompatible, and chemically inert semiconductor. The device support was micromachined from p-type SiC with conductors created from n-type SiC, simultaneously providing electrical isolation through the resulting p-n junction. Electrodes possessed geometric surface area (GSA) varying from 496 to 500 K μm^2. Electrical characterization showed high-performance p-n diode behavior, with typical turn-on voltages of ~2.3 V and reverse bias leakage below 1 nArms. Current leakage between adjacent electrodes was ~7.5 nArms over a voltage range of -50 V to 50 V. The devices interacted electrochemically with a purely capacitive relationship at frequencies less than 10 kHz. Electrode impedance ranged from 675 ± 130 kΩ (GSA = 496 μm^2) to 46.5 ± 4.80 kΩ (GSA = 500 K μm^2). Since the all-SiC devices rely on the integration of only robust and highly compatible SiC material, they offer a promising solution to probe delamination and biological rejection associated with the use of multiple materials used in many current INI devices.

Keywords: neural interface; silicon carbide; robust microelectrode

---

1. Introduction

Neuro-engineering is an emerging field which not only seeks to develop engineered therapeutic treatments for a variety of nervous system injuries and disorders, but also looks to understand the functionality of the nervous system. One promising application of neurotechnology is the brain-machine interface (BMI), also known as the brain-computer interface (BCI) [1–5]. Many BCI systems target neuronal electrophysiological signals which interact with signal transducing systems and processing algorithms so they can control external electromechanical devices, such as computers or robotic assistants/limbs [6]. Stimulating BCI systems have modulated the electrochemical environment around neurons to inhibit their activity, as has been demonstrated for Parkinson's, epilepsy, and pain management; more recently they have been used to replace lost sensory information, as seen with commercial implants like the Cochlear and Argus II [7–9]. Using BCI as a bi-directional pathway between electrically active cells and an external device would provide an optimal platform which could utilize closed-loop control, enabling adaptive therapeutic functionality and providing full sensory response for robotic limb replacements.

While many BCI systems operate using noninvasive physiological interfaces, for example, the electroencephalogram (EEG), invasive devices allow intimate contact with cellular populations, thus increasing spatial and temporal resolution as well as signal-to-noise ratio (SNR). The intracortical neural implant (INI) is an emerging technology which targets neurons in the motor cortex, but has also demonstrated applications in the sensory and visual cortex [1,2]. INI can extract high-quality electrophysiological signals, such as action potentials for the control of complicated external mechanical devices [4,10].

Unlike current state-of-the-art implantable neural devices with macro-electrodes, e.g., deep-brain and spinal cord stimulators, cortical INI devices have experienced major issues which have prevented their increased acceptance and use in clinical therapeutic applications. One of the foremost problems is a questionable long-term reliability, which has manifested itself as signal degradation leading to complete loss of device functionality [11–13]. The reliability issue has been attributed to both biotic and abiotic sources. While many INI are initially tolerated by the brain after surgical implantation, the inflammatory response progresses in a pattern akin to neural degenerative diseases, silencing nearby neural signals and eventually encapsulating the device in scar tissue [14,15]. Abiotic mechanisms have been attributed to chemical interactions, such as oxidation, leading to corrosion of the device material [16–18]. Water absorption has also played a part and has been linked to physical degradation, swelling, delamination, and cracking in multiple-material-layer devices [12,16,17,19,20]. These issues must be addressed with the goal of extending the viability of these devices from only a few years to multiple decades so that they can be sanctioned for widespread use in humans.

One approach to addressing abiotic mechanisms has been the materials required to fabricate the INI [21]. Many state-of-the-art INI devices are constructed using stacks of multiple materials, such as silicon (Si), titanium (Ti), platinum (Pt), parylene C, and polyimide [5,22–24]. Not only must each material tolerate the biological environment without exacerbating the inflammatory response, each of the materials used must physically withstand the environment as well as interact well with each other. Our group believes an alternative material strategy may address both issues simultaneously. The device would be constructed exclusively of one material which has a demonstrated track record of physical robustness, chemical inertness, and a great degree of biological tolerance: crystalline silicon carbide (SiC) [25–31]. Additionally, the amorphous form of SiC (*a*-SiC) has also been demonstrated as an effective insulating coating which does not take up water and is very compatible with neural cells [25,32,33].

Here we report on the development, fabrication, and characterization of monolithic SiC microelectrode arrays (MEAs). These arrays were composed completely of one material, SiC. Hexagonal crystalline SiC (4H-SiC) served as both the substrate and conductive electrode elements. Use of alternate polarity SiC, i.e., n- and p-type regions, creates a p-n diode to provide isolation. *a*-SiC served as a conformal, top-side insulator coating to prevent the electrochemical environment from shorting the p-n diode. The novel idea behind an all-SiC device is the concept that a single-material system would be inherently more robust since it does not rely on the heterogeneous integration of multiple dissimilar materials. Another benefit is that SiC uses the same well-established processing techniques developed within the silicon device industry. The result of this study shows that all-SiC microelectrodes interact with an electrochemical environment primarily through capacitive mechanisms with an impedance comparable to gold electrodes. Furthermore, while it cannot deliver charge as efficiently as other conventionally used microelectrode materials, like iridium oxide, the expanded water window of SiC increases the capacitive charge delivery to levels on par with that necessary to evoke physiological activity.

2. Materials and Methods

2.1. All-SiC Device Fabrication Process

The all-SiC neural devices reported here were developed using standard semiconductor device fabrication processes. SiC epitaxial wafers were grown at Linköping University (Linköping, Sweden) via hot-wall chemical vapor deposition (CVD) [34,35]. A ~5 μm thick, low-doped (aluminum) p-type epitaxial layer of 4H-SiC was homoepitaxially grown on a quarter wafer of 4° off-axis 4H-SiC (0001) [36]. The doping density of the p-type base epitaxial layer was ~1×10^{16} cm^{-3}. This was followed by the deposition of an opposite polarity 2.5 μm thick, heavily doped (nitrogen) n$^+$ film which is known to display semi-metallic conduction [36]. The two layers form a pn junction diode, which provided electrical isolation between adjacent electrode mesa traces and offered minimal leakage current.

An insulating *a*-SiC film providing conformal surface insulation was deposited using a PlasmaTherm model 730 Plasma-Enhanced Chemical Vapor Deposition (PECVD) system. The plasma field frequency was set to 13.56 MHz, substrate temperature to 250 °C, and pressure to 900 mTorr. Silane (SiH$_4$) and Methane (CH$_4$) were used as the reactive gas species at flow rates of 360 sccm and 12 sccm, respectively [25]. Argon (Ar) was used as the carrier gas with a flow rate of 500 sccm. Kapton™ tape was placed on a blank Silicon (Si) companion wafer prior to *a*-SiC deposition for thickness measurement of the deposited film using a Dektak D150 profilometer. The scans additionally allowed determination of film stress by scanning the deposited wafer pre and post *a*-SiC deposition and utilizing the Stoney equation [37].

The fabrication sequence to realize the all-SiC microelectrode devices was detailed in Bernardin et al. [38]; however, it has since been refined as explained here. Figure 1a shows the mask design used to produce the single-ended all-SiC electrodes (top) and the test structures (bottom). The as-grown p-n$^+$ epiwafers' surfaces were first functionalized with HMDS (Hexamethyldisilazane Microchemicals GmBH, Ulm, Germany) followed by 15–18 μm of AZ-12XT-20PL positive photoresist (Microchemicals GmBH). The photoresist was patterned by UV exposure (110 mJ/cm^2) using a Quintel Mask Aligner and developed using the AZ300 developer (Microchemicals GmBH). The thicker photoresist layer than previously reported allowed the Adixen AMS 100 deep reactive ion etcher (DRIE) to etch through 3 μm of the n$^+$-doped epilayer, ensuring p base layer exposure and n$^+$ conductive trace isolation. The DRIE etched at an approximate rate of 1 μm per minute of SiC with a 0.5:1 mask selectivity. The samples were then placed in the PECVD chamber for the deposition of 200 nm of *a*-SiC as previously described. AZ-12XT (Microchemicals GmBH) was used to define windows in the *a*-SiC film, thus allowing access to the contact pads for device packaging, as well as to expose the active recording sites. The windows were then opened by removing the exposed *a*-SiC layer via reactive ion etching (RIE) in a PlasmaTherm etcher. The process gases used for the RIE steps were 37 sccm of CF$_4$ and 13 sccm of O$_2$. The process ran for 210 s, with power set to 200 W and pressure at 50 mTorr. The formed window recesses were ~210 nm deep as measured via stylus profilometry.

High-quality ohmic contacts are necessary to transfer signals to and from the semiconductor and the external circuitry [36]. Therefore, the process to create metal contact pads which allow connection to commercial connectors has been optimized to improve device electrical connectivity. The metal lift-off process was defined using a two-layer photoresist step as follows: A 2 μm lift-off resist (LOR10B MicroChem Corp., Westborough, MA, USA), followed by 5 μm of AZ-12XT-20PL, a positive resist. Once exposed to UV and developed, a thin film of titanium (Ti), followed by Nickel (Ni), was deposited in sequence via RF sputtering without breaking vacuum. Liftoff was performed in a Microposit™ Remover 1165 bath. The contacts were then annealed in a rapid thermal processor (RTP) at 1000 °C for 30 s to form a Ti/Ni silicide. A secondary metal lift-off process was performed using Ti and Gold (Au) deposited onto the annealed Ti/Ni stack. The final stack was annealed at 450 °C for 30 min and ohmic contact confirmed via IV measurements.

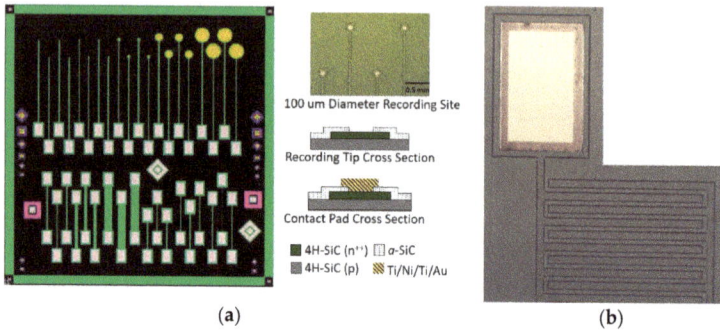

(a)   **(b)**

Figure 1. All-SiC planar device used for electrical and electrochemical testing. (**a**) Single-ended electrodes (top) with various recording areas (diameters of 25, 50, 100, 400, and 800 µm) and test structures (bottom) consisting of p-n diodes and resistor mesas of various length and width. An optical micrograph of fabricated all-SiC single-ended electrodes, with 100 µm diameter active recording sites, is provided (top right). Bright areas are windows in the *a*-SiC insulator. (**b**) One end of the all-SiC interdigitated electrode (IDE) showing a metal contact pad (top) and a portion of the two interdigitated 50 µm wide mesas of n$^+$ on p base layer with a pitch of 25 µm.

2.2. All-SiC Evaluation Devices

Two structures were fabricated to characterize the electrical capabilities of the all-SiC devices. In Bernardin et al. [38], all of the electrodes tested were of a single size with a 25 µm recording tip diameter, but varied in lead length from 4 to 10 mm. While we established that trace length did not significantly affect the overall electrical impedance, it has been shown that the geometrical surface area (GSA) of an electrode can be an important factor in overall performance [24]. Therefore, 20 single-ended planar electrodes were constructed with different recording tip diameters of 25, 50, 100, 400, and 800 µm to extract performance as a function of GSA, as shown in Figure 1a. Four (4) planar electrodes of each GSA were fabricated per die. All electrodes had the same lead wire (i.e., the n$^+$-doped mesa) length of 3.5 mm and were ~3 µm thick and 50 µm wide.

An important consideration for any electrical device is signal leakage and cross-talk between traces. While many of the INI devices use an insulating material as the basis for metal trace isolation, the semiconductor properties of our single crystal material allow the use of p-n junction isolation to serve this function. Furthermore, the surface coating of *a*-SiC prevents the p-doped substrate and n-doped trace regions from being shorted together when immersed in electrolytic media. To evaluate the efficacy of this insulation strategy, interdigitated electrode (IDE) devices were fabricated to evaluate the insulating properties and reliability of the *a*-SiC coating and p-n isolation between adjacent traces. The IDE devices consisted of two electrodes which were 50 µm wide and 3 µm high. Each of the electrodes contained 22 digits with a length of 1 mm and were spaced 100 µm away from their adjacent digit. Both electrodes were fitted within each other at a spacing (pitch) of 25 µm, with a total enclosed interaction length between both electrodes of 4.5 cm.

2.3. SiC Doping and PN Isolation Evaluation

The doping density of the conductive electrode layer was calculated through the characterization of a Schottky diode using the method described by Schroder [39]. Briefly, capacitance/voltage (C/V) and current/voltage measurements (IV) were used on the epitaxial stack prior to device fabrication. An LEI 2017b Mercury (Hg) Probe (Lehighton Electronics, Inc., Lehighton, PA, USA) created a Schottky junction when the Hg came into contact with the top n$^+$ epitaxial layer of the wafer. The Hg probe is equipped with a Schottky dot diameter of 0.64 mm and a 3.81 mm diameter Hg return contact. IV measurements were initially performed, sweeping the voltage from −5 V to 5 V at a rate of 0.5 V/s with a Keithley 2400 SourceMeter (Tektronix, Inc., Beaverton, OR, USA) to extract the forward bias turn-on voltage of the Schottky diode. C/V measurements were then made using a Keithley 590 CV Analyzer (Tektronix, Inc.) The C/V measurements were performed by sweeping the voltage 1 V under the reverse bias of the Schottky junction. Measurements were taken at a frequency of 1 MHz and at a rate of 150 mV/s. The C/V measurements were then used to calculate doping density.

As previously described, p-n junctions formed during 4H-SiC epitaxial growth were used to provide electrical isolation between electrodes. PN diodes characteristically pass current in only one direction after a potential is provided, known as the turn-on voltage, while they resist current flow in the opposite direction until a second potential is achieved, known as the reverse breakdown voltage. IV measurements were utilized to establish the turn-on potential, characteristic reverse leakage current, and reverse breakdown voltage. PN diode test devices were included on the all-SiC single-ended electrode die (Figure 1a bottom) consisting of a square, n-doped epilayer mesa with a metal contact which was surrounded by a second metal contact to the p-doped base epilayer separated by 10 µm. The Keithley 2400 SourceMeter was used to facilitate IV measurements from potential limits of −20 V to 5 V at a rate of 0.5 V/s. Turn-on voltage was estimated by plotting current vs voltage on a semi-logarithmic current scale, and extrapolating the linear forward current to where it intersects the voltage axis. The reverse breakdown voltage occurs at the point where the diode's current increases rapidly with the applied reverse voltage and we used 1 nA as our quantitative measure of reverse breakdown voltage for comparative purposes. The reverse leakage current was estimated from the root mean square of the current between the turn-on and breakdown potentials.

The IDE devices (Figure 1b) were evaluated to examine the isolation between distinct traces. In this case, complete isolation consisted of two back-to-back p-n junction diodes, both requiring large biases to surpass. The IDEs were characterized using the Keithley 2400 SourceMeter. The source contact was connected to one of the two outer electrodes of the IDE, and the return contact was connected to the center, or common, electrode. IV measurements were performed from potential limits of −50 to 50 V at a rate of 5 V/s. Device failure was marked using the same criteria as used for the junction diode evaluation (i.e., when the current exceeded 1 nA). We tested a total of 10 IDE structures.

2.4. Electrochemical Characterization of 4H-SiC Material

All electrochemical evaluations were performed in phosphate-buffered solution (PBS) of composition 137 mMol NaCl, 27 mMol KCl, 100 mMol Na_2HPO_4, and 17.6 nMol KH_2PO_4. The pH was titrated using HCl to reach 7.4 pH. All measurements were taken at laboratory temperature of ~22 °C. A model 604E Series Electrochemical Analyzer/ Workstation (CH Instruments Inc., Austin, TX, USA) and vendor-provided software were used to characterize the 4H-SiC electrodes using cyclic voltammetry (CV) and electrochemical impedance spectroscopy (EIS). A three-electrode system was used consisting of a 127 µm diameter, ~5 cm wide Pt wire (A-M Systems, Sequim, WA, USA), a 5 cm long Ag | AgCl reference electrode of 254 µm diameter, and the all-SiC electrode working electrode.

The EIS and CV measurements were performed on four (4) die containing 20 electrodes of five different sizes (N = 16 for each electrode size). EIS measurements consisted of the application of a 10-mV root mean square (rms) sinusoidal wave at a frequency range between 0.1 Hz and 100 KHz, and recording of the returned current response 12 times per decade. A circuit model representation for the 4H-SiC electrochemical interface was selected from [40,41] as a basis for interpreting electrochemical impedance spectroscopy data. This model was used in ZSimpWin software (Amtek Scientific Instruments Inc., Austin, TX, USA) in an iteration mode to calculate values for the circuit components.

The initial CV measurement started at the open circuit potential, swept to the negative potential of −0.6 V at a rate of 50 mV/s, reversed direction to the positive potential of 0.8 V, and returned to the negative potential, repeating the cycle three times. The potential limits of −0.6 to 0.8 V, which correspond to the limits reported for Pt, were chosen to allow direct comparison with previously published results [24,42]. A second CV measurement was performed using the same boundary conditions, but the potential limit was widened 0.1 V after each complete scan. Once it was noticed that the onset of a large current occurred, which was a typical marker of water electrolysis, that potential became that electrode's extended limit. The sweeps were performed until both oxidation and reduction potential limits were established, after which the final three CV sweeps were performed.

3. Results

3.1. Device Characterization

Capacitance versus voltage measurements of Schottky contacts to the n^+ layer verified that the doping on the n^+ epi layer was on the order of 3.45×10^{18} cm^{-3} which was consistent with our epi-doping estimates of ~3 × 10^{18} cm^{-3} from prior growth runs using the same level of intentional nitrogen doping [38]. Typical doping of the p-type base epitaxial layer was ~1 × 10^{16} cm^{-3}. Figure 2a displays a semi-log IV plot from a selected p-n junction diode. The p-n diode measurements showed a high-performing p-n diode with a typical turn-on voltage of ~2.3 V and a reverse bias leakage that fell below our equipment limit of less than 1 nA. The turn-on voltage value is comparable to values reported in the literature [36,43,44].

The n-p-n junction, which isolates adjacent leads through the substrate, was also tested by repeating the IV measurements using the contact pad of one device to the contact pad of its neighboring device. This test helped demonstrate the effectiveness of the n-p-n junction in isolating individual electrodes (and devices) from one another. These measurements were performed under dry (air) conditions at a voltage range of −50 to 50 V. Figure 2b shows that the n-p-n diode has a slight current leakage of less than 7.5 nA$_{rms}$ over the measured voltage range.

Of the 20 IDE devices tested (Figure 2c), only 2 demonstrated a significant current flow at the turn-on potential for the junction diodes (2.3 V) and 4 IDEs showed current flow at cathodic potentials between −16 V to −50 V. The remaining 14 forward-biased electrodes continued to block currents to at least −50. Under reverse bias, 5 IDEs experienced leakage currents of more than 1 nA between 6 V to 35 V, while the remaining 15 continued to block up to 50 V.

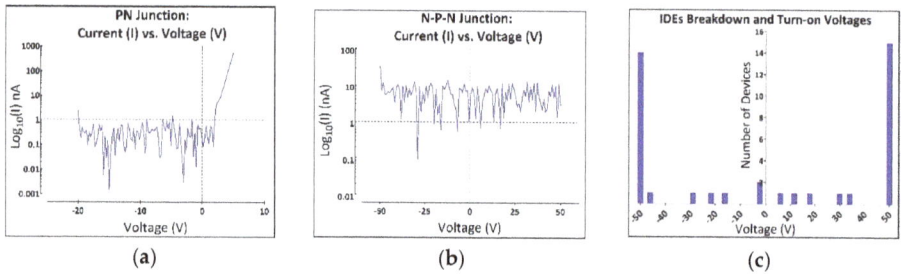

Figure 2. All-SiC device electrical characterization. The electrical properties of the device were first tested by performing current vs voltage (IV) measurements on the fabricated test structures. (**a**) IV measurements were performed over a range of −20 V to 5 V on the p-n diodes post fabrication. The results, shown on a semi-log plot, demonstrate a typical forward-biased turn-on voltage of ~2.3 V and a leakage current well below 1 nA out to −20 V. (**b**) Conductive trace mesa isolation measurements via IV sweeping from −50 to 50 V in air. Note that the long p-n junctions provided excellent isolation with a slight current leakage of less than 7.5 nA$_{rms}$ over the measured voltage range. (**c**) Histogram from the insulation/isolation measurements performed on 20 IDE structures of Figure 1b. IV characterization for 20 IDE devices were taken from −50 V to 50 V. Of the 20 devices, only 2 showed significant current flow at the p-n junction's turn-on voltage (−2.3 V), while 4 IDEs showed current flow at cathodic potentials between −16 V to −50 V and the remaining 14 continued to block to at least −50 V. Under reverse bias conditions, 5 IDEs experienced leakage current between 6 V to 35 V, while the remaining 15 continued to block up to 50 V.

3.2. Electrochemical Characterization

The results from the EIS performed on the 4H-SiC electrodes in 7.4 pH aerated PBS are shown in Figure 3a. The electrode interaction with the electrolyte displayed a nearly purely capacitive property at frequencies less than 10 kHz, as is displayed by the phase angle of ~80 °C for the electrodes with less than 7.85 K μm² geometrical surface area. Another notable trend was that the impedance decreased with an increase in electrode area. Figure 3b displays the impedance and phase obtained from the electrodes when measured at 1 kHz, the frequency associated with the action potential associated with cortical neural processes. The smallest electrode (496 μm²) had an average impedance of 675 ± 130 kΩ, which decreased to 46.5 ± 4.80 kΩ for the largest, 500 K μm² area electrodes. The trend lines added to the graph show a relative linearity associated with all the electrodes.

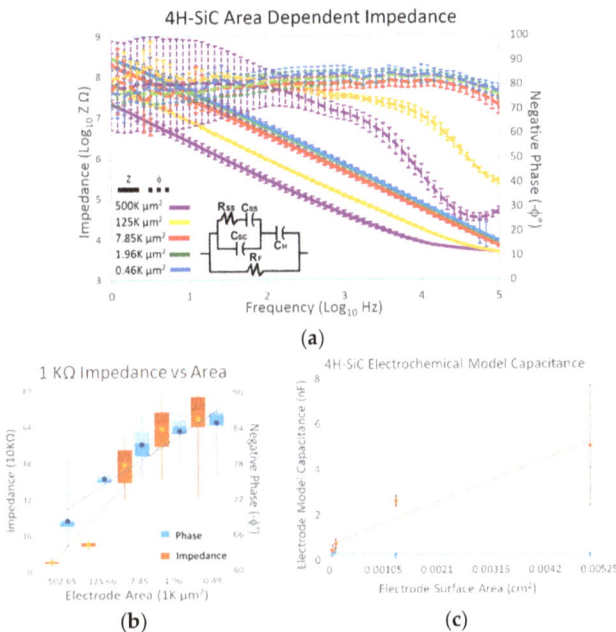

Figure 3. (a) Electrochemical impedance spectroscopy (EIS) performed on 4H-SiC electrodes of varying geometrical surface areas (GSA). The error bars represent the standard deviation. The inset shows the basic circuit model which produced an impedance profile which was similar to that which was obtained in experimental investigation. (b) A box and whiskers plot for the impedance and phase of the 4H-SiC electrodes at the frequency of 1 kHz across the 5 tested areas. The mean impedance and phase is represented with a dot. (c) The value of the space charge capacitance (CSC) obtained through the electrochemical modeling of the EIS for the 4H-SiC electrodes divided by the geometric surface area of each electrode. All tests were performed in PBS that was naturally aerated (i.e., no N_2/Ar gas bubbling to remove dissolved O_2) and possessed a pH of 7.4.

The inset in Figure 3a shows the circuit model which was used in the ZSimpWin software to predict the impedance response similar to the data obtained from our actual electrodes. The circuit model consists of the Helmholtz double-layer capacitance (C_H) and Faradaic resistance (R_F) normally seen in a Randles circuit model, but includes an additional component exclusive to semiconductors [40,41]. The additional component models the capacitance of the space charge region (C) and the accompanying charging component corresponding to the speed of the change in surface state (R_{SS} and C_{SS}). These components are directly derived from the metal/semiconductor junction, where the interaction of the electrolyte and semiconductor leads to the fixation of the Fermi level and a bending of the conduction and valence energy bands which, in turn, drive the semiconductor surface into depletion. The Faradaic impedance (R_F) started near 1 GΩ for the largest electrode, increasing to approximately 6 GΩ for the smallest electrodes. The Helmholtz double capacitance (C_H) was on the order of 3 nC for the large-scale electrodes and approached 0.5 nC for the small electrodes. The surface state resistance (R_{SS}) was in the hundreds of kΩ with the smallest electrodes and was only in the tens of kΩ for the largest electrodes.

Figure 4a displays select representative CV curves for each of the electrodes reported in this study taken across the potential water limit for Pt. Figure 4a, on the other hand, shows select curves using the extended water window from the all-SiC electrodes. Both micrographs demonstrate a decrease in the hysteresis cycle when the area is decreased. Once again, CV data supports a dominant capacitive interaction mechanism with the electrolytic ions. The current remains constant for the CV sweep, until it nears the potential limit on either side of the test. At this point, the charge potential is reversed, leading to a large influx of current which follows the resistor-capacitor (RC) charging process. After the charging, the current once again remains constant until the next potential ramp shift. While many of the devices produced curves that were strictly capacitive, a few of the electrodes show increased Faradaic oxidation currents. These oxidation reactions were noticed exclusively on the tests where the potential limits were being evaluated, and an example can be seen in Figure 4b on the 7.85 K μm^2 area electrode. A second observation was that the coupled reduction current was not present on the same electrodes. While these electrodes posed an electrochemical difference, the overall interaction was relatively consistent. This is seen in the variability lower than 5% for the potential limits. The cathodic potential limit was observed to be -1.98 ± 0.08 V while the anodic limit was 2.77 ± 0.07 V.

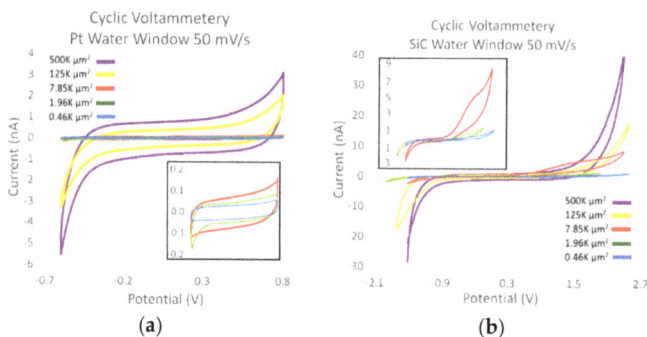

Figure 4. (a) CV plot showing a single curve from the cyclic voltammetry evaluation of a select 4H-SiC electrode. The curves were bounded at the potentials typically used for platinum or iridium electrodes of -0.6 V and 0.8 V. The inset shows detail for the three smallest electrodes. (b) A plot of the second CV curve from a select electrode. The ramp rate was the same as for (a), but the potential limits were extended to the onset of a large current flux. All tests were performed in PBS that was naturally aerated (i.e., no application of gas bubbling) and possessed a pH of 7.4.

The difference between the electrodes is more apparent when evaluating the overall charge storage capacity (CSC) and charge delivered per phase. Table 1 displays the mean and standard deviation of the mean for all the tested electrodes. The electrodes once again demonstrate a simple area relationship. The smaller electrodes have the largest values for CSC, which decreases with the increase in area. The largest electrodes deliver the largest amount of charge per phase, which decreases with a decrease in area.

Table 1. Cathodic and anodic charge storage capacity and charge per phase *.

Electrode Area (μm^2)	Cathodic				Anodic			
	Charge Storage Capacity (mC/cm²)		Charge Per Phase (nC)		Charge Storage Capacity (mC/cm²)		Charge Per Phase (nC)	
	−0.6 to 0.8 V	−2.0 to 2.8 V	−0.6 to 0.8 V	−2.0 to 2.8 V	−0.6 to 0.8 V	−2.0 to 2.8 V	−0.6 to 0.8 V	−2.0 to 2.8 V
502,651	4.38×10^{-3} (1.24×10^{-4})	8.00×10^{-2} (0.644)	22 (0.625)	380 (0.642)	3.70×10^{-3} (4.81×10^{-5})	0.257 (0.52)	18.4 (0.242)	1340 (0.520)
125,663	1.18×10^{-2} (1.42×10^{-3})	8.61×10^{-2} (1.60×10^{-2})	14.8 (1.78)	108 (20.1)	7.02×10^{-3} (2.9×10^{-4})	0.115 (2.28×10^{-2})	8.82 (0.369)	144 (28.7)
7854	2.98×10^{-2} (2.60×10^{-3})	1.01 (0.185)	2.34 (0.204)	79.5 (14.5)	6.22×10^{-2} (3.10×10^{-3})	1.29 (0.113)	4.89 (0.244)	102 (8.87)
1964	6.46×10^{-2} (2.07×10^{-3})	1.51 (0.167)	1.27 (4.06×10^{-2})	29.6 (3.27)	0.177 (9.22×10^{-3})	1.37 (0.187)	3.48 (0.181)	27 (3.66)
491	0.194 (5.67×10^{-3})	5.53 (1.38)	0.953 (2.78×10^{-2})	30.4 (6.63)	0.406 (2.22×10^{-2})	5.42 (0.666)	2.00 (0.109)	41.7 (3.81)

* Data displayed for both the standard Pt water window as well as for the water window empirically derived for SiC. Standard deviation of the mean is shown in parentheses.

4. Discussion

Both the neuroscience and biomedical communities have been focused on improving the overall reliability of implantable microelectrode systems. Complications have been demonstrated to arise from both biotic and abiotic mechanisms. Biotic systems have been connected to the inflammatory response, which has been linked to material modulus mismatch and foreign body response, resulting in a tissue response on par with neural degeneration [45–47]. Material degeneration, oxidation, water absorption, swelling, stress fractures, and delamination have all been associated with abiotic mechanisms [12,20,48–50].

For many implantable neural interface (INI) devices, the electrical interaction with the physiological environment has been an electrode. While electrodes are in their simplest form devices composed of at least one conductive material and one insulating material, overall device reliability remains complicated. The fact that the device needs to be fabricated from at least two materials raises concern on dissimilar material surface interaction in order to minimize delamination [12,51–53]. The materials are constantly exposed to a harsh, oxidizing environment with large variation in pH, which has required a careful evaluation of chemical resistivity to avoid degeneration and production of chemical species which are toxic or exacerbation of the inflammatory response [45,54]. Another consideration has been the characterization of the electrochemical interface, where Faradaic reactions have required careful consideration to avoid the generation of harmful reactive species and hydrogen/oxygen gasses [55,56]. Finally, a recent focus has been on material hardness and flexibility as there has been evidence showing that a mismatch between the mechanics of the material and soft tissues which are in constant micromotion has generated additional biological damage [47,48,57]. For clarity it should be noted that the all-SiC concept presented here does not address the micromotion issue.

While conductors and insulators are normally the materials of choice for electrode fabrication, another class of materials, semiconductors, offers an interesting fabrication methodology that allows electrode construction from a single-material system. The advantage of this method is that delamination is highly improbable. Semiconductors, unlike conductors, require a certain amount of applied potential to promote electrons from the valence band, over the forbidden energy band gap and into the conduction band where they can move freely; however, while this energy level is much smaller than that required for insulators, it still is much larger than the potential found in neuronal signals. This issue has been solved by the fact that semiconductors have been modified into a much more conductive state through the addition of atoms into their crystalline matrix, referred to as dopants. Unlike traditional metallic conductors, these dopant atoms enable conduction through either the donation of an electron into the conduction band of the semiconductor, thus producing n-type "electron-rich" material, or by accepting valence band electrons, thus creating "holes" to create a p-type, or positively charged, semiconductor. By switching the dopant type (donors for n-type or acceptors for p-type) during semiconductor growth, a junction is created between the n- and p-type materials. At this PN junction, electrons from the n side diffuse to the p side, while holes from the p side of the junction diffuse in the opposite direction. This creates a region devoid of mobile carriers which then blocks the flow of further mobile charge carriers. This rectifying junction thus blocks current flow and only through the application of a bias potential, called forward bias, may appreciable diffusion current flow again. In a silicon PN diode this potential is ~0.7 V, whereas in 4H-SiC it is ~2.3 V. Thus, a wide-bandgap semiconductor is advantageous since the diode remains in its off state at considerably higher potentials.

Semiconductor junction electrode isolation was demonstrated in the Utah intracortical array, now known as the Blackrock microelectrode array [58,59]. Although the feasibility of the method was demonstrated, p-dopant thermo-migration shorted multiple electrodes together and a large surface contamination required silicon dioxide surface passivation. One important factor which was mentioned concerned stimulation. At voltages above 0.7 V, the silicon junction forward turn-on voltage, the diode turned on and injected current into the substrate, thus shorting all of the electrodes together. Later reports have shown that silicon and its related material derivatives (SiO_2 and Si_3N_4) have been connected to chronic neuroinflammation, most likely due to chemical reactivity and physical modulus mismatch [11–13,60]. Many other semiconductor materials demonstrate traits that would not allow their use in reliable INIs, such as gallium arsenide, and have demonstrated biological toxicity [61]. Diamond and gallium nitride have demonstrated elements of anodic oxidation and subsequent material corrosion [62,63]. Boron nitride has demonstrated an extremely low electron mobility, leading to increased resistivity and signal attenuation [64]. While these issues from many semiconductor materials limit their ability for use in INI applications, one semiconductor material, silicon carbide (SiC), appears ideally suited for reasons which will now be explained.

Silicon carbide is a semiconductor which possesses extreme resistance to corrosive chemistries, experiences only limited oxidation, and has demonstrated no appreciable toxicity [65–68]. We have demonstrated that hexagonal silicon carbide junction isolation electrode devices have a much higher forward bias turn-on potential than Si (2.3 V vs. 0.7 V). The Utah microelectrode array was driven into forward bias conditions during the application of anodic potential stimulation, at levels of nominally ~0.8 V, which ensures that the device remains within the safe water window for Pt. While our device used a similar junction isolation technique, there are major differences which enhanced our successful application of a single-material electrode. First, our electrodes are composed of heavily doped n-type 4H-SiC, while our substrate is lightly doped p-type 4H-SiC, which forms the junction isolation bias. The 4H-SiC device isolation would actively pass minority carrier current into the substrate with cathodic stimulation greater than −2.3 V, which thus represents the upper limit in applied bias. This junction configuration also required the application of potentials well in excess of 50 V to bias the junction into reverse breakdown. While 5 electrodes (25%) demonstrated a failure to sufficiently block reverse potentials between 6 V and 50 V and demonstrated significant breakdown current, this failure was well above the anodic water window of 2.8 V. Therefore, we conclude the possibility of device failure due to anodic bias to be very small.

It was noticed that the devices were not functioning in the same way as reported in the Utah investigation once the turn-on potential was reached. Application of cathodic potential to the IDE electrodes revealed that only two (2) demonstrated a significant current flow at potentials above −2.3 V, the turn-on potential for the junction diodes. Only 4 more electrodes showed current flow, and that happened at cathodic potentials between −16 V and −50 V. The remaining 14 forward-biased electrodes continued to block current to at least −50 V. At forward junction potential, the current was offered two parallel pathways. One was a large surface area, essentially the entire 2-dimensional contact area enclosed within the electrode and the trace added together, with a very short length that connected to the entire device surface area of the n-type substrate. The second path consisted of a surface area composed of the 5 μm thick p-type layer and the length of one side of the electrode (1 mm). The spacing between the electrodes was 100 μm. The substrate provides a good sink (<1 Ω resistance) which is more favorable than the pathway to the neighboring adjacent electrodes (>10 KΩ resistivity). Of course, the further away the electrodes are, the greater the signal attenuation. Unfortunately, one issue exists with injecting current into the substrate in that it is potentially in contact with the electrochemical environment. The substrate would have to be totally encapsulated in *a*-SiC to safely operate (i.e., the backside and edge of the device would need to be coated with *a*-SiC).

It should be noted that while our device is constructed from a single material, SiC, it was not a single piece of material. *a*-SiC has demonstrated excellent insulating capability, both in vitro and in vivo, and does not allow diffusion of metal ions (Na, K, Fe) as has been observed with SiO_2 [33,69]. The *a*-SiC coating that we chose was extremely thin, at ~200 nm, increasing the chance to reduce its insulating properties, which would potentially short both sides of the junction diode together. A thicker insulating film can be used in next-generation devices. We have shown that the pn junctions provide excellent substrate isolation, but this single junction isolation showed issues 20–30% of the time. The solution to both issues would be to bury the n^+ conductor layer under a p-type epitaxial layer and then form an n^+ conductive via through the p-type film to the device surface by use of ion implantation, which is a common process step in SiC power electronic devices. An added benefit of this increase in complexity would be that this could add active negative bias on the innermost layer, thus ensuring a counter bias against an active junction [70].

Many commonly used electrode materials use dual mechanisms to exchange charge within an electrochemical environment. These materials have a Faradaic element, wherein the charge is transferred through a surface oxidation or reduction reaction [71–73]. Materials that rely heavily on this charge transfer mechanism are the noble metals and iridium oxide (IrOx). The secondary method is through capacitive means, normally due to the absorption of water—which is an excellent insulator—across the surface of the electrode; this essentially leads to a separation of the charged ions in the electrolyte and electrons in the electrode, giving rise to a parallel plate capacitance [74]. Titanium nitride (TiN) and carbon materials have been associated with this capacitive mechanism to transfer charge [75–77]. With materials that primarily rely on capacitive charge transfer, large surface areas are desired to achieve increased charge transfer.

Five all-SiC electrodes of increasing geometrical surface area, via doubling electrode diameter from 25 to 800 μm (200 μm was left out to save real estate), were characterized electrochemically in PBS. Our previous investigation evaluated only 25 μm diameter electrodes and demonstrated capacitive interaction with little Faradaic activity [38]. That study demonstrated that 4H-SiC fits the same electrochemical model as reported for semiconductor electrodes [41,78]. 4H-SiC is extremely chemically resistant, only possessing limited surface oxidation for Faradaic chemical electron transfer, thereby increasing overall impedance and resulting in a reduced current transfer path. Instead, SiC demonstrated charge transfer through a parallel capacitive pathway. Unlike metallic conductors which rely mainly on double-layer capacitance for charge transfer, semiconductors possess an additional capacitive element. Charged ions on the surface of the semiconductor form a Schottky barrier, where the Fermi energy level equalizes, resulting in bending of the valence and conduction bands. Just as with the junction diode, majority carriers deplete through electron-hole annihilation, resulting in the presence of a space charge region [41,78]. This space charge region creates a large distance between the semiconductor bulk charge and the ions on the surface when compared with the double layer, leading to much smaller capacitances. At levels of doping below 10^{19} cm^{-3}, the space charge capacitance, which is in series with the double-layer capacitance, dominates the overall electrode capacitance [41,78].

Electrochemical characterization allowed us to evaluate the electrical functionality for the various 4H-SiC electrodes with respect to area. The electrochemical impedance of 4H-SiC electrodes versus geometric surface area, obtained at a frequency of 1 kHz, has been indicated in the box plots displayed in Figure 3b. The semiconductor electrochemical circuit model described earlier was used to calculate the resistive and capacitive elements for the electrodes, and the space charge capacitance and double-layer capacitance are displayed in Figure 3c. The overall resistance of the electrodes, modeling the electron exchange through chemical interaction between the electrode surface and the ionic media, increases exponentially with increasing surface area. This finding is in line with chemical reactions which are surface limited.

The differences between the two capacitive elements show that our devices possessed irregularities that need to be investigated. While the double-layer capacitance showed that an increase in capacitance accompanied increasing area, the capacitance associated with the space charge, or depletion, region of the semiconductor does not show an appreciable increase with surface area but stays nearly constant. Close examination of the electrodes with 7.85 K μm^2 or less showed an increasing capacitance with increasing surface area, while the electrodes of 125 K μm^2 or greater showed an inverse relationship. The static capacitance has also been displayed through individual CV micrographs where Figure 4a showed an increasing current saturation for each electrode size, from smallest to largest. However, Figure 4b shows that electrodes larger than 125 K μm^2 surface area possess nearly the same level of current saturation throughout the potential ramp. If the Helmholtz double-layer capacitance increases with surface area, and the potential rate remains the same, the lack of increased current associated with increased electrode diameter could be attributed to an issue with the space charge capacitance (C_{SC}). Research has indicated that increasing Schottky interface area does not change depletion depth, but instead leads to increased effects due to edge effects [79–81]. Additionally, while fringing effects usually increase the effective capacitance, resistive shunts are formed at the edge of Schottky barriers which effectively reduce current [81]. It should also be noted that decreased capacitance has been reported due to crystalline defects [82]. Epitaxial growth defects known as carrots (or comet trails) defects, island growth, and step bunching have been directly associated with Schottky rectification [83]. Although reported defect densities are low for 4H-SiC (10–20 per cm^2), our large-area electrodes increase the chance of containing at least one defect per device. To overcome some of these issues, double-trench isolation, consisting of multiple layers of alternating p- and n-type material, along with the addition of semi-insulating or intrinsic layers around the devices could provide additional leakage isolation and guard rings to counter edge effects [70]. As with all solutions, the process would require additional device complexity, with additional epitaxial growth stages, masking, and processing stages. However, it would also allow one additional benefit in that the double-trenched electrodes would not require an external *a*-SiC coating, making the device truly monolithic, composed of a single crystalline material, eliminating the possibility of insulation delamination altogether.

Microelectrode neural implantation devices normally have electrodes with areas in the thousands of μm^2, or even smaller. Issues were discovered with the 4H-SiC electrodes with geometric area larger than 8000 μm^2 used as comparison when evaluating the capabilities of these electrodes concerning cathodic charge storage capacity (CSC_c). The CSC_c for 4H-SiC electrodes with a potential limit of -0.6 V was 64 $\mu C/cm^2$ for electrodes of 7854 μm^2 area, increasing to 194 $\mu C/cm^2$ for 490 μm^2. Increasing the potential window to -2.0 V, the CSC_c was 1.51 mC/cm^2 for an area of 7854 μm^2 and 5.53 mC/cm^2 for a 490 μm^2 area. Comparatively, these electrodes demonstrate charge storage comparable to that reported for Pt electrodes (0.8–1.6 mC/cm^2 for 6500 μm^2) [84], and only slightly lower than that reported for TiN (2.47 mC/cm^2 for 4000 μm^2) [85]. 4H-SiC has demonstrated an electrochemical interaction dominated through capacitive electron transfer, much like TiN. Materials like poly(3,4-ethylenedioxythiophene) (PEDOT) (11.4 mC/cm^2 for 4000 μm^2) [86], activated iridium oxide (AIROF) (24.0 mC/cm^2 for 1000 μm^2) [87], and electrodeposited iridium oxide (EIROF) (48.7 mC/cm^2 for 385 μm^2) [33] achieve electron transfer through Faradaic chemical reaction mechanisms, leading to larger CSCc values exceeding capacitive 4H-SiC by at least a factor of 10.

However, there are many improvements that can be made to put SiC on a slightly better stimulation footing. The first is to increase the doping density. A boron-doped diamond coating (2×10^{21} cm^{-3}) was used on a 5000 μm^2 area electrode with a CSC_c of 10 mC/cm^2, which is comparable to the value reported for PEDOT [88]. The increased charge storage required multiple improvements, but 4H-SiC can use the same methods. Like 4H-SiC, the diamond required an extended potential of -2 to 1.5 V to increase its capacitive charge delivery. An increase in the doping levels of 4H-SiC to at least 10^{20} cm^{-3} will decrease the resistance of the electrode through an increase of majority charge carriers. The hole mobility of boron p-type doping in diamond was 50 cm^2/Vs at 300 K for 10^{21} cm^{-3} [89]. Achieving a doping level of 10^{20} cm^{-3}, an order of magnitude lower, would be more realistic for 4H-SiC as it requires ion implantation and subsequent dopant activation to achieve levels of doping above 10^{19} cm^{-3}. The electron mobility for n-type 4H-SiC would be comparable to the reported level for diamond, around 30 to 50 cm^2/Vs [90]. The diamond reported in [88] was highly nanostructured, producing a large increase in surface area. The SiC electrodes reported here were relatively flat. Many methods have been reported that can increase the surface area of SiC, like the formation of surface nanostructures or creating a more porous surface [91–93]. However, as we have demonstrated with our large-area electrodes, increasing the surface area of SiC may not produce a straightforward increase in electrochemical interaction and would require more investigation.

We have demonstrated a 4H-SiC electrode composed of single crystal, n-type semi-metallic material grown on a p-type base and reported on the suitability of this material system for biological utilization. Here we show that 4H-SiC interacts within an electrochemical environment primarily through a capacitive mechanism, dominated by a Schottky depletion capacitance instead of the classic double-layer capacitance. Additionally, the two-layer doping junction provided excellent, low-leakage isolation through the substrate, superior to that demonstrated by silicon devices. It is interesting to note that while PN junction isolation did perform as expected, there is the possibility of AC signal coupling across the junction for large signal amplitudes if the junction is not DC biased into reverse bias. Since we are able to control the potential between the p base layer and the n$^+$ semi-metallic layer (and, thus, the electrochemical environment) such that the PN diodes are in reverse bias, we do not anticipate that this will be an issue, but it certainly is an important issue that must be accounted for during device operation. Finally, the impedance of the material is comparable to those of many of the noble metals, like gold and platinum, but the charge storage capacity was lower than those of commonly used materials like iridium oxide and PEDOT. The electrodes have demonstrated adequate functionality and should be able to interact within the physiological environment and interface with electrically active tissue and cells.

5. Conclusions

A monolithic all-SiC MEA has been fabricated, where 4H-SiC served as the base (substrate), as well as the conducting traces (electrodes) of the device, while *a*-SiC was used as the insulating layer. Conventional silicon photolithographic processing techniques where employed in the design and fabrication of the all-SiC device. Electrical testing of the p-n$^+$ junction demonstrated that the 4H-SiC device is capable of blocking a forward-biased voltage up to 2.3 V and a reverse voltage of more than 10 V. Furthermore, electrochemical results show that the 4H-SiC microelectrodes interact with an electrochemical environment primarily through capacitive mechanisms and have impedance comparable to that of gold electrodes. However, the 4H-SiC devices cannot deliver charge as efficiently as other conventionally used microelectrode materials, such as iridium oxide. Using the already established silicon processing techniques, a variety of different forms of monolithic SiC neural devices are possible such as the single- or multiple-shank planar neural probes. All studies and data collected thus far indicate that the monolithic SiC neural device can aid in the advancement of chronic INI use in clinical settings. However, to demonstrate a fully functional INI device, further studies must be performed. Future work includes conducting accelerated aging experiments with our all-SiC device to test the performance and stability of the insulating *a*-SiC film. This future study will evaluate whether our insulator adheres to the all-SiC device or delaminates under physiological conditions. In addition, extensive in vivo studies will be conducted to determine the extent to which the neural probes will function post implant.

Author Contributions: Conceptualization, S.E.S. and C.L.F.; Methodology, E.K.B., R.E., J.U.-H., and C.L.F.; Validation, E.K.B. and C.L.F.; Formal Analysis, E.K.B. and C.L.F.; Investigation, E.K.B., R.E., J.U.-H., and C.L.F.; Resources, S.E.S.; Data Curation, E.K.B. and C.L.F.; Writing—Original Draft Preparation, E.K.B. and C.L.F.;

Writing—Review & Editing, S.E.S.; Visualization, E.K.B.; Supervision, S.E.S., and C.L.F.; Project Administration, S.E.S.

Funding: Partial funding was provided by the University of South Florida via a Proposal Enhancement Grant and by the Swedish Energy Agency project number 43611-1.

Acknowledgments: Matthew Hopper of the USF SiC Group is acknowledged for his assistance to Evans K. Bernardin in the taking of IV and CV data. The Florida Education Fund's McKnight Doctoral Fellowship Program and the Alfred P. Sloan Foundation University Center of Exemplary Mentoring (UCEM) are gratefully acknowledged for providing financial support to Evans K. Bernardin during this research.

Conflicts of Interest: Christopher L. Frewin and Stephen E. Saddow are part of a United States Patent 9,211,401 B2, 15 December 2015 for which this work contributes to the proof-of-concept.

References

1. Donoghue, J.P. Bridging the brain to the world: A perspective on neural interface systems. *Neuron* **2008**, *60*, 511–521. [CrossRef] [PubMed]
2. Lebedev, M.A.; Nicolelis, M.A.L. Brain-machine interfaces: Past, present and future. *Trends Neurosci.* **2006**, *29*, 536–546. [CrossRef] [PubMed]
3. Wolpaw, J.R.; Birbaumer, N.; McFarland, D.J.; Pfurtscheller, G.; Vaughan, T.M. Brain-computer interfaces for communication and control. *Clin. Neurophysiol.* **2002**, *113*, 767–791. [CrossRef]
4. Lobel, D.A.; Lee, K.H. Brain machine interface and limb reanimation technologies: Restoring function after spinal cord injury through development of a bypass system. *Mayo Clin. Proc.* **2014**, *89*, 708–714. [CrossRef] [PubMed]
5. Maynard, E.M.; Nordhausen, C.T.; Normann, R.A. The Utah intracortical electrode array: A recording structure for potential brain-computer interfaces. *Electroencephalogr. Clin. Neurophysiol.* **1997**, *102*, 228–239. [CrossRef]
6. Jorfi, M.; Skousen, J.L.; Weder, C.; Capadona, J.R. Progress towards biocompatible intracortical microelectrodes for neural interfacing applications. *J. Neural Eng.* **2015**, *12*, 011001. [CrossRef] [PubMed]
7. Luo, Y.H.-L.; da Cruz, L. The argus® II retinal prosthesis system. *Prog. Retin. Eye Res.* **2016**, *50*, 89–107. [CrossRef] [PubMed]
8. Markowitz, M.; Rankin, M.; Mongy, M.; Patino, B.E.; Manusow, J.; Devenyi, R.G.; Markowitz, S.N. Rehabilitation of lost functional vision with the argus ii retinal prosthesis. *Can. J. Ophthalmol.* **2018**, *53*, 14–22. [CrossRef] [PubMed]
9. Clark, G.M. The multi-channel cochlear implant: Multi-disciplinary development of electrical stimulation of the cochlea and the resulting clinical benefit. *Hear. Res.* **2015**, *322*, 4–13. [CrossRef] [PubMed]
10. Aziliz, L.; Emeline, D.; Christian, B. A review on mechanical considerations for chronically-implanted neural probes. *J. Neural Eng.* **2018**, *15*, 031001.
11. Rousche, P.J.; Normann, R.A. Chronic recording capability of the utah intracortical electrode array in cat sensory cortex. *J. Neurosci. Methods* **1998**, *82*, 1–15. [CrossRef]
12. Barrese, J.C.; Aceros, J.; Donoghue, J.P. Scanning electron microscopy of chronically implanted intracortical microelectrode arrays in non-human primates. *J. Neural Eng.* **2016**, *13*, 026003. [CrossRef] [PubMed]
13. Barrese, J.C.; Rao, N.; Paroo, K.; Triebwasser, C.; Vargas-Irwin, C.; Franquemont, L.; Donoghue, J.P. Failure mode analysis of silicon-based intracortical microelectrode arrays in non-human primates. *J. Neural Eng.* **2013**, *10*, 066014. [CrossRef] [PubMed]
14. Griffith, R.W.; Humphrey, D.R. Long-term gliosis around chronically implanted platinum electrodes in the rhesus macaque motor cortex. *Neurosci. Lett.* **2006**, *406*, 81–86. [CrossRef] [PubMed]
15. Kotov, N.A.; Winter, J.O.; Clements, I.P.; Jan, E.; Timko, B.P.; Campidelli, S.; Pathak, S.; Mazzatenta, A.; Lieber, C.M.; Prato, M.; et al. Nanomaterials for neural interfaces. *Adv. Mater.* **2009**, *21*, 3970–4004. [CrossRef]
16. Prasad, A.; Xue, Q.S.; Sankar, V.; Nishida, T.; Shaw, G.; Streit, W.J.; Sanchez, J.C. Comprehensive characterization and failure modes of tungsten microwire arrays in chronic neural implants. *J. Neural Eng.* **2012**, *9*, 056015. [CrossRef] [PubMed]
17. Massey, L.K. *Permeability Properties of Plastics and Elastomers: A Guide to Packaging and Barrier Materials*, 2nd ed.; William Andrew: Norwich, NY, USA, 2002.
18. Jones, D. *Principles and Prevention of Corrosion*, 2nd ed.; Prentice-Hall: Upper Saddle River, NJ, USA, 1996.
19. Deiasi, R.; Russell, J. Aqueous degradation of polyimides. *J. Appl. Polym. Sci.* **1971**, *15*, 2965–2974. [CrossRef]

20. Rubehn, B.; Stieglitz, T. In vitro evaluation of the long-term stability of polyimide as a material for neural implants. *Biomaterials* **2010**, *31*, 3449–3458. [CrossRef] [PubMed]

21. Polikov, V.S.; Tresco, P.A.; Reichert, W.M. Response of brain tissue to chronically implanted neural electrodes. *J. Neurosci. Methods* **2005**, *148*, 1–18. [CrossRef] [PubMed]

22. Nordhausen, C.T.; Maynard, E.M.; Normann, R.A. Single unit recording capabilities of a 100 microelectrode array. *Brain Res.* **1996**, *726*, 129–140. [CrossRef]

23. Kipke, D.R.; Vetter, R.J.; Williams, J.C.; Hetke, J.F. Silicon-substrate intracortical microelectrode arrays for long-term recording of neuronal spike activity in cerebral cortex. *IEEE Trans. Neural Syst. Rehabil. Eng.* **2003**, *11*, 151–155. [CrossRef] [PubMed]

24. Cogan, S.F. Neural stimulation and recording electrodes. *Annu. Rev. Biomed. Eng.* **2008**, *10*, 275–309. [CrossRef] [PubMed]

25. Saddow, S.E.; Frewin, C.L.; Nezafati, M.; Oliveros, A.; Afroz, S.; Register, J.; Reyes, M.; Thomas, S. 3C-SiC on Si: A bio- and hemo-compatible material for advanced nano-bio devices. In Proceedings of the 2014 IEEE 9th Nanotechnology Materials and Devices Conference (NMDC), Aci Castello, Italy, 12–15 October 2014; pp. 49–53.

26. Frewin, C.L.; Locke, C.; Saddow, S.E.; Weeber, E.J. Biocompatibility of sic for neurological applications. In *Silicon Carbide Biotechnology: A Biocompatible Semiconductor for Advanced Biomedical Devices and Applications*, 1st ed.; Saddow, S.E., Ed.; Elsevier: Oxford, UK, 2011.

27. Frewin, L.C.; Coletti, C.; Register, J.J.; Nezafati, M.; Thomas, S.; Saddow, E.S. Silicon carbide materials for biomedical applications. In *Carbon for Sensing Devices*; Demarchi, D., Tagliaferro, A., Eds.; Springer: Cham, Switzerland, 2015; pp. 153–207.

28. Lei, X.; Kane, S.; Cogan, S.; Lorach, H.; Galambos, L.; Huie, P.; Mathieson, K.; Kamins, T.; Harris, J.; Palanker, D. Sic protective coating for photovoltaic retinal prosthesis. *J. Neural Eng.* **2016**, *13*, 046016. [CrossRef] [PubMed]

29. Saddow, S.E.; Frewin, C.; Reyes, M.; Register, J.; Nezafati, M.; Thomas, S. 3C-SiC on Si: A biocompatible material for advanced bioelectronic devices. *ECS Trans.* **2014**, *61*, 101–111. [CrossRef]

30. Zorman, C.A. Silicon carbide as a material for biomedical microsystems. In Proceedings of the 2009 Symposium on Design, Test, Integration & Packaging of MEMS/MOEMS, Rome, Italy, 1–3 April 2009; pp. 1–7.

31. Frewin, C.L.; Locke, C.; Mariusso, L.; Weeber, E.J.; Saddow, S.E. Silicon carbide neural implants: In vivo neural tissue reaction. In Proceedings of the 2013 6th International IEEE/EMBS Conference on Neural Engineering (NER), San Diego, CA, USA, 6–8 November 2013; pp. 661–664.

32. Cogan, S.F.; Edell, D.J.; Guzelian, A.A.; Ping Liu, Y.; Edell, R. Plasma-enhanced chemical vapor deposited silicon carbide as an implantable dielectric coating. *J. Biomed. Mater. Res. A* **2003**, *67*, 856–867. [CrossRef] [PubMed]

33. Deku, F.; Cohen, Y.; Joshi-Imre, A.; Kanneganti, A.; Gardner, T.J.; Cogan, S.F. Amorphous silicon carbide ultramicroelectrode arrays for neural stimulation and recording. *J. Neural Eng.* **2018**, *15*, 016007. [CrossRef] [PubMed]

34. Henry, A.; ul Hassan, J.; Bergman, J.P.; Hallin, C.; Janzén, E. Thick silicon carbide homoepitaxial layers grown by cvd techniques. *Chem. Vapor Depos.* **2006**, *12*, 475–482. [CrossRef]

35. Hassan, J.; Bae, H.T.; Lilja, L.; Farkas, I.; Kim, I.; Stenberg, P.; Sun, J.W.; Kordina, O.; Bergman, P.; Ha, S.Y.; Janzén, E. Fast growth rate epitaxy on 4° off-cut 4-inch diameter 4H-SiC wafers. *Mater. Sci. Forum* **2014**, *778–780*, 179–182. [CrossRef]

36. Saxena, V.; Steckl, A.J. Chapter 3 building blocks for sic devices: Ohmic contacts, schottky contacts, and p-n junctions. In *Semiconductors and Semimetals*; Soo Park, Y., Ed.; Elsevier: New York, NY, USA, 1998; Volume 52, pp. 77–160.

37. Feng, X.; Huang, Y.; Rosakis, A.J. On the stoney formula for a thin film/substrate system with nonuniform substrate thickness. *J. Appl. Mech.* **2007**, *74*, 1276–1281. [CrossRef]

38. Bernardin, E.; Frewin, C.L.; Dey, A.; Everly, R.; ul Hassan, J.; Janzén, E.; Pancrazio, J.; Saddow, S.E. Development of an all-sic neuronal interface device. *MRS Adv.* **2016**, *1*, 3679–3684. [CrossRef]

39. Schroder, D.K. Semiconductor material and device characterization. In *Carrier and Doping Density*, 3rd ed.; John Wiley and Sons, Inc.: Hoboken, NJ, USA, 2006; p. 779.

40. Allongue, P.; Cachet, H. Band-edge shift and surface-charges at illuminated n-GaAs aqueous electrolyte junctions. Surface state analysis and simulation of their occupation rate. *J. Electrochem. Soc.* **1985**, *132*, 45–52. [CrossRef]

41. Peter, L.M. Semiconductor electrochemistry. In *Photoelectrochemical Solar Fuel Production*; Giménez, S., Bisquert, J., Eds.; Springer: Cham, Switzerland, 2016.

42. Rose, T.L.; Robblee, L.S. Electrical-stimulation with pt electrodes. VIII. Electrochemically safe charge injection limits with 0.2 ms pulses. *IEEE Trans. Biomed. Eng.* **1990**, *37*, 1118–1120. [CrossRef] [PubMed]

43. Peters, D.; Schorner, R.; Holzlein, K.-H.; Friedrichs, P. Planar aluminum-implanted 1400 V 4h silicon carbide p-n diodes with low on resistance. *Appl. Phys. Lett.* **1997**, *71*, 2996–2997. [CrossRef]

44. Mitlehner, H.; Friedrichs, P.; Peters, D.; Schorner, R.; Weinert, U.; Weis, B.; Stephani, D. Switching behaviour of fast high voltage sic pn-diodes. In Proceedings of the 10th International Symposium on Power Semiconductor Devices and ICs (ISPSD'98), Kyoto, Japan, 3–6 June 1998; pp. 127–130.

45. McConnell, G.C.; Rees, H.D.; Levey, A.I.; Gutekunst, C.A.; Gross, R.E.; Bellamkonda, R.V. Implanted neural electrodes cause chronic, local inflammation that is correlated with local neurodegeneration. *J. Neural Eng.* **2009**, *6*, 056003. [CrossRef] [PubMed]

46. Prasad, A.; Xue, Q.-S.; Dieme, R.; Sankar, V.; Mayrand, R.; Nishida, T.; Streit, W.; Sanchez, J. Abiotic-biotic characterization of pt/ir microelectrode arrays in chronic implants. *Front. Neuroeng.* **2014**, *7*. [CrossRef] [PubMed]

47. Simon, D.M.; Charkhkar, H.; St. John, C.; Rajendran, S.; Kang, T.; Reit, R.; Arreaga-Salas, D.; McHail, D.G.; Knaack, G.L.; Sloan, A.; et al. Design and demonstration of an intracortical probe technology with tunable modulus. *J. Biomed. Mater. Res. A* **2017**, *105*, 159–168. [CrossRef] [PubMed]

48. Reit, R.; Zamorano, D.; Parker, S.; Simon, D.; Lund, B.; Voit, W.; Ware, T.H. Hydrolytically stable thiol-ene networks for flexible bioelectronics. *ACS Appl. Mater. Interfaces* **2015**, *7*, 28673–28681. [CrossRef] [PubMed]

49. Teo, A.J.T.; Mishra, A.; Park, I.; Kim, Y.-J.; Park, W.-T.; Yoon, Y.-J. Polymeric biomaterials for medical implants and devices. *ACS Biomater. Sci. Eng.* **2016**, *2*, 454–472. [CrossRef]

50. Kozai, T.D.Y.; Catt, K.; Li, X.; Gugel, Z.V.; Olafsson, V.T.; Vazquez, A.L.; Cui, X.T. Mechanical failure modes of chronically implanted planar silicon-based neural probes for laminar recording. *Biomaterials* **2015**, *37*, 25–39. [CrossRef] [PubMed]

51. Kip, A.L.; Jeffrey, D.U.; Junyan, Y.; David, C.M.; Daryl, R.K. Chronic neural recordings using silicon microelectrode arrays electrochemically deposited with a poly(3,4-ethylenedioxythiophene) (pedot) film. *J. Neural Eng.* **2006**, *3*, 59–70.

52. Wilks, S.; Richardson-Burn, S.; Hendricks, J.; Martin, D.; Otto, K. Poly(3,4-ethylene dioxythiophene) (pedot) as a micro-neural interface material for electrostimulation. *Front. Neuroeng.* **2009**, *2*, 7. [CrossRef] [PubMed]

53. Aqrawe, Z.; Montgomery, J.; Travas-Sejdic, J.; Svirskis, D. Conducting polymers for neuronal microelectrode array recording and stimulation. *Sens. Actuat. B Chem.* **2018**, *257*, 753–765. [CrossRef]

54. Block, M.L.; Hong, J.S. Microglia and inflammation-mediated neurodegeneration: Multiple triggers with a common mechanism. *Prog. Neurobiol.* **2005**, *76*, 77–98. [CrossRef] [PubMed]

55. McHardy, J.; Geller, D.; Brummer, S.B. An approach to corrosion control during electrical stimulation. *Ann. Biomed. Eng.* **1977**, *5*, 144–149. [CrossRef] [PubMed]

56. Cogan, S.F.; Ludwig, K.A.; Welle, C.G.; Takmakov, P. Tissue damage thresholds during therapeutic electrical stimulation. *J. Neural Eng.* **2016**, *13*, 021001. [CrossRef] [PubMed]

57. Do, D.-H.; Ecker, M.; Voit, W.E. Characterization of a thiol-ene/acrylate-based polymer for neuroprosthetic implants. *ACS Omega* **2017**, *2*, 4604–4611. [CrossRef] [PubMed]

58. Jones, K.E.; Campbell, P.K.; Normann, R.A. Interelectrode isolation in a penetrating intracortical electrode array. In Proceedings of the Twelfth Annual International Conference of the IEEE Engineering in Medicine and Biology Society, Philadelphia, PA, USA, 1–4 November 1990; pp. 496–497.

59. Jones, K.E.; Campbell, P.K.; Normann, R.A. A glass/silicon composite intracortical electrode array. *Ann. Biomed. Eng.* **1992**, *20*, 423–437. [CrossRef] [PubMed]

60. Branner, A.; Stein, R.B.; Fernandez, E.; Aoyagi, Y.; Normann, R.A. Long-term stimulation and recording with a penetrating microelectrode array in cat sciatic nerve. *IEEE Trans. Biomed. Eng.* **2004**, *51*, 146–157. [CrossRef] [PubMed]

61. Tanaka, A. Toxicity of indium arsenide, gallium arsenide, and aluminium gallium arsenide. *Toxicol. Appl. Pharmacol.* **2004**, *198*, 405–411. [CrossRef] [PubMed]

62. Pakes, A.; Skeldon, P.; Thompson, G.E.; Fraser, J.W.; Moisa, S.; Sproule, G.I.; Graham, M.J.; Newcomb, S.B. Anodic oxidation of gallium nitride. *J. Mater. Sci.* **2003**, *38*, 343–349. [CrossRef]

63. Kashiwada, T.; Watanabe, T.; Ootani, Y.; Tateyama, Y.; Einaga, Y. A study on electrolytic corrosion of boron-doped diamond electrodes when decomposing organic compounds. *ACS Appl. Mater. Interfaces* **2016**, *8*, 28299–28305. [CrossRef] [PubMed]

64. Pan, M.; Liang, L.; Lin, W.; Kim, S.M.; Li, Q.; Kong, J.; Dresselhaus, M.S.; Meunier, V. Modification of the electronic properties of hexagonal boron-nitride in bn/graphene vertical heterostructures. *2D Mater.* **2016**, *3*, 045002. [CrossRef]

65. Saddow, S.E. SiC biotechnology for advanced biomedical applications. In *Second Workshop on Advanced Cybernetics*; University of Sao Paulo: Sao Carlos, Brasil, 2013.

66. Saddow, S.E. *Silicon Carbide Biotechnology: A Biocompatible Semiconductor for Advanced Biomedical Devices and Applications*; Elsevier: Amsterdam, The Netherlands, 2011.

67. Kordina, O.; Saddow, S.E. Silicon carbide overview. In *Advances In Silicon Carbide Processing and Applications*, 1st ed.; Saddow, S.E., Agarwal, A., Eds.; Artech House, Inc.: Boston, MA, USA, 2004; pp. 2–3.

68. Frewin, C.L.; Oliveros, A.; Locke, C.; Filonova, I.; Rogers, J.; Weeber, E.; Saddow, S.E. The development of silicon carbide based electrode devices for central nervous system biomedical implants. *Mater. Res. Soc. Symp. Proc.* **2009**, *1236E*. [CrossRef]

69. Osburn, C.M.; Raider, S.I. Effect of mobile sodium ions on field enhancement dielectric breakdown in SiO_2 films on silicon. *J. Electrochem. Soc.* **1973**, *120*, 1369–1376. [CrossRef]

70. Jansz, P.; Hinckley, S. Double boundary trench isolation effects on a stacked gradient homojunction photodiode array. In Proceedings of the 2008 Conference on Optoelectronic and Microelectronic Materials and Devices, Sydney, NSW, Australia, 28 July–1 August 2008; pp. 156–159.

71. Meyer, R.D.; Cogan, S.F.; Nguyen, T.H.; Rauh, R.D. Electrodeposited iridium oxide for neural stimulation and recording electrodes. *IEEE Trans. Neural Syst. Rehabil. Eng.* **2001**, *9*, 2–11. [CrossRef] [PubMed]

72. Cogan, S.F.; Ehrlich, J.; Plante, T.D.; Smirnov, A.; Shire, D.B.; Gingerich, M.; Rizzo, J.F. Sputtered iridium oxide films for neural stimulation electrodes. *J. Biomed. Mater. Res. Part B Appl. Biomater.* **2009**, *89B*, 353–361. [CrossRef] [PubMed]

73. Cogan, S.F.; Ehrlich, J.; Plante, T.D.; Gingerich, M.D.; Shire, D.B. Contribution of oxygen reduction to charge injection on platinum and sputtered iridium oxide neural stimulation electrodes. *IEEE Trans. Biomed. Eng.* **2010**, *57*, 2313–2321. [CrossRef] [PubMed]

74. Randles, J.E.B. Kinetics of rapid electrode reactions. *Discuss. Faraday Soc.* **1947**, *1*, 11–19. [CrossRef]

75. Stoner, B.R.; Raut, A.S.; Brown, B.; Parker, C.B.; Glass, J.T. Graphenated carbon nanotubes for enhanced electrochemical double layer capacitor performance. *Appl. Phys. Lett.* **2011**, *99*, 183104. [CrossRef]

76. Aryan, N.P.; Asad, M.I.H.B.; Brendler, C.; Kibbel, S.; Heusel, G.; Rothermel, A. In vitro study of titanium nitride electrodes for neural stimulation. In Proceedings of the 2011 Annual International Conference of the IEEE Engineering in Medicine and Biology Society, Boston, MA, USA, 30 August 2011–3 September 2011; pp. 2866–2869.

77. Meijs, S.; Alcaide, M.; Sørensen, C.; McDonald, M.; Sørensen, S.; Rechendorff, K.; Gerhardt, A.; Nesladek, M.; Rijkhoff, N.J.M.; Pennisi, C.P. Biofouling resistance of boron-doped diamond neural stimulation electrodes is superior to titanium nitride electrodes in vivo. *J. Neural Eng.* **2016**, *13*, 056011. [CrossRef] [PubMed]

78. Krishnan, R. Fundamentals of semiconductor electrochemistry and photoelectrochemistry. In *Encyclopedia of Electrochemistry*; Wiley-VCH Verlag GmbH & Co. KGaA: Weinheim, Germany, 2007.

79. Clarke, R.A.; Green, M.A.; Shewchun, J. Contact area dependence of minority-carrier injection in schottky barrier diodes. *J. Appl. Phys.* **1974**, *45*, 1442–1443. [CrossRef]

80. Ilatikhameneh, H.; Ameen, T.; Chen, F.; Sahasrabudhe, H.; Klimeck, G.; Rahman, R. Dramatic impact of dimensionality on the electrostatics of p-n junctions and its sensing and switching applications. *IEEE Trans. Nanotechnol.* **2018**, *17*, 293–298. [CrossRef]

81. Willis, A.J. Edge effects in schottky diodes. *Solid State Electron.* **1990**, *33*, 531–536. [CrossRef]

82. Moon, B.H.; Han, G.H.; Kim, H.; Choi, H.; Bae, J.J.; Kim, J.; Jin, Y.; Jeong, H.Y.; Joo, M.-K.; Lee, Y.H.; et al. Junction-structure-dependent schottky barrier inhomogeneity and device ideality of monolayer MoS_2 field-effect transistors. *ACS Appl. Mater. Interfaces* **2017**, *9*, 11240–11246. [CrossRef] [PubMed]

83. Neudeck, P.G. Electrical impact of sic structural crystal defects on high electric field devices. *Mater. Sci. Forum* **2000**, *338–342*, 1161–1166. [CrossRef]

84. McCreery, D.B.; Agnew, W.F.; Yuen, T.G.H.; Bullara, L. Charge density and charge per phase as cofactors in neural injury induced by electrical stimulation. *IEEE Trans. Biomed. Eng.* **1990**, *37*, 996–1001. [CrossRef] [PubMed]

85. Weiland, J.D.; Anderson, D.J.; Humayun, M.S. In vitro electrical properties for iridium oxide versus titanium nitride stimulating electrodes. *IEEE Trans. Biomed. Eng.* **2002**, *49*, 1574–1579. [CrossRef] [PubMed]

86. Jan, E.; Hendricks, J.L.; Husaini, V.; Richardson-Burns, S.M.; Sereno, A.; Martin, D.C.; Kotov, N.A. Layered carbon nanotube-polyelectrolyte electrodes outperform traditional neural interface materials. *Nano Lett.* **2009**, *9*, 4012–4018. [CrossRef] [PubMed]

87. Stuart, F.C.; Philip, R.T.; Julia, E.; Christina, M.G.; Timothy, D.P. The influence of electrolyte composition on the in vitro charge-injection limits of activated iridium oxide (AIROF) stimulation electrodes. *J. Neural Eng.* **2007**, *4*, 79–86.

88. Piret, G.; Hébert, C.; Mazellier, J.-P.; Rousseau, L.; Scorsone, E.; Cottance, M.; Lissorgues, G.; Heuschkel, M.O.; Picaud, S.; Bergonzo, P.; et al. 3d-nanostructured boron-doped diamond for microelectrode array neural interfacing. *Biomaterials* **2015**, *53*, 173–183. [CrossRef] [PubMed]

89. Pernot, J.; Volpe, P.N.; Omnès, F.; Muret, P.; Mortet, V.; Haenen, K.; Teraji, T. Hall hole mobility in boron-doped homoepitaxial diamond. *Phys. Rev. B* **2010**, *81*, 205203. [CrossRef]

90. Vasilevskiy, K.V.; Roy, S.K.; Wood, N.; Horsfall, A.B.; Wright, N.G. On electrons mobility in heavily nitrogen doped 4H-SiC. *Mater. Sci. Forum* **2017**, *897*, 254–257. [CrossRef]

91. Bieber, J.A.; Saddow, S.E.; Moreno, W.A. Synthesis of nanoscale structures in single crystal silicon carbide by electron beam lithography. In Proceedings of the Fifth IEEE International Caracas Conference on Devices, Circuits and Systems, Punta Cana, Dominican Republic, 3–5 November 2004; pp. 158–163.

92. Rosenbloom, A.J.; Nie, S.; Ke, Y.; Devaty, R.P.; Choyke, W.J. Columnar morphology of porous silicon carbide as a protein-permeable membrane for biosensors and other applications. *Mater. Sci. Forum* **2006**, *527–529*, 751–754. [CrossRef]

93. Saddow, S.E.; Melnychuk, G.; Mynbaeva, M.; Nikitina, I.; Vetter, W.M.; Jin, L.; Dudley, M.; Shamsuzzoha, M.; Dmitriev, V.; Wood, C.E.C. Structural characterization of sic epitaxial layers grown on porous sic substrates. *MRS Proc.* **2011**, *640*, H2.7. [CrossRef]

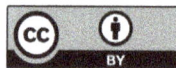

micromachines

MDPI

Article

Remote Stimulation of Sciatic Nerve Using Cuff Electrodes and Implanted Diodes

Arati Sridharan, Sanchit Chirania, Bruce C. Towe and Jit Muthuswamy *

School of Biological & Health Systems Engineering, Ira A. Fulton School of Engineering, Arizona State University, Tempe, AZ 85287, USA; asridhar@asu.edu (A.S.); Sanchit.Chirania@asu.edu (S.C.); bruce.towe@asu.edu (B.C.T.)
* Correspondence: jit@asu.edu; Tel.: +1-480-965-1599

Received: 29 August 2018; Accepted: 12 November 2018; Published: 14 November 2018

Abstract: We demonstrate a method of neurostimulation using implanted, free-floating, inter-neural diodes. They are activated by volume-conducted, high frequency, alternating current (AC) fields and address the issue of instability caused by interconnect wires in chronic nerve stimulation. The aim of this study is to optimize the set of AC electrical parameters and the diode features to achieve wireless neurostimulation. Three different packaged Schottky diodes (1.5 mm, 500 μm and 220 μm feature sizes) were tested in vivo ($n = 17$ rats). A careful assessment of sciatic nerve activation as a function of diode–dipole lengths and relative position of the diode was conducted. Subsequently, free-floating Schottky microdiodes were implanted in the nerve ($n = 3$ rats) and stimulated wirelessly. Thresholds for muscle twitch responses increased non-linearly with frequency. Currents through implanted diodes within the nerve suffer large attenuations (~100 fold) requiring 1–2 mA drive currents for thresholds at 17 μA. The muscle recruitment response using electromyograms (EMGs) is intrinsically steep for subepineurial implants and becomes steeper as diode is implanted at increasing depths away from external AC stimulating electrodes. The study demonstrates the feasibility of activating remote, untethered, implanted microscale diodes using external AC fields and achieving neurostimulation.

Keywords: wireless; implantable; microstimulators; neuromodulation; peripheral nerve stimulation; neural prostheses; microelectrode; neural interfaces

---

1. Introduction

Neuromodulation for peripheral nerve stimulation (PNS) applications is increasingly being used to treat and manage chronic diseases (i.e., epilepsy, micturition, pain, etc. [1–4]). A major problem with chronic neurostimulation of peripheral nerve for purposes of neural interfacing is that of lead wires tugging on microelectrodes penetrating into the body of a nerve. This becomes a more severe problem when large numbers of wires are used for advanced multichannel neural interface systems needed for both sensory and motor control of prosthetics [5]. Such systems require more channels than can be provided by most nerve cuff systems and need to contact or stimulate nerves lying deeper at the fascicular and subfasicular level. Penetrating needle electrode arrays such as the Utah array (USEA), flat interface nerve electrodes (FINE), transverse intrafascicular multi-channel electrodes (TIME), and longitudinal intrafascicular electrodes (LIFE) [6,7], are increasingly being used to make this connection but lead wire ribbon cables create differential inertia during sudden movement and the potential for damaging nerves during normal nerve movement with the limb. Wireless systems using RF, optical, heat, magnetic and ultrasound energy are increasingly being considered for neuromodulation [8–15]. The present work suggests the potential use of free-floating, stimulating, diode-electrode systems that are wholly implanted within the nerve and the use of strong electric field gradients produced by extraneural electrodes to achieve channel selection.

Excitable tissues of the body are not generally stimulated by short pulses of zero-mean, high frequency (>100 kHz) electric alternating currents (AC) at typically used amplitudes (10 µA–10's of mA). In fact, classic strength-duration curves reflect that nerve excitation at lower durations (corresponding to high frequency) of stimulus require exponentially increasing monophasic current amplitudes for stimulation. Recent nerve stimulation studies using transdermal amplitude modulated signals (TAMS) using computational models and in vivo experiments indicate that sinusoidal carrier waves of frequencies >20 kHz (variable amplitudes) do not significantly enhance the activation of neurons [16].

However, it is known that high-frequency, pulsed, monophasic (half wave-rectified) or partially rectified currents can stimulate a nerve and do so in ways that depend more on the envelope of the pulse rather than its carrier frequency [17]. Such stimulation currents can be achieved by diodes that rectify high frequency AC currents driven in tissues by remote electrodes that behave according to induced field distributions of volume conductors. Diodes placed in tissue rectify the fraction of high-frequency currents that pass through them relative to that passing through the tissue and can cause local neural activation, as we demonstrate in this study. Different diode placements on the nerve elicited selective electromyogram (EMG) responses in different muscle groups. The differential motor responses suggest the potential for the employment of many very small diodes dispersed around and within nerve to achieve a multichannel configuration driven by combinations of remote electrodes.

This approach to using volume-conducted currents to power implanted diodes and other devices in tissue was first explored by Palti [17] and others more recently [18–21] for direct stimulation of muscles [18] and nerves [19–21]. But a careful assessment of nerve activation using smaller microscale diodes as a function of the AC stimulation parameters such as frequency, peak-to-peak voltage amplitudes and diode parameters such as diode–dipole lengths, feature size and relative position of the diodes with respect to the stimulation electrodes has not yet been done. We find that non-stimulatory AC currents can be remotely driven in the conductivity of the nerve and a small diode with attached microelectrodes will allow intra-neural placement. In this situation, there is the potential for highly localized neurostimulation because of the short dipole spacing of the electrodes on the diode. Therefore, the key aspects of this design are the electric field gradient in tissue and the geometric factors of the diode and its electrodes.

The effect of diodes in a volume-conducted AC field has been modeled for various dipolar configurations in prior modeling studies [22,23]. This study models specific geometric relationships between the diode's electrodes, the remote activation electrodes, their proximity, and orientation. There is particularly a strong dependence on the anode–cathode length of the diode and the distance of remote activation electrodes. In general, volume conduction of significant amounts of current is limited by the roughly cubic expanding region of reduced current density around the stimulation electrodes as a function of separation distance. Even so, relatively high amplitude pulsed AC currents at high frequencies are well tolerated by tissues and so offer a way to help overcome path losses. We investigate the potential for energy transfer within constraints acceptable for local power transfer from outside a nerve epineurium to inside the nerve. The focus of the study here is to partly understand the limitations on the scheme of placing very short, but untethered diode–dipoles within a nerve cuff and then using differences in volume conduction and electrode current path lengths to define diode activation. This is proposed in order to reduce the need for penetrating electrodes and their potential for damage by lead wires. It is this key aspect of 'wirelessness' at this point in the chain of electrical pulse generators and lead wires that offers an advantage to the development of advanced nerve interfaces. The concept we are testing is the potential to achieve multichannel stimulation of a compound nerve by inserting or placing multiple small diodes within or on the nerve such that each responds to specific combinations of remote electrodes providing different configurations of electrical fields. Such diodes will not be connected by wires. This concept is enabled for experimentation by the availability of commercially available Schottky diodes in formats such as the Skyworks CDC-7630 having a 1.5 mm length and unpackaged silicon diode die of 220 μm square, but we note that diodes are easily made by modern photolithography at much smaller sizes.

2. Materials and Methods

2.1. In Vivo Rodent Sciatic Nerve Model

All animal procedures were done with the approval of the Institute of Animal Care and Use Committee (IACUC) of Arizona State University and in accordance with the National Institute of Health (NIH) guidelines. All efforts were made to minimize animal suffering and to use only the number of animals necessary to produce reliable scientific data. In all, 17 rats were used in total for all experiments.

Briefly, 300–600 g male Sprague–Dawley (*Rattus norvegicus*) rats ($n = 17$ rats total) were anesthetized (induction) using 50 mg/mL ketamine, 5 mg/mL xylazine, and 1 mg/mL acepromazine administered via intraperitoneal injection and maintained with 0.5–1% isoflurane. The left hind legs were shaved and residual hair was removed using hair removal cream. The animal was mounted on a stereotaxic frame and heart rate (~280–350 beats/min) and breathing (~60 breaths/min) were monitored using SurgiVet™ (Smith Medical Systems, Dublin, OH, USA). Aseptic techniques to disinfect the skin (i.e., application of isopropyl alcohol or betadiene) were used to ensure sterility. After skin incision and dissection of the muscle planes, the sciatic nerve was identified and isolated. Connective tissue surrounding the nerve was gently removed using iris microscissors at least 1 cm distal from the trifurcation point. The nerve cuff described previously was placed approximately 1 cm distal from the trifurcation point where the sural, peroneal and tibial bundles split. The cuff was placed such that the insulating silicone bottom under the rings as the only contact point with the rat body to ensure no contact with surrounding muscle groups to prevent potential off-target stimulation effects. A total of 10 (out of 17) animals were used for characterizing the performance of remote diodes with a stimulation threshold as a function of AC stimulation parameters (i.e., frequency, AC burst duration, measurements of diode current amplitudes based on relative position of remote diodes from stimulating electrodes, diode–dipole length and implantation depth).

To demonstrate that modified, implanted mini-, and micro-diodes can stimulate the nerve, needle-based electromyography (EMG) was used. Disposable monopolar needle electrodes (Rhythmlink™, Columbia, SC, USA) were placed in digit 5 of the rat hind leg paw (either left or right) for nerve cuff based experiments. The animal was grounded with a needle electrode in the opposite hind leg. EMGs were recorded using Intan™ recording system (Intan, Los Angeles, CA, USA) and analyzed in MATLAB offline. The recordings were digitally filtered on the Intan™ system using a bandpass filter from 100–3000 Hz to remove motion artifacts. EMG recordings were analyzed for 10 repetition trials of each stimulation condition.

Large SC-79 package diodes were also used to test selectivity. Multiple EMG electrodes at different sites (ankle/plantar, biceps femoris, and tibialis anterior) were placed in 3 (out of the total of 17) additional animals to test for muscle selectivity using AC excitation at 300 kHz or 1 MHz. Muscle response was recorded using needle-based EMGs.

Mean ± standard deviation of the EMG amplitude was calculated and muscle recruitment curves were plotted for nerve stimulation using diodes placed subepineurally and diodes implanted in the sciatic nerve. A total of 4 additional animals (out of the total 17) were used for the in vivo validation (2 for subepineurial and 2 for deep nerve implants). For stimulus threshold voltage measurements, mean ± standard error (SE) was plotted and statistical analysis was performed using one-way analysis of variance (ANOVA) and if found significant, the maximum and minimum values were evaluated for significance ($\alpha = 0.01$) using the Student's *t*-test.

2.2. Diode Packaging and Modification

Ultra-small, commercially-available Schottky diodes (Skyworks 7630, Woburn, MA, USA) were purchased in three different packages (SC-79, 0201 SMT, and bare die CDC7630)). The diode lengths were 1.5 mm, 0.5 mm and 0.22 mm respectively, with the first diode capable of stimulation on or outside the nerve, while the second and third diode packages offered intraneural, implantable sizes. The implantable 0201 SMT and bare die (hereafter referred to as mini- and micro-diodes respectively) were connected with 50 µm diameter platinum leads for nerve tissue contact that could be trimmed to desired diode–dipole lengths. Mini- and micro-diodes were dipped in a fluorosilane-based coating (3M-Novec EGC-1720) for 2 min and dried at room temperature for insulating electrically sensitive portions of the device. An additional, ethyl-cyanoacrylate based layer (Gorilla™ impact tough super glue) was added to strengthen the bond between the platinum leads and the diode bond pads to withstand mechanical stresses from the animal for durable implantation. The three packaged diodes are shown against the tip of smallest finger of a human hand in Figure 1.

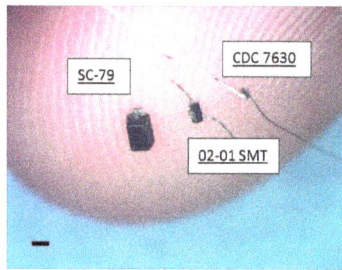

Figure 1. Pictures of the modified Skyworks 7630 diodes placed on an adult (digit 5) finger that were used for wireless neuromodulation. Images of the mini- and micro-diodes are prior to lead trimming and subsequent implantation into the peripheral nerve. The mini-diode is capable of placement under the epineurium, while the micro-diode is capable of both subepineurial and deep nerve tissue placement. Scale bar is 0.5 mm.

Current–voltage characteristic (I-V) curves of all three packages shown in Figure 2 were generated (10 kHz–1 MHz) using a Siglent™ function generator and oscilloscope to ensure that post-modifications did not affect diode characteristics such as threshold voltage as a function of frequency. Typical thresholds ranged from 150–180 mV at different frequencies, which is comparable to manufacturer datasheets.

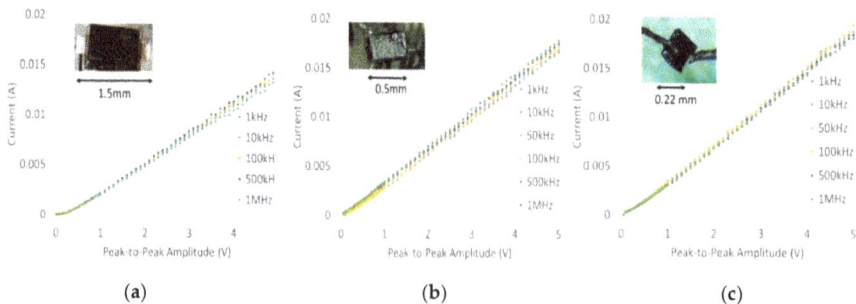

Figure 2. Current–voltage (I-V) characterization of modified, mini- and micro-diode packages—(**a**) SC-79, (**b**) 02-01SMT, (**c**) CDC 7630–for 10 kHz–1 MHz expectedly showed no significant electrical deviations due to frequency. Peak-to-peak, rectified current was measured across a load of 1.1 kΩ resistor.

2.3. Nerve Cuff Testing Platform

A cuff-electrode was used as a platform to generate AC fields in the sciatic nerve. A nerve cuff with 100 μm diameter platinum electrodes with 9 rings spaced 250 μm apart as shown in Figure 3a was custom fabricated by Microprobes (Gaithersburg, MD, USA). The total distance between the inner edge of electrode rings '1' and '9' was 2.7 mm. Each ring on the cuff had an impedance of ~2 kΩ at 1 kHz. This set-up was used to measure currents through a diode that is superficially placed on the sciatic nerve between two electrodes with AC excitation.

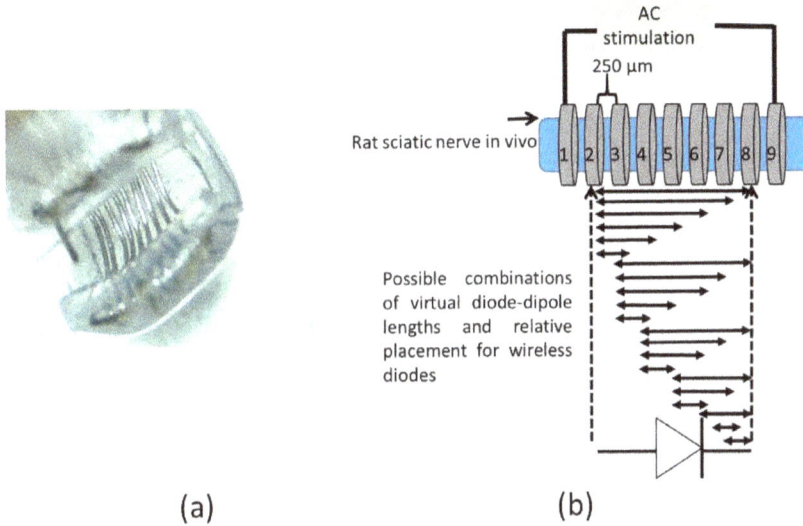

(a)   (b)

Figure 3. Nerve cuff-based platform was used to test currents through a diode placed superficially on a nerve for different diode–dipole lengths and placement of diodes relative to the external alternating current (AC) excitation voltages. (**a**) Image of a 9-ring nerve cuff with 100 μm diameter platinum leads spaced 250 μm apart. (**b**) Rings '1' and '9' were used to supply AC stimulus drive voltage (10 kHz–1 MHz) on the nerve. Rings '2' through '8' were used to test different combinations of diode–dipole lengths and the position relative to the AC drive voltages.

To study the impact of diode–dipole length and placement of the diodes relative to the excitation electrodes on nerve excitation, the outer rings '1' and '9' were used to deliver AC stimulation (peak-to-peak voltage of 0–20 V sine waveform) to the sciatic nerve in vivo. The mini- or micro-diode was wired to any 2 of the remaining rings (rings 2 through 8). Different combinations of the inner rings were used to test different diode–dipole lengths with the externally attached, mini- or micro-diode as illustrated in Figure 3b. A 510 Ω resistor was placed in series with the diode for current measurements through the diode and in series with the function generator for current measurements through rings '1' and '9' in the cuff for comparison (Figure 4a). The AC stimulation leads were electrically isolated using a custom-built transformer with a broad frequency range (10 kHz–2 MHz) to prevent ground loops. At 10 kHz, the output was slightly attenuated by 25% and was adjusted in current calculations. Figure 4a shows the setup for drive current measurements with a 510 Ω resistor placed in series with AC input. As seen in Figure 5, the current through the nerve was between 1–2 mA and fairly stable across frequencies. At lower frequencies (10–20 kHz), a marginal dependence on frequency was observed.

To measure typical currents through a microdiode that is implanted in a nerve, the anode and the cathode of the diodes were connected to Teflon-insulated platinum wires (~110 μm diameter, A–M Systems) spaced 1 mm apart as shown in Figure 4a,b. The diode was then mounted on a micromanipulator and the ends of the platinum wires were then used as probes to measure current through different depths in the nerve, namely (a) on the surface of the epineurium, (b) subepineurial placement (c) ~500 μm deep in the sciatic nerve, and (d) ~1 mm deep inside the nerve. Two different diode positions—'edge' which is ~250 μm away from the stimulating electrode, and 'center' which is 1 mm away from the stimulating electrode)—were assessed for current flow. Examples of partially rectified output for a 1 Vpp (peak-to-peak amplitude) input AC burst at 50 kHz and 500 kHz are shown in Figure 4c.

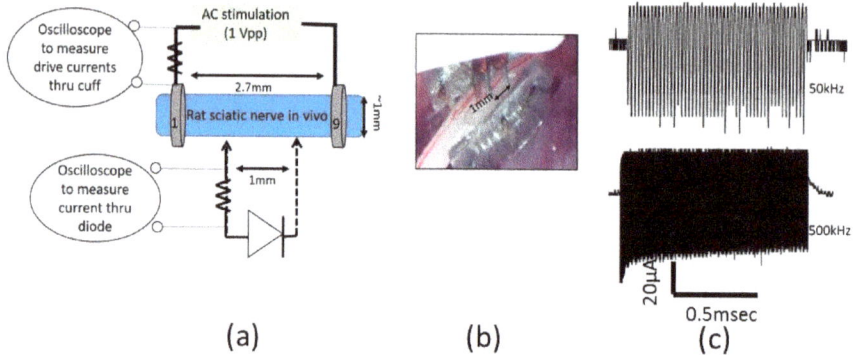

Figure 4. Experimental setup to measure current through remote mini-diodes whose cathode and anode are implanted at different depths (0, ~500 μm, ~1 mm) inside the sciatic nerve. (**a**) An AC stimulus (1 Vpp, peak-to-peak amplitude) is placed on rings '1' and '9' spaced 2.7 mm apart. (**b**) Insulated, platinum microwires (~110 μm diameter) spaced 1 mm apart and externally connected to a mini-diode are placed on the 'edge' (~250 μm) away from a stimulus ring electrode or near the 'center', which is ~1 mm away from the stimulus electrode. In this image, the probe is placed at the edge. The output is recorded via an oscilloscope and the current is calculated from voltage measurements across a 510 Ω resistor. (**c**) Examples of the partially rectified diode output for 50 kHz and 500 kHz waveforms with 1 msec burst.

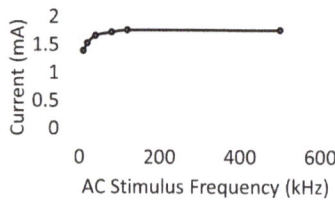

Figure 5. Representative currents measured through a sciatic nerve with a cuff in vivo. Variability in current amplitudes across animals was within ~15%. Currents were measured through a 510 Ω resistor for a 1 Vpeak-to-peak (1 Vpp) input voltage.

3. Results

3.1. Stimulus Voltage Threshold for the Muscle Increases Non-Linearly with Frequency of Alternating Current (AC) Stimulation but the Presence of the Diode Microstimulator on the Nerve Lowers the Stimulus Voltage Threshold

Large (1.5 mm diode–dipole length) diodes placed on nerve tissue rectify the fraction of high frequency currents that pass through them and can cause local neural activation, an example of which is shown in Figure 6. EMG responses recorded via needle electrodes placed downstream in three muscle locations (ankle, biceps femoris, tibialis) (Figure 6g) showed different amplitudes at a stimulus required for 50% of maximum response (Figure 6a–f). The diode was placed close to platinum hook electrodes, as seen in Figure 6. In additional animal experiments (Figure 7a), placement of the diode in a different location between the hook electrodes resulted in variable responses at the three muscle locations (ankle, biceps femoris, tibialis), with the ankle/plantar location showing no EMG response. Increasing the diode length by placing two diodes in tandem resulted in increased EMG amplitudes and a differential activation pattern (Figure 7b). Although the largest responses were seen in the biceps femoris muscle group, the tibial and plantar showed different activation patterns (Figures 6 and 7) depending on location and form factor of diodes.

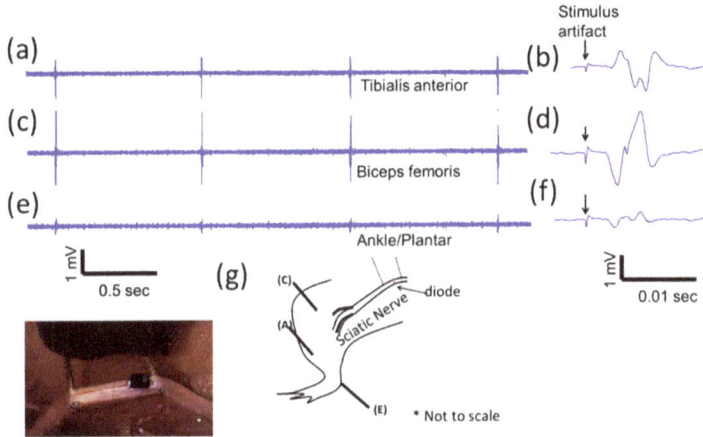

Figure 6. Representative electromyographic (EMG) responses from different muscle groups due to a single, remote, SC-79 packaged Skyworks diode stimulated with a high frequency (1 MHz) AC field by platinum hook electrodes. (**a,c,e**) are EMG responses at 1 Hz repetition rate. (**b,d,f**) are close-up of waveforms in (**a,c,e**) showing single EMG response with stimulus artifact indicated by an arrow. (**g**) Locations of EMG electrodes for the measurements in (**a,c,e**) in the hind limb. Inset shows a picture of a remote diode in free-floating placement on top of the nerve between two platinum based hook electrodes. Scale bar is 1 mm.

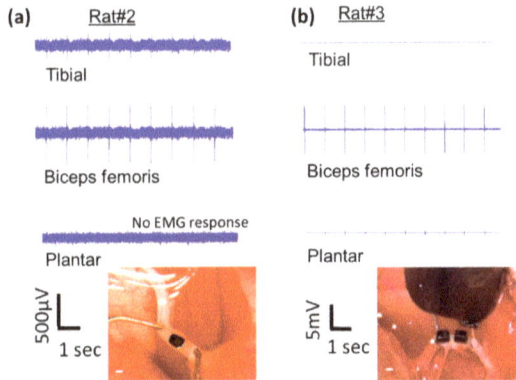

Figure 7. Variable EMG responses from different muscle groups due to (**a**) single, free-floating, SC-79 packaged Skyworks diode stimulated with a high frequency (300 kHz) AC field by platinum hook electrodes and (**b**) two, free-floating SC-79 packaged Skyworks diode stimulated at 1 MHz. The burst repetition rate was 1 Hz for both diode configurations. Relative locations of diodes are shown below the respective EMG responses. Scale bar is 1 mm.

To better understand the ability to activate remote diodes, a nerve cuff-based platform was utilized. The outer rings of the nerve cuff platform was used to deliver an AC stimulation burst with varying frequencies (0–500 kHz) and durations (33 µsec–1 msec) to an in vivo sciatic nerve preparation with a repetition rate of 1 burst/second in 2 animals. As frequency of the AC stimulation increases, the stimulation drive voltage for muscle twitch threshold increases exponentially as shown in Figure 8a. For increasing burst durations of AC, the threshold for muscle twitch decreases monotonically as shown in Figure 8b. When diodes are wired between two rings closest to the stimulation electrodes (rings '2' and '8') as illustrated in Figure 3b, the stimulus voltage threshold decreases over all frequencies 20–50 kHz as shown in Figure 8c. Interestingly, the stimulus threshold plateaus for frequencies >100 kHz ranging 1.5–5 V stimulus drive voltage as shown in Figure 8d. In contrast, the stimulus threshold in the absence of the diode continues to increase exponentially reaching ~45 V for 500 kHz bursts. This significant decrease in stimulus voltage threshold in the presence of a diode in the current paths in the nerve will be the key property that will help us achieve a spatially selective neural stimulation that is localized in the vicinity of the diodes themselves. Switching the anode–cathode orientation of the diode between the same 2 cuff rings results in only a marginal change in the stimulus voltage threshold as shown in Figure 8d.

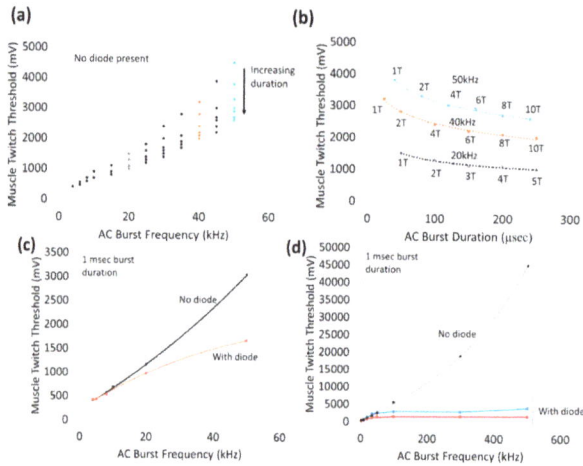

Figure 8. Representative stimulus voltage thresholds for different frequencies of AC stimulation. (a) and (b) show that the stimulus voltage threshold is dependent on the AC frequency and the burst duration, which is generated by variation in the number of periods (T) or full cycles as seen for 20, 40, and 50 kHz in (b). At 20 kHz, increasing burst duration from 50 µsec (1 T) to 1 msec (c) decreased the threshold stimulus by 45–55%. The trends observed in the curves in (b) are best fit to a power relationship ($R^2 > 0.99$). (c) The presence of the diode decreases stimulus voltage threshold in a frequency-dependent manner (≥ 20 kHz). At higher frequencies (d), the stimulus voltage threshold increases non-linearly with the input AC frequency in the absence of a diode. The blue (forward bias away from cathode) and red (forward bias toward cathode) lines indicate the presence of a diode in two different orientations.

The best fit suggests a quadratic relationship ($y = 0.1199x^2 + 28.829x + 371.27$, $R^2 > 0.99$). However, with the introduction of a diode in the current paths (between rings '2' and '8'), the stimulus voltage thresholds are significantly reduced, particularly for frequencies >100 kHz (1.5–5 V drive stimulus). While noting the stimulus is AC, switching the diode orientation toward the cathode (defined as the lead that connects to instrument ground) only changed the stimulus voltage threshold marginally (red versus blue line). Note that the stimulus voltage threshold 500 kHz in the absence of a diode was determined using an additional amplifier to the input signal to achieve high voltages.

3.2. Diode–Dipole Length, Relative Position to the Stimulation Electrodes, and Implantation Depth within the Nerve Are Major Factors in Determining Stimulation Thresholds

The stimulus voltage threshold for a visible muscle twitch was assessed as a function of diode–dipole length (based on the setup illustrated in Figure 3b) in 4 additional animals (n = 6 sciatic nerves for 20 and 500 kHz and n = 5 sciatic nerves for 50 kHz). The average stimulus voltage threshold was inversely proportional to the diode–dipole length. In negative control experiments without diodes, stimulus voltage thresholds were 876 ± 94 mV at 20 kHz and 2.85 ± 0.5 V at 50 kHz. At 500 kHz, the stimulus voltage threshold exceeded instrumentation range. Previous work in Figure 8d suggested the stimulus voltage threshold for 500 kHz to be approximately ~45 V.

Stimulus voltage thresholds decreased with increasing diode–dipole lengths as shown in Figure 9a–c. At 20 kHz, the change in stimulus voltage threshold with respect to dipole length was less pronounced (~20% decrease at 2 mm diode–dipole length) and was found not statistically significant (one way-ANOVA) as shown in Figure 9a. At 50 kHz, the stimulus voltage threshold for a diode–dipole length of 2 mm was ~55% of that during control AC stimulation (without a diode) and were found to be statistically significant ($p < 0.01$) as shown in Figure 9b. At 500 kHz, the effects of diode–dipole lengths were more pronounced were found to be statistically significant ($p < 0.01$). Even the smallest diode–dipole length (250 μm) at 500 kHz resulted in stimulus voltage threshold that is ~20–50% of that of control experiments with no diode. The larger dipole lengths (>500 μm) resulted in stimulus voltage thresholds that were <10% of that of control experiments with no diodes as shown in Figure 9c.

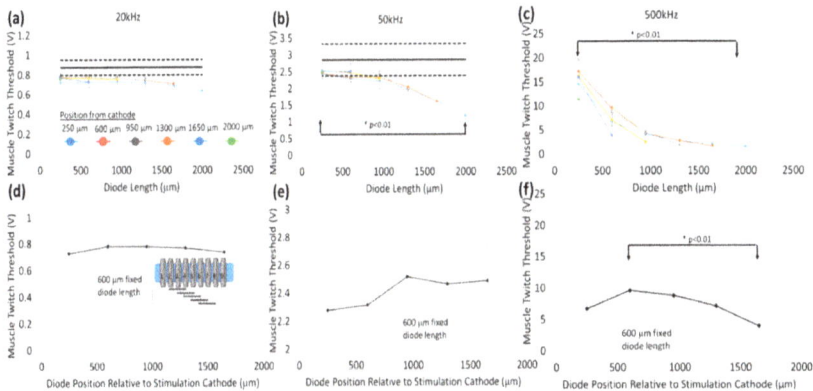

Figure 9. Stimulus voltage thresholds as a function of diode–dipole lengths for different frequencies −20 kHz in (**a**), 50 kHz in (**b**) and 500 kHz in (**c**) and relative position of the diode with respect to the stimulus cathode. Stimulus AC input was delivered on rings '1' and '9' (2.7 mm distance). Stimulus thresholds for conditions with no diodes are shown as the mean (solid black line) with 95% confidence levels (dashed, black lines) in (**a,b**). Stimulus voltage thresholds in control experiments with no diodes at 20 kHz (n = 6 sciatic nerves, 3 left and 3 right nerves from hind limb) and 50 kHz (n = 5 sciatic nerves 2 left and 3 right side) are 876 ± 94 mV and 2.85 ± 0.5 V respectively. At 500 kHz no visible muscle response was observed up to 20 V (instrument limit) (**d–f**) show the change in stimulus voltage thresholds due to relative position of the diode with respect to the stimulating electrodes when the diode–dipole length was fixed at 600 μm. The illustrative inset in (**d**) shows the change in position of the fixed diode length relative to the stimulating electrodes. All experiments were conducted with 1 msec AC burst duration. All data are expressed as mean ± SE. Significance was assessed by one-way analysis of variance (ANOVA), followed by Student's t-test (α = 0.01) between the maximum and minimum in (**a–f**).

In addition to the diode lengths, diode position and relative placement with respect to the stimulating electrodes played a role in determining threshold stimulus value. In Figure 9a–c, multiple data points at each diode length correspond to different positions of the diode relative to the stimulus electrode. Figure 9d–f shows a representative example of how stimulus threshold changes as a function of diode position for different frequencies when the diode–dipole length is fixed at 600 μm. A schematic of the relative diode position with respect to the cuff leads is shown in the inset in Figure 9d. At all three frequencies (20, 50, 500 kHz), the proximity of the diode to the stimulus electrodes decreases stimulus threshold, while diode placement toward the center increases the stimulus threshold maximally by ~10% and was not found to be significantly different for 20–50 kHz. At higher diode lengths (>1 mm), the relative change in threshold due to position was minimal. At 500 kHz, the minimum (near stimulation electrodes) and maximum values (closer to center) were found to be statistically significant for diode position in an AC field. It should be noted while the differential trends due to diode position are evident at 500 kHz, there is large variation between samples, suggesting the field lines within the nerve are variable. At 20 and 50 kHz, the contributions of the AC field from the external electrodes towards stimulating the nerve diminish the effect of diode position within the AC field.

In an effort to assess the typical currents that flow through the diode, a total of 3 animals were used to test different diode–dipole length configurations in Figures 10 and 11. To better understand the currents that flow through a diode using remote AC stimulating electrodes, current through the diode was measured for different diode lengths and positions (Figure 10a) for a 1 V (peak-to-peak amplitude) AC drive voltage through rings '1' and '9'. Interestingly, the current flowing through the diode was generally invariant in the employed frequency range (up to 500 kHz), suggesting that interactions of diode–electrode impedance and tissue impedances were responsible for this effect.

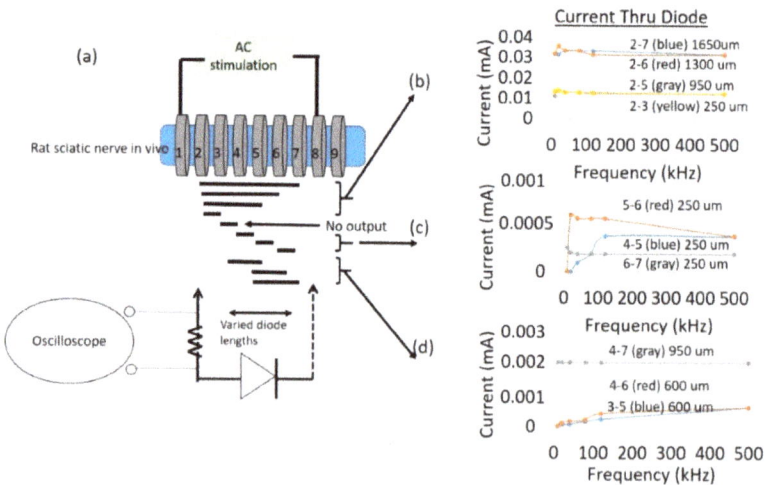

Figure 10. Typical current measurements through the diode for different diode lengths and positions for a 1 V (peak-to-peak amplitude) AC drive voltage. The experimental setup and the different diode lengths and positions that were tested are shown in (**a**). The diode was externally attached to different cuff leads as indicated to emulate different diode length and position relative to stimulating electrodes. (**b**) Larger diode–dipole lengths and placement within 250 μm of a stimulating AC electrode resulted in larger measured currents. (**c**) Shorter diode–dipole lengths of 250 μm and placement >250 μm away from the stimulating electrodes showed 20–60 fold less current through the diode. (**d**) Current measurements for diode–dipole lengths of 600 μm and 950 μm and placement >250 μm away from the stimulating electrodes.

While the experiments in Figure 10 represented currents through ring electrodes with large surface areas, the experimental setup described in Figure 4 measured currents through a 'remote' microdiode with a small electrode surface area (cross-sectional face of ~110 µm diameter wire) at various positions and implantation depths. The platinum leads spaced 1 mm apart (for a diode–dipole length of 1 mm) were placed at the "edge" and "center" of the nerve encompassed by the nerve cuff are shown in Figure 11 for 2 animals for a peak-to-peak excitation voltage of 1 V applied across rings '1' and '9' of the cuff electrode. In one of the animals, measured currents through the diode placed on top of the epineurium (0+) was marginally higher than the currents measured from implanted diodes. Similarly, only marginal differences were observed between currents through diodes placed at the "edge" (or closer to the excitation electrodes) versus currents through diodes placed at the "center" of the cuff.

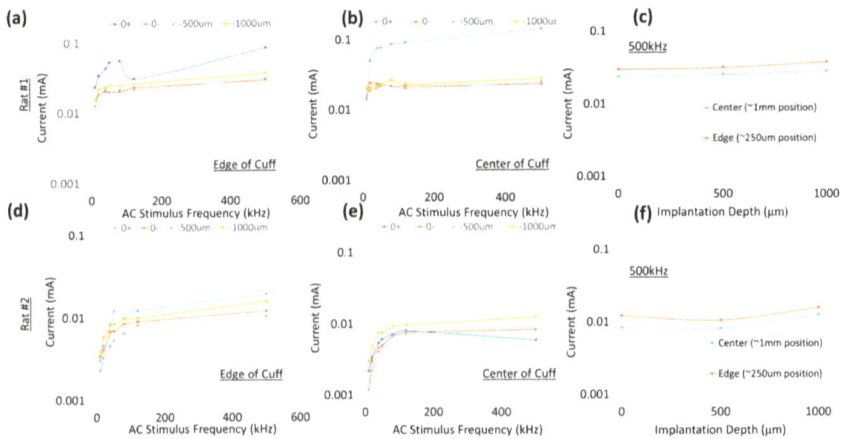

Figure 11. Characterization of current through a remote diode at 3 different implantation depths and 2 different lateral positions along the cuff. All currents were measured in response to a peak-to-peak excitation voltage of 1 V applied across rings '1' and '9' of the cuff electrode. (**a,d**) Current through diodes placed at the 'edge' of the cuff in 2 different animals and (**b,e**) 'center' of the cuff for 3 different depths—above the epineurium (0+), just below the epineurium (0−), at 500 µm and 1 mm implantation depths. (**c,f**) Representative currents through the diodes at 500 kHz are shown for different implantation depths and position. The highest currents were attained closer to the epineurium (0 or 1 mm depth) of the nerve and closest to the stimulating electrodes.

Experiments were also conducted in one animal to test the minimum monophasic current pulse through the diode required to achieve the stimulus current threshold. The stimulus current threshold for the diode was 17 µA at 10 kHz frequency for 1 msec burst duration. Similar experiments at 900 mV drive voltage at 10 kHz frequency with 1 msec burst duration showed that 19.6 µA would be required to reach stimulus threshold. In an additional separate control animal using hook electrodes spaced 3–4 mm apart, 15 µA was required to achieve stimulus threshold at 500 kHz, 500 µsec burst duration. The currents through the remote diode in Figure 10 for the different implantation depths have similar µA range, suggesting remote neurostimulation is feasible for microscale diode implants. Low µA range currents are also reported for stimulators placed close to the nerve [24,25].

3.3. Validation of Remote Neurostimulation Using Implanted Mini- and Micro-Diodes Using the Optimal Stimulation Frequency, Diode Dimensions and Placement Determined

Remote, free-floating, implanted mini- and micro-diodes with modified lead lengths to match the length of the stimulating nerve cuff (~3 mm) were demonstrated to stimulate the sciatic nerve. Figure 12 shows representative micro-diodes implanted deep into the nerve and hence not visible in the images (Figure 12a,b) and mini-diodes placed subepineurially (Figure 12d,e), where the outer sheath held the diode in place even when subjected to mild shear forces.

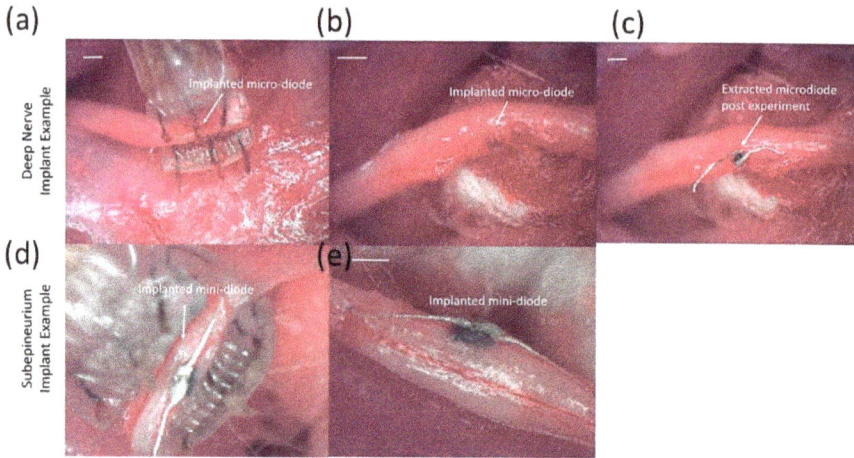

Figure 12. Representative images of implanted micro- and mini-diodes. (**a–c**) represent an example of a diode with a 220 μm feature size and lead lengths to match the length of the cuff implanted deep inside the nerve. (**d,e**) show an example of a diode with 0.5 mm feature size with 3 mm long leads, the entirety of which is implanted subepineurally.

When a diode was placed on the nerve or implanted in the nerve between the two stimulating electrodes and activated using the ring electrodes '1' and '9' of the cuff electrode at 500 kHz and 1 msec pulse duration, a visible muscle twitch was visually observed and a corresponding, typically biphasic EMG response was recorded (Figure 13). Representative EMG signals in response to activation of a deeply implanted diode and another subepineurial diode are shown in Figure 13. Control AC stimulations in the absence of any implanted diodes showed only the stimulus artifact, which has a duration of 1 msec. Needles for EMG recordings were placed in digit 5 of the hind paw. A similar range of latencies was seen across 3 implanted animals (5.8 ± 1.3 msec) in response to activation of both subepineurially implanted diodes and diodes implanted deep in the nerve. The EMG waveform has a peak-to-peak duration of 2.6 ± 0.55 msec in all animals.

Muscle EMG recruitment curves for subepineurial diode implants and deep nerve diode implants ($n = 4$ additional animals for all implants) are shown in Figure 14. Subepineurial implants in 2 animals had thresholds in the range ~2.8–3.0 V and had recruitment curves comparable to those obtained for diodes just placed on the nerve implants with 1.5–2.8 V threshold stimulus. It was noted that during the recording of the second recruitment curve for the subepineurial implant #2, the stimulus was selective to movement of only digit 5 suggesting recruitment of localized axonal fibers; whereas with the placement of the diode on the nerve in the same animal or in the case of the subepineurial implant #1 a larger recruitment was seen, causing the whole hind leg to move at higher stimulus voltages. Deep nerve implants in 2 animals had a higher stimulus voltage threshold (6.0 V in one case and 20 V in the second case). The EMG recruitment curve for the first diode implanted deep in the nerve is shown in Figure 14. The recruitment curves for the second implanted diode could not be obtained due to high activation voltages that were needed. EMGs for this animal had a large peak-to-peak amplitude (~12 mV) for the diodes implanted deep in the nerve (data not shown).

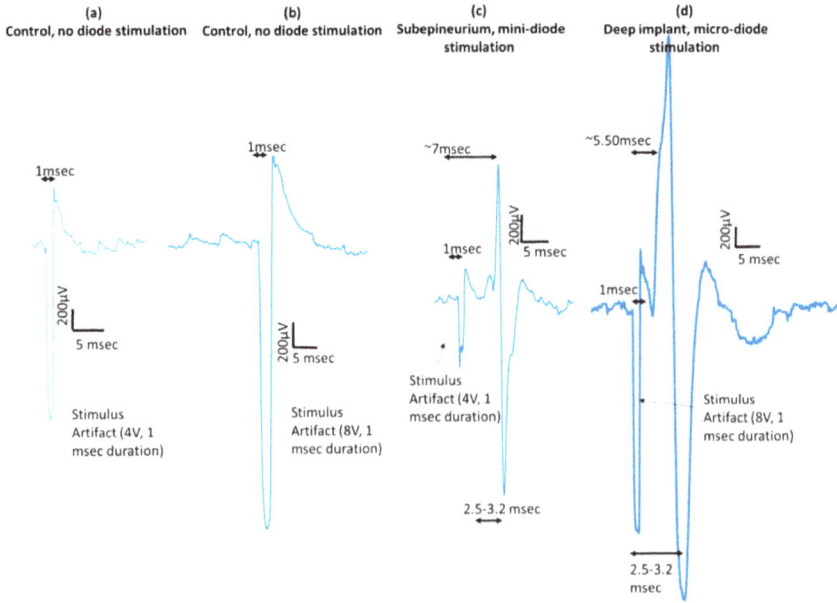

Figure 13. Activation of remote diodes using AC stimulation waveforms induces distinct dose-dependent EMG responses. (**a,b**) EMG responses are not observed in the absence of any diodes to AC stimulation of 4 V and 8 V. (**c**) Distinct EMG peak amplitudes are seen ~7 msec after the stimulus artifact in response to activation of diodes placed subepineurially and ~5.5 msec after stimulus artifact in response to activation of diodes placed deep in the nerve (**d**). These representative EMGs were recorded in response to an AC stimulus of 500 kHz frequency with a 1 msec stimulus duration.

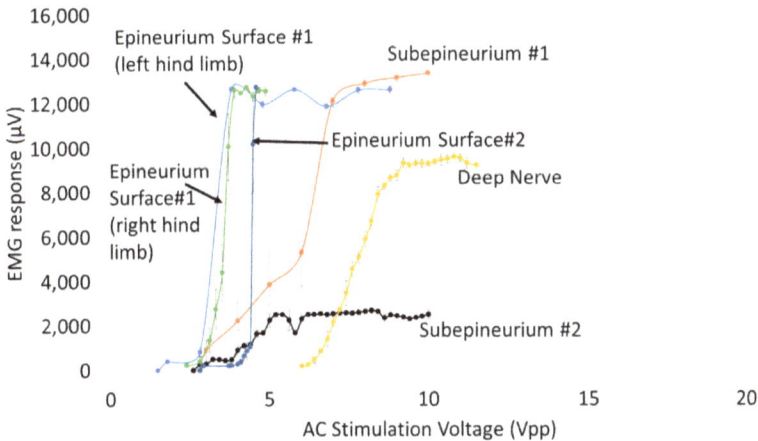

Figure 14. EMG recruitment curves for diodes implanted that are implanted subepineurially (2 animals) and deep in the sciatic nerve (one animal shown). A second animal with a deep nerve implant showed a response only at 20 Vpp (not shown). In addition, EMG recruitment curves of three diodes placed on the sciatic nerve is also shown labeled "epineurium surface #1' and 'epineurium surface #2'. Each data point is represented by the mean ± standard deviation of EMG responses to 10 stimulations at a given amplitude.

4. Discussion

The primary goal of this study was to determine the set of stimulation parameters, diode dimensions and placement that would enable microscale, implantable diodes to function as wireless neuromodulators. The working principle was to use the volume conduction properties of tissue as a method of transferring power from non-contacting but nearby electrodes to free-floating diodes placed on or inside the nerves. The initial concept of using a rectifier (germanium diodes with silver leads (1–3 cm long) to stimulate external organs was demonstrated by Palti in 1966 [17]. Recent work reiterated the concept by placing leads from a full-wave bridge rectifying circuit prototype (eAxon) into selected muscle fibers that are stimulated using a 1 MHz sinusoidal input [18]. In this study, we demonstrated remote neurostimulation using microscale, silicon diodes directly implanted in the nerve in at least 13 animals (Figures 6–9, 12 and 13). This approach allowed neurostimulation without wires traversing the epineurium to contact electrodes. Thus, there is a wireless bridging of the last millimeter of distance between the local environment outside of the nerve body and its interior. Using different feature sizes (1.5 mm, 0.5 mm, and 0.22 mm) off-the-shelf, commercially-available, Schottky diodes (Skyworks 7630), we assessed the parameters of the external stimulating AC signal (such as frequency 10–500 kHz, drive voltages, and currents), diode dimensions and relative position of the diode with respect to the external AC stimulating electrodes that would be required to achieve wireless neurostimulation for microdiodes implanted in the sciatic nerve. We found AC stimulating frequency and diode length to be major factors in diode performance in vivo, followed by proximity of the diode to the stimulating electrodes and implantation depth.

Application of 1 msec bursts of zero-offset, sinusoidal AC waveforms via a nerve cuff platform by itself stimulated the sciatic nerve in a frequency-dependent manner from 10–500 kHz (Figure 8). The non-linearly increasing thresholds required to achieve a visible muscle twitch at higher frequencies can perhaps be explained by earlier observations of classic strength–duration relationships for nerve stimulation. Such strength–duration curves for nerves have demonstrated a non-linear, hyperbolic relationship between strength and duration required to achieve threshold. High frequencies correspond to lower durations and hence threshold for AC stimulation of nerves can be expected to increase non-linearly with frequency. In addition, high frequency AC stimulation that exceed the kinetics of the ion channels in the cell membrane, will result in significantly higher voltage thresholds (such as ~45 Vpp at 500 kHz). In fact, pure sinusoidal AC continuous waveforms up to 40 kHz have been used effectively in nerve conduction block applications, such as relief from phantom limb pain [26–28].

Placement of a wireless, remote diode in AC electric field is expected to fully or partially rectify the input sinusoidal wave and generate a DC component that is proportional to input Vrms and large enough to stimulate a nerve. Above 20 kHz, the addition of a wireless diode between the stimulus electrodes achieved increasing reductions in the stimulus voltage threshold. For instance, the stimulation voltage thresholds at 20 kHz and 50 kHz were ~700 mV and ~1.5 V with a wireless diode compared to ~900 mV, ~3 V without diode, respectively. Beyond 100 kHz, the stimulus voltage threshold plateaued (<5 V) and was fairly independent of frequency. We speculate that between 20–100 kHz, the rectified signals of the diode augmented the neurostimulation of the applied external AC signal in achieving the threshold. Below 20 kHz, the augmentation effect of the diode presence was not significant, suggesting the neurostimulation was dominated primarily by the external AC stimulation. Frequency-dependent effects are not expected from diodes since current-voltage (I-V) characterization of modified diodes show similar diode threshold values and rectification properties across a range of frequencies (10 kHz–1 MHz, Figure 2).

In this study, the measured currents through the diode were at least 100-fold less (Figure 10) than the currents through the rings '1' and '9' of the cuff electrode (Figure 5), suggesting high levels of volume conduction loss. Increasing the diode–dipole length from 250 μm to 2 mm reduced the threshold by ~10–20% and ~55% at 20 kHz and 50 kHz, respectively, as shown in Figure 9. Significant improvements in stimulus voltage thresholds were seen for diode–dipole lengths >1 mm at 50 kHz, while the effect of diode length was only marginal at 20 kHz. The effects of diode–dipole lengths were more pronounced for 500 kHz stimulation frequency. The stimulus voltage threshold lowered 10-fold at 500 kHz as the diode–dipole length changed increased from 250 µm to 2 mm. The smaller diode–dipole lengths have relatively lower energy transfer efficiency due to less volume-conducted currents being intercepted by diode–electrodes. At high frequencies, only the current through the diode that is rectified would be useful for neurostimulation. The results are in agreement with [23], who theorized that diode designs with long, thin geometry that maximize separation distance with short electrode leads would have maximum energy transfer efficiency. Sahin et al. [22] showed that separation distance of remote electrodes more than two times the diode anode–cathode separation distances (or diode–dipole length) entails high volume conductor losses. The stimulating electrode in the cuff were separated by 2.7 mm and, indeed, at 500 kHz where the augmentation of the diode would be most dominant, a diode–dipole length of >1 mm resulted in the lowest voltage thresholds.

For a fixed diode–dipole length, increasing the diode proximity to the stimulating electrodes reduced the stimulus voltage threshold value by ~10% compared to positions more central between the stimulating electrodes (Figure 9d,e). Measured currents through a diode reduced 20–60 times when the diode was placed >250 µm away from the stimulating electrode (Figure 10). A remote diode with a smaller contact surface area also reduced by up to 2-fold toward the central position between two stimulating ring electrodes and toward ~500 µm implantation depth (Figure 11). In the case of implanted microdiodes, a large contact surface area between the anode/cathode and the tissue is attained via an additional 1 mm extension of bare, uninsulated platinum wire (total length of the microdiode and wire extension ~3 mm). The larger contact surface area allowed for a lower interfacial impedance and hence a more conducive current path compared to the typically higher tissue impedance surrounding the implant. The feasibility of obtaining recruitment curves from implanted microdiode stimulators (Figure 14) confirmed that having lower contact impedances is an important design parameter in addition to diode–dipole length and placement in the AC field.

An interesting point was that diodes placed on the nerve and diodes embedded just underneath the epineurium had similar threshold values, suggesting the epineurium did not impede in the energy transfer between the stimulating electrode and the diode. It is well known that at high frequencies (such as 500 kHz) the impedance of electrodes placed above the epineurium and those implanted just beneath in the nerve (sub-epineurium) would converge, essentially eliminating any impedance mismatches for energy transfer. However, implants placed deeper in the peripheral nerve tissue would be expected to have a higher threshold due to higher tissue path impedance. Indeed when comparing EMG recruitment curves of diodes implanted deep in the nerve and that of subepineurial diodes for similar diode lengths at 500 kHz input frequency (Figure 14), the stimulus voltage threshold increased by 2–3 fold from 2.8–3 V to 6 V. In fact, one diode implanted deep in the nerve required a stimulus voltage threshold of 20 V, suggesting steep recruitment curves (data not shown). It should be noted that the minimum current needed to achieve the threshold were similar for a monophasic, square pulse with a 1 msec duration (17 µA) compared to the minimum current through a diode at the threshold (19.6 µA). Therefore, deep implants require more drive to achieve similar performance. It should be emphasized the repeatability and robustness of the diode placement would be an important experimental variable in potential application of this kind of neurostimulation strategy. The repeatability/robustness of the nerve responses from the diodes from trial to trial is governed partly by surgical technique and animal-to-animal variations in electrophysiological response. The primary focus of this study was not to characterize known biological responses to pulsed monophasic but rather the ability to stimulate them remotely by electric field manipulation. Strategies to optimize positioning and manipulation of diode lengths will be needed in the future for modulation of deep fibers. Volume conduction models that assume homogenous and isotropic tissue properties with uniform conduction would predict the highest threshold to be at the midpoint. However, the data in Figure 8d–f suggested that while stimulus thresholds trended higher in the region between the edges of the stimulus electrodes, there was a large variance in the exact position where least current and higher thresholds occur. Considering that tissue properties have in reality more inhomogeneous composition [29], and the nerve itself has a non-spherical, oblong geometry, better mapping of conduction properties inside the nerve would be needed in the future for the optimal placement of diodes. It should be noted that variance in current properties outside the nerve epineurium (Figure 10) was possibly due to the presence and effective concentrations of body fluids over the time course of the experiment. It should be made clear that the study is not proposing the placing of commercial diodes in nerves, since even at the smallest feature size of 220 μm, they may cause significant tissue damage due to relative tissue motion. However, assessment of the biocompatibility of the current remote diode–dipole chips is beyond the scope of this work since the primary motivation here was to investigate the possibility of inter-neurally, implantable microstimulators to be remotely activated. The potential advantages of this approach are selective targeting and decoupling of the physical wire connectivity to mitigate the relative motion between implanted devices and the nerve tissue. The disadvantages are relatively higher currents applied to nerve cuffs (currents in the cuffs are in the order of a few mAs to 10's of mA which are ~100 times higher than currents through the remote diodes) and limitations in placement of multiple diodes due to the need for diode electrode lengths in the order of 1 mm.

This often affects the performance of tethered implants in terms of energy usage, targeting precision and optimal performance since it may require frequent recalibration. This work did not examine issues of nerve damage due to diode placement. However, we note that to mitigate the tissue damage due to diode implant itself, design modifications such the use of materials that are mechanically matched to the tissue, flexible designs and miniaturization may be used to improve chronic functional performance.

5. Conclusions

We observe that small 220 μm, free-floating, Schottky micro-diodes placed free-floating inside a rat sciatic nerve can reduce thresholds and stimulate action events using high frequency AC bursts with 1 msec duration. The advantage is that no chronic trans-epineurial wires to individual nerve fibers are needed to locally stimulate fibers. This work suggests that free-floating diodes placed internal to the nerve in combination with nerve cuffs thus can act similarly to penetrating electrodes in achieving selective (focal) sites of nerve stimulation but without penetrating wires implanted intraneurally. Experiments show, however, strong sensitivity to diode–dipole length with the minimum values of in the order of 1 mm, frequency of AC carriers, limits on the distance of diodes from stimulation electrodes, and thus implantation depths at practical AC drive currents. This places significant limits on extrapolations of this approach to multiple channels. Currents through implanted diodes within the nerve suffer large attenuations (~100 fold) compared to AC burst currents requiring relatively high (1–2 mA) drive currents. Muscle EMG curves with implanted free-floating diodes are intrinsically steep and get steeper as a diode is placed at increasing depths away from external AC stimulating electrodes.

Author Contributions: Conceptualization, A.S., S.C., B.C.T. and J.M.; Methodology, A.S., S.C., B.C.T. and J.M.; Validation, A.S., S.C., B.C.T. and J.M.; Formal Analysis, A.S., B.C.T. and J.M.; Writing—Original Draft Preparation, A.S., B.C.T. and J.M.; Writing—Review and Editing, A.S., B.C.T. and J.M.; Supervision, A.S., B.C.T. and J.M.; Project Administration, B.C.T. and J.M.; Funding Acquisition, B.C.T. and J.M.

Funding: This research was funded by Defense Advanced Research Projects Agency (DARPA), grant No. HR0011-16-2-0023 under the Electrical Prescriptions (ElectRx) program and a seed grant from the Fulton Schools of Engineering at Arizona State University, Tempe, AZ, USA.

Acknowledgments: The authors thank Siddharath Kulasekaran for custom fabrication and donation of transformers. The authors also thank Swathy Sampath Kumar for valuable discussions into experimental design. In addition, we acknowledge the role of student volunteers Dania Keller, University of Miami, Biomedical Engineering undergraduate program; and Tyler Mitchell, Arizona State University, BME undergraduate program; for their assistance in characterizing the diodes.

Conflicts of Interest: The authors declare no conflict of interest.

References

1. Le, N.-B.; Kim, J.H. Expanding the Role of Neuromodulation for Overactive Bladder: New Indications and Alternatives to Delivery. *Curr. Bladder Dysfunct. Rep.* **2011**, *6*, 25–30. [CrossRef] [PubMed]
2. Holtzheimer, P.E.; Mayberg, H.S. Neuromodulation for treatment-resistant depression. *F1000 Med. Rep.* **2012**, *4*, 22. [CrossRef] [PubMed]
3. Goroszeniuk, T.; Pang, D. Peripheral neuromodulation: A review. *Curr. Pain Headache Rep.* **2014**, *18*, 5. [CrossRef] [PubMed]
4. Krahl, S.E. Vagus nerve stimulation for epilepsy: A review of the peripheral mechanisms. *Surg. Neurol. Int.* **2014**, *3*, S47–S52. [CrossRef] [PubMed]
5. Pena, A.; Kuntaegowdanahalli, S.; Abbas, J.J.; Patrick, J.; Horch, K.W.; Jung, R. Mechanical fatigue resistance of an implantable branched lead system for a distributed set of longitudinal intrafascicular electrodes. *J. Neural Eng.* **2017**, *14*, 1–10. [CrossRef] [PubMed]
6. Eggers, T.E.; Dweiri, Y.M.; McCallum, G.A.; Dominique, M. Durand. Recovering motor activation with chronic peripheral nerve computer interface. *Sci. Rep.* **2018**, *8*, 141419. [CrossRef] [PubMed]
7. Jung, R.; Abbas, J.J.; Kuntaegowdanahalli, S.; Thota, A.K. Bionic intrafascicular interfaces for recording and stimulating peripheral nerve fibers. *Bioelectron. Med.* **2018**, *1*, 55–69. [CrossRef] [PubMed]
8. Weber, M.J.; Bhat, A.; Chang, T.C.; Charthad, J.; Arbabian, A. A miniaturized ultrasonically powered programmable optogenetic implant stimulator system. In Proceedings of the 2016 IEEE Topical Conference on Biomedical Wireless Technologies, Networks, and Sensing Systems (BioWireleSS), Austin, TX, USA, 24–27 January 2016; pp. 12–14.
9. Lee, J.; Jang, J.; Song, Y.K. A review on wireless powering schemes for implantable microsystems in neural engineering applications. *Biomed. Eng. Lett.* **2016**, *6*, 205–215. [CrossRef]
10. Hannan, M.A.; Mutashar, S.; Samad, S.A.; Hussain, A. Energy harvesting for the implantable biomedical devices: Issues and challenges. *Biomed. Eng. Online* **2014**, *13*, 79. [CrossRef] [PubMed]
11. Luan, S.; Williams, I.; Nikolic, K.; Constandinou, T.G. Neuromodulation: Present and emerging methods. *Front. Neuroeng.* **2014**, *7*, 27. [CrossRef] [PubMed]
12. Carmo, J.P.; Correia, J.H. Wireless microsystems for biomedical applications. *J. Microwav. Optoelectron. Electromagn. Appl.* **2013**, *12*, 492–505. [CrossRef]
13. Ho, J.S.; Yeh, A.J.; Neofytou, E.; Kim, S.; Tanabe, Y.; Patlolla, B.; Beygui, R.E.; Poon, A.S. Wireless power transfer to deep-tissue microimplants. *Proc. Natl. Acad. Sci. USA* **2014**, *111*, 7974–7979. [CrossRef] [PubMed]
14. Lovik, R.D.; Abraham, J.P.; Sparrow, E.M. Potential tissue damage from transcutaneous recharge of neuromodulation implants. *Int. J. Heat Mass Transf.* **2009**, *52*, 3518–3524. [CrossRef]
15. Rossini, P.M.; Rossini, L.; Ferreri, F. Brain-behavior relations: Transcranial magnetic stimulation: A review. *IEEE Eng. Med. Biol. Mag.* **2010**, *29*, 84–95. [CrossRef] [PubMed]
16. Medina, L.E.; Grill, W.M. Nerve excitation using an amplitude-modulated signal with kilohertz-frequency carrier and non-zero offset. *J. Neuroeng. Rehabil.* **2016**, *13*, 63. [CrossRef] [PubMed]
17. Palti, Y. Stimulation of Internal Organs by Means of Externally Applied Electrodes. *J. Appl. Physiol.* **1966**, *21*, 1619–1624. [CrossRef] [PubMed]
18. Becerra-Fajardo, L.; Ivorra, A. In vivo demonstration of addressable microstimulators powered by rectification of epidermically applied currents for miniaturized neuroprostheses. *PLoS ONE* **2015**, *10*. [CrossRef] [PubMed]
19. Celinskis, D.; Towe, B.C. Characterization of the implantable neurostimulator-based wireless bioimpedance measurement technique. In Proceedings of the 2016 IEEE EMBS International Student Conference (ISC), Ottawa, ON, Canada, 29–31 May 2016.
20. Larson, P.J.; Towe, B.C. Miniature ultrasonically powered wireless nerve cuff stimulator. In Proceedings of the 2011 5th International IEEE/EMBS Conference on Neural Engineering, Cancun, Mexico, 27 April–1 May 2011; pp. 265–268.
21. Gulick, D.W.; Towe, B.C. Characterization of simple wireless neurostimulators and sensors. In Proceedings of the 2014 36th Annual International Conference of the IEEE Engineering in Medicine and Biology Society, Chicago, IL, USA, 26–30 August 2014; pp. 3130–3133.
22. Sahin, M.; Ur-Rahman, S.S. Finite Element Analysis of a Floating Microstimulator. *IEEE Trans. Neural Syst. Rehabil. Eng.* **2007**, *15*, 227–234. [CrossRef] [PubMed]

23. Schuder, J.C.; Gold, J.H. Localized DC Field Produced by Diode Implanted in Isotropic Homogeneous Medium and Exposed to Uniform RF Field. *IEEE Trans. Biomed. Eng.* **1974**, *21*, 152–163. [CrossRef] [PubMed]
24. Grill, W.M.; Mortimer, J.T. Stimulus waveforms for selective neural stimulation. *IEEE Eng. Med. Biol. Mag.* **1995**, *14*, 375–385. [CrossRef]
25. Mortimer, J.T.; Agnew, W.F.; Horch, K.; Citron, P.; Creasey, G.; Kantor, C. Perspectives on New Electrode technology for stimulating peripheral nerves with implantable motor prostheses. *IEEE Trans. Rehabil. Eng.* **1995**, *3*, 145–154. [CrossRef]
26. Bhadra, N.; Kilgore, K.L. High-frequency electrical conduction block of mammalian peripheral motor nerve. *Muscle Nerve* **2005**, *32*, 782–790. [CrossRef] [PubMed]
27. Soin, A.; Syed, S.N.; Fang, Z.-P. High-Frequency Electrical Nerve Block for Postamputation Pain: A Pilot Study. *Neuromodulation Technol. Neural Interface* **2015**, *18*, 197–206. [CrossRef] [PubMed]
28. Soin, A.; Fang, Z.-P.; Velasco, J.; Shah, N.; Guirguis, M.; Mekhail, M. High-frequency peripheral electric nerve block to treat postamputation pain. *Tech. Reg. Anesth. Pain Manag.* **2014**, *18*, 156–162. [CrossRef]
29. Lubba, C.H.; Le Guen, Y.; Jarvis, S.; Jones, N.S.; Cork, S.C.; Eftekhar, A.; Schultz, S.R. PyPNS: Multiscale Simulation of a Peripheral Nerve in Python. *Neuroinformatics* **2018**, 1–19. [CrossRef] [PubMed]

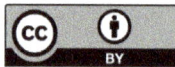

micromachines

MDPI

Article

Characterizing Longitudinal Changes in the Impedance Spectra of In-Vivo Peripheral Nerve Electrodes

Malgorzata M. Straka [1,*]**, Benjamin Shafer** [2]**, Srikanth Vasudevan** [2]**, Cristin Welle** [3] **and Loren Rieth** [1,4]

1   Center for Bioelectronic Medicine, Feinstein Institute for Medical Research, Northwell Health, Manhasset, NY 11030, USA; lrieth@northwell.edu
2   U.S. Food and Drug Administration, Center for Devices and Radiological Health (CDRH), Office of Science and Engineering Laboratory (OSEL), Division of Biomedical Physics (DBP), Silver Spring, MD 20993, USA; benshafer92@gmail.com (B.S.); Srikanth.Vasudevan@fda.hhs.gov (S.V.)
3   Departments of Neurosurgery and Bioengineering, University of Colorado, Aurora, CO 80045, USA; cristin.welle@ucdenver.edu
4   Departments of Electrical Engineering and Bioengineering, University of Utah, Salt Lake City, UT 84112, USA
*   Correspondence: mstraka@northwell.edu; Tel.: +1-516-562-3638

Received: 6 October 2018; Accepted: 5 November 2018; Published: 12 November 2018

Abstract: Characterizing the aging processes of electrodes in vivo is essential in order to elucidate the changes of the electrode–tissue interface and the device. However, commonly used impedance measurements at 1 kHz are insufficient for determining electrode viability, with measurements being prone to false positives. We implanted cohorts of five iridium oxide (IrOx) and six platinum (Pt) Utah arrays into the sciatic nerve of rats, and collected the electrochemical impedance spectroscopy (EIS) up to 12 weeks or until array failure. We developed a method to classify the shapes of the magnitude and phase spectra, and correlated the classifications to circuit models and electrochemical processes at the interface likely responsible. We found categories of EIS characteristic of iridium oxide tip metallization, platinum tip metallization, tip metal degradation, encapsulation degradation, and wire breakage in the lead. We also fitted the impedance spectra as features to a fine-Gaussian support vector machine (SVM) algorithm for both IrOx and Pt tipped arrays, with a prediction accuracy for categories of 95% and 99%, respectively. Together, this suggests that these simple and computationally efficient algorithms are sufficient to explain the majority of variance across a wide range of EIS data describing Utah arrays. These categories were assessed over time, providing insights into the degradation and failure mechanisms for both the electrode–tissue interface and wire bundle. Methods developed in this study will allow for a better understanding of how EIS can characterize the physical changes to electrodes in vivo.

Keywords: impedance; Utah electrode arrays; electrode–tissue interface; peripheral nerves

1. Introduction

Impedance measurements are one of the most widely used techniques to evaluate neural electrodes, both on the benchtop and in vivo. Single frequency impedance measures (e.g., 1 kHz) can be obtained rapidly, used to diagnose open and short circuit failures, and confirm that impedances are compatible with electrical stimulation. Impedance measurements have the possibility of conveying information regarding other key factors of electrode performance, including the (1) degradation of neural electrodes, (2) changes in the electrode–tissue interface, and a (3) correlation to the quality of the acquired neural data. However, the direct interpretation of impedance changes of Utah arrays has remained elusive, despite the development of sophisticated impedance models [1,2]. This is, in part, due to the complexity of the external circuit, compounded by the limited range of the frequencies collected to form the impedance spectra, as well as the compromises in the impedance measurement methods. In addition, for microelectrode arrays such as the Utah electrode array (UEA), abiotic and biotic changes at the electrode tissue interface can drive both increases and decreases in impedance, such that the competition between these mechanisms can result in complex changes in impedance over time [3]. The impedance changes due to abiotic sources are from the changes in the material and surface area of the electrode, whereas the biotic changes result from alterations in the tissue and physiological environment between the electrode and the counter electrode. Moreover, even profound physical damage, such as broken lead wires, can sometimes result in fairly modest changes in the measured 1 kHz impedance. Circuit models for these individual changes have been thoroughly discussed in the literature [1,2]. However, the diversity of the factors that influence impedance, often simultaneously in opposite valences, makes the characterization of the electrode/tissue interface and the identification of failure modes complex. This work combines elements of several models [1,2,4], and enables the categorization of spectra from Utah arrays based on common characteristics.

The sheer volume of data generated by repeated broad-spectrum EIS measurements from high channel-count interfaces also adds to the difficult process of interpreting data. As part of a larger effort to investigate the failure mechanisms of Utah arrays in-vivo, this work was intended to provide a resource-efficient method so as to characterize impedance dynamics and pinpoint failure mechanisms. With this aim, impedance spectra were collected from 1 to 10^6 Hz, from 16 channel UEAs implanted in the sciatic nerve relative to platinum/iridium reference (aka counter or ground) wires in the adjacent tissue of rat models ($N = 11$), for up to 12 weeks. The spectra were classified using an algorithm that we developed to distinguish commonly observed trends in the magnitude and phase spectra. The results of this classification were supervised by our team, and on rare occasions, the classification was manually corrected. Both the performance of the classification, its impact on error analysis in aggregated spectra, and its representation of long-term trends were analyzed. Portions of the spectra up to 10^4 Hz were fitted with a simple Randles circuit model to quantify their electrical characteristics, and to perform quantitative statistical comparisons between them. Furthermore, these fits provided additional insight in to changes of the circuit over time, as well as likely failure modes.

These results provide a high-throughput approach to quantifying changes in impedance spectra under in-vivo conditions. The algorithm significantly increases the ability to diagnose specific failure modes, both biotic and abiotic, in order to provide insight into the real-time integrity of the implanted electrode and biological response.

2. Materials and Methods

The surgical implantation and data collection of the impedance spectra occurred at the Food and Drug Administration. This study was approved by the Institutional Animal Care and Use Committee (IACUC) at the Food and Drug Administration, White Oak campus (protocol number WO2014-145, approved April 2014). Female Lewis rats were purchased from Charles River Laboratories International Inc., for the experiments described in this manuscript. The experiments were conducted on animals weighing between 200 and 280 g at the time of surgery. The animals were single housed in plastic cages with 12-h light and dark cycles throughout the experiments. The animals were randomly assigned to one of the following two groups: (1) IrOx Utah arrays ($N = 5$) and (2) Pt Utah arrays ($N = 6$). Six iridium oxide arrays were originally planned for the study, but one broke during surgical implantation and was removed from the data analysis. Impedance data was collected as part of a different study for evaluating nerve and electromyography (EMG) activity (not presented here).

Sixteen channel (16 recording) Blackrock microelectrode arrays with shanks arranged in a 4×4 configuration were used in this study. Each shank was 1 mm in length with a 0.4 mm pitch between electrodes. The Utah arrays with platinum electrode contacts and Parylene-C insulation were purchased from Blackrock Microsystems. The Iridium Oxide Utah electrode arrays (UEAs), which had a low impedance tip metallization relative to Pt, were provided by Rohit Sharma, Ryan Caldwell, Brian Baker, and Dr. Loren Rieth. The production of these arrays has been described previously [5–7]. Briefly, iridium oxide arrays were fabricated from *p*-type silicon with trenches diced into the backside, and were back-filled with glass for electrical isolation. Subsequently, the front side was diced to the glass and the resulting shanks were etched to form needle-shaped electrodes. The backside bond pads were sputter-deposited from Pt and Ir, and the frontside metallization was sputter-deposited from Pt/Ir/IrOx. The electrodes were encapsulated with 6 μm of Parylene-C and the tips were de-insulated using an oxygen plasma process. The electrodes were wire-bonded to the circuit-board and the bond pads were encapsulated using silicone. The electrodes and the connector (A79026-001, Omnetics Connector Corporation, Minneapolis, MN, USA) were linked via a 55 mm long lead wire bundle, as shown in Figure 1a,b. A 2.5 cm long silicone tube starting at the connector level was added to protect the leads wires from high mechanical stress. Custom-designed EMG arrays were purchased from Microprobes for Life Science, with eight insulated stainless-steel wires of 110 mm length and 0.1 mm diameter arranged into four bipolar pairs, attached to an Omnetics connector (A79038-001) (not shown).

The connector mounts were designed using SolidWorks (2014, Dassault Systèmes SolidWorks Corp., Waltham, MA, USA). Two types of connector mounts were used in this study, the first of which was 3D printed with bronze infused stainless-steel (Figure 1a), which was used in two Pt Utah arrays. The second mount had the bottom part 3D printed with Nylon and the top part with bronze infused stainless steel (Shapeways.com) (Figure 1b). A 35 mm × 30 mm Mersiline mesh was attached to the bottom part of the connector mount using epoxy (Loctite Hysol Epoxy). Connectors from the nerve microelectrode array (and the EMG electrode array were inserted into their respective places inside the connector mount and were bonded with epoxy and, finally, Kwik-cast (World Precision Instruments, Sarasota, FL, USA) were thoroughly applied to the bottom portion of the connector mount to provide a softer tissue contacting surface.

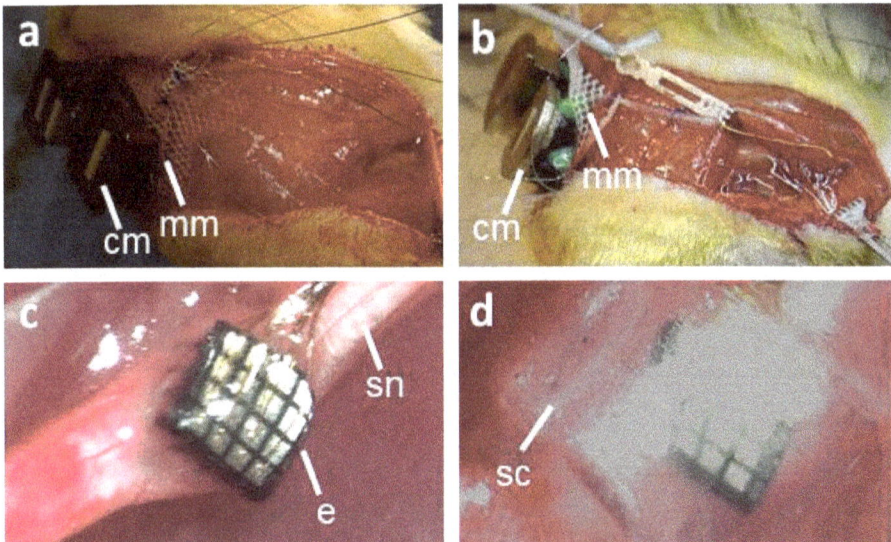

Figure 1. Surgical procedure for the implantation of a nerve electrode array. (**a**) Bronze infused stainless-steel connector mount secured to the lumbar fascia. (**b**) Two-part connector mount secured to the lumbar fascia. (**c**) Electrode array implanted into the sciatic nerve. (**d**) Silicone cuff used to secure the electrode array inside the sciatic nerve. cm—connector mount; mm—mersilene mesh, e—electrode array, sn—sciatic nerve; sc—silicone cuff.

2.1. Surgical Procedure

The animals were anesthetized with an intraperitoneal injection of a ketamine (75 mg·kg^{-1}) and Dexmedetomidine (0.25 mg·kg^{-1}) cocktail. After confirming the lack of a toe pinch reflex, the surgical site was shaved starting from the thoracic region down to the right leg, and was sterilized with betadine and alcohol. An ocular lubricant was applied to prevent drying, and 3 mL of warm sterile saline was administered subcutaneously to prevent dehydration.

A skin incision was made over the thoracic/upper lumbar fascia, and which extended to the right biceps femoris. The connector mount was secured to the fascia with sutures (4-0, Prolene, Polypropylene suture, Med-Vet International, Mettawa, IL, USA), as shown in Figure 1a,b. Mersilene mesh was gently tucked under the skin after dissecting the underlying connective tissue. The sciatic nerve was exposed using blunt dissection techniques described elsewhere [8–10]. The nerve was freed from the surrounding connective tissue, and a piece of sterile silicone block (~10 mm × 8 mm × 1 mm sylgard 184 silicone elastomer kit, Dow Corning, Midland, MI, USA) was placed underneath the nerve. A small sheet of sterile parafilm was placed between the nerve and the silicone block. The UEA array was carefully positioned over the nerve and inserted using a pneumatic impactor (Blackrock Microsystems, Salt Lake City, UT, USA) set at 10 psi. The electrode was gently tapped with the impactor ~5–6 times, so as to achieve insertion. Once the shanks were inside the nerve, a few drops of a two-part fibrin sealant (TISSEEL, Baxter Healthcare Corporation, Deerfield, IL, USA) were applied to stabilize the construct, as shown in Figure 1c. After the fibrin sealant was cured, the silicone block and parafilm were removed from underneath the nerve, followed by the placement of a 4 mm long, 3.2 mm inner diameter silicone cuff around the nerve and electrode. The lumen of this silicone tube was filled with a fibrin sealant, as shown in Figure 1d (cloudy inside silicone tube). The muscle incision over the nerve was closed. The delaminated ground and reference leads were threaded and secured at two different locations inside the muscle over the sciatic nerve implant site using a 21 G needle serving as a cannula.

To implant the EMG arrays, a skin incision was made between the right gastrocnemius and the tibialis anterior muscle. EMG wires were tunneled under the skin, and two pairs of EMG wires for the gastrocnemius and two pairs for the tibialis anterior were inserted into the muscles for redundancy using a 25 G needle serving as a cannula. The wires were then secured in place using sutures (4-0, Prolene, OASIS). Finally, all of the skin incisions were closed using a combination of sutures (4-0, Prolene, OASIS) and the application of gluture. The animals were then administered Atipamezole (0.5 mg kg^{-1}, i.p. (intraperitoneal)) for anesthesia reversal, Meloxicam (2 mg kg^{-1}, s.c. (subcutaneous)) for analgesia, and Gentamycin (8 mg kg^{-1}, s.c.) for antibiotic treatment. Meloxicam (1 mg kg^{-1}, s.c.) per day for two days was administered following surgery.

2.2. Impedance Measurements

The broadband impedance measurements of the individual channels with respect to the ground wire were recorded using electrochemical impedance spectroscopy (1–10^6 Hz, Gamry Instruments Inc., Warminster, PA, USA). To record the pre-implant measurements of a given channel, the electrode array and the ground wires were immersed in 0.15 M phosphate buffered saline. For the post-implant measurements, the impedance of the arrays was measured immediately (~1 h) after the surgery, to confirm the device function, and again, weekly, starting two weeks, for 12 weeks or until device failure.

2.3. Visualization of Spectra

The magnitude and phase of the impedance was loaded into MATLAB (2017b, Mathworks, Natick, MA, USA) for further analysis. As seen in Figure 2, a custom graphical user interface (GUI), called PlotEISGUI, was designed for the visualization of data (code available, see Supplementary Materials). This was also used to correct any categorization errors that were identified visually.

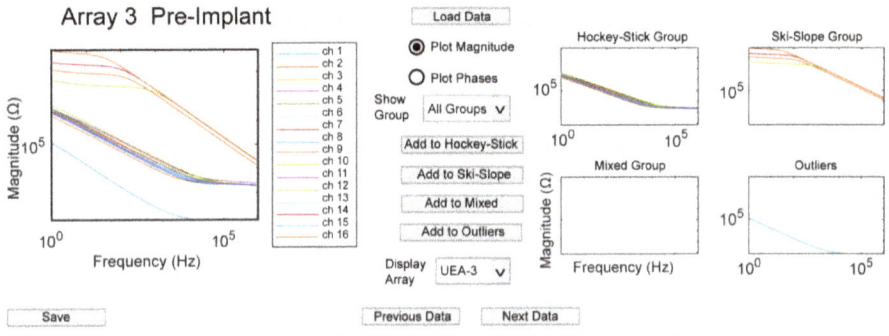

Figure 2. PlotEISGUI with a sample of the iridium oxide Utah electrode array (UEA). In the left plot, the magnitude spectra are plotted for all 16 channels. In the figures on the right, the spectra are divided based on the categories, where Groups 1–3 are the hockey-stick, ski-slope, and mixed groups, respectively.

2.4. Categorization Algorithm

A categorization algorithm was developed to separate the spectra for each channel into distinct groups named hockey-stick, ski-slope, mixed, and outliers. A typical example for each group can be seen in Figure 3, along with the inclusion criteria (detailed below) in the shaded boxes. The hockey-stick group has spectra shape common to that of IrOx [4,11,12] and other low impedance materials (e.g., poly(3,4-ethylenedioxythiophene) (PEDOT)), with the magnitude spectra shape being flat at lower impedances occurring at high frequencies. The ski-slope group, named for the shape of the magnitude spectra, which is flat at high impedances occurring at low frequencies. This shape is likely indicative of a parasitic leakage pathway, resulting in a large impedance that is primarily real (and not imaginary), because of the encapsulation damage at the electrode or lead. This also occurs more readily when the electrode impedance is high, because of tip metal degradation or lead wire breakage. The mixed group, with a complex shape with multiple inflections points, is common in all platinum arrays as well as IrOx electrodes after aging and likely associated degradation. The outliers group had very high, often linear impedance spectra that were likely due to site failure or lead-wire breakage in a location, resulting in a higher impedance pathway to the electrolyte.

The default category was a mixed group for both types of arrays. This group consisted a magnitude spectrum with a gradual, consistent slope with no distinct features, and a phase spectrum that had multiple, small inflection points at various frequencies. The intermediate to more negative phases are indicative of a more capacitive character, but these do sometimes have phases closer to $0°$, and are associated with more real resistances. The less characteristic fluctuations of this category suggest that it represents a larger diversity of conduction pathways.

For Iridium oxide arrays, some spectra were grouped into a hockey-stick Group. The criteria for the hockey-stick group include all four of the following conditions:

(1) $mean(Z_{<100Hz}) < 8 \times 10^6 \ \Omega$
(2) $-80° < mean(\varphi_{<100Hz}) < -40°$
(3) $Max(\varphi_{0.1-50kHz}) > -30°$
(4) $|Max(\varphi_{0.1-10kHz}) - mean(\varphi_{<100Hz})| > 25°$

where Z is the impedance magnitude and φ is the phase magnitude, with the mean or maximum value found for frequencies in the subscript. Condition 1 ensured that the impedance at low frequencies was within a typical range, which was lower for a given geometric surface area, because of the use of IrOx. Conditions 2 and 3 evaluated the characteristics of the phase spectrum, where the phase was highly negative at low frequencies and increased with frequency. The phase at lower frequencies is associated with the combination of Faradaic and capacitive characters of the electrodes. In addition, the small phase angle at high frequencies is associated with the access resistance (i.e., the resistance associated with the electrolyte, the path through the electrolyte, the geometry of the electrode, and the geometric surface area of the electrode) behaving more like a pure resistive element. Condition 4 was designed to reflect that a large increase in slope was present, namely, that the phases at low and high frequencies differed more than 25°. This reflects the distinct transition from the spectrum being dominated by the more capacitive electrode–electrolyte interface at low frequencies, to being dominated by the access resistance at high frequencies.

Iridium oxide arrays were also categorized into a ski-slope group, as the magnitude spectrum was flat at low frequencies and decreased at higher frequencies. The phase spectrum was similar to a decreasing sigmoidal function, with small phases at low frequencies and highly negative phases at large frequencies. The criteria for the ski-slope group included the following:

(1) $mean(\varphi_{>10\text{kHz}}) < -80°$

or all of the following conditions:

(1) $mean(\varphi_{<100\text{Hz}}) > -35°$
(2) $mean(\varphi_{>50\text{kHz}}) < -70°$
(3) $max(\Delta_\varphi) > 25°$

where Δ_φ refers to the slope of the phase (i.e., the difference in values between successive frequencies). Condition 1 is associated with the highly capacitive behavior that occurs at the higher frequencies for these electrodes; whereas, condition 2 is associated with a relatively high impedance (on the order of 10^7 Ω) parasitic leakage pathway through the encapsulation. Condition 3 again indicates that a relatively large change in phase angle occurs between low frequencies and higher frequencies, as the impedance transitions from more resistive at low frequencies to capacitive at higher frequencies.

The final group was designated as outliers. For platinum arrays, the channels were categorized as outliers when the average impedance magnitude at <100 Hz exceeded 1×10^8 Ω. For iridium oxide arrays, the channels were categorized as outliers when the average impedance magnitude at <100 Hz exceeded 2×10^9 Ω. The high impedances of these electrodes are at the limits of the impedances that can be accurately measured, and likely represent a failure in the connector system or lead wires near the connector, with the failures having only a high impedance path through the electrolyte associated with failure that is more isolated from the physiological environment.

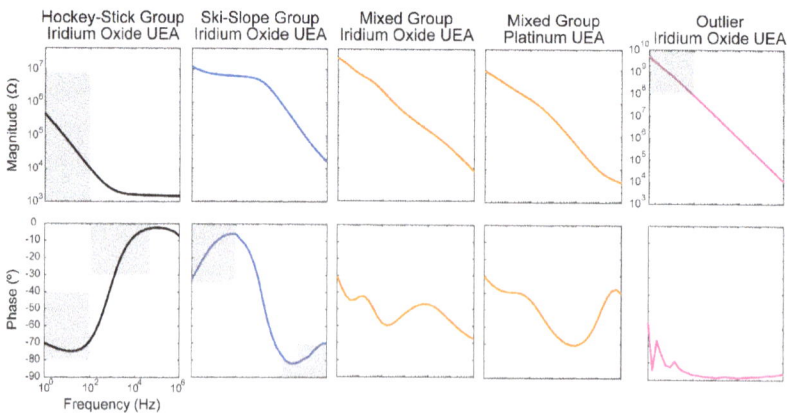

Figure 3. Impedance spectra were classified into groups based on the characteristics of the magnitude and phases. Examples of groups are shown along with categorization criteria (grey boxes; see Section 2.4). Note that the *y*-axis for outliers is scaled to include much higher magnitudes.

2.5. Equivalence Circuit Model

The impedance spectra were fitted to a modified Randles equivalence circuit model, seen in Figure 4a [13]. This circuit comprises of an electrolyte resistance R_s (i.e., access resistance), electrode charge transfer resistance R_E, and constant phase element (Z_{CPE}) representing imperfect capacitance at the electrode/electrolyte interface. Z_{CPE} is defined as

$$Z_{CPE}(w) = \frac{1}{Q(jw)^n},$$

where Q is the admittance of the constant phase element and thus a measure of the magnitude, w is the frequency, and n is a constant between 0 and 1 that describes resistive or capacitive characteristics. The Randles model, which as Z_{CPE} in parallel with R_E, with these elements in series with R_S. Thus, the equation to fit the impedance spectra is:

$$Z_{EIS}(w) = R_s + \frac{R_E}{1 + R_E Q(jw)^n}.$$

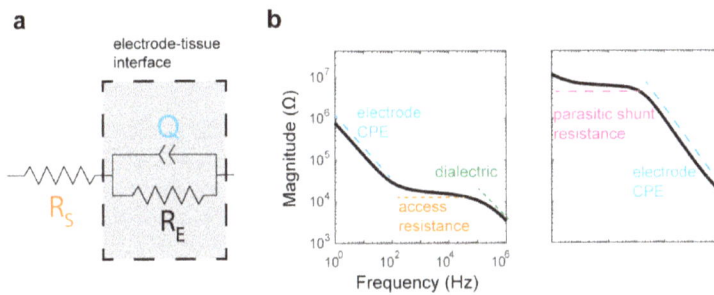

Figure 4. The Randles equivalence circuit used to model an electrode in solution (**a**). The solution resistance, R_S, is in series with the elements denoting the electrode–electrolyte interface, including the electrode transfer resistance, R_E, and the admittance of the constant phase element (CPE), Q. Elements have different contributions to the impedance spectra (**b**), as highlighted by examples classified as hockey-stick (**left**) and ski-slope (**right**). In addition to the electrode CPE, Q, and access resistance, R_S, parasitic shunt resistance may also be present at low frequencies, as well as coupling through a dielectric capacitance at high frequencies.

Each spectrum was fit in MATLAB using Zfit (v1.2.0, 2005, written by Jean-Luc Dellis). The real and imaginary impedances at frequencies of up to 10 kHz were used to create the fit. Higher frequencies were not included in these fits because aging iridium oxide arrays often have a high-frequency roll-off, likely associated with capacitive coupling at a relatively large surface area. This could be from demetallized regions, or areas of silicon exposed by Parylene-C degradation. The initial parameters into the equations were estimated for R_E as 6×10^7 Ω, Q as 5×10^{-7} S s^{-n}, n as 0.8, and R_S as the real component of the impedance measured at 10 kHz. For the lower and upper bounds, the parameter boundary conditions included 1×10^4–1×10^{11} Ω for R_E, 1×10^{-15}–1×10^{-5} for Q, 0–1 for n, and 10–infinity Ω for R_S.

2.6. Machine Learning Algorithm

Using the Classification Learner App in MATLAB, we developed a support vector machine (SVM) algorithm with a fine Gaussian kernel to evaluate the automated categorization for each array type. In this SVM model, the response was the group and predictors included the phase, magnitude, time, and channel for each frequency. Using five-fold validation to protect against overfitting, the algorithm was trained and the prediction accuracy was found.

161

2.7. Statistics

The statistical analyses were performed in MATLAB, with the data reported as mean ± standard error of mean (SEM), unless otherwise noted. The mean and SEM were calculated if more than three channels were present within a specific group at a given time. Unless otherwise specified, the multi-way analysis of variance (ANOVA) was calculated using time, groups, and the log of the impedance magnitude (to normalize values) to detect for significant factors. Significance was determined if $p < 0.05$ after a Bonferroni correction.

To determine predictors for the fit parameters of the equivalent circuit, we created a repeated measures model with the fitrm command in MATLAB. With this repeated measure model, the responses were the fit parameters (n, and the logarithm of R_E, Q, and R_S to normalize the ranges), and the predictors included the groups, times, and channels. Repeated measures ANOVA (using the MATLAB command ranova) were then used to determine which predictors have a significant effect in the model. Wilcoxon signed-rank tests were then used to compare the parameters between groups, with significance determined if $p < 0.05$ after a Holm–Bonferroni correction.

3. Results

The primary goal of the study was to evaluate the longitudinal changes in electrode integrity post implantation. Cohorts of 16-channel Utah arrays were implanted into the sciatic nerve of rats, and the frequency spectra were collected weekly for up to 12 weeks. The implanted arrays were either iridium oxide ($N = 5$) or platinum ($N = 6$) arrays. During the initial analysis, the spectra for each electrode type were averaged to evaluate changes over time. However, it was evident that elucidating trends was problematic because of the large error bars associated with the different spectra shapes that obscured the trends (data not shown). To visualize the individual spectra at specific time points, we developed PlotEISGUI, and observed distinct patterns of the impedance spectra that formed the basis of the categories described below.

3.1. Description of Classes

Each site was classified based on select features in the magnitude and phase impedance spectra (see Section 2.4 for details). The electrode sites were categorized into four groups, hockey-stick, ski-slope, mixed, and outliers (Figure 3).

The hockey-stick category spectra look similar to the spectra from the iridium oxide electrodes previously observed in a variety of in vitro studies [4,11,12]. This category was named for the shape of the magnitude spectrum, which has a large negative slope at low frequencies, associated with more capacitive or mixed capacitive, and a Faradaic character that flattened at higher frequencies, behaving like a real resistance. The phase spectrum also had a characteristic shape of either an increasing sigmoid or inverted-U shape, which results from the transition from the dominant impedance transitioning from capacitive/Faradaic to the real impedance. Specifically, a highly negative phase was present at low frequencies, and the phase increased with frequency and either remained high (i.e., closer to zero) or returned to a more negative phase. The hockey-stick group was always associated with iridium oxide arrays for these UEAs and their associated surface area of 4000 μm^2, including baseline in vitro measurements and some in vivo measurements.

Some of the spectra were categorized in the ski-slope group, where the magnitude spectrum had a consistent, flat slope at low frequencies, which became consistently negative at high frequencies. The Randles equivalent circuit parameters and flat slope of the curve indicate that the electrode was primarily resistive at lower frequencies (see Table 1 and Section 3.3, below). This is likely due to the damage at the wire-bundle lead or to encapsulation, resulting in a parasitic path (Figure 4b), as well as significant tip metal degradation to drive the increased impedance that then reveals the presence of the higher impedance parasitic pathway. The phase spectrum was similar to a decreasing sigmoidal function, with small phases at low frequencies and highly negative phases at large frequencies.

Table 1. Summary of the circuit parameters' fits to Randles equations. The mean +/− standard error of mean (SEM) of each variable is shown both in-vivo and in-vivo past two weeks implantation. No outliers were present for in-vitro conditions for either array.

Array Type	Group	Condition	Number Spectra	R_E (10^{10} Ω)	Q (10^{-8} S s^{-n})	n	R_S (kΩ)
Iridium Oxide	Hockey-stick	In vitro	67	2.0 ± 0.4	22 ± 1	0.81 ± 0.01	2.17 ± 0.07
		In vivo	205	6.2 ± 0.3	30 ± 2	0.64 ± 0.01	138 ± 12
	Ski-slope	In vitro	9	2.1 ± 1.2	7.4 ± 3.2	0.68 ± 0.11	156 ± 90
		In vivo	99	1.0 ± 0.3	1.1 ± 0.3	0.85 ± 0.02	76 ± 28
	Mixed	In vitro	4	4.5 ± 2.6	43 ± 34	0.75 ± 0.09	0.15 ± 0.12
		In vivo	299	3.0 ± 0.2	11 ± 2	0.61 ± 0.01	59 ± 7
	Outliers	In vitro	0				
		In vivo	17	6.8 ± 1.0	0.53 ± 0.35	0.89 ± 0.05	416 ± 245
Platinum	Mixed	In vitro	96	0.46 ± 0.18	0.72 ± 0.08	0.74 ± 0.01	7.3 ± 1.3
		In vivo	854	5.0 ± 0.1	11 ± 1	0.55 ± 0.01	25 ± 2
	Outliers	In vitro	0				
		In vivo	42	1.1 ± 0.3	0.064 ± 0.062	0.96 ± 0.01	93 ± 20

The third group was the mixed group, where the magnitude spectrum decreased with a constant slope and the phase spectrum, and had multiple, small inflection points. For the IrOx arrays, these spectra were similar to one that have been chronically implanted for at least 30 days [11], or to the uncoated sputtered iridium oxide films (SIROF) sites [12], and are thus likely aging sites, with the iridium oxide flaking off, damage to the tips, and/or a complex interaction with the encapsulation sheath. For the platinum arrays, the mixed category was the most prevalent group for all of the timepoints, and the spectra were similar to those previously characterized in vitro [14,15].

Finally, outliers were identified by high impedance magnitudes at low frequencies. These spectra had a very high impedance (see Table 1 and Section 3.3 below), and were likely due to wire failures in the lead that were also well isolated from physiological electrolytes, such as in or near the connector system.

After classification using the automated algorithm, each spectrum was visually assessed using PlotEISGUI. Upon visual inspection, 4.5% ($N = 35/764$) of the classifications were changed for the iridium oxide arrays, with the most common change being from mixed group to outliers ($N = 32$ changes). For the platinum arrays, 3.5% ($N = 17/1087$) of the classifications were adjusted, with mixed group sites being reclassified as ski-slope ($N = 23$) or outliers ($N = 15$). Further analysis was not performed on the hockey-stick or ski-slope groups for the platinum arrays, because of the low number (≤ 3 channels) of channels at any point of time. For both array types, the algorithm correctly grouped the sites for over 95% of the channels.

To evaluate the strength of the categorization based on the spectra, we employed a machine learning algorithm to determine the power of the classification. We fit a five-fold cross-validation fine-Gaussian SVM to the log of the impedance magnitude, log of the frequency, phase, channel, time, and group. The predictive accuracy is 95% for the IrOx arrays and 98.9% for the Pt arrays, with the confusion matrices as seen in Figure 5. Thus, this machine learning approach is comparable or slightly better (for Pt arrays) than the performance of the categorization algorithm, but at the cost of being more computationally complex.

3.2. Longitudinal 1 kHz Impedances

A common method of evaluating electrode integrity is determining the impedance magnitude at 1 kHz. For both the iridium oxide and platinum arrays, we found that groups were a significant predictor of impedances (Kruskal-Wallis, $p < 1 \times 10^{-40}$), with differences between the groups at all timepoints after the implantation highlighted in Figure 6b. Outliers could not be differentiated from mixed groups for the IrOx arrays, and from the ski-slope group for the Pt arrays, although all of the other group comparisons were significantly different ($p < 3 \times 10^{-4}$, with Bonferroni correction). Thus, the impedance magnitude at 1 kHz is insufficient to distinguish between all of the groups, and importantly, cannot distinguish between aging, besides the intact electrodes (mixed group) and putative open circuits (outliers) for the IrOx arrays.

Depending on the category, the impedances change in unique ways, as seen in Figure 6a. For the IrOx arrays, the impedances either increase (as in the hockey-stick group) or decrease (as in the ski-slope group) immediately after implantation, in comparison to the impedances measured in vitro. Interestingly, it appears that the impedances for the mixed group of Pt arrays stay similar for 1 h after implantation, compared to the in vitro impedances, although they slowly appear to decrease over time.

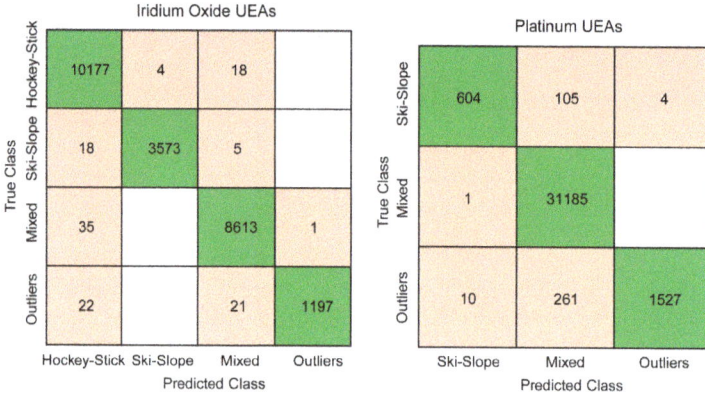

Figure 5. Confusion matrices of the trained SVM algorithm for the iridium oxide (**left**) and platinum arrays (**right**). The numbers refer to the data points within the impedance spectrum, with each spectrum consisting of 31 frequencies collected per channel for each point in time.

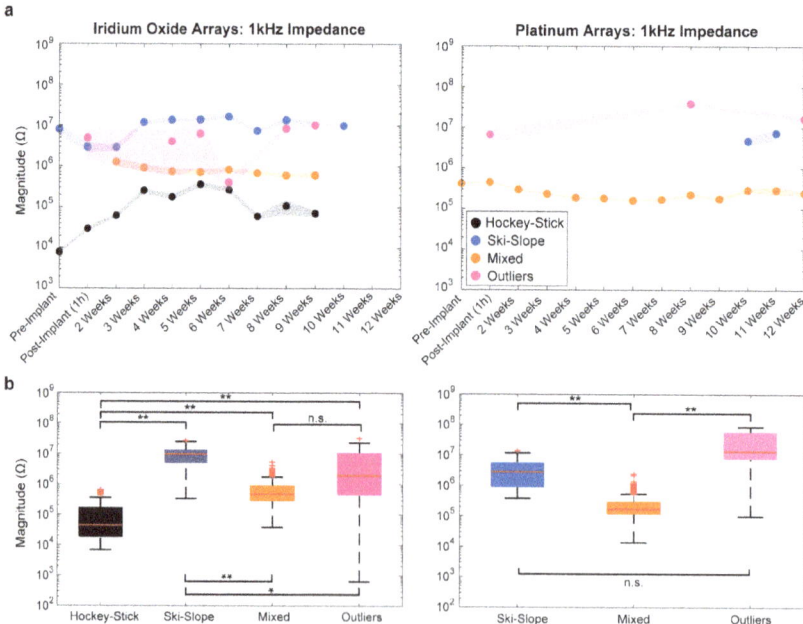

Figure 6. Impedance at 1 kHz for iridium oxide (**left**) and platinum (**right**) arrays vary per group. The mean and standard error of mean (SEM) can be seen at all timepoints (**a**), and the boxplots show the medians for all of the timepoints after implantation (i.e., 1 h through site failure) (**b**) (* refers to $p < 3 \times 10^{-4}$, and ** $p < 1 \times 10^{-13}$, after the Holm–Bonferroni correction).

3.3. Fitting Categories to Randles Model

While the algorithm separated groups based on frequency-specific criteria, fitting the spectra to a Randles equivalent circuit (see Section 2.5 for details) revealed that these differences correlated to the physical properties of the array. For the iridium oxide and platinum arrays, a repeated measured analysis of variance found significant effects for groups ($p < 2 \times 10^{-29}$), times ($p < 4.1 \times 10^{-19}$), and channels ($p < 9 \times 10^{-5}$) (see Section 2.7 for details).

Upon inspection, most of the in vitro parameters typically varied dramatically after implantation and then stabilized after the two-week time point. This surgical recovery period is typical to those in previous studies [1,3,16,17], allowing for the encapsulation of electrodes. Thus, we summarized the average fit values for each group for in vitro and in vivo plus two weeks in Table 1, and plotted boxplots of the fit parameters for the in-vivo plus two weeks in Figure 7. The group most reflective of typical IrOx spectra, the hockey-stick group, demonstrated significantly different values for in vivo verses in vitro for the resistance through the electrolyte, R_S; the electrode–tissue interface resistance, R_E; and for the constant phase element, n. Similarly, the Pt mixed group, the most prevalent group for this array, had Randles fit equation values that differed for all four parameters ($p < 2 \times 10^{-13}$) for in vivo in comparison to in vitro. This suggests the critical influence of the in vivo environment on impedance metrics. For both array types, the R_S significantly increased, indicating that either the effective impedance of the electrolyte increased and/or the effective area of the electrode decreased, likely because of biofouling. In addition, both arrays demonstrated a significantly decreased n value, indicating that the electrode was acting more resistive, potentially because of an increase in the effective area. For the Pt arrays, the constant phase element admittance, Q, value significantly increased, likely because of the decrease of impedance, especially at low frequencies. For the IrOx arrays, there was no significant difference with the Q value over time, although the distribution of values became increasingly skewed with time (data not shown), indicating that the mean is less representative of the population. Finally, both the R_E values increased for both of the arrays, although this is likely from noise, because some in vivo values matched the upper limitations of the model, set at 1×10^{11} Ω to mimic the measurement limitations of the Gamry.

Next, we wanted to determine whether these Randles circuit parameters reflect the differences between groups by determining whether comparisons are significant. For the in vitro spectra of the iridium oxide arrays, the hockey-stick group had a significantly different Q value than the ski-slope group ($p < 0.003$, Wilcoxon signed-rank tests with Holm–Bonferroni correction). In addition, the hockey-stick group had a different in vitro R_S from the mixed group ($p < 0.003$). The differences between the groups became more prevalent when looking at the plus two weeks in vivo values. The hockey-stick group was different from the ski-slope for all four of the parameters ($p < 4 \times 10^{-6}$); different from the mixed group for R_E, Q, and R_S ($p < 2 \times 10^{-9}$); and different from the outliers for Q and n ($p < 2 \times 10^{-5}$). In addition, the ski-slope group had different values for Q and n than the mixed group ($p < 3 \times 10^{-24}$) and a different R_E value from the outliers ($p < 3 \times 10^{-7}$). Finally, the mixed group had significantly different R_E, Q, and n values than the outlier group ($p < 3 \times 10^{-4}$). For the Pt arrays implanted for at least two weeks, the values for the mixed group were all significantly different than the outliers ($p < 8 \times 10^{-5}$). Together, this demonstrates that the groups differ because of the physical features at the electrode and electrode–electrolyte interface.

The Randles circuit n-value, which represents how capacitive or resistive the electrode is behaving, had stark differentiation between groups. By definition, the n-values range from 0 to 1, depending on whether the constant phase element in the Randles circuit behaves more like a capacitor or resistor, respectively. For the chronically implanted iridium oxide arrays, the hockey-stick and mixed groups had n-values that averaged approximately 0.6, indicative of a leaky capacitor common to that of IrOx. In contrast, the ski-slope and outliers for both of the array types had much higher n-values of 0.85 or more, indicating a leakage path of a shunt resistor. This is likely due to breakage in the wire bundle, allowing for the current to flow directly to the environment. For the ski-slope group, this is also demonstrated by the lower R_E values, indicative of a greater charge transfer to tissue.

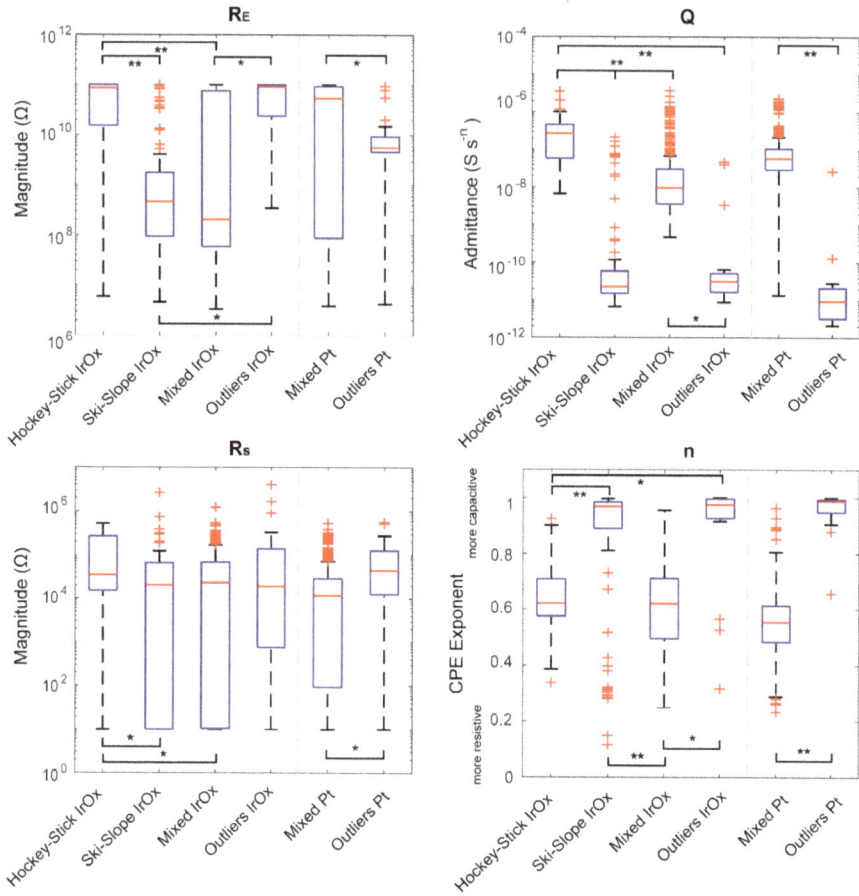

Figure 7. Boxplots of fit Randles equation fit values for in vivo impedance spectra. Boxplots show median values, and comparisons were tested with Wilcoxon sign-rank tests (* refers to $p < 3 \times 10^{-4}$, ** $p < 8 \times 10^{-11}$, after a Holm–Bonferroni correction). Note that the upper bound of R_E values were 1×10^{11} Ω, as a result of limitations of the Gamry instrument.

The constant phase element admittance, Q, also greatly varied between groups. The hockey-stick groups had the highest values at approximately 30×10^{-8} S s^{-n}, with the mixed groups having slightly lower values at 11×10^{-8} S s^{-n}. In contrast, the groups that likely demonstrate damaged sites/wire bundle, the ski-slope and outlier groups, have values of 1×10^{-8} S s^{-n} or lower.

The shunt resistance, R_E, also reveals differences between the categories, with the exception of the hockey-stick to outliers, and ski-slope to mixed. However, this may not be representative, because the value is near or at the upper bound of 10^{11} Ω defined in the Randles model, a limitation incorporated because this is the limit of the impedance that the spectrometer can measure. In addition, this may further be limited, because we did not collect frequencies lower than 1 Hz. Collecting impedances at lower frequencies may illuminate further difference between the categories.

The access resistance, R_S, is associated with the effective impedance of the tissue/electrolyte between the electrode and reference, as well as the effective geometry and geometric surface area of the electrode, and is often observed to increase during in vitro and in vivo studies as a function of tissue encapsulation or fouling (e.g., [18]). The increases in impedance can also occur as metallization is lost, and thus the effective electrode area is decreased. Because of the particularly large difference in impedance between silicon and IrOx, this value can be sensitive to the loss of metallization with resulting exposure of Si, which has been reported [4]. It also depends on the effective conductance of the physiological environment, which can be modulated by the types of tissue or the foreign-body response associated with the electrode. For mixed and outlier groups, there is no flat region of the spectra associated with the access resistance, indicating that the categories are always limited by the impedance of the electrode/electrolyte interface, where the "electrode" might be a broken, but it encapsulates the wire in the lead, particularly for the case of the outliers.

The Randles model also highlights the differences between the types of arrays. Comparing the values between the hockey-stick group and the mixed Pt group (i.e., the channels most like typical IrOx and Pt sites), all of the plus two week in vivo fit values were significantly less for the Pt sites ($p < 1 \times 10^{-10}$, Wilcoxon sign-rank tests). In addition, the R_E, Q, and R_S values were also lower in vitro for the Pt mixed group ($p < 0.005$). Given that higher n-values indicate that the model is acting more as a capacitor, it is unexpected for the n-values to be lower for the mixed Pt group. This may be due to the n-values for the Pt mixed group being lower here than in the previously published in vitro results [1], although it is important to note that these values are from planar electrodes. However, given that IrOx is known to have lower impedances than Pt sites, it is unsurprising that the values are lower for Q, with lower Q values being consistent with a lower impedance magnitude of the constant phase element.

3.4. Longitudinal Changes of Categories

The distribution of groups changes over time, as seen in Figure 8. For the iridium oxide arrays, the sites are primarily hockey-stick in shape, until three weeks post-implantation. The mixed groups become more prevalent starting at two weeks, and continuously increase through to week eight. The spectra for the IrOx mixed group appear similar to the IrOx arrays implanted for at least 30 days, tested by Cogan et al. [11]; the Pt electrodes from this and other UEA studies; uncoated SIROF (i.e., just the gold metallization for planar electrodes) sites [12]; and the analysis of impedance as a function of the materials and surface area [4]. The lower impedance expected for IrOx suggests that the transition from the hockey-stick to mixed arrays is likely attributable to a loss of surface area resulting from IrOx delamination and/or fouling associated with adsorption and glial encapsulation during aging. This results in the impedances remaining above the access resistance associated with the flat part of the hockey-stick curve only potentially occurring at higher frequencies (e.g., Figure 4b). Starting at week eight, many sites stop being measured because of device failure, with the last sites being measured at week ten. For the Pt arrays, the mixed group is the predominant group until week 11, at which point 50% of the sites have failed. Overall, there are few sites that belong to other groups until week eight, when over 30 sites become outliers. Thus, the Pt arrays demonstrate more stable impedance spectra than the IrOx arrays. This is possibly, in part, due to the higher starting impedance values for the Pt electrodes, decreasing the changes in impedance associated with metal delamination. A careful SEM evaluation of the metal degradation would be required to discriminate these.

Within a group, the impedance spectra change over time in complex ways, as seen in Figure 9. For the iridium oxide arrays, the hockey-stick group has a phase spectrum that initially looks like an increasing sigmoid function (dark blue in Figure 9a, bottom panel). After implantation, the peak phase shifts to lower frequencies and forms a maximum at approximately 1 kHz, by approximately nine weeks (yellow shades in Figure 9a). As time progresses, the curve maximum occurs at incrementally lower frequencies. This maximum is associated with phase angles closer to zero, and therefore resistive impedance character. When associated with the magnitude spectra, an incrementally increasing resistance for the flat part of the curve is observed, which we associate with the access resistance. This increase in resistance causes this component of the curve to intersect the sloped region at lower frequencies, resulting in the concomitant propagation of the maximum to lower frequencies. The results are consistent with an increasing impedance for the physiological electrolyte or a decreased surface area for the electrode. These could be associated with the foreign body response and tissue healing process, and tip metal degradation, respectively. For each hockey-stick spectrum, we found f_{peak}, the frequency at which the maximum phase occurred, and found that time has a significant effect ($p < 7 \times 10^{-49}$, Kruskal–Wallis test). Using Wilcoxon signed-rank tests to compare across timepoints, we found the f_{peak} to be progressively lower up to week six. After approximately six weeks, this f_{peak} value becomes similar. This phase peak is reflected in the magnitude spectrum via the high-frequency roll-off (i.e., the elevated magnitude at approximately 10 kHz). This roll-off is thought to be due to the degradation of the Parylene-C and current leakage through the silicon or even capacitive coupling through the dielectric [4] (see Figure 4b).

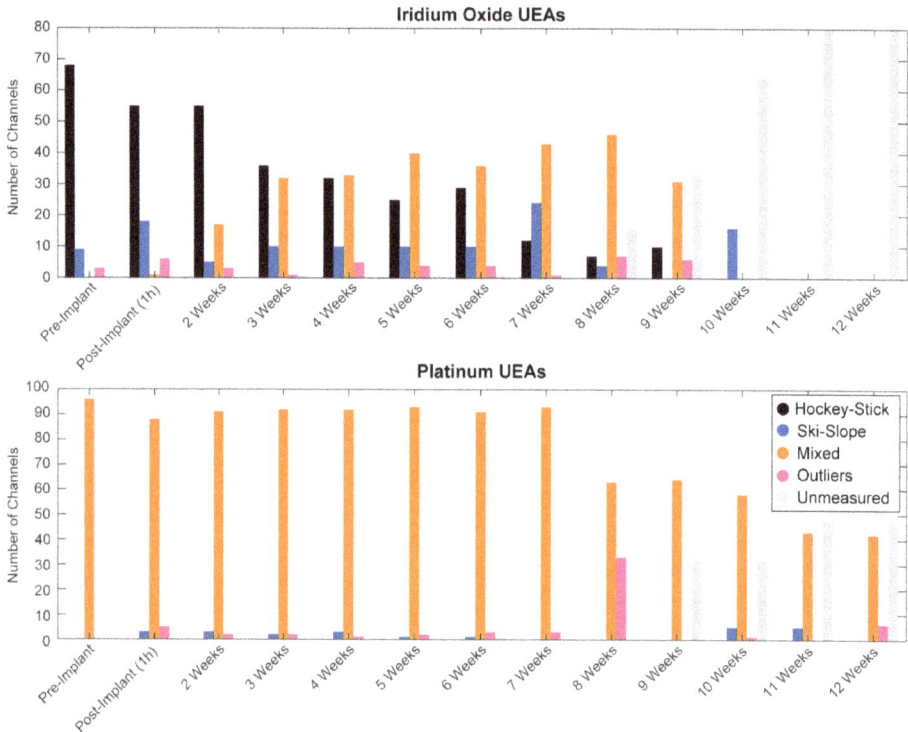

Figure 8. Summary of population changes for groups over time for iridium oxide (**top**) and platinum (**bottom**) arrays. After the failure of all sites in an array, the impedance spectra were no longer collected and are designated as unmeasured.

For the iridium oxide arrays belonging in the Ski-Slope group (Figure 9b), the phase spectrum appears as a decreasing sigmoid. Immediately after implantation, the inflection point of this sigmoid (i.e., greatest slope) occurs at a higher frequency. In the successive weeks, the inflection point occurs at progressively lower frequencies, without statistical significance ($p > 0.05$).

For the platinum arrays, the phase spectrum for the predominant mixed group initially presented with a U-shaped minimum in middle frequencies, similar to that of Pt UEAs previously shown in vitro [14,15]. As time progresses, this minimum flattens out and a high-frequency peak develops. When similar electrodes age in a saline bath, the size of this minimum decreases, although it does not become as flat as those observed here at approximately seven weeks. Thus, these changes are likely due the foreign body response, although the aging of the electrode may also contribute. The magnitude spectra are similar [14,15] or much lower than a previous study [19], with the latter difference potentially arising from the large error bars presented with the mean. Over time, we found that the impedance decreased at low frequencies (<100 Hz) and increased at very high frequencies (1 MHz).

Electrodes aging in a PBS bath decreased in impedance at low frequencies, but remained similar at high frequencies [14]. In contrast, reactive accelerated aging via exposure to reactive oxygen species decreased the impedance across all of the frequencies [19]. These differences are likely attributed to factors arising from glial response in vivo.

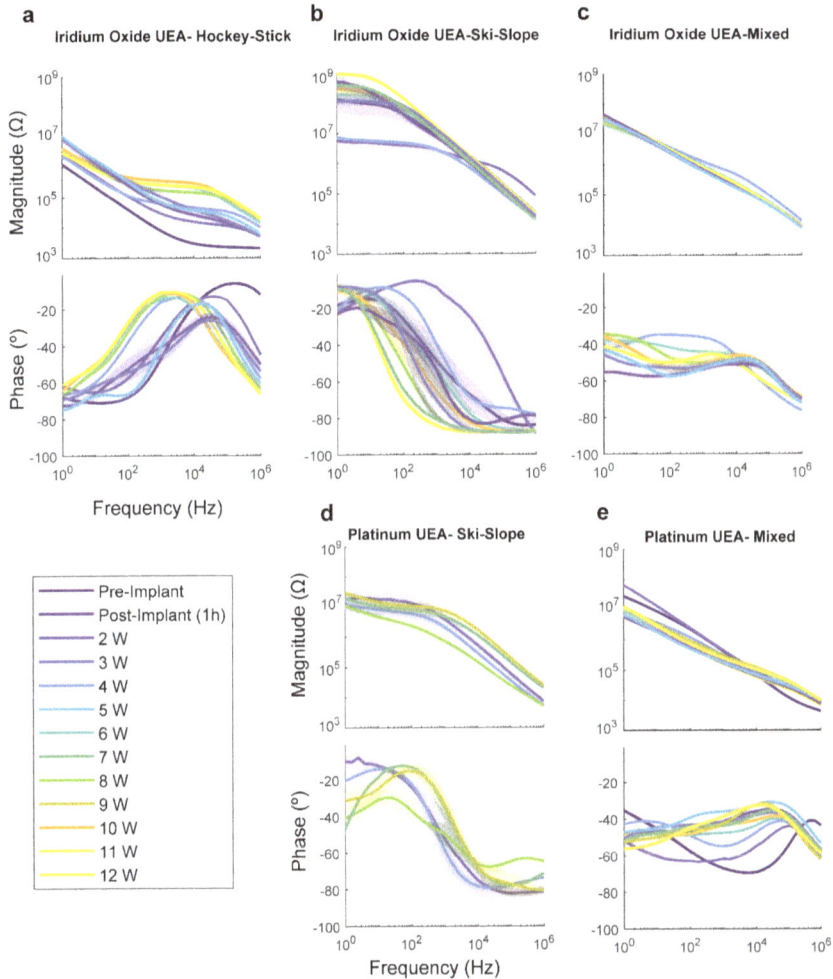

Figure 9. Mean magnitude and phase spectra for iridium oxide (**a–c**) and platinum (**d,e**) UEAs (shaded areas are SEM) over time.

4. Discussion

We developed a simple categorization algorithm for the impedance spectra that can enable a more thorough longitudinal analysis of the implanted electrodes. We also created a visualization GUI, called PlotEISGUI, to display the categories and enable corrections with visual inspection. We found this algorithm to be robust and it correctly categorized 95% of the spectra, with correction required for approximately 5% of the spectra. This performance was comparable to a fine-Gaussian SVM algorithm, which had a prediction accuracy of 95% for iridium oxide arrays and 98.9% for platinum arrays. The advantages of the algorithm over the SVM included its simplicity, which allows it to classify an individual electrode's spectra at one point in time with computation efficiency and without expensive toolboxes. The groups are further distinguished by the difference in fit parameters when modeling each spectrum to a Randles equivalence circuit, further demonstrating the distinctiveness of each category.

4.1. Physical Characteristics Underlying Groups

The hockey-stick shape described here is common to the spectra previously observed in the iridium oxide arrays [4,11,12]. As the IrOx electrodes age, the hockey-stick group develops a characteristic flattening, with an increased impedance with time at approximately 100 Hz–10 kHz, similar to the previously observed spectra of the implanted electrodes [16]. This flat aspect is associated with the access resistance, which is controlled by the geometric surface area of the electrode, the geometry of the electrode (including the length), and the effective impedance of the path through the (physiological) electrolyte (e.g., Figure 4b). The impedance of the physiological environment can change because of the formation of the glial scar around the electrodes, or other tissue healing or responses for the tissue between the electrodes. In unpublished studies, we have observed that this increase in access resistance begins within minutes after implantation. This effect is not observed for the Pt arrays, which actually have a small yet significant decrease in 1 kHz impedance after implantation (comparing in vitro to week three and following time points, $p < 1 \times 10^{-6}$ after Bonferroni correction). The Pt impedance is higher than IrOx, and typically has a smoother surface, making increases in impedance with in-dwelling time smaller. Also, implantation can decrease the impedances through encapsulation degradation and water ingress. Additionally, Pt microelectrodes, with their associated small surface area (~4000 μm^2), do not demonstrate a flat region associated with the access resistance. Comparing the in vitro values of the Randles fit equations to those of the IrOx arrays found by Caldwell et al. [4], the latter reported a n of 0.87, which is within one standard deviation of the value presented here. They also reported Q$_0$ of 27 × 10^{-6} S s^{-n} mm^{-2}, which when multiplied by our size electrode (i.e., 4000 μm^2), would be equivalent to 1.1 × 10^{-7} S s^{-n}, a value approximately one standard deviation from our mean of 2.2 × 10^{-7} S s^{-n}. In addition, aging electrodes in the hockey-stick group also developed a high-frequency roll-off, which is thought to be associated with leakage through the dielectric capacitance [2].

The ski-slope group for IrOx is likely a result of lead wire breakage or a significant loss of tip metallization, and the presence of a parasitic leakage path responsible for the flat region at low frequencies (e.g., Figure 4b). The parasitic leakage path often occurs at very high impedances of 10^8 to 10^9 Ω, and therefore can only be observed when the impedance of the channel is high enough that it can be appreciated. The individual gold lead wires are overmolded by silicone; therefore, when these wires break, their impedance can increase modestly if the break is in a way that results in a lower impedance path, or with a significantly higher impedance because of poor communication to the electrolyte. The flat region at low frequencies has a resistive character, suggesting that this is a small/high impedance leakage path, potentially associated with encapsulation degradation. This is supported by Randles circuit models, where the in vivo n-values are 0.85, and the R_E values are below that of the other groups, indicative of a leakage path due to a shunt resistance and greater charge transfer to tissue. The increase in R_E values suggests that either tissue remodeling or further material degradation results in an increased impedance for the shunt pathway. The mechanism of wire breakage is further supported by the fact changes in group categorization to the ski-slope group were often global across the array. Specifically, for two IrOx arrays, at least 15 of the 16 of sites became designated as ski-slope at the same point in time.

For the iridium oxide arrays, the mixed group interpretation of the impedance spectra is more difficult and would benefit from the physical characterization of the electrodes using SEM, optical microscopy, and other failure analysis techniques. The impedance magnitudes are similar to the hockey-stick group at high frequencies (>10^5 Hz, especially for hockey-stick sites after approximately six weeks), but is ~2 to 10 times higher than the hockey-stick sites at 1 Hz. The higher impedances at low frequencies for the mixed group electrodes result in R_S not dominating the impedance spectra at intermediate or high frequencies. In addition, there is a large difference in the phase curves between these two groups. The phase curve for the hockey-stick indicates a relatively capacitive coupling at low frequencies, because of more negative phase values, which increase towards values closer to zero, indicative of a resistive character. In contrast, the mixed electrodes maintain a relatively consistent phase angle across the spectra from low to intermediate values. This is similar in character and magnitude to the spectra from the Pt electrodes. The loss of the flat region characteristic of the hockey-stick spectrum indicates that the impedance of the electrode interface dominates the spectra across the measured range. This can result from a loss of geometric surface area for the metallization, or a decrease in effective capacitance, resulting in an increased impedance. The former would result from metal delamination, or the effective surface area being decreased by the foreign body response. The increase in effective capacitance could result from a change in the surface material; to the underlayers of Pt and Ir if the IrOx delaminates, leaving those layers behind; or even the silicon surface of the shank. In principle, fouling of the IrOx surface could also result in a decreased capacitance, but this is at odds with the behavior of the aged IrOx that maintains the hockey-stick character.

The platinum arrays were most commonly assigned as the mixed group. Compared to the Pt UEAs in saline, these spectra were similar [14,15] or lower [19] in impedance to those previously observed. For the data with a higher impedance, the study found large error bars when averaging across the 16 channels [19], which makes interpretations more challenging. In addition, the spectra summarized here were similar in magnitude but not phase to planar black Pt microelectrode arrays with a tip size of 900 μm^2 [1]. For the planar electrodes, the Randles equivalence circuit parameters were as follows: Q was $0.89 \pm 0.52 \times 10^{-9}$ $s\Omega^{-1/n}$, n was 0.86 ± 0.02, R_S was 7.38 ± 1.74 kΩ, and R_E was $2.7 \pm 1.31 \times 10^9$ Ω (mean $\pm$ standard deviation). The R_E and n values were similar to the ones presented here, at approximately 0.1 and 1.4 standard deviations from our determined values, respectively. Given that R_S reflects the size of the electrode, we divided this value by the ratio of sizes, assuming that our Pt UEAs were approximately 4000 μm^2. This results in a corrected mean of 1.7 kΩ, which is approximately half a standard deviation from the mean found here. To compare Q values, we converted the units by multiplying to the power of n, with a value for Q of 1.6×10^{-8} (S s^{-n}), which is approximately 1.5 standard deviations of the mean values presented here. The mixed group for the Pt array also showed a pronounced phase shift over time, with a high-frequency maxima developing several weeks post implantation. This is consistent with previous work suggesting the development of moderate encapsulation around Utah electrode arrays implanted in rodent cortex [20].

The ski-slope group for the Pt electrodes was different than for IrOx, in particular, with lower impedances for the flat aspect of the spectra. This suggests that the impedance associated with the parasitic shunt pathway had a lower impedance (Figure 4b), and therefore had a large area. This suggests a greater degree of encapsulation degradation for the electrodes, as a roll-off at low frequencies has been consistently found as an early hallmark for this degradation across both test structures and for electrodes.

4.2. Categorization Algorithms

The elegance of this approach allows for the differential categorization of electrodes within a given array—providing electrode-by-electrode information on interface dynamics. This categorization can be accomplished with a simple equation, and does not require large datasets, complicated machine learning algorithms, or expensive toolboxes. Importantly, this approach allows for the improved characterization of array dynamics over time. The dual inclusion of magnitude and phase characteristics can separate resistive and capacitive evolution over the course of in vivo implantation.

Interestingly, the categorization criteria relied heavily on the phase values, and supplemental on impedance magnitude at frequencies <100 Hz. This is consistent with the data from in vitro accelerated aging studies incorporating reactive species, which demonstrated that the largest changes in the aged electrodes were in frequencies <100 Hz, regardless of the initial electrode materials, form factor, or impedance spectra characteristics [19].

In contrast, the information at 1 kHz, as commonly used to describe the electrodes, was less informative. Impedance at 1 kHz could not differentiate between the outlier and mixed groups for the IrOx arrays, and between the outlier and ski-slope groups for the Pt arrays, with the outlier groups likely being broken electrodes. In addition, the 1 kHz measurement showed little temporal variation, and stayed relatively similar between the in vivo and in vitro measurement environments. Interestingly, we did not observe marked increases in impedance at 1 kHz in the first several weeks post-implantation, in contrast with other measurements of devices implanted in the central nervous system [2,5,17,21–23]. This may be a feature of implantation in the peripheral nerve stimulation (PNS) or, the implantation method using a silicone cuff and fibrin sealant, which may change the immediate physiological environment and itself be degraded over time. Alternately, this may suggest minimal edema following implantation, as transient increases in impedance have been tied to transient biofouling, edema, and neuroinflammation in the central nervous system (CNS) [23–25].

However, the evaluation of the full spectrum EIS showed robust temporal dynamics over the course of implantation. This more accurately matches what is known regarding the time-evolving tissue response [26–30], and the gradual degradation in electrode materials known to occur in vivo [17,31]. For instance, the population of the hockey-stick group declined following three weeks in vivo, representing dynamic changes to the electrodes following implantation. These changes likely result from increased impedances associated with metal delamination or from significant fouling of the IrOx, possibly counterbalanced by water penetration through the Parylene-C dielectric [19,32], as evidenced by the roll-off seen at high frequencies (e.g., Figure 4b).

Anecdotally, we found that changes in the assignment of categorization for an individual electrode was often reflective of changes throughout the array. For one iridium oxide array, 15 of 16 electrodes were designated as hockey-stick before implantation. During implantation, one electrode became an outlier, and the remaining 14 were categorized as hockey-stick until week eight, when all of the sites became Ski-Slope. The following week, the array was no longer measured because of failure. A similar change happened for another IrOx array, when at 1 h post implantation, 15 sites were hockey-stick, and all 15 sites became mixed group at week three. The sites remained at the mixed group until array failure at week 10. A third array was more variable, all of the electrodes were hockey-stick both in-vitro and immediately post implantation, and at two weeks, 14 sites were hockey-stick and two sites were mixed group. By week five, three sites were outliers, five sites were mixed, and the eight remained hockey-stick. This remained varied until week 10, when all of the sites became hockey-stick, regardless of their previous category. For the remaining two iridium oxide arrays, the sites were more varied in the categories from the in-vitro tests. Platinum arrays similarly have universal changes to sites. For two platinum arrays, at least 15 sites were in a mixed group until week eight, when all of the sites became outliers. In another two arrays, at least 15 sites were mixed until week 12. Perhaps these global changes result from abiotic factors such as damage to lead wires, delamination at the bond pad, connectors, or abrupt biological changes, such as bleeding.

4.3. Future Work

The data presented here analyzes the changes to the impedance spectra over time, creating categories to allow for the analysis of trends over time. It will be critical to correlate those changes with the physical changes of the electrode tips. At the completion of the study, the arrays were harvested and imaged using scanning electrode microscopy (data not presented here). The results will further illuminate whether these categories correlate to specific physical changes or damage to the electrode.

This work shows changes in electrode spectra when implanted chronically in the peripheral nerve of a rat. It will be informative to determine whether similar effects are found for similar electrodes implanted in the central nervous system, as well as within different animals. In addition, collecting spectra from a wider range, including frequencies down to 0.01 Hz, may provide further information about nonlinear effects at low frequencies. For iridium oxide electrodes, relating cyclic voltammetry to the different groups may provide further information about the charge density and health of the site.

5. Conclusions

These data represent a new approach to characterizing broad spectrum EIS from electrodes implanted in vivo. Utilizing EIS provides meaningful information that cannot be conveyed with a single frequency impedance measurement. Critically, a 1 kHz impedance was not able to differentiate between functional and presumed broken channels. We found that the key characteristics for defining the variability of in vivo electrodes were shifts in the phase and impedance magnitude at <100 Hz. The classification algorithm that we developed is a rapid, resource-efficient classification tool to evaluate longitudinal, broad spectrum EIS data. The application of this algorithm to Utah arrays implanted in the rat sciatic nerve demonstrated that iridium oxide electrodes rapidly alter their properties in vivo, while the platinum arrays had greater stability. This difference may be due to the lower impedance of the iridium oxide sites, which make the changes in aging arrays more easily observed, in contrast to platinum, which has a more similar impedance to Silicon, and thus the changes could be more difficult to elucidate. The relatively low impedances of the IrOx, and the fact that the access resistance is the limiting resistance for these, might result in the aging of the electrodes being more easily observed. In addition, abrupt categorization changes often preceded array failure, and seemed to implicate lead wire breakage as a major failure mechanism. Future work will relate these classifications to alterations in the physical properties of the device materials and to the quality of the detected neural signal.

Supplementary Materials: The code for PlotsEISGUI and the categorization algorithm are available online at: https://bitbucket.org/MargoS/eis-analysis.git.

Author Contributions: Conceptualization, L.R., C.W., and S.V.; methodology, M.M.S., L.R., C.W., and S.V.; software, M.M.S.; investigation, S.V. and B.S.; resources, S.V., L.R., and C.W.; supervision, S.V. and C.W.; formal analysis, M.M.S., S.V., C.W., and L.R.; visualization, M.M.S.; writing (original draft preparation, review, and editing), M.M.S., B.S., L.R., S.V., and C.W.; funding acquisition, L.R., C.W., and S.V.

Funding: This research project was funded by the Defense Advanced Research Projects Agency (DARPA), the Biotechnology Technology Office (BTO), and the Hand Proprioception and Touch Interfaces (HAPTIX) Program, through an Interagency Agreement with the United States Food and Drug Administration (DARPA-FDA IAA 224-14-6009).

Disclaimer: The mention of commercial products, their sources, or their use in connection with the material reported herein is not to be construed as either an actual or implied endorsement of such products by the Department of Health and Human Services.

Conflicts of Interest: The authors declare no conflict of interest. The funders had no role in the design of the study; in the collection, analyses, or interpretation of data; in the writing of the manuscript; or in the decision to publish the results.

References

1. Franks, W.; Schenker, I.; Schmutz, P.; Hierlemann, A. Impedance Characterization and Modeling of Electrodes for Biomedical Applications. *IEEE Trans. Biomed. Eng.* **2005**, *52*, 1295–1302. [CrossRef] [PubMed]
2. Mercanzini, A.; Colin, P.; Bensadoun, J.-C.; Bertsch, A.; Renaud, P. In Vivo Electrical Impedance Spectroscopy of Tissue Reaction to Microelectrode Arrays. *IEEE Trans. Biomed. Eng.* **2009**, *56*, 1909–1918. [CrossRef] [PubMed]
3. Prasad, A.; Xue, Q.-S.; Dieme, R.; Sankar, V.; Mayrand, R.C.; Nishida, T.; Streit, W.J.; Sanchez, J.C. Abiotic-Biotic Characterization of Pt/Ir Microelectrode Arrays in Chronic Implants. *Front. Neuroeng.* **2014**, *7*, 2. [CrossRef] [PubMed]
4. Caldwell, R.; Sharma, R.; Takmakov, P.; Street, M.G.; Solzbacher, F.; Tathireddy, P.; Rieth, L. Neural Electrode Resilience against Dielectric Damage May Be Improved by Use of Highly Doped Silicon as a Conductive Material. *J. Neurosci. Methods* **2018**, *293*, 210–225. [CrossRef] [PubMed]
5. Rousche, P.J.; Normann, R.A. Chronic Recording Capability of the Utah Intracortical Electrode Array in Cat Sensory Cortex. *J. Neurosci. Methods* **1998**, *82*, 1–15. [CrossRef]
6. Jones, K.E.; Campbell, P.K.; Normann, R.A. A Glass/Silicon Composite Intracortical Electrode Array. *Ann. Biomed. Eng.* **1992**, *20*, 423–437. [CrossRef] [PubMed]

7. Bhandari, R.; Negi, S.; Rieth, L.; Solzbacher, F. A Wafer-Scale Etching Technique for High Aspect Ratio Implantable MEMS Structures. *Sens. Actuators A Phys.* **2010**, *162*, 130–136. [CrossRef] [PubMed]
8. Vasudevan, S.; Huang, J.; Botterman, B.; Matloub, H.S.; Keefer, E.; Cheng, J. Detergent-Free Decellularized Nerve Grafts for Long-Gap Peripheral Nerve Reconstruction. *Plast. Reconstr. Surg. Glob. Open* **2014**, *2*, e201. [CrossRef] [PubMed]
9. Vasudevan, S.; Patel, K.; Welle, C. Rodent Model for Assessing the Long Term Safety and Performance of Peripheral Nerve Recording Electrodes. *J. Neural Eng.* **2017**, *14*, 016008. [CrossRef] [PubMed]
10. Vasudevan, S.; Yan, J.-G.; Zhang, L.-L.; Matloub, H.S.; Cheng, J.J. A Rat Model for Long-Gap Peripheral Nerve Reconstruction. *Plast. Reconstr. Surg.* **2013**, *132*, 871–876. [CrossRef] [PubMed]
11. Kane, S.R.; Cogan, S.F.; Ehrlich, J.; Plante, T.D.; McCreery, D.B. Electrical Performance of Penetrating Microelectrodes Chronically Implanted in Cat Cortex. In Proceedings of the 2011 Annual International Conference of the IEEE Engineering in Medicine and Biology Society, Boston, MA, USA, 30 August–3 September 2011; IEEE: Piscataway, NJ, USA, 2011; Volume 2011, pp. 5416–5419.
12. Cogan, S.F.; Ehrlich, J.; Plante, T.D.; Smirnov, A.; Shire, D.B.; Gingerich, M.; Rizzo, J.F. Sputtered Iridium Oxide Films for Neural Stimulation Electrodes. *J. Biomed. Mater. Res. Part B Appl. Biomater.* **2009**, *89B*, 353–361. [CrossRef] [PubMed]
13. Randles, J.E.B. Kinetics of Rapid Electrode Reactions. *Discuss. Faraday Soc.* **1947**, *1*, 11. [CrossRef]
14. Leber, M.; Bhandari, R.; Mize, J.; Warren, D.J.; Shandhi, M.M.H.; Solzbacher, F.; Negi, S. Long Term Performance of Porous Platinum Coated Neural Electrodes. *Biomed. Microdevices* **2017**, *19*, 62. [CrossRef] [PubMed]
15. Leber, M.; Shandhi, M.M.H.; Hogan, A.; Solzbacher, F.; Bhandari, R.; Negi, S. Different Methods to Alter Surface Morphology of High Aspect Ratio Structures. *Appl. Surf. Sci.* **2016**, *365*, 180–190. [CrossRef] [PubMed]
16. Weiland, J.D.; Anderson, D.J. Chronic Neural Stimulation with Thin-Film, Iridium Oxide Electrodes. *IEEE Trans. Biomed. Eng.* **2000**, *47*, 911–918. [CrossRef] [PubMed]
17. Prasad, A.; Sanchez, J.C. Quantifying Long-Term Microelectrode Array Functionality Using Chronic In Vivo Impedance Testing. *J. Neural Eng.* **2012**, *9*, 026028. [CrossRef] [PubMed]
18. Newbold, C.; Richardson, R.; Millard, R.; Huang, C.; Milojevic, D.; Shepherd, R.; Cowan, R. Changes in Biphasic Electrode Impedance with Protein Adsorption and Cell Growth. *J. Neural Eng.* **2010**, *7*, 056011. [CrossRef] [PubMed]
19. Takmakov, P.; Ruda, K.; Scott Phillips, K.; Isayeva, I.S.; Krauthamer, V.; Welle, C.G. Rapid Evaluation of the Durability of Cortical Neural Implants Using Accelerated Aging with Reactive Oxygen Species. *J. Neural Eng.* **2015**, *12*, 026003. [CrossRef] [PubMed]
20. Cody, P.A.; Eles, J.R.; Lagenaur, C.F.; Kozai, T.D.Y.; Cui, X.T. Unique Electrophysiological and Impedance Signatures between Encapsulation Types: An Analysis of Biological Utah Array Failure and Benefit of a Biomimetic Coating in a Rat Model. *Biomaterials* **2018**, *161*, 117–128. [CrossRef] [PubMed]
21. Simeral, J.D.; Kim, S.-P.; Black, M.J.; Donoghue, J.P.; Hochberg, L.R. Neural Control of Cursor Trajectory and Click by a Human with Tetraplegia 1000 Days after Implant of an Intracortical Microelectrode Array. *J. Neural Eng.* **2011**, *8*, 025027. [CrossRef] [PubMed]
22. Barrese, J.C.; Rao, N.; Paroo, K.; Triebwasser, C.; Vargas-Irwin, C.; Franquemont, L.; Donoghue, J.P. Failure Mode Analysis of Silicon-Based Intracortical Microelectrode Arrays in Non-Human Primates. *J. Neural Eng.* **2013**, *10*, 066014. [CrossRef] [PubMed]
23. Malaga, K.A.; Schroeder, K.E.; Patel, P.R.; Irwin, Z.T.; Thompson, D.E.; Nicole Bentley, J.; Lempka, S.F.; Chestek, C.A.; Patil, P.G. Data-Driven Model Comparing the Effects of Glial Scarring and Interface Interactions on Chronic Neural Recordings in Non-Human Primates. *J. Neural Eng.* **2016**, *13*, 016010. [CrossRef] [PubMed]
24. Williams, J.C.; Hippensteel, J.A.; Dilgen, J.; Shain, W.; Kipke, D.R. Complex Impedance Spectroscopy for Monitoring Tissue Responses to Inserted Neural Implants. *J. Neural Eng.* **2007**, *4*, 410–423. [CrossRef] [PubMed]
25. McConnell, G.C.; Rees, H.D.; Levey, A.I.; Gutekunst, C.-A.; Gross, R.E.; Bellamkonda, R.V. Implanted Neural Electrodes Cause Chronic, Local Inflammation That Is Correlated with Local Neurodegeneration. *J. Neural Eng.* **2009**, *6*, 056003. [CrossRef] [PubMed]

26. Szarowski, D.H.; Andersen, M.D.; Retterer, S.; Spence, A.J.; Isaacson, M.; Craighead, H.G.; Turner, J.N.; Shain, W. Brain Responses to Micro-Machined Silicon Devices. *Brain Res.* **2003**, *983*, 23–35. [CrossRef]

27. Polikov, V.S.; Tresco, P.A.; Reichert, W.M. Response of Brain Tissue to Chronically Implanted Neural Electrodes. *J. Neurosci. Methods* **2005**, *148*, 1–18. [CrossRef] [PubMed]

28. Spataro, L.; Dilgen, J.; Retterer, S.; Spence, A.J.; Isaacson, M.; Turner, J.N.; Shain, W. Dexamethasone Treatment Reduces Astroglia Responses to Inserted Neuroprosthetic Devices in Rat Neocortex. *Exp. Neurol.* **2005**, *194*, 289–300. [CrossRef] [PubMed]

29. Nolta, N.F.; Christensen, M.B.; Crane, P.D.; Skousen, J.L.; Tresco, P.A. BBB Leakage, Astrogliosis, and Tissue Loss Correlate with Silicon Microelectrode Array Recording Performance. *Biomaterials* **2015**, *53*, 753–762. [CrossRef] [PubMed]

30. Jorfi, M.; Skousen, J.L.; Weder, C.; Capadona, J.R. Progress towards Biocompatible Intracortical Microelectrodes for Neural Interfacing Applications. *J. Neural Eng.* **2015**, *12*, 011001. [CrossRef] [PubMed]

31. Kozai, T.D.Y.; Catt, K.; Li, X.; Gugel, Z.V.; Olafsson, V.T.; Vazquez, A.L.; Cui, X.T. Mechanical Failure Modes of Chronically Implanted Planar Silicon-Based Neural Probes for Laminar Recording. *Biomaterials* **2015**, *37*, 25–39. [CrossRef] [PubMed]

32. Davis, E.M.; Benetatos, N.M.; Regnault, W.F.; Winey, K.I.; Elabd, Y.A. The Influence of Thermal History on Structure and Water Transport in Parylene C Coatings. *Polymer* **2011**, *52*, 5378–5386. [CrossRef]

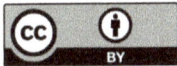

micromachines

MDPI

Article

Integrity Assessment of a Hybrid DBS Probe that Enables Neurotransmitter Detection Simultaneously to Electrical Stimulation and Recording

Danesh Ashouri Vajari [1,2,*], Maria Vomero [1,2], Johannes B. Erhardt [1,2], Ali Sadr [1], Juan S. Ordonez [1,3], Volker A. Coenen [2,5,6] and Thomas Stieglitz [1,2,4]

[1]   Laboratory for Biomedical Microtechnology, Department of Microsystems Engineering (IMTEK), University of Freiburg, Georges-Kohler-Allee 102, 79110 Freiburg, Germany; maria.vomero@imtek.uni-freiburg.de (M.V.); johannes.erhardt@imtek.uni-freiburg.de (J.B.E.); ali.sadr.63@gmail.com (A.S.); jsordonez@posteo.net (J.S.O.); thomas.stieglitz@imtek.uni-freiburg.de (T.S.)
[2]   BrainLinks-BrainTools Cluster of Excellence, University of Freiburg, Georges-Kohler-Allee 79, 79110 Freiburg, Germany; volker.coenen@uniklinik-freiburg.de
[3]   Indigo Diabetes N.V., Bollebergen 2B box 5, B-9052 Gent, Belgium
[4]   Bernstein Center Freiburg, University of Freiburg, Hansastrasse 9a, 79104 Freiburg, Germany
[5]   Department of Stereotactic and Functional Neurosurgery, University Medical Center Freiburg, Breisacher Strasse 64, 79106 Freiburg, Germany
[6]   Faculty of Medicine, University of Freiburg, 79110 Freiburg, Germany
*   Correspondence: danesh.ashouri@imtek.uni-freiburg.de

Received: 15 September 2018; Accepted: 5 October 2018; Published: 10 October 2018

Abstract: Deep brain stimulation (DBS) is a successful medical therapy for many treatment resistant neuropsychiatric disorders such as movement disorders; e.g., Parkinson's disease, Tremor, and dystonia. Moreover, DBS is becoming more and more appealing for a rapidly growing number of patients with other neuropsychiatric diseases such as depression and obsessive compulsive disorder. In spite of the promising outcomes, the current clinical hardware used in DBS does not match the technological standards of other medical applications and as a result could possibly lead to side effects such as high energy consumption and others. By implementing more advanced DBS devices, in fact, many of these limitations could be overcome. For example, a higher channels count and smaller electrode sites could allow more focal and tailored stimulation. In addition, new materials, like carbon for example, could be incorporated into the probes to enable adaptive stimulation protocols by biosensing neurotransmitters in the brain. Updating the current clinical DBS technology adequately requires combining the most recent technological advances in the field of neural engineering. Here, a novel hybrid multimodal DBS probe with glassy carbon microelectrodes on a polyimide thin-film device assembled on a silicon rubber tubing is introduced. The glassy carbon interface enables neurotransmitter detection using fast scan cyclic voltammetry and electrophysiological recordings while simultaneously performing electrical stimulation. Additionally, the presented DBS technology shows no imaging artefacts in magnetic resonance imaging. Thus, we present a promising new tool that might lead to a better fundamental understanding of the underlying mechanism of DBS while simultaneously paving our way towards better treatments.

Keywords: deep brain stimulation; fast scan cyclic voltammetry; dopamine; glassy carbon electrode; magnetic resonance imaging

1. Introduction

Deep brain stimulation (DBS) is a widely used treatment for neurologic disorders such as Parkinson's disease, tremor, dystonia, and epilepsy [1–3]. Promising research is performed in other psychiatric disorders like depression and others [2–5]. In principle, DBS mainly activates nerve cells in certain brain regions (specified by the application and thus the anatomical placement) by delivering an electrical stimulus through conductive sites (Figure 1) [5]. Precision in stimulating the target area—and therefore having a defined volume of activated tissue—plays an essential role in the success of the treatment. However, the current technology used for DBS is relatively outdated and comes down to some limitations. The rather large size of the contact sites (annular electrode contacts; 1.27 mm diameter, 1.5 mm height; i.e., 6.0 mm^2 surface area) and hence, the large volume of activated tissue in the case of conventional DBS probes, can cause the flow of current to reach outside of the target regions and also sometimes high stimulus intensities and/or misplaced leads can increase the chance of inadvertently stimulating the functional environment and hence, result in unwanted stimulation-related side effects [6,7].

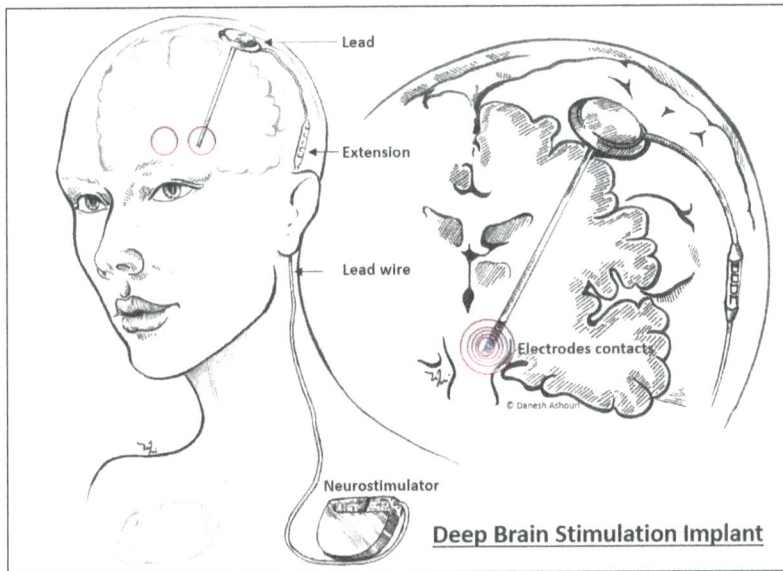

Figure 1. Illustration of a deep brain stimulation device implanted in a patient. A deep brain stimulation implant consists of four main components; electrode contacts, lead, lead wire, extension part and the implantable pulse generator (IPG or neurostimulator). A conventional DBS probe is featured with four annular active sites/contacts to deliver electrical current to the target tissue (diagram by D. Ashouri Vajari).

One approach to improve precision in stimulation is by decreasing the dimension of the stimulating electrodes accompanied by a higher channel count, in order to minimize the desired tissue volume to be excited [5,8–10]. Recently some efforts have been made to increase the channel density of DBS probes (Table 1) associated with spatial selectivity; e.g., Toader et al. (Sapiens probe)—to minimize side effects by optimizing the specificity and reducing the volumes of activated tissue [11,12]. A higher channel density enables the activation of single miniaturized sites (individually or in combination with other contacts) and can provide a higher degree of freedom by facilitating asymmetrical stimulation and steering the stimulation field [12,13].

While the accuracy of DBS outcome is supported by imaging [14], modeling [15], navigation [16,17], and microelectrode recording [18], feedback of the awake patient during surgery is requested [19] in some implantation paradigms. Even though no statistical significant differences have been reported in clinical output between electrode placement in awake and anaesthetized patients, this topic is discussed highly controversially [20–22]. In addition to verbal feedback, which lacks accurate informative features of the undergoing biological events, acquiring more quantitative information, for example, monitoring the neurotransmitter levels can be beneficial to further advance our understanding of the applied methodology. Fast scan cyclic voltammetry (FSCV) is an electrochemical method that provides information about the relative changes of the electroactive neurochemicals in a sub-second range, both in vitro and in vivo [23]. The most commonly used electrodes for this measurement are carbon fibers microelectrodes (CFMs) because they provide high sensitivity and selectivity in detection of neurotransmitters [24]. However, CFMs are brittle and applicable for intrasurgical application only and therefore [25,26], cannot be incorporated into current DBS probes.

Table 1. Comparison of the DBS lead parameters.

Parameter	Conventional DBS [1]	DBS-Array Sapiens [1]	Hybrid Probe
Diameter of the Lead	1.27 mm	1.27 mm	1.19 mm
Individual Contact Shape	ring	disc	disc
Individual Contact Size	1.50 mm	0.50 mm	50 µm
Circumferential Pitch	N.A.	90°	90°
Total Length of Array	7.5–10.5 mm	12.0 mm	10 mm
Total Number of Contacts	4	64	16
Biosensing Capability	no	no	yes

[1] Data adapted from [11].

Precise implantation is another essential aspect of a successful treatment that is assisted by utilizing a stereotactic frame and imaging techniques. Magnetic resonance imaging (MRI) is considered as the gold standard for post implantation electrode placement verification [27]. However, the magnetic susceptibility artefacts of the conventional DBS probes can impede a precise localization [28]. Besides, there is great interest in the combination of DBS and functional MRI (fMRI) to acquire more data and a deeper understanding of the brain [29,30]. fMRI is more sensitive to susceptibility artefacts than standard MRI, hence the diagnostic value in the vicinity of conventional DBS probes is limited due to signal voids [31].

In recent years many efforts have been made to address multiple limitations in (a) the development of reliable small devices and (b) having access to biomarkers such as neurotransmitter activities. However, yet in the field of neuromodulation, there is a lack of probes that combine such multi-modalities to enable a comprehensive coverage of the known biological informative features (e.g., neural activity and neurotransmitter levels) in order to further investigate the underlying mechanisms of brain disorders. Aligned with these challenging aspects, we have previously presented the application of both polyimide thin-film devices [32–37] as well as silicone rubber based electrodes in the field of neural prosthesis. Furthermore, the usage of carbon-based material (e.g., glassy carbon [38–40] and laser induced carbon [41,42]) as a multimodal interface that enables electrical stimulation, monitoring neural activity in addition to neurochemical detection, was also introduced. The presented technologies on sight can potentially give new directions in various fields of brain research. However, yet there has not been a device which combines these advances reliably and in compliance with the conventional technologies. The presented work focuses on deep brain stimulation (DBS) as a widely used clinical technique and aims to further advance its capabilities by addressing the main associated limitations.

In this study we present a design of a hybrid DBS probe, a combination of a polyimide based thin-film devices and a silicone rubber substrate, which in addition to the basic modalities (i.e., electrical stimulation and local field potentials (LFP) recording) offers the possibility of performing FSCV to monitor the relative changes of the in situ neurotransmitter levels. The fabrication of the probe was realized by utilizing the previously published Carbon-Microelectromechanical systems (C-MEMS) technology [39,40] that allows the incorporation of glassy carbon (GC) electrodes onto a PI substrate [33–35,43] and combining the fabricated thin-film device with the flexible silicone rubber tubing.

2. Materials and Methods

2.1. Electrode Fabrication

2.1.1. C-MEMS Technology and Fabrication of Glassy Carbon

The thin-film device with GC electrodes was fabricated using a method previously described elsewhere [38–40]. In short, the high aspect ratio photoresist SU-8 (MicroChem, Westborough, MA, USA) was used as a precursor for 50 um-diameter glassy carbon electrodes, which was resulted from pyrolyzation in a nitrogen atmosphere at 1000 °C. Then a layer of polyimide (PI, U-Varnish-S, UBE Industries, Ltd., Ube, Japan) was spun onto the carrier wafers and subsequently, the PI layer was etched above these electrodes to provide access. Metallization of the conducting tracks and a second layer of PI for insulation followed. This process yielded 8 µm-thick devices (Figure 2). Zero insertion force (ZIF) connector was the used interconnection technology, which facilitates a simple and quick usage for on-bench measurements.

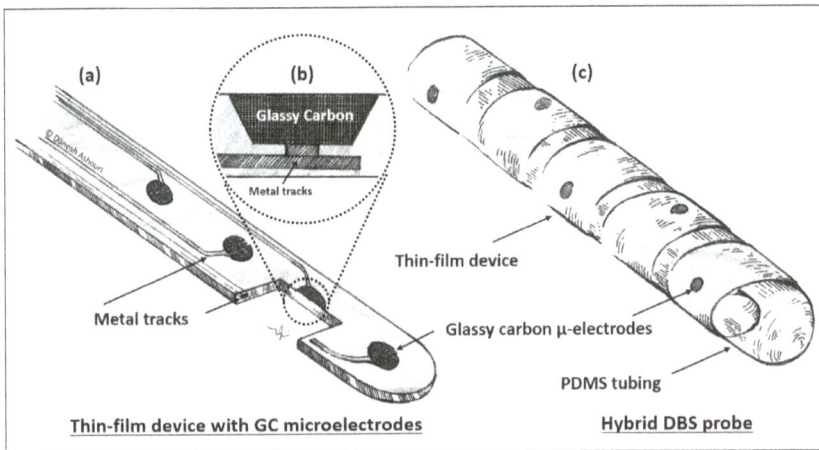

Figure 2. Schematic of the hybrid deep brain stimulation (DBS) probe. (**a**) Thin-film device with glassy carbon (GC) microelectrodes (50 um in diameter) embedded into a polyimide substrate. The active sites are distributed homogeneously along the length of the foil; (**b**) Cross-sectional view of the interface between the glassy carbon and the metal tracks (**c**) Assembled hybrid probe showing the spiral design of the wrapped thin-film device shown in (**a**) around the silicone-rubber tubing (diagram by D. Ashouri Vajari).

2.1.2. Assembly of the Hybrid Probe

The assembly of the hybrid probe consisted of two steps: first, the thin-film device was released from the wafer and rinsed in isopropanol and DI water, together with a silicone tubing featuring an outer diameter of 1.19 mm. Then the thin film device tip was fixed to the open end of the silicone tubing using silicone rubber adhesive (silicone rubber, DC 3140, RTV coating, Dow Corning, Midland, MI, USA) which was then left to cure for six hours. A tungsten rod was used as a stylet to keep the tubing straight. A thin layer of silicone rubber adhesive was applied onto the surface of the tubing to ease the assembly of the probe. The thin-film device was held at a 45° angle with respect to the tubing and carefully wrapped around (by turning the tubing clockwise around its longitudinal axis). The assembled probes were then left to cure at room temperature for 24 h.

2.2. Electrochemical Characterization

The electrochemical performance of all the fabricated electrodes was evaluated by means of cyclic voltammetry (CV) and electrochemical impedance spectroscopy (EIS). For both measurements, a three electrode configuration was used where a silver | silver-chloride electrode and a standard Pt electrode were utilized as the reference and counter electrode, respectively [44]. For the CV measurements, a conventional triangular waveform was used in which the vertex potential was swept in between −0.9 V to 1.1 V at a scan rate of 50 mV/s. Prior to each CV characterization, a cleaning step (6 cycles using the same parameters at a scan rate of 250 mV/s) was introduced. Following the CV, in order to study the impedance behavior of the electrodes under test, all the samples were subjected to EIS measurements. To perform the EIS measurements, a sinusoidal excitation of 10 mV$_{pp}$ between 1 Hz and 100 kHz was applied. Both methods were realized by utilizing a potentiostat in combination with a frequency analyzer (Solartron 1260–1287 by Solartron Analytical, Farnborough, Hampshire, UK). After each measurement, the working electrode was rinsed in DI water.

2.3. Electrical Stimulation

Electrical stimulation was used to study the performance of the hybrid DBS probe when subjected to the clinically relevant stimulation paradigms. The used stimulation parameters were adapted from a used set for treating Parkinson's disease. A charge balanced, rectangular, cathodic first stimulation waveform at 130 Hz repetition rate was used to conduct the electrical stimulation. This experiment was performed using a Plexon stimulator (Neurotechnology Research Systems) and an in-built circuit to subtract the voltage drop over the access resistance. The needed charge density for the hybrid probe (electrode size: 50 µm in diameter) was 7.2 µC/cm^2 charge density/phase (adapted from the Parkinson's treatment). Phosphate buffered saline (PBS with pH = 7.4) was used as the carrier electrolyte. For this experiment, a two electrode configuration was used in which a large area (~1 cm^2) stainless steel electrode served as the counter electrode.

2.4. Neurochemical Measurements

Fast scan cyclic voltammetry is an electrochemical method which facilitates high-resolution real-time analyte measurements; e.g., dopamine [45,46]. FSCV was realized using a potentiostat (Invilog systems Ltd., Kuopio, Finland) providing a triangular waveform in which the vertex potential was swept between −0.4 V and 1.3 V at 10 Hz repetition rate with a scan rate of 300 V/s (Figure 3). The two electrode configuration was used to form the electrochemical cell where a chlorinated silver wire served as the reference electrode [46]. In FSCV, the applied triangular waveform at the sensing electrode causes the electroactive compounds in the vicinity of the electrode surface to undergo oxidation/reduction [47]. The applied potential results in oxidizing the dopamine molecule to dopamine-o-quinone by delivering two electrons which is then followed by the reduction of the remaining dopamine-o-quinone back to dopamine by sweeping the voltage in the opposite direction [48]. The occurred oxidation-reduction (redox) reactions generate a current that is linearly proportional to the amount of electroactive compounds in the vicinity of the surface of the sensing electrode. Assuming the sensing electrode stays consistent in its properties, the potential ranges in which the generated redox current appear to differ depending on the neurochemical of interest [49,50]. Therefore, using the magnitude of the generated oxidation peak and its potential range, an estimation on the nature of the present electroactive compounds and their concentration can be obtained. The temporal resolution of this detection system is limited by the applied delay time in between two FSCV scans (in the order of 100 ms) which covers a big range of both the low frequency (1–5 Hz) tonic activity and the high frequency (≥ 20 Hz) phasic activity modes of the dopaminergic neurons [51,52]. In this study, glassy carbon was the material of choice used as the sensing interface.

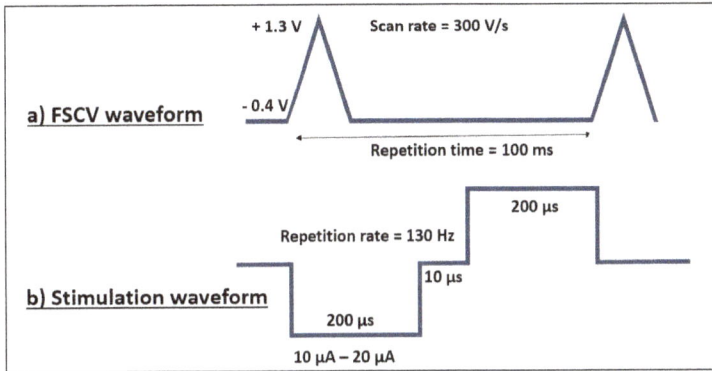

Figure 3. Schematic of the used waveform for electrical stimulation and for fast scan cyclic voltammetry; (**a**) Fast scan cyclic voltammetry (FSCV) waveform, the 100 ms delay with the −0.4 V holding potential increases the possibility of accumulation of the dopamine molecules prior each scan, the temporal resolution of the detection system is limited by the delay time between two scans; (**b**) biphasic, charged balanced, cathodic first waveform used for the pulse test.

The collected data were digitally subtracted to eliminate the impact of the capacitive component of the redox reactions. All the data processing needed for this experiment was done using MATLAB (MATLAB and Statistics Toolbox Release 2012b, The MathWorks, Inc., Natick, MA, USA). Prior to and after each experiment, all the under study active sites were electrochemically characterized (see Section 2.2). After the initial characterization of electrodes, all the testing sites were cycled for 20 min using the given setup (Figure 3.). This baseline measurement was essential to improve the signal quality by decreasing the fluctuations of the background current (μA range) and therefore, to bring more stability and visibility to the faradic components of the signal (in some tens of nA range). The calibration was then realized by applying the known concentration of the prepared dopamine stock solution to the under-test electrochemical cell. The applied concentrations were ranged in a manner that would cover both the fundamental and the application targeted purposes. Six different concentrations were used to perform the calibration: 100 nM, 500 nM, 1 μM, 2 μM, 3 μM, and 5 μM. After each registration of dopamine, a 40 s delay was introduced before proceeding with the next injection. After each calibration, the tested sites were initially rinsed with DI water and cycled in PBS using given waveforms in order to ensure having no residues of the solution left on the surface of the electrode. The cleaned electrodes were then taken to the next characterization step by means of EIS and CV.

2.5. Magnetic Resonance Imaging

A hybrid probe and a 3389 DBS lead (Medtronic®, Minneapolis, MN, USA) were cast in a 1% agarose phantom, mimicking the MRI contrast of grey matter [53,54]. The sample was then placed in a receive only head coil of a 1.5 T MRI system (MAGNETOM Tim Symphony, Siemens Healthcare GmbH, Erlangen, Germany) where the leads were oriented along the axis of the bore while coiling excess length of the DBS lead in the transversal plane similar to the arrangement recommended by the manufacturer. The samples were then imaged employing the following three standard imaging sequences: Turbo Spin Echo (spatial resolution $0.7 \times 0.7 \times 2$ mm^3; repetition time 2000 ms; echo time 9.3 ms; 4 averages), Inversion Recovery (spatial resolution $0.7 \times 0.7 \times 3$ mm^3; repetition time 4000 ms; echo time 74 ms; 4 averages) and Gradient Echo (coronal and transversal: spatial resolution $0.75 \times 0.75 \times 2$ mm^3; repetition time 10 ms; echo time 5.1 ms; 32 averages). Additionally, images were taken using Echo Planar Imaging (spatial resolution $0.9 \times 0.9 \times 3.2$ mm^3; repetition time 145 ms; echo time 15 ms; 32 averages) to illustrate the imaging artefacts that would have to be taken into account during fMRI.

3. Results

3.1. Fabrication and Assembly of the Hybrid Probe

Fabrication and assembly of the hybrid (DBS) probes were successful (Figure 4). The thin-film devices with GC microelectrodes smoothly followed the curvature of the silicone tubing and adhered to it. Silicone rubber was applied around the tubing before wrapping the thin-film component, and to fix the thin-films in place and fill the eventual voids between the polyimide and the tubing. No sharp edges remained. The final result was thus a uniform and solid composite device with GC electrodes and PI on the external 'shell' and soft silicone rubber in the core.

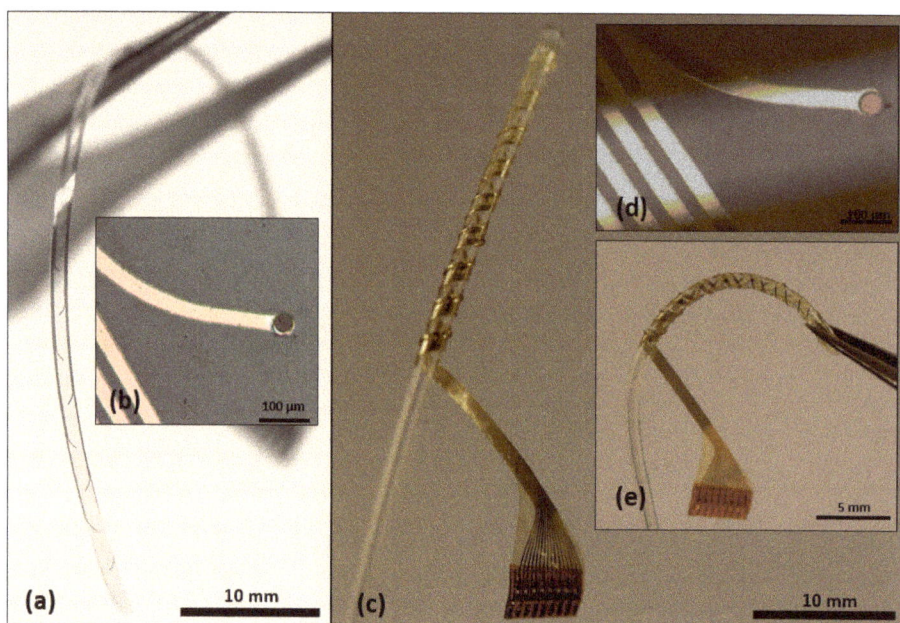

Figure 4. Representation of the fabricated thin-film device and the assembled hybrid probe; (a) cleanroom fabricated GC thin-film electrode featuring 16 active channels and zero insertion force (ZIF) interconnection in hybrid assembly; (b) a close-up of the thin-film device and the GC sites:, the dark disk-shaped site represent a glassy carbon interface present at the end of the metal tracks; (c) the assembled hybrid DBS probe; (d) a representative image of the electrode surface after wrapping the thin-film device around the silicone rubber tubing—no deformation/delamination on the glassy carbon interface was observed; (e) the hybrid assembly offering a higher stability to the thin-film device by not only introducing more flexibility and also by allowing for stretch without damage.

3.2. Electrochemical Characterization

The performed EIS measurements on the thin-film devices and the hybrid probes revealed an impedance value of 67 kΩ (@1 kHz) and 13.9 kΩ (@1 kHz), respectively. The presented data were obtained by calculating the average values and the standard deviation of the characterized electrodes (n = 10). The averaged phase value was found to be −64° (@1 kHz) and −56° (@1 kHz), respectively (Figure 5a). CVs of both, thin-film device and the hybrid probe (Figure 5b), exhibit comparable shape with no oxygen/hydrogen evolution at the two edges of the vertex potentials (i.e., −0.9 and 1.1 V (Figure 5b)) but increased in area under the curve, indicating more redox reactions during cycling and more capacitive behavior during EIS at frequencies above 100 Hz.

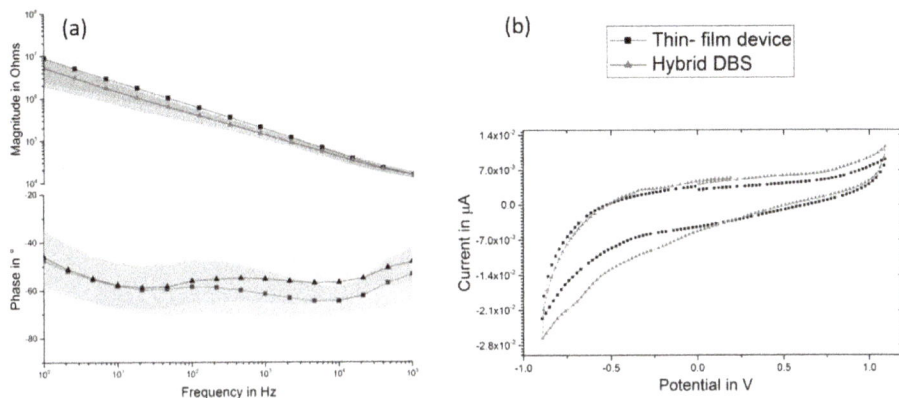

Figure 5. Electrochemical characterization of the fabricated glassy carbon electrodes prior to and after the wrapping: (**a**) The conducted electrochemical impedance spectroscopy (EIS) showing the influence of the wrapping on the performance of the electrodes in comparison to the un-wrapped electrode; (**b**) The representative CV diagram presenting the resulted characterizations of the thin-film device and hybrid probe.

3.3. Influence of Electrical Stimulation

The performed electrical stimulation (the stimulation parameters are given in Figure 3b) resulted in a voltage across the phase boundary with a magnitude of 500.6 mV (averaged for n = 10). To further evaluate the performance of the hybrid probe, active sites were subjected to 81 $\mu C/cm^2$ charge density per phase, which resulted in a phase boundary potential of 1.9 V.

3.4. Neurochemical Measurements

All the samples underwent the same baseline measurements in the FSCV experiment in which electrodes were cycled for 20 min using the given waveform (Figure 3) in order to obtain a stable background current. After reaching a relatively stable current value over time, different dopamine concentrations were applied and by averaging the generated oxidation peak, the calibration values for single electrode were calculated. The overall sensitivity was then obtained by applying the linear regression over the calculated average values including the standard deviation values of the grouped samples prior to and after wrapping. The calibration of the device prior to wrapping revealed a sensitivity of 18.28 nA/μM (n = 3 probes). The calibration of the individual single electrodes, however, delivered slight deviations in the sensitivity value (Figure 6, standard deviation). The calibration of the hybrid probe (after wrapping) resulted in a sensitivity of 34.23 nA/μM. Regardless of the observed differences in the absolute sensitivity values, all samples were found sensitive to the changes of applied concentration of dopamine.

3.5. Magnetic Resonance Imaging of a DBS Probe and the Hybrid Probe

The performed MRI showed the hybrid probe in all four employed MRI sequences clearly visible without any image distortions or signal losses due to its metal components. By contrast, the conventional DBS probe showed susceptibility artefacts around the electrode active sites where the image is distorted and signal voids occur (Figure 7). In the coronal acquired images (b–d), the lateral dimension of the commercial DBS lead tip appears three times as wide as its dimensions. The Echo Planar Imaging sequence (Figure 7f) showed twofold larger artefacts for the conventional DBS lead as compared to the previous sequences. The cross-section in Figure 7e shows the conventional DBS lead tip as an area fourfold of its dimensions.

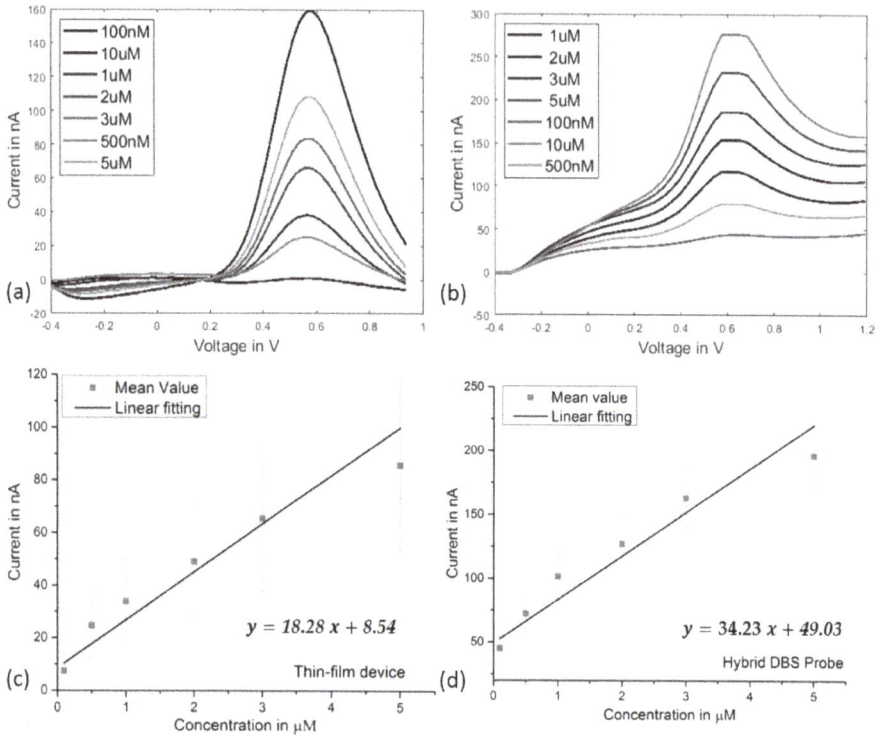

Figure 6. In vitro calibration curves of the conducted FSCV experiments for the thin-film devices as well as the hybrid probes; (**a**) representative FSCV diagram using thin-film device; (**b**) representative FSCV diagram of one of the calibrated hybrid probes with the calculated standard deviations; (**c**) linear fitting of the calibration curve for the thin-film device (n = 3); (**d**) linear fitting of the calibration values based on the calculated average for the hybrid assembly (with the calculated standard deviations ; n = 6).

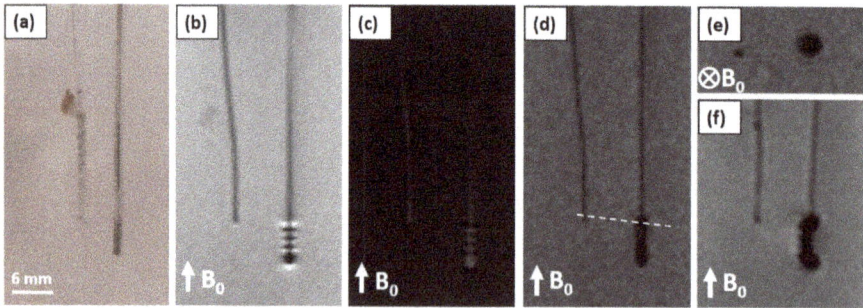

Figure 7. Comparison of the hybrid probe with a conventional DBS probe with respect to implant localization and imaging artefacts due to the electrode material in common MRI sequences using a 1.5 T scanner; (**a**) Photograph of the hybrid probe (left) and the conventional 3389 Medtronic® DBS probe (right) in a 1% agarose phantom; (**b**) Coronal view using a Turbo Spin Echo sequence; (**c**) Coronal view using an Inversion Recovery sequence; (**d**) Coronal view using a Gradient Echo sequence; (**e**) Transversal view along dashed line in (**d**) using a Gradient Echo sequence; (**f**) Coronal view using an Echo Planar Imaging sequence. Both devices have a similar diameter range (hybrid probe 1.19 mm; conventional DBS 1.27 mm) the displayed diameter at the tip of the conventional DBS probe, however, appears larger due to susceptibility artefacts.

4. Discussion

In this manuscript, we have combined technologies to design and manufacture a prototype of a multimodal DBS probe. Used technologies are all state of the art in microsystems engineering. Therefore, the reduction of electrode size and increase in channel count goes hand in hand with the opportunity to transfer this study into a medical device. This would increase manufacturing readiness level together with the technology readiness level in preclinical studies and clinical trials with few iterations, only. We were able to manufacture a proof-of-concept prototype and to characterize the hybrid probe in vitro. Since glassy carbon is a relatively stiff and brittle material [55], special attention has been laid on the influence of wrapping on the thin-film electrode integrity and its performance during electrochemical characterization.

4.1. Fabrication and Assembly of the Probe

Cleanroom fabrication steps were successfully carried out and the final devices met the expectations in terms of optical appearance and electrochemical properties. The suggested design in this work targets an exemplary probe architecture. Nevertheless, having the advantage of cleanroom fabrication, the hybrid probe can be tailored for different applications. Furthermore, glassy carbon as the interface of the probe enables a multimodality of every active site to conduct electrical stimulation, record from neural activity, and also monitor neurotransmitters like dopamine. For this proof-of-concept probe, a manual fabrication technique was used, however, the development of an automated production would be an essential step for increasing the manufacturing readiness level of the concept on its way to a medical device.

4.2. Fast Scan Cyclic Voltammetry

According to our FSCV experiments, both sample types, i.e., the unwrapped and wrapped thin-film devices, showed sensitivity towards the applied concentration of dopamine in the calibration experiment. The sensitivity value was calculated to be 18.28 nA/μM and 34.23 nA/μM for the thin-film device and the hybrid probe, respectively. Among all the calibrated samples, the sensitivity trend towards the applied concentration was clear. However, the magnitude of the generated oxidation peaks varied slightly in between different electrodes. Nevertheless, individual sensing sites showed consistent performance in sensing dopamine considering their peak potential and the magnitude of oxidation current. Differences in performance among the carbon electrodes can be due to different surface porosity achieved during pyrolysis. The samples, in fact, were not polished or treated (i.e., activated) in any way before conducting the dopamine detection experiments and thus differences in surface morphology and surface oxidation are expected [38,39]. Nevertheless, the overall performance of the hybrid probe in the given configuration was found promising and opens new directions in neurochemical monitoring during neurosurgical interventions and treatments using DBS.

4.3. Electrical Stimulation

The performed electrical stimulation showed that the hybrid probes are capable of delivering a similar charge as the conventional DBS probes without exceeding their water window. The result of voltage transient in response to the applied waveform was found in between the water window of glassy carbon interface and even by increasing the delivered charge by a factor of ~11, the potential across the phase boundary remained within water window [38,40] and no adverse reaction was observed. This suggests the functionality of the hybrid probes for the used stimulation paradigms in clinical applications.

4.4. Magnetic Resonance Imaging

The side by side comparison of the hybrid probe and a conventional DBS probe in MRI standard sequences showed imaging artefacts that exceeded the dimensions of the DBS probe by a factor between three and six and thus conceals the region of most interest. The hybrid probe, on the contrary, was displayed clearly and within its dimensions, without showing artefacts nor decreasing the imaging value in its vicinity. As has been reported earlier, these MR-imaging artefacts are eccentric of the electrode sites [28,56], which makes the localization of the electrodes imprecise and may affect the validation of the correct position negatively. The echo-planar imaging sequence commonly used for fMRI applications shows imaging artefacts twice the size of the other shown sequences, which is expected due to the higher sensitivity to image distortions caused by metal [31]. The here reported artefact size agrees with a report on artefacts extending approximately 1 cm from the DBS probe imaged in fMRI using a 3 T scanner [57]. Cunningham and co-workers claimed that the development of artifact-free electrodes would increase the applicability of fMRI [57]. Consequently, this highlights another advantage of the hybrid probe for studies aiming at gaining a better understanding of the brain where DBS is combined with fMRI. Further imaging of the hybrid probe should be performed in tissue to validate its visibility for localization purposes in vivo.

4.5. Limitations and Challenges

One may ask how these pilot results might serve in the development towards early clinical proof-of-concept/feasibility trials and what the next development steps should be. As the channel counts increases the task of interconnecting single channels to the implantable pulse generator (IPG) becomes more challenging. On the one hand, the aim is to miniaturize the dedicated space to the connection sides and on the other hand, the integrity of the connector (by means of mechanical and electrical aspects) should be kept intact. For the prototyped hybrid probes, the thin-film device was featured with 16 channels and the interconnection was realized using ZIF connectors. This approach can be followed up for acute clinical trials during surgical intervention. However, for chronic implantation, implementing more advanced interconnection technologies [58] is mandatory. These technologies require not only the compatibility with the hybrid probe but also they have to be in compliance with the changes in the interconnection technology to actual IPGs. Thin-film electrodes have proven their applicability and reliability in clinical trials [59,60] and so have the PDMS based electrodes in cardiac pacemakers [61] and all neuromodulation devices [62]. The hybrid probe is designed to benefit from both of these promising technologies. However, it must be mentioned that for a reliable manufacturing of the hybrid probe the interface between the PI and PDMS—as presented in this paper—is only suited for acute studies and has to be modified for enhanced adhesion and longevity in case of chronic applications. We have previously investigated the interface stability of the hybrid probe by applying a graded interface made out of silicon carbide and silicon dioxide to increase the adhesion strength of the polyimide to the underlying PDMS substrate [36,37]. The focus of this work was to investigate the influence of the spiral assembly in the hybrid design, introducing bending forces on the thin-film device on the performance of the incorporated glassy carbon. As a following step towards the clinical applications, besides addressing the needed technological improvements given in the discussion section, it is essential to evaluate the performance of the hybrid probe in the biological host environment in order to evaluate its longevity under the influence of the acute and chronic experiments.

5. Conclusions

The prototyped hybrid probe shows potential development pathways to increase channel count, reduce electrode size for higher spatial selectivity, and opens a window to integrate electrochemical neurotransmitter detection in addition to electrical recording and stimulation capabilities. Microsystems engineering offers the materials, technologies, and processes to manufacture functional structures. If combined it can be utilized in clinically implantable devices by using mandrels and hollow silicone rubber tubes. New diagnostic and treatment options can be further investigated and hence, structure and function of the brain can be further explored, not only on an anatomical but also on a multimodal/functional level. The way from technical designs studies and in vitro investigations to clinical trials and medical device approval is long and expensive. Applicability, functionality, and reliability have to be proven step by step in order to deliver novel tools and therapies using the latest technologies. Therefore, it is necessary to take advantage of the established materials and methods which are applicable to address the existing limitations and as a result, to bring innovative instruments as fast as possible into clinical applications.

Author Contributions: Conceptualization, D.A. and J.O.; Methodology, D.A.; M.V, J.B.E.; Software, D.A. and A.S.; Writing-Original Draft Preparation, D.A., M.V., J.B.E.; Writing-Review & Editing, D.A., M.V., J.O., J.B.E., T.S.; Visualization, D.A.; Supervision and scientific advice, T.S., V.A.C.; Project Administration, T.S.

Funding: This work was supported by BrainLinks-BrainTools Cluster of Excellence funded by the German Research Foundation (DFG, grant number EXC 1086).

Acknowledgments: The authors would like to thank Thomas Lottner for his help on MRI acquisition. The article processing charge was funded by the German Research Foundation (DFG) and the University of Freiburg in the funding programme Open Access Publishing.

Conflicts of Interest: The authors declare no conflict of interest. The funders had no role in the design of the study; in the collection, analyses, or interpretation of data; in the writing of the manuscript, and in the decision to publish the results.

References

1. Benabid, A.L. Deep brain stimulation for Parkinson's disease. *Curr. Opin. Neurobiol.* **2003**, *13*, 696–706. [CrossRef] [PubMed]
2. Williams, N.R.; Okun, M.S. Deep brain stimulation (DBS) at the interface of neurology and psychiatry. *J. Clin. Investig.* **2013**, *123*, 4546–4556. [CrossRef] [PubMed]
3. Schlaepfer, T.E.; Bewernick, B.H.; Kayser, S.; Mädler, B.; Coenen, V.A. Rapid effects of deep brain stimulation for treatment-resistant major depression. *Biol. Psychiatry* **2013**, *73*, 1204–1212. [CrossRef] [PubMed]
4. Nemeroff, C.B. Prevalence and management of treatment-resistant depression. *J. Clin. Psychiatry* **2007**, *68*, 17–25. [PubMed]
5. Coenen, V.A.; Amtage, F.; Volkmann, J.; Schläpfer, T.E. Deep Brain Stimulation in Neurological and Psychiatric Disorders. *Dtsch. Arztebl. Int.* **2015**, *112*, 519–526. [CrossRef] [PubMed]
6. Buhmann, C.; Huckhagel, T.; Engel, K.; Gulberti, A.; Hidding, U.; Poetter-Nerger, M.; Goerendt, I.; Ludewig, P.; Braass, H.; Choe, C.-U.; et al. Adverse events in deep brain stimulation: A retrospective long-term analysis of neurological, psychiatric and other occurrences. *PLoS ONE* **2017**, *12*, e0178984. [CrossRef] [PubMed]
7. Bewernick, B.H.; Kayser, S.; Gippert, S.M.; Switala, C.; Coenen, V.A.; Schlaepfer, T.E. Deep brain stimulation to the medial forebrain bundle for depression- long-term outcomes and a novel data analysis strategy. *Brain Stimul.* **2017**, *10*, 664–671. [CrossRef] [PubMed]
8. Connolly, A.T.; Vetter, R.J.; Hetke, J.F.; Teplitzky, B.A.; Kipke, D.R.; Pellinen, D.S.; Anderson, D.J.; Baker, K.B.; Vitek, J.L.; Johnson, M.D. A Novel Lead Design for Modulation and Sensing of Deep Brain Structures. *IEEE Trans. Biomed. Eng.* **2016**, *63*, 148–157. [CrossRef] [PubMed]
9. Mavridis, I.N. Anatomic guidance for stereotactic microneurosurgery: A modern necessity and the example of Mavridis' area. *Surg. Radiol. Anat.* **2015**, *37*, 119–120. [CrossRef] [PubMed]
10. Butson, C.R.; McIntyre, C.C. Role of electrode design on the volume of tissue activated during deep brain stimulation. *J. Neural Eng.* **2006**, *3*, 1–8. [CrossRef] [PubMed]
11. Toader, E.; Decre, M.M.J.; Martens, H.C.F. Steering deep brain stimulation fields using a high resolution electrode array. In Proceedings of the 2010 Annual International Conference of the IEEE Engineering in Medicine and Biology, Buenos Aires, Argentina, 31 August–4 September 2010; IEEE: Piscataway, NJ, USA, 2010.
12. Martens, H.C.F.; Toader, E.; Decré, M.M.J.; Anderson, D.J.; Vetter, R.; Kipke, D.R.; Baker, K.B.; Johnson, M.D.; Vitek, J.L. Spatial steering of deep brain stimulation volumes using a novel lead design. *Clin. Neurophysiol.* **2011**, *122*, 558–566. [CrossRef] [PubMed]
13. Alonso, F.; Latorre, M.A.; Göransson, N.; Zsigmond, P.; Wårdell, K. Investigation into Deep Brain Stimulation Lead Designs: A Patient-Specific Simulation Study. *Brain Sci.* **2016**, *6*, 39. [CrossRef] [PubMed]

14. Uitti, R.J.; Tsuboi, Y.; Pooley, R.A.; Putzke, J.D.; Turk, M.F.; Wszolek, Z.K.; Witte, R.J.; Wharen, R.E. Magnetic Resonance Imaging and Deep Brain Stimulation. *Neurosurgery* **2002**, *51*, 1423–1431. [CrossRef] [PubMed]

15. Chaturvedi, A.; Butson, C.R.; Lempka, S.F.; Cooper, S.E.; McIntyre, C.C. Patient-specific models of deep brain stimulation: Influence of field model complexity on neural activation predictions. *Brain Stimul.* **2010**, *3*, 65–67. [CrossRef] [PubMed]

16. Shahlaie, K.; Larson, P.S.; Starr, P.A. Intraoperative computed tomography for deep brain stimulation surgery: Technique and accuracy assessment. *Neurosurgery* **2011**, *68*, 114–124. [CrossRef] [PubMed]

17. Guo, T.; Finnis, K.W.; Parrent, A.G.; Peters, T.M. Visualization and navigation system development and application for stereotactic deep-brain neurosurgeries. *Comput. Aided Surg.* **2006**, *11*, 231–239. [CrossRef] [PubMed]

18. Kinfe, T.M.; Vesper, J. The impact of multichannel microelectrode recording (MER) in deep brain stimulation of the basal ganglia. *Acta Neurochir.* **2013**, *117*, 27–33. [CrossRef]

19. Kochanski, R.B.; Sani, S. Awake versus Asleep Deep Brain Stimulation Surgery: Technical Considerations and Critical Review of the Literature. *Brain Sci.* **2018**, *8*, 17. [CrossRef] [PubMed]

20. Saleh, S.; Swanson, K.I.; Lake, W.B.; Sillay, K.A. Awake Neurophysiologically Guided versus Asleep MRI-Guided STN DBS for Parkinson Disease: A Comparison of Outcomes Using Levodopa Equivalents. *Stereotact. Funct. Neurosurg.* **2015**, *93*, 419–426. [CrossRef] [PubMed]

21. LaHue, S.C.; Ostrem, J.L.; Galifianakis, N.B.; San Luciano, M.; Ziman, N.; Wang, S.; Racine, C.A.; Starr, P.A.; Larson, P.S.; Katz, M. Parkinson's disease patient preference and experience with various methods of DBS lead placement. *Parkinsonism Relat. Disord.* **2017**, *41*, 25–30. [CrossRef] [PubMed]

22. Chen, T.; Mirzadeh, Z.; Chapple, K.M.; Lambert, M.; Shill, H.A.; Moguel-Cobos, G.; Tröster, A.I.; Dhall, R.; Ponce, F.A. Clinical outcomes following awake and asleep deep brain stimulation for Parkinson disease. *J. Neurosurg.* **2018**, 1–12. [CrossRef] [PubMed]

23. Clark, J.J.; Sandberg, S.G.; Wanat, M.J.; Gan, J.O.; Horne, E.A.; Hart, A.S.; Akers, C.A.; Parker, J.G.; Willuhn, I.; Martinez, V.; et al. Chronic microsensors for longitudinal, subsecond dopamine detection in behaving animals. *Nat. Methods* **2010**, *7*, 126–129. [CrossRef] [PubMed]

24. Huffman, M.L.; Venton, B.J. Electrochemical Properties of Different Carbon-Fiber Microelectrodes Using Fast-Scan Cyclic Voltammetry. *Electroanalysis* **2008**, *20*, 2422–2428. [CrossRef]

25. Chang, S.-Y.; Kim, I.; Marsh, M.P.; Jang, D.P.; Hwang, S.-C.; van Gompel, J.J.; Goerss, S.J.; Kimble, C.J.; Bennet, K.E.; Garris, P.A.; et al. Wireless fast-scan cyclic voltammetry to monitor adenosine in patients with essential tremor during deep brain stimulation. *Mayo Clin. Proc.* **2012**, *87*, 760–765. [CrossRef] [PubMed]

26. Takmakov, P.; Zachek, M.K.; Keithley, R.B.; Walsh, P.L.; Donley, C.; McCarty, G.S.; Wightman, R.M. Carbon microelectrodes with a renewable surface. *Anal. Chem.* **2010**, *82*, 2020–2028. [CrossRef] [PubMed]

27. Zrinzo, L.; Yoshida, F.; Hariz, M.I.; Thornton, J.; Foltynie, T.; Yousry, T.A.; Limousin, P. Clinical safety of brain magnetic resonance imaging with implanted deep brain stimulation hardware: Large case series and review of the literature. *World Neurosurg.* **2011**, *76*, 164–172; discussion 69–73. [CrossRef] [PubMed]

28. Pinsker, M.O.; Herzog, J.; Falk, D.; Volkmann, J.; Deuschl, G.; Mehdorn, M. Accuracy and distortion of deep brain stimulation electrodes on postoperative MRI and CT. *Zentralblatt fur Neurochirurgie* **2008**, *69*, 144–147. [CrossRef] [PubMed]

29. Carmichael, D.W.; Pinto, S.; Limousin-Dowsey, P.; Thobois, S.; Allen, P.J.; Lemieux, L.; Yousry, T.; Thornton, J.S. Functional MRI with active, fully implanted, deep brain stimulation systems: Safety and experimental confounds. *Neuroimage* **2007**, *37*, 508–517. [CrossRef] [PubMed]

30. Min, H.-K.; Hwang, S.-C.; Marsh, M.P.; Kim, I.; Knight, E.; Striemer, B.; Felmlee, J.P.; Welker, K.M.; Blaha, C.D.; Chang, S.-Y.; et al. Deep brain stimulation induces BOLD activation in motor and non-motor networks: An fMRI comparison study of STN and EN/GPi DBS in large animals. *Neuroimage* **2012**, *63*, 1408–1420. [CrossRef] [PubMed]

31. Erhardt, J.B.; Fuhrer, E.; Gruschke, O.G.; Leupold, J.; Wapler, M.C.; Hennig, J.; Stieglitz, T.; Korvink, J.G. Should patients with brain implants undergo MRI? *J. Neural Eng.* **2018**, *15*, 41002. [CrossRef] [PubMed]

32. Badia, J.; Boretius, T.; Pascual-Font, A.; Udina, E.; Stieglitz, T.; Navarro, X. Biocompatibility of chronically implanted transverse intrafascicular multichannel electrode (TIME) in the rat sciatic nerve. *IEEE Trans. Biomed. Eng.* **2011**, *58*. [CrossRef] [PubMed]

33. Hassler, C.; Boretius, T.; Stieglitz, T. Polymers for neural implants. *J. Polym. Sci. B Polym. Phys.* **2011**, *49*, 18–33. [CrossRef]

34. Stieglitz, T.; Beutel, H.T.; Schuettler, M.; Meyer, J.-U. Micromachined, Polyimide-Based Devices for Flexible Neural Interfaces. *Biomed. Microdevices* **2000**, *2*, 283–294. [CrossRef]

35. Stieglitz, T.; Boretius, T.; Navarro, X.; Badia, J.; Guiraud, D.; Divoux, J.-L.; Micera, S.; Rossini, P.M.; Yoshida, K.; Harreby, K.R.; et al. Development of a neurotechnological system for relieving phantom limb pain using transverse intrafascicular electrodes (TIME). *Biomed. Tech. Biomed. Eng.* **2012**, *57*, 457–465. [CrossRef] [PubMed]

36. Vajari, D.A.; Ordonez, J.S.; Furlanetti, L.; Dobrossy, M.; Coenen, V.; Stieglitz, T. Hybrid multimodal Deep Brain probe (DBS array) for advanced brain research. In Proceedings of the 2015 7th International IEEE/EMBS Conference on Neural Engineering (NER), Montpellier, France, 22–24 April 2015; IEEE: Piscataway, NJ, USA, 2015; pp. 280–283.

37. Ordonez, J.; Schuettler, M.; Boehler, C.; Boretius, T.; Stieglitz, T. Thin films and microelectrode arrays for neuroprosthetics. *MRS Bull.* **2012**, *37*, 590–598. [CrossRef]

38. Vomero, M.; Castagnola, E.; Ordonez, J.S.; Carli, S.; Zucchini, E.; Maggiolini, E.; Gueli, C.; Goshi, N.; Fadiga, L.; Ricci, D.; et al. Improved long-term stability of thin-film glassy carbon. In Proceedings of the 2017 8th International IEEE/EMBS Conference on Neural Engineering (NER), Shanghai, China, 25–28 May 2017; IEEE: Piscataway, NJ, USA, 2017; pp. 288–291.

39. Vomero, M.; Castagnola, E.; Ordonez, J.S.; Carli, S.; Zucchini, E.; Maggiolini, E.; Gueli, C.; Goshi, N.; Ciarpella, F.; Cea, C.; et al. Incorporation of Silicon Carbide and Diamond-Like Carbon as Adhesion Promoters Improves In Vitro and In Vivo Stability of Thin-Film Glassy Carbon Electrocorticography Arrays. *Adv. Biosyst.* **2018**, *2*, 1700081. [CrossRef]

40. Vomero, M.; Castagnola, E.; Ciarpella, F.; Maggiolini, E.; Goshi, N.; Zucchini, E.; Carli, S.; Fadiga, L.; Kassegne, S.; Ricci, D. Highly Stable Glassy Carbon Interfaces for Long-Term Neural Stimulation and Low-Noise Recording of Brain Activity. *Sci Rep.* **2017**, *7*, 40332. [CrossRef] [PubMed]

41. Oliveira, A.; Ordonez, J.S.; Vajari, D.A.; Eickenscheidt, M.; Stieglitz, T. Laser-Induced Carbon Pyrolysis of Electrodes for Neural Interface Systems. *Eur. J. Trans. Myol.* **2016**, *26*, 6062. [CrossRef] [PubMed]

42. Vomero, M.; Oliveira, A.; Ashouri, D.; Eickenscheidt, M.; Stieglitz, T. Graphitic Carbon Electrodes on Flexible Substrate for Neural Applications Entirely Fabricated Using Infrared Nanosecond Laser Technology. *Sci. Rep.* **2018**, *8*, 14749. [CrossRef] [PubMed]

43. Rubehn, B.; Stieglitz, T. In vitro evaluation of the long-term stability of polyimide as a material for neural implants. *Biomaterials* **2010**, *31*, 3449–3458. [CrossRef] [PubMed]

44. Cogan, S.F. Neural stimulation and recording electrodes. *Ann. Rev. Biomed. Eng.* **2008**, *10*, 275–309. [CrossRef] [PubMed]

45. Grahn, P.J.; Mallory, G.W.; Khurram, O.U.; Berry, B.M.; Hachmann, J.T.; Bieber, A.J.; Bennet, K.E.; Min, H.-K.; Chang, S.-Y.; Lee, K.H.; et al. A neurochemical closed-loop controller for deep brain stimulation: Toward individualized smart neuromodulation therapies. *Front. Neurosci.* **2014**, *8*, 169. [CrossRef] [PubMed]

46. Takmakov, P.; McKinney, C.J.; Carelli, R.M.; Wightman, R.M. Instrumentation for fast-scan cyclic voltammetry combined with electrophysiology for behavioral experiments in freely moving animals. *Rev. Sci. Instrum.* **2011**, *82*, 74302. [CrossRef] [PubMed]

47. Covey, E.; Carter, M. *Basic Electrophysiological Methods (DRAFT)*; Oxford University Press: Oxford, UK, 2015.

48. Phillips, P.E.M.; Wightman, R.M. Critical guidelines for validation of the selectivity of in-vivo chemical microsensors. *TrAC Trends Anal. Chem.* **2003**, *22*, 509–514. [CrossRef]

49. Rodeberg, N.T.; Sandberg, S.G.; Johnson, J.A.; Phillips, P.E.M.; Wightman, R.M. Hitchhiker's Guide to Voltammetry: Acute and Chronic Electrodes for in Vivo Fast-Scan Cyclic Voltammetry. *ACS Chem. Neurosci.* **2017**, *8*, 221–234. [CrossRef] [PubMed]

50. Robinson, D.L.; Hermans, A.; Seipel, A.T.; Wightman, R.M. Monitoring rapid chemical communication in the brain. *Chem. Rev.* **2008**, *108*, 2554–2584. [CrossRef] [PubMed]

51. Wenzel, J.M.; Cheer, J.F. Endocannabinoid-dependent modulation of phasic dopamine signaling encodes external and internal reward-predictive cues. *Front. Psychiatry* **2014**, *5*, 118. [CrossRef] [PubMed]

52. Grace, A.A.; Bunney, B.S. The control of firing pattern in nigral dopamine neurons: Burst firing. *J. Neurosci.* **1984**, *4*, 2877–2890. [CrossRef] [PubMed]

53. Mitchell, M.D.; Kundel, H.L.; Axel, L.; Joseph, P.M. Agarose as a tissue equivalent phantom material for NMR imaging. *Magn. Reson. Imaging* **1986**, *4*, 263–266. [CrossRef]

54. Hellerbach, A.; Schuster, V.; Jansen, A.; Sommer, J. MRI phantoms—Are there alternatives to agar? *PLoS ONE* **2013**, *8*, e70343. [CrossRef] [PubMed]

55. Kassegne, S.; Vomero, M.; Gavuglio, R.; Hirabayashi, M.; Özyilmaz, E.; Nguyen, S.; Rodriguez, J.; Özyilmaz, E.; van Niekerk, P.; Khosla, A. Electrical impedance, electrochemistry, mechanical stiffness, and hardness tunability in glassy carbon MEMS μECoG electrodes. *Microelectron. Eng.* **2015**, *133*, 36–44. [CrossRef]

56. Schenck, J.F. The role of magnetic susceptibility in magnetic resonance imaging: MRI magnetic compatibility of the first and second kinds. *Med. Phys.* **1996**, *23*, 815–850. [CrossRef] [PubMed]

57. Cunningham, C.B.J.; Goodyear, B.G.; Badawy, R.; Zaamout, F.; Pittman, D.J.; Beers, C.A.; Federico, P. Intracranial EEG-fMRI analysis of focal epileptiform discharges in humans. *Epilepsia* **2012**, *53*, 1636–1648. [CrossRef] [PubMed]

58. Khan, S.; Ordonez, J.S.; Stieglitz, T. Dual-sided process with graded interfaces for adhering underfill and globtop materials to microelectrode arrays. In Proceedings of the 2017 8th International IEEE/EMBS Conference on Neural Engineering (NER), Shanghai, China, 25–28 May 2017; IEEE: Piscataway, NJ, US, 2017; pp. 247–250.

59. Raspopovic, S.; Capogrosso, M.; Petrini, F.M.; Bonizzato, M.; Rigosa, J.; Di Pino, G.; Carpaneto, J.; Controzzi, M.; Boretius, T.; Fernandez, E.; et al. Restoring natural sensory feedback in real-time bidirectional hand prostheses. *Sci. Trans. Med.* **2014**, *6*, 222ra19. [CrossRef] [PubMed]

60. Ibáñez, J.; González-Vargas, J.; Azorín, J.M.; Akay, M.; Pons, J.L. Converging Clinical and Engineering Research on Neurorehabilitation II. In Proceedings of the 3rd International Conference on NeuroRehabilitation (ICNR2016), Segovia, Spain, 18–21 October 2016; Springer: Cham, Switzerland, 2017.

61. Aguilera, A.L.; Volokhina, Y.V.; Fisher, K.L. Radiography of cardiac conduction devices: A comprehensive review. *Radiographics* **2011**, *31*, 1669–1682. [CrossRef] [PubMed]

62. Amon, A.; Alesch, F. Systems for deep brain stimulation: Review of technical features. *J. Neural Trans.* **2017**, *124*, 1083–1091. [CrossRef] [PubMed]

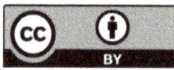

![micromachines logo] *micromachines*

MDPI

Communication

Design Choices for Next-Generation Neurotechnology Can Impact Motion Artifact in Electrophysiological and Fast-Scan Cyclic Voltammetry Measurements

Evan N. Nicolai [1], Nicholas J. Michelson [2,3], Megan L. Settell [1], Seth A. Hara [4],
James K. Trevathan [1], Anders J. Asp [1], Kaylene C. Stocking [2], J. Luis Lujan [5,6],
Takashi D.Y. Kozai [2,7,8,9,10,*,†] and Kip A. Ludwig [11,12,*,†]

[1]   Mayo Clinic Graduate School of Biomedical Sciences, Rochester, MN 55905, USA;
      nicolai.evan@mayo.edu (E.N.N.); settell.megan@mayo.edu (M.L.S.); trevathan.james@mayo.edu (J.K.T.);
      asp.anders@mayo.edu (A.J.A.)
[2]   Department of Bioengineering, University of Pittsburgh, Pittsburgh, PA 15213, USA;
      njm89@pitt.edu (N.J.M.); kcs58@pitt.edu (K.C.S.)
[3]   Department of Psychiatry, University of British Columbia, Vancouver, BC V6T 1Z3, Canada
[4]   Division of Engineering, Mayo Clinic, Rochester, MN 55905, USA; hara.seth@mayo.edu
[5]   Department of Neurologic Surgery, Mayo Clinic, Rochester, MN 55905, USA; lujan.luis@mayo.edu
[6]   Department of Physiology and Biomedical Engineering, Mayo Clinic, Rochester, MN 55905, USA
[7]   Center for the Neural Basis of Cognition, University of Pittsburgh and Carnegie Mellon University,
      Pittsburgh, PA 15213, USA
[8]   McGowan Institute for Regenerative Medicine, University of Pittsburgh, Pittsburgh, PA 15213, USA
[9]   NeuroTech Center of the University of Pittsburgh Brain Institute, Pittsburgh, PA 15213, USA
[10] Center for Neuroscience, University of Pittsburgh, Pittsburgh, PA 15213, USA
[11] Department of Bioengineering, University of Wisconsin, Madison, WI 53706, USA
[12] Department of Neurological Surgery, University of Wisconsin, Madison, WI 53706, USA
*   Correspondence: tdk18@pitt.edu (T.D.Y.K.); kip.ludwig@wisc.com (K.A.L.); Tel.: +1-608-265-3544 (K.A.L.)
†   These authors have contributed equally to this work.

Received: 15 August 2018; Accepted: 21 September 2018; Published: 27 September 2018

Abstract: Implantable devices to measure neurochemical or electrical activity from the brain are mainstays of neuroscience research and have become increasingly utilized as enabling components of clinical therapies. In order to increase the number of recording channels on these devices while minimizing the immune response, flexible electrodes under 10 μm in diameter have been proposed as ideal next-generation neural interfaces. However, the representation of motion artifact during neurochemical or electrophysiological recordings using ultra-small, flexible electrodes remains unexplored. In this short communication, we characterize motion artifact generated by the movement of 7 μm diameter carbon fiber electrodes during electrophysiological recordings and fast-scan cyclic voltammetry (FSCV) measurements of electroactive neurochemicals. Through in vitro and in vivo experiments, we demonstrate that artifact induced by motion can be problematic to distinguish from the characteristic signals associated with recorded action potentials or neurochemical measurements. These results underscore that new electrode materials and recording paradigms can alter the representation of common sources of artifact in vivo and therefore must be carefully characterized.

Keywords: electrode; artifact; electrophysiology; electrochemistry; fast-scan cyclic voltammetry (FSCV); neurotechnology; neural interface; neuromodulation; neuroprosthetics; brain-machine interfaces

1. Introduction

Implantable neural interface devices can be used to examine chemical or electrical activity within the brain, making them critical tools for conducting neuroscience research [1–7]. The information recorded from these instruments can also enable state-of-the-art therapeutic or rehabilitative strategies [8]. For example, extracellular neuronal signal information recorded from implanted microelectrode arrays (i.e., single units, multiunits, or local field potentials) may be used to decode intended movements and control assistive devices [1,9–12]. Similarly, measurements of phasic changes in the extracellular concentration of dopamine taken by small electrodes placed within the brain have been proposed as a feedback signal to titrate levels of deep brain stimulation (DBS) to alleviate tremors associated with Parkinson's Disease [13–15].

The utility of a neural interface device depends on how well one can differentiate the measured physiological signal of interest from other sources of physiological signals (electromyogram (EMG), electrooculogram (EOG)), noise (shot noise, flicker noise, etc.), and artifact signals [16]. Artifact signals that resemble physiological signals—caused by motion [17], stimulation [18], or changes in ambient radiofrequency (RF) noise [19]—are a known problem for in vivo electrophysiological recordings. Motion artifacts are particularly troublesome because they can be highly variable in amplitude across time, making them difficult to remove with standard filtering techniques and therefore potentially difficult to distinguish from the measurands of interest [17,20].

There are three primary mechanisms by which a motion artifact can be generated. First, motion experienced during free behavior is often transferred to connection points, such as where external instrumentation is plugged into a head-stage on the animal. Atoms interact at the boundary point where two objects touch each other, generating a charge at both material interfaces. When these objects move relative to each other, an electrostatic voltage is generated known as the triboelectric effect [21]. Second, motion of the wire induces an artifact current if the wire is subject to intrinsic or extrinsic magnetic fields [22]. Lastly, artifact can be introduced by motion of the electrode with respect to the neural tissue at the electrode/electrolyte interface [20]. When an electrode is placed in an electrolytic solution, a multitude of events takes place. Solvent molecules adsorb to the surface, resulting in the formation of an electric double-layer; non-specifically adsorbed ions also form a diffuse layer, which is dependent on the ionic concentration of the solution. A potential difference between the electrode and electrolyte is also generated by oxidation/reduction electrochemical reactions occurring at the surface of the electrode [17,23]. Electrochemical reactions continue until the potential difference between the electrode and the electrolyte drives an equal balance between oxidation and reduction reactions to generate no net current at the interface [23,24]. When an electrode is moved with respect to the electrolyte, equilibrium at the electrode/electrolyte interface is disturbed and must be reestablished, creating an artifact current [25].

Recently, there has been increased interest in developing 7 µm diameter carbon fiber electrodes for chronic electrophysiological recordings and measurements of electroactive neurochemicals in vivo using fast-scan cyclic voltammetry (FSCV) [26–44]. The small diameter limits the amount of tissue displaced during implantation, mitigating local neurodegeneration and damage to synaptic sources of neurotransmitters of interest [30,44,45]. Moreover, carbon fibers can be manufactured to be flexible post-implantation, improving the mechanical match with surrounding brain tissue and thereby decreasing chronic inflammation [28–30,32,33,40]. Although initial results utilizing ultra-small, flexible carbon fiber electrodes are promising, the impact of these design changes on the representation of motion artifact during recording remains largely unexplored.

Here we demonstrate on the benchtop and in vivo that motion of carbon fibers while recording can generate artifact signals that are nearly indistinguishable from neural electrophysiological or neurochemical signals. In addition, classical signal processing techniques can exacerbate the similarity of these artifact signals to physiological signals. These findings highlight that one must carefully consider how neural interface design changes impact unwanted artifact signals in behaving neural recordings, which ultimately may lead to novel neural interface designs that minimize the impact of these artifacts [20,28].

2. Materials and Methods

2.1. Electrophysiological Recordings

All experimental protocols were approved by the University of Pittsburgh Division of Laboratory Animal Resources and Institutional Animal Care and Use Committee, in accordance with the standards for humane animal care as set by the Animal Welfare Act and the National Institutes of Health Guide for the Care and Use of Laboratory Animals.

Benchtop data was collected from a single channel microwire, placed in a three-electrode electrochemical cell (1× phosphate buffered saline (PBS), AgCl reference, Pt Counter electrode). Recordings were conducted with the microwire within a fully electrically isolated Faraday cage. To simulate motion, the wire was moved three times using a non-conductive zip tie over the course of the recording duration (approximately 8 s). To compare benchtop data with in vivo results, C57BL/6 mice (22–28 g) were implanted with a planar, silicon microelectrode array (A-1×16-3 mm-100-703-CM16LP, Neuronexus Technologies. Ann Arbor, MI, USA) in left monocular visual cortex [6,20,32,46,47]. Additionally, artifacts were compared between flexible carbon fiber arrays and rigid silicon arrays, with simultaneous recordings from an adult male Long Evans rat implanted with a 16 channel carbon fiber array in right primary motor cortex, and a single shank silicon electrode array in left primary motor cortex [29,40]. In each recording session, animals were awake, non-behaving, and non-restrained [20,29,40]. Recordings were conducted from within a fully electrically isolated Faraday cage. Data was sampled at 24,414 Hz, with a pre-amplifier high pass filter at 2.2 Hz and an anti-aliasing filter at 7.5 kHz. The raw data was then filtered using a 2nd order Butterworth filter (300–5000 Hz) to produce spike streams. A threshold set at 3.5 standard deviations below the mean of each channel's spike stream data was established for the detection of single or multiunit activity. Putative electrophysiological artifacts were identified using a custom MATLAB script (MATLAB R2016b, MathWorks, Inc., Natick, MA, USA), as previously described [20]. Briefly, artifacts were defined as incidents in which threshold crossing events occurred simultaneously (±0.05 ms) across at least three channels. As the voltage of the extracellular action potential decays substantially with distance [28,48], threshold crossing events which occurred simultaneously across three channels are unlikely to be caused by a single neuron, given the 100 μm spacing between electrode sites [49]. As expected, in corresponding anesthetized studies, threshold crossings were not detected on multiple channels within 0.05 ms of each other [5–7,20,32,46,47,50]. Additionally, although certain neurophysiologic events such as spindle activity [51] may be observed across such distances, lower frequency activity (<300 Hz) was filtered before analyzing spike trains.

2.2. Electrochemical Recordings

Carbon fiber FSCV microelectrodes were built in-house, based on the electrodes described by Clark et al. [44]. Briefly, a single 7 μm diameter carbon fiber was placed within a silica tube of 100 μm diameter and one end was sealed with polyimide. The other end was connected to an extension wire of 300 μm diameter nitinol using an equal parts 99% pure silver powder and polyimide mixture. The exposed carbon fiber was trimmed to a final length of 100 μm. Reference electrodes (Ag-AgCl) were constructed using a silver wire immersed in 0.9% NaCl solution and applying a current using a 9 V battery to form a chlorinated electrode.

To test the carbon fiber electrodes in vitro, multiple experiment vessels—50 mL Falcon tubes— were filled with 0.6% agarose in tris-buffered saline (140 mM NaCl, 1.25 mM NaH_2PO_4, 3.25 mM KCl, 1.2 mM $CaCl_2$, 15 mM Trizma Base, 1.2 mM $MgCl_2$, 2 mM Na_2SO_4) to create an agarose gel solution that mimics the viscoelastic properties of the brain [52,53]. The concentrations of dopamine in each gel were varied to characterize motion artifact during FSCV recordings as a function of dopamine concentration in solution. All chemicals were purchased from Sigma-Aldrich (St. Louis, MO, USA).

A novel experimental set-up was devised to generate controlled movement of the carbon fiber in the agarose solution without the use of a power source which might also induce artifact. A stereotactic manipulator knob controlling movement in the vertical plane was connected to a weight hanging from a pulley (Figure 1a). This was done such that when the weight was released, the stereotactic knob would turn and move the electrode down a set distance. A non-conductive zip tie was used to turn the stereotactic knob, which lifted the electrode up through the solution. Releasing the weight would then lower the electrode a set distance via free fall acceleration by gravity. Carbon fiber microelectrodes were placed in a holder secured to this stereotactic manipulator, then initially lowered into the gel solution such that the electrode tip was centered and at approximately the 25 mL mark on the Falcon tube (half the depth).

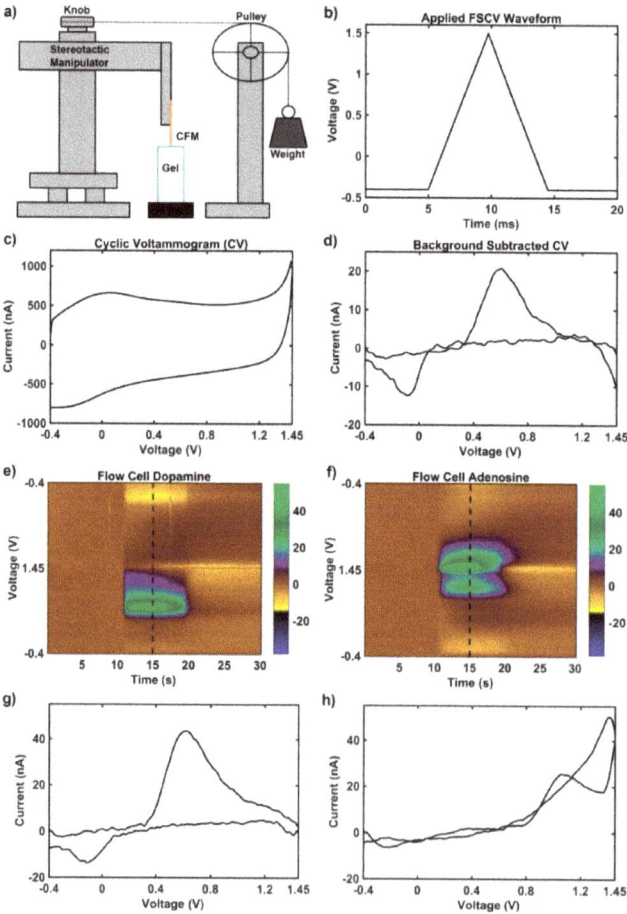

Figure 1. Experimental setup and fast scan cyclic voltammetry methodology. (**a**) Schematic of the mechanism used to produce motion of the carbon fiber microelectrode through agar solution without generating electromagnetic interference. (**b**) Example triangular voltage waveform applied to carbon fiber microelectrode vs. the Ag-AgCl reference electrode. (**c**) Example current obtained at all voltage points during application of triangle waveform (cyclic voltammogram) in (**b**). The current generated includes both capacitive and faradaic components. (**d**) Example cyclic voltammogram obtained via background subtraction during a transient dopamine concentration change, which emphasizes faradaic changes such as the oxidation near 0.6 V and the reduction near −0.2 V. (**e–h**) Known signals for dopamine and adenosine obtained via measurement in a benchtop flow cell (different than the setup in Figure 1A) using the methodology described by Shon et al. [54]. Briefly, a flow cell passes buffer solution by the electrode continuously with transient boluses of electrochemical in order to produce

a phasic signal. High concentrations (1 µM dopamine and 5 µM adenosine) were passed by the carbon fiber microelectrode in pure buffer to produce large, idealistic—low noise—signals to emphasize the characteristic faradaic components (**e**) Dopamine signal with characteristic oxidation at 0.6 V and reduction at −0.2 V. (**g**) Characteristic cyclic voltammogram of dopamine signal from (**e**) (collected at dotted vertical line). (**f**) Adenosine signal with characteristic primary oxidation at 1.4 V and secondary oxidation at 1.0 V. (**h**) Characteristic cyclic voltammogram of adenosine signal from (**f**) (collected at dotted vertical line).

All experiments were performed in a fully electrically isolated Faraday cage. Data was collected using the Universal Electrochemical Instrument (UEI, University of North Carolina, Chapel Hill, NC, USA) starting with a gel solution that had no neurochemicals, and proceeding through multiple gel solutions containing various concentrations of neurochemical in a randomized order (2, 5, 10 µM dopamine, n = 6 electrodes and n = 3 of these electrodes included 1 µM dopamine; 10, 20, 50 µM adenosine, n = 1 electrode). The applied voltage waveform was held at −0.4 V with triangular excursions to 1.3 V and back at a 400 V/s scan rate every 100 milliseconds for measurements of dopamine; a similar waveform was used for measurements of adenosine, except the peak voltage was 1.5 V instead of 1.3 V. Within each solution, the carbon fiber microelectrode was subjected to a slow upward motion lasting approximately 3 s, a 30 s motionless period, and then a fast downward motion (~0.250 s) resulting from the free fall of a hanging weight (147 g). Duration of the motion was measured using a slow motion camera, and the duration (0.25 s) and distance traveled (1 mm) were used to calculate the acceleration (0.032 m/s^2). A minimum of six measurements were collected per concentration; three measurements were taken during 100 µm movements and three during 1 mm movements to mimic the distance traveled by the brain during behavior in rodents and non-human primates, respectively [46].

Data was analyzed using HDCV Analysis (University of North Carolina, Chapel Hill, NC, USA). Filtering and automatic averaging were turned off. The average of five cyclic voltammograms occurring one second before motion occurred was used for background subtraction. A background subtracted cyclic voltammogram collected 200 milliseconds after the start of the motion was used to determine location of peak oxidation potential. An average of the peak current at the oxidation potential and the two data points before and after the peak following application of motion was recorded as the magnitude of the artifact response.

3. Results

Movement can generate robust electrical artifact signal through (1) the triboelectric effect, (2) electromagnetic flux magnified by active electronics, and (3) disruption of the electrochemical interface. In the following section, motion artifact is first characterized during electrophysiological recordings, where active electronics are used to minimize current flow. Then, the impact of motion artifact is characterized during FSCV neurochemical recordings for comparison. During FSCV a triangle waveform is applied to oxidize/reduce neurochemicals adsorbed to the carbon fiber electrode surface, adding additional complexity to the recording system.

3.1. Motion Artifact During Electrophysiological Recordings

Electrophysiological recordings are susceptible to contamination by artifacts, which can appear as high amplitude voltage deflections that occur simultaneously across multiple channels (Figure 2a). These non-neural signals demonstrate high variability in shape and amplitude, and in some cases, may share similar temporal characteristics to single unit or multiunit signals (Figure 2b). These similarities may result in the misclassification of those artifacts as neural signals. In our awake free-moving mouse recordings, principal component analysis and k-means clustering failed to separate all artifacts from action potentials, resulting in the grouping of some artifact signals with single units (Figure 2c red and blue snippets, respectively). For comparison with in vivo data recordings, artifacts were also generated on the benchtop without an animal, using an un-implanted single channel microwire connected through the same headstage preamplifier and amplifier in a three electrode electrochemical cell in 1× PBS placed in a fully electrically isolated Faraday cage. The electrode was moved with a non-conductive zip tie held outside of the Faraday cage. This ensured that electrical artifacts or line noise originating from outside of the cage did not influence the signal obtained from within the cage. Movement of the electrode three times generated high amplitude artifacts (Figure 2d) [20]. In awake free-moving rats, recordings were conducted simultaneously from a 16 channel carbon fiber array and a single shank silicon electrode array implanted into the right and left primary motor cortex, respectively [29]. Here, artifacts were more prominent on the carbon fiber array (Figure 2e,f, red traces) than the silicon array (Figure 2e,f, blue traces), suggesting that differences in the design of the carbon fiber array contributed to the representation of motion artifact.

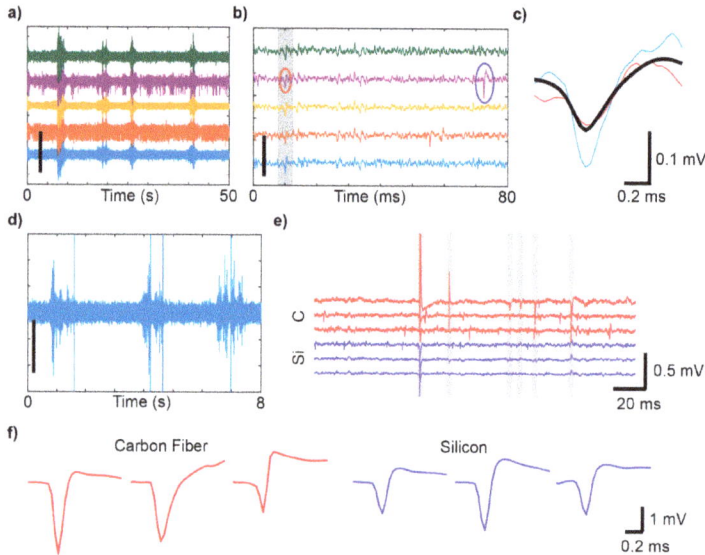

Figure 2. Animal movement creates artifacts that contaminate electrophysiological recordings. (**a**) Sample recordings from a silicon electrode array implanted in an awake, freely moving mouse. (**b**) Same as (**a**), over 80ms. Gray shading highlights artifacts. A true action potential is circled in blue, while an artifact recorded on the same channel is circled in red. (**c**) Example spike and artifact waveforms from (**b**). In this case, principal component analysis (PCA) and *k*-means clustering failed to separate the highlighted artifact (red) from the action potential (blue). The cluster average (black), as isolated with PCA and *k*-means clustering, is shown for comparison. (**d**) Brief recordings from an un-implanted microwire, where the electrode was moved three times with a non-conductive zip tie. (**e**) Sample recording data taken simultaneously from a carbon fiber array (red) and a silicon array (blue) implanted in right and left primary motor cortex in a rat, respectively. Gray shading highlights artifacts that were flagged using the detection method described previously. (**f**) Examples of artifacts from the carbon fiber array (red) and silicon array (blue). Scalebars: (**a**,**b**) 400 µV, (**c**,**d**) 100 µV. (**a**–**e**): © IOP Publishing. Adapted with permission from [20]. All rights reserved.

3.2. Motion Artifact During FSCV Recordings

The representation of motion artifact during FSCV recordings has not previously been characterized. As described in the methods, it was important to ensure that electromagnetic radiation from motors and pumps did not influence the motion artifact; therefore, a pulley and weight system was used to generate the motion. Phasic changes in dopamine concentration in vivo generate corresponding changes in currents measured at 0.6 V and −0.2 V during FSCV recordings, due to the oxidation and reduction of dopamine respectively. During motion, transient signals were reliably produced with current changes observed at the characteristic oxidation and reduction potentials for dopamine (DA), but only when dopamine was in solution (Figure 3, center column). Without DA in solution, changes in current due to motion were often not detectable or appeared as low amplitude, broad changes that bear no resemblance to neurochemicals of interest (Figure 3, right column). FSCV data was also collected in the absence of motion, and does not contain apparent artifacts (Figure 3, left column). The amplitude of the artifact signal was dependent on both the concentration of dopamine in the experiment vessel (Figure 4a) and the distance traveled by the microelectrode (Figure 4b).

To determine whether the artifact signal was specific to dopamine, similar motion in the presence of adenosine was also evaluated (Figure 5). In contrast to dopamine, adenosine adsorbed to the surface of the electrode generates a primary oxidation peak at 1.4 V and a secondary oxidation peak at 1.0 V during FSCV (Figure 1f) [55]. Due to the kinetics of the reaction, the secondary oxidation peak is often delayed from the onset of the primary oxidation peak by 0.5 s during a phasic change in adenosine [55]. Notably, the motion artifact in dopamine gel solution (Figure 3, center column) strongly resembles phasic change in dopamine concentration (Figure 1e). In contrast, the motion artifact in adenosine gel solution (Figure 5, center column) has an increase in current at 1.4 V matching the primary oxidation peak observed during phasic change in adenosine concentration, but an apparent decrease in current near 1.0 V. This is the opposite direction of current changes expected at the secondary oxidation peak during phasic changes of adenosine (Figure 1f).

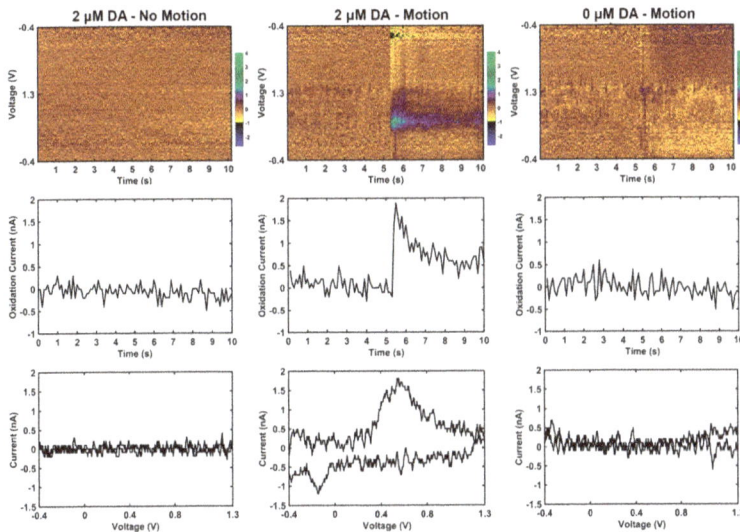

Figure 3. Motion causes dopamine-like artifact signal in vitro only in the presence of dopamine (DA); data is from one representative carbon fiber microelectrode. **Top row:** Pseudo color plots where x, y, and z are time (s), voltage (V), and current (nA) respectively. **Middle row:** Current vs. time plots at the known 0.6 V oxidation potential of dopamine. **Bottom row:** Current vs. voltage plots (cyclic voltammograms) collected 200 µs following initiation of motion. For the no-motion condition, the cyclic voltammogram was collected at the 5 s mark. **Left column:** Example carbon fiber microelectrode FSCV recordings in 0.6% agarose with 2 µM dopamine in solution when no motion is applied. There are no artifact signals apparent in the color plot. **Middle column:** Example of the same electrode in the same solution as the left column data but with a 1 mm motion downward at the 5 s mark that lasts approximately 0.25 s. Note the presence of a transient signal following motion that has the characteristic oxidation and reduction potential changes of dopamine. **Right column:** Example of the same electrode as the other columns in a gel solution with no dopamine and a 1 mm motion downward at the 5 s mark that lasts approximately 0.25 s. There is a transient, broad band disturbance in the color plot at the time of motion, but with no apparent changes at specific voltages.

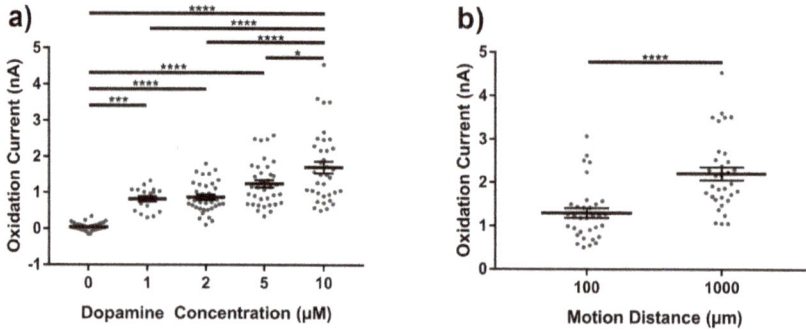

Figure 4. Characterization of fast-scan cyclic voltammetry (FSCV) motion artifacts in vitro in gel solutions of dopamine. (**a**) Effect of gel solution dopamine concentration on motion evoked artifact current at the dopamine oxidation potential 0.6 V (all data points shown as grey dots, mean ± standard error of the mean shown as horizontal black lines and error bars); 0 μM–0.044 ± 0.018 nA (mean ± standard error, $n = 6$ electrodes, 36 measurements), 1 μM–0.816 ± 0.075 nA ($n = 3$ electrodes, 18 measurements), 2 μM–0.865 ± 0.071 nA ($n = 6$ electrodes, 36 measurements), 5 μM–1.241 ± 0.103 nA ($n = 6$ electrodes, 36 measurements), 10 μM–1.706 ± 0.164 nA ($n = 6$ electrodes, 36 measurements); * indicates p-value < 0.05, *** p-value < 0.005, **** p-value < 0.0001, 1 μM vs. 2 μM was non-significant (p-value > 0.999), 2 μM vs. 5 μM was non-significant (p-value = 0.082), 1 μM vs. 5 μM was non-significant (p-value = 0.145), one way ANOVA with post-hoc Bonferroni's multiple comparisons test). (**b**) Effect of motion distance on motion evoked artifact current at the dopamine oxidation potential 0.6 V in gel solutions containing 10 μM dopamine (all data points shown as grey dots, mean ± standard error of the mean shown as horizontal black lines and error bars); 100 μm–1.294 ± 0.112 nA (mean ± standard error, $n = 6$ electrodes, 33 measurements), 1000 μm–2.206 ± 0.148 nA ($n = 6$ electrodes, 33 measurements); **** indicates p-value < 0.0001, t-test with Welch's correction).

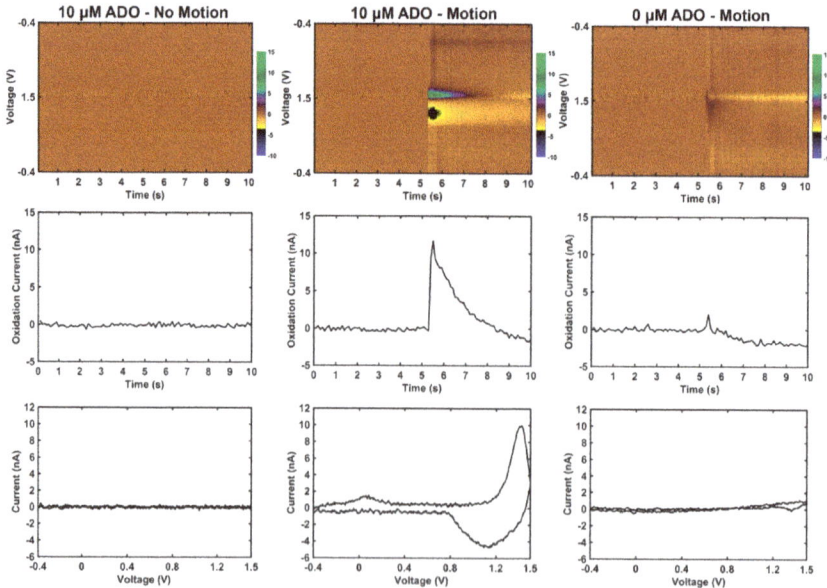

Figure 5. Motion causes adenosine-like artifact signal in vitro only in the presence of adenosine (ADO) that is different than motion induced artifact produced in the presence of dopamine; data is from one representative carbon fiber microelectrode. **Top row:** Pseudo color plots where x, y, and z are time (s),

voltage (V), and current (nA) respectively. **Middle row:** Current vs. time plots at the known 1.4 V primary oxidation potential of adenosine. **Bottom row:** Current vs. voltage plots (cyclic voltammograms) collected 200 µs following initiation of motion. For the no-motion condition, the cyclic voltammogram was collected at the 5 s mark. **Left column:** Example carbon fiber microelectrode FSCV recordings in 0.6% agarose with 10 µM adenosine in solution when no motion is applied. There are no artifact signals apparent in the color plot. **Middle column:** Example of the same electrode in the same gel solution as the left column but with a 1 mm motion downward at the 5 s mark that lasts approximately 0.25 s. Note the increase in current at 1.4 V resembling that of the known primary oxidation for ADO signal (Figure 1f), and a decrease in current near the known secondary oxidation for ADO. **Right column:** Example of the same electrode as the other columns in a gel solution containing no adenosine and a 1 mm motion downward at the 5 s mark that lasts approximately 0.25 s. There is a transient, broad band change at the time of motion, but the signal possesses no apparent changes at specific voltages.

4. Discussion

The data presented in this short communication show that motion can generate electrophysiological and electrochemical artifacts resembling signals traditionally associated with physiological changes of interest. Movement can generate robust artifact signal through numerous potential mechanisms. While the current work does not isolate the individual contribution of each potential mechanism, this work highlights the necessity and importance of device and experimental design to accurately interpret the detected signals. The present work characterizes the impact of motion artifact signals on electrophysiological and neurochemical recordings, as well as emphasizes the existence of an unexpected trade-off—potentially enhanced motion artifact—inherent to developing flexible devices for electrophysiological and neurochemical sensing.

4.1. Motion Artifact During Electrophysiological Recordings Using Flexible Carbon Fibers

The electrode system used for recordings in this study may have impacted the manifestation of motion artifact in several ways. First, in contrast to comparatively more rigid silicon arrays, small diameter carbon fibers are manufactured with geometries that give them greater compliancy [30]. More compliant electrodes are more likely to bend when subjected to stress [26,31,35–39]. The bending of the wire can in turn generate electrostatic and electromagnetic artifact current that can be exacerbated by active electronics [22,56].

Electrophysiological recordings require the use of preamplifier headstage/amplifier stages, which may also be a source of motion artifact signals [16]. In an ideal recording system, small electrical potentials are amplified by the preamplifier headstage and amplifier prior to digitization [56]. The preamplifier is placed as close to the electrode as possible to minimize the length of wire prior to amplification, which minimizes noise introduced by coupling between extrinsic noise sources and the length of wire. Often a small bundle of wire within the headstage still connects the preamplifier output to the amplifier input for subsequent analog to digital conversion. Because the wire is part of the active electronics of the headstage, electrical current is being maintained through the headstage, electrode, the reference, and ground. Each point of connection represents a potential source of triboelectric artifact. These results have implications for integrated multiplexers (MUX) on high-channel recording arrays and on-array powered electronics. Switching across MUX channels requires changes in current to switch channels, which capacitively couples with and leads to charge injection in the analog signal path [57]. Switching also disturbs the equilibrium potential of the electrode/electrolyte interface as a previously floating electrode is connected to the measurement circuit [57]. This issue has the potential to limit the frequency at which channels can be sampled when using multiplexers for electrophysiological and neurochemical signal detection.

Signal processing techniques can alter the temporal characteristics of artifacts and thus further confound the detection and removal of non-neuronal signals. Application of a Butterworth filter to remove local field potentials, for example, may change the shape of movement artifacts via ringing of the filter such that they more closely resemble neuronal action potentials (Figure 6). This issue is particularly noteworthy as some pre-amplifiers are configured with a hardware high pass filter to eliminate slow fluctuations (<2 Hz) that may saturate the amplifier.

Lastly, changing the electrode material at the electrode/electrolyte interface has been shown to affect the magnitude of the artifact created when the electrode/electrolyte interface is disturbed [17,18,58]. For example, Kahn et al. noted only a 1 mV offset potential when flowing a stream of saline solution across a non-polarizable Ag-AgCl electrode, whereas they observed a 30 mV offset potential when using a polarizable pure silver electrode of similar dimensions [16]. Similarly, it has been demonstrated in vivo in chronic rodent studies that electrode sites coated with poly(3,4-ethylenedioxythiophene) polystyrene sulfonate (PEDOT:PSS) [53] or PEDOT nanotubes [59] exhibit notably less low frequency artifact when compared to control iridium or gold electrode sites in the same animal.

The data presented here demonstrates that artifact signals may share similar temporal characteristics with relevant neuronal signals and can be erroneously classified as single unit or multiunit events during standard spike sorting operations [20,60] (e.g., thresholding and clustering in principal component space). As the number and timing of neuronal signals has important implications for the transmission of information within the brain, the misclassification of motion artifacts as single or multiunit signals may influence our interpretation of the data, and ultimately our understanding of the underlying neurophysiological processes.

4.2. Potential Impact of Differential Recording Strategies

Motion artifact is often minimized in vivo through differential recordings [25]. In a differential recording set-up, the measurements taken from a reference electrode are subtracted from the measurements taken by the working electrode [57]. To eliminate motion artifact, the reference electrode ideally needs to be in a similar location as the working electrode and consist of similar dimensions and material to observe a similar 'common' representation of motion artifact for subsequent subtraction [57]. This subtraction is often known as 'common-mode' rejection. Electrophysiological recordings in vivo have historically used rigid multi-electrode arrays or tethered microwire systems [9–11,25,53,59,61,62], which have several advantages with respect to minimizing motion artifact. First, the rigid structures minimize electrical artifacts by resisting bending, and therefore limit artifacts described above [25]. Second, there are multiple electrodes of similar dimension and electrode material located in the same area of tissue that move in tandem with respect to motion [25]. This maximizes the similarity of recorded motion artifact for subsequent subtraction via common-mode rejection/common average reference strategies [25].

As electrodes on a flexible array can potentially move independently of each other, the representation of artifact on each electrode may differ. For example, electrodes at the most shallow contact and at the deepest contact on a single-shank electrode array would presumably experience different stresses with respect to motion of the brain due to tethering [63]. In turn, the motion artifact on the two contacts would also be different. In this case a common median reference (CMR) [64] may avoid creating spurious artifacts on channels without signal, or a small Laplacian (sLAP) referencing strategy could be employed consisting of electrodes with the most similar representation of motion artifact [20]. Nevertheless, due to the extensive variability in artifact amplitude across channels (Figures 1 and 6), neither common average referencing (CAR), CMR, nor sLAP are likely to be sufficient to completely eliminate the misclassification of artifacts as units.

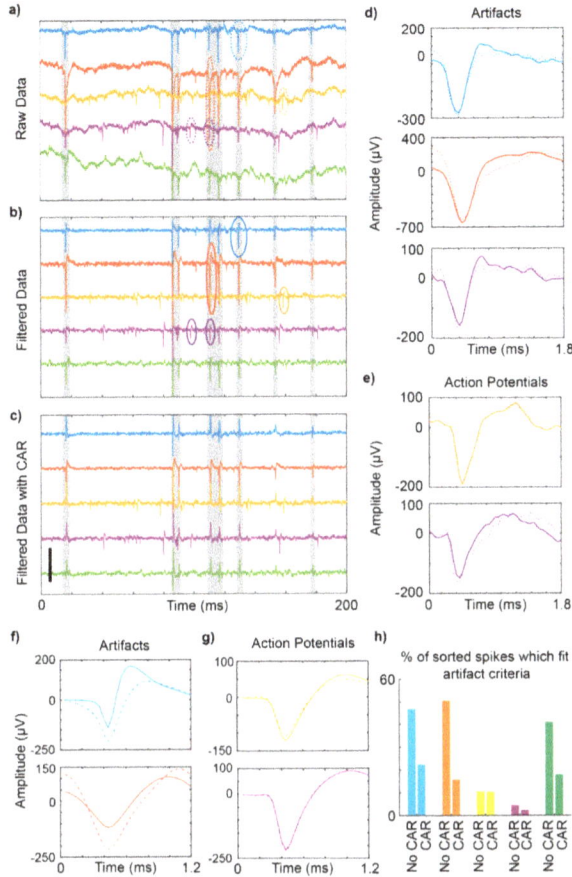

Figure 6. Common average referencing (CAR) helps to reduce motion artifact misclassification. (a–c) Example data (200 ms) from an awake moving rat, implanted with a linear silicon microelectrode array. Application of a high frequency band pass filter (2nd order Butterworth filter, passband 0.3–1 kHz) can cause artifacts (a) to resemble action potentials (b). Grey shading highlights artifacts. (d,e) Circled artifacts and action potentials from (a,b), shown before and after filtering (dashed and solid lines, respectively). (f,g) Mean waveforms for clustered artifacts (d) and action potentials (e) from each channel without CAR (dashed line) and with CAR (solid line). (h) Percentage of sorted units which fit the criteria for artifacts defined in the methods. Scalebar: (a–c) 500 µV. (a–g) © IOP Publishing. Adapted with permission from [20]. All rights reserved.

To minimize spike sorting errors associated with common noise across channels, algorithms that compare signals across channels have been proposed. For example, evaluation of inter-electrode correlation between candidate spike segments as an additional criteria for spike sorting has been shown to improve clustering in principal component space [60,65]. Although this technique reduces the instances of correlated noise impacting the signal, actual units may be discarded with this operation, such as when artifacts occur coincidentally with action potentials or if a neuron's soma is equidistant from two electrode sites. Additionally, simply removing the corrupted data surrounding artifacts will also eliminate detection of coincident spiking activity. Thus, the problem of successfully identifying and discarding artifactual signals remains an important problem for future investigation. In our data, the principal component of sorted single units maintained their eigenvalues before and after applying a common average reference, while noise typically exhibited dramatic changes in eigenvectors, signal shape, and even signal amplitude (Figure 6f,g). This discrepancy may therefore represent an additional strategy to identify artifacts and is currently under further investigation.

4.3. Motion Artifact During Fast Scan Cyclic Voltammetry Measurements Using Carbon Fibers

Like electrophysiological recordings, FSCV neurochemical recordings are also susceptible to motion artifact issues. FSCV recordings are predicated on sweeping a voltage potential through a very small, polarizable carbon fiber electrode in reference to a much larger non-polarizable Ag-AgCl reference electrode to generate a triangle waveform that is repeated at regular intervals [46,47]. The reference electrode must be very large in comparison to guarantee that the impedance of the reference is trivial with respect to the carbon fiber/tissue interface; this in turn guarantees that almost all of the voltage drop occurs at the carbon fiber/tissue interface to drive the oxidation/reduction reaction with electroactive neurochemicals adsorbed to the carbon fiber surface [29,32,40]. The reference is traditionally a non-polarizable electrode to avoid distorting the applied triangle waveform by a change of the potential during the FSCV pulse [20].

During FSCV in vivo, the carbon fiber 'working electrode' is implanted in a brain region of interest whereas the Ag-AgCl 'reference electrode' is normally placed above cortex. The triangle waveform voltage pulse applied to the carbon fiber electrode with respect to the Ag-AgCl electrode causes electroactive neurochemicals adsorbed to the surface of the carbon fiber to oxidize and reduce, generating a faradaic current. As the carbon fiber is a polarizable electrode, a non-faradaic capacitive current is also generated. The voltage at which oxidation/reduction currents are observed in combination with the magnitude of those currents can be used to infer the specific electroactive neurochemical and the approximate concentration of that neurochemical in the vicinity of the carbon fiber electrode. As the neurochemical concentration undergoes phasic changes, the faradaic current changes while the non-faradaic current remains relatively constant. Therefore, the real-time FSCV waveform can be subtracted by an FSCV measurement at an earlier point in time—known as background subtraction—to minimize the non-faradaic portion of the observed current. This helps isolate faradaic changes in current putatively associated with phasic changes in local neurochemical concentration.

The idea that spurious signals may contaminate even background subtracted FSCV recordings is not new. The preliminary studies performed by Adams in the 1970s demonstrated that neurotransmitters are only a percentage of species within the brain able to oxidize/reduce when at the electrode surface [30]. This led Mark Wightman and his colleagues to propose a set of guidelines often referred to as the 'Five Golden Rules' of electroanalytical chemistry in vivo [28,66]. In brief, these rules include (1) electrochemical verification of the FSCV signal generated by specific concentrations of the neurotransmitter of interest in vitro, (2) anatomical verification that the electrode is placed in a region of the brain in the vicinity of post-synaptic terminals where the neurotransmitter of interest would be found, (3) physiological verification through behavioral manipulation that would be anticipated to change the extracellular concentration of the neurotransmitter of interest, for example electrical stimulation of the pre-synaptic pathway, (4) pharmacological manipulation—e.g., a reuptake inhibitor specific to the neurotransmitter of interest—that would elicit changes in the measured concentrations specific to the neurotransmitter of interest, and (5) independent confirmation with a secondary measure such as microdialysis. Note these rules are predicated on the assumption that measurements of the neurochemical of interest are primarily confounded by interfering signal caused by the adsorption of other electroactive molecules in the brain to the surface of the electrode. In general artifacts due to motion, sources of radio frequency radiation, or electrical/optical stimulation in vivo have previously been thought to create 'broad-band' changes in observed currents. These broad-band changes are assumed to be roughly uniformly distributed across all voltages applied during the FSCV pulse [67], instead of changes at the characteristic voltages stereotypical of the oxidation/reduction potentials of a specific electroactive neurochemical. Consequently, datasets contaminated by motion or other artifacts are traditionally identified by a trained operator through visual inspection for broad-band changes and are removed.

Here we have demonstrated that motion can generate an artifact signal during FSCV that resembles phasic neurochemical concentration changes regularly measured in vivo if that neurochemical is present in the recording medium. Motion of the electrode in solution with no electroactive molecules—buffer solution with only salt ions—produces broad band artifact currents that bear no resemblance to specific electroactive molecules. Importantly, changes in current at the oxidation and reduction potential of a neurochemical is defined as a change in concentration of that neurochemical when using FSCV as a measurement tool, therefore measurement of those oxidation/reduction potential current changes during motion is unexpected given the concentration of neurochemical did not change during the motion.

Motion of the electrode/electrolyte interface during FSCV disturbs the established electric double layer and thus may lead to changes in the capacitive charging current as well as the distribution of charged species, such as dopamine near the FSCV electrode surface [68,69]. In addition, movement of the electrode could change the equilibrium concentrations of dopamine and dopamine-o-quinone (oxidation product of dopamine) near the electrode that is formed as a result of oxidation/reduction, mass transfer, and adsorption dynamics near the electrode [68,70]. Upon motion, the electrode might be leaving the equilibrium formed by those dynamics and entering the bulk concentration that has a higher ratio of dopamine to dopamine-o-quinone, thus resulting in a measured transient increase that decays back to baseline as equilibrium re-establishes. Finally, disturbing either the working or reference electrode transiently alters their respective half-cell potentials. As a voltage is actively being applied between the working and reference electrode to drive redox reactions, disturbing the electrode/electrolyte interface of either may alter the effective voltage being applied between them.

The finding that motion artifact during FSCV closely resembles phasic changes of electroactive neurochemicals in the solution may be particularly problematic when inferring in vivo concentrations from pre and post-operative calibrations performed in vitro. This issue is compounded by the observation that different neurochemicals produce different motion artifacts, and the magnitude of the motion artifact depends on the tonic concentration of neurochemical in the recording environment. Consequently, commonly used reuptake inhibitors for pharmacological validation—which increase the concentration of the neurochemical of interest in the extracellular environment—may inadvertently also increase the magnitude of motion artifacts that resemble the neurochemical of interest.

It is important to note the motion artifact produced during these experiments does not always exactly resemble the neurochemical's characteristic redox potentials. For example, a decrease in current was observed at the stereotypical adenosine secondary oxidation peak (1.0 V) during motion (Figure 5, compare to increase at secondary peak for known adenosine in Figure 1). In addition, the magnitude of motion artifact was highly variable given multiple electrodes of the same active site dimensions in a controlled in vitro condition (Figure 4). This suggests motion artifacts may be difficult to predict in magnitude, especially in vivo. It is also important to note that the lowest neurochemical concentrations of dopamine and adenosine used in these experiments are at the high end of what would be anticipated in vivo, with the resulting motion induced current deflections typically in the 1–4 nA ranges. Consequently, the impact of motion artifact on interpreting FSCV becomes more significant in chronic studies where the observed signal is reduced due to biofouling and may be only in the 1 nA range [71–73].

The findings presented here serve to underscore the necessity of following Wightman's "Five Golden Rules" when interpreting in vivo FSCV recordings. This includes independent confirmation with a secondary measure, ideally one capable of measuring changes in concentration of the neurochemical of interest, albeit at slower temporal resolution. Other common sources of artifact that disturb the electrode/electrolyte interface, such as electrical stimulation or extrinsic sources of electromagnetic radiation were also preliminarily tested during the execution of these studies (data not shown). Under the right conditions these traditional sources of electrophysiological artifacts also generate characteristic waveforms normally associated with phasic changes of electroactive neurochemicals during FSCV measurements. These perturbations should be explored in future work.

5. Conclusions

Both the electrophysiological recording and FSCV motion artifact data presented in this short communication suggest that any change to design or usage-context of a neural interface needs to be carefully evaluated to determine if meaningful neurological signals can be detected and separated from sources of artifact. Validation of meaningful neurological signals ideally includes evaluating a physiological input to drive peri-stimulus neural activity [6,20,31,32,46,47,50,74]. In addition, the stimulus needs to be evaluated on the benchtop or in a post-mortem control to ensure that the stimulus itself does not generate an artifactual signal. Moreover, active shielding and signal processing needs to be carefully evaluated to better identify and remove motion related artifacts as increasingly flexible devices are developed.

Author Contributions: Conceptualization, E.N.N., N.J.M., T.D.Y.K. and K.A.L.; Methodology, E.N.N., N.J.M., T.D.Y.K. and K.A.L.; Software, E.N.N. and N.J.M.; Validation, E.N.N., N.J.M., M.L.S., S.A.H., J.K.T., A.J.A., J.L.L., T.D.Y.K. and K.A.L.; Formal Analysis, E.N.N., N.J.M., J.K.T., A.J.A.; Investigation, E.N.N., N.J.M., M.L.S., S.A.H.; Resources, J.L.L., T.D.Y.K. and K.A.L.; Data Curation, E.N.N., N.J.M., J.K.T., A.J.A., K.C.S.; Writing-Original Draft Preparation, E.N.N., N.J.M., T.D.Y.K. and K.A.L.; Writing-Review & Editing, E.N.N., N.J.M., M.L.S., S.A.H., J.K.T., A.J.A., K.C.S., J.L.L., T.D.Y.K. and K.A.L.; Visualization, E.N.N., N.J.M., J.K.T., A.J.A.; Supervision, J.L.L., T.D.Y.K. and K.A.L.; Project Administration, J.L.L., T.D.Y.K. and K.A.L.; Funding Acquisition, J.L.L., T.D.Y.K. and K.A.L.

Funding: This research was funded by National Institutes of Health (NIH) National Institute of Neurological Disorders and Stroke (NINDS) (Grants R01NS062019, R01NS094396, R01NS089688, and R21NS108098), The Defense Advanced Research Projects Agency (DARPA) Biological Technologies Office (BTO) Targeted Neuroplasticity Training Program under the auspices of Doug Weber and Tristan McClure-Begley through the Space and Naval Warfare Systems Command (SPAWAR) Systems Center with (SSC) Pacific grants no. N66001-17-2-4010., and The Grainger Foundation.

Acknowledgments: The authors would like to thank Pavel Takmakov for his advice on the interpretation of the FSCV data presented. The authors would also like to thank Paras R. Patel for sharing the rat electrophysiology data.

Conflicts of Interest: The authors declare no conflict of interest.

References

1. Schwartz, A.B. Cortical neural prosthetics. *Annu. Rev. Neurosci.* **2004**, *27*, 487–507. [CrossRef] [PubMed]
2. Schwartz, A.B.; Cui, X.T.; Weber, D.J.; Moran, D.W. Brain-controlled interfaces: Movement restoration with neural prosthetics. *Neuron* **2006**, *52*, 205–220. [CrossRef] [PubMed]
3. Kipke, D.R.; Shain, W.; Buzsaki, G.; Fetz, E.; Henderson, J.M.; Hetke, J.F.; Schalk, G. Advanced Neurotechnologies for Chronic Neural Interfaces: New Horizons and Clinical Opportunities. *J. Neurosci.* **2008**, *28*, 11830–11838. [CrossRef] [PubMed]
4. Brandman, D.M.; Cash, S.S.; Hochberg, L.R. Review: Human Intracortical recording and neural decoding for brain-computer interfaces. *IEEE Trans. Neural Syst. Rehabil. Eng.* **2017**, *25*, 1687–1696. [CrossRef] [PubMed]
5. Iordanova, B.; Vazquez, A.L.; Kozai, T.D.Y.; Fukuda, M.; Kim, S.G. Optogenetic investigation of the variable neurovascular coupling along the interhemispheric circuits. *J. Cereb. Blood Flow Metab.* **2018**, *38*, 627–640. [CrossRef] [PubMed]
6. Michelson, N.J.; Kozai, T.D.Y. Isoflurane and Ketamine Differentially Influence Spontaneous and Evoked Laminar Electrophysiology in Mouse V1. *J. Neurophysiol.* **2018**. [CrossRef] [PubMed]
7. Golabchi, A.; Wu, B.; Li, X.; Carlisle, D.L.; Kozai, T.D.Y.; Friedlander, R.M.; Cui, X.T. Melatonin improves quality and longevity of chronic neural recording. *Biomaterials* **2018**, *180*, 225–239. [CrossRef] [PubMed]
8. Mosier, E.M.; Wolfson, M.; Ross, E.; Harris, J.; Weber, D.; Ludwig, K.A. The Brain Initiative—Implications for a Revolutionary Change in Clinical Medicine via Neuromodulation Technology. *Neuromodulation* **2018**, 55–68. [CrossRef]
9. Gage, G.J.; Ludwig, K.A.; Otto, K.J.; Ionides, E.L.; Kipke, D.R. Naive coadaptive cortical control. *J. Neural Eng.* **2005**, *2*, 52–63. [CrossRef] [PubMed]

10. Gage, G.J.; Otto, K.J.; Ludwig, K.A.; Kipke, D.R. Co-adaptive Kalman filtering in a naive rat cortical control task. In Proceedings of the 26th Annual International Conference of the IEEE Engineering in Medicine and Biology Society, San Francisco, CA, USA, 1–5 September 2004; pp. 4367–4370.

11. Ludwig, K.A.; Miriani, R.M.; Langhals, N.B.; Marzullo, T.C.; Kipke, D.R. Use of a Bayesian maximum-likelihood classifier to generate training data for brain-machine interfaces. *J. Neural Eng.* **2011**, *8*, 046009. [CrossRef] [PubMed]

12. Bowsher, K.; Civillico, E.; Coburn, J.; Collinger, J.; Contreras-Vidal, J.; Denison, T.; Donoghue, J.; French, J.; Getzoff, N.; Hochberg, L. Brain–computer interface devices for patients with paralysis and amputation: A meeting report. *J. Neural Eng.* **2016**, *13*, 023001. [CrossRef] [PubMed]

13. Trevathan, J.K.; Yousefi, A.; Park, H.O.; Bartoletta, J.J.; Ludwig, K.A.; Lee, K.H.; Lujan, J.L. Computational modeling of neurotransmitter release evoked by electrical stimulation: nonlinear approaches to predicting stimulation-evoked dopamine release. *ACS Chem. Neurosci.* **2017**, *8*, 394–410. [CrossRef] [PubMed]

14. Grahn, P.J.; Mallory, G.W.; Khurram, O.U.; Berry, B.M.; Hachmann, J.T.; Bieber, A.J.; Bennet, K.E.; Min, H.K.; Chang, S.Y.; Lee, K.H.; et al. A neurochemical closed-loop controller for deep brain stimulation: Toward individualized smart neuromodulation therapies. *Front. Neurosci.* **2014**, *8*, 169. [CrossRef] [PubMed]

15. Covey, D.P.; Garris, P.A. Using fast-scan cyclic voltammetry to evaluate striatal dopamine release elicited by subthalamic nucleus stimulation. In Proceedings of the 2009 Annual International Conference of the IEEE Engineering in Medicine and Biology Society, Minneapolis, MN, USA, 3–6 September 2009; Volume 2009, pp. 3306–3309.

16. Webster, J. *Medical Instrumentation: Application and Design*; John Wiley & Sons: Hoboken, NJ, USA, 2009.

17. Tam, H.; Webster, J.G. Minimizing electrode motion artifact by skin abrasion. *IEEE Trans. Biomed. Eng.* **1977**, 134–139. [CrossRef] [PubMed]

18. Stecker, M. Factors Affecting Stimulus Artifact: Solution Factors. *EC Neurol.* **2017**, *5*, 52–61.

19. Heffer, L.F.; Fallon, J.B. A novel stimulus artifact removal technique for high-rate electrical stimulation. *J. Neurosci. Methods* **2008**, *170*, 277–284. [CrossRef] [PubMed]

20. Michelson, N.J.; Vazquez, A.L.; Eles, J.R.; Salatino, J.W.; Purcell, E.K.; Williams, J.J.; Cui, X.T.; Kozai, T.D.Y. Multi-scale, multi-modal analysis uncovers complex relationship at the brain tissue-implant neural interface: New Emphasis on the Biological Interface. *J. Neural Eng.* **2018**, *15*, 033001. [CrossRef] [PubMed]

21. Wartzek, T.; Lammersen, T.; Eilebrecht, B.; Walter, M.; Leonhardt, S. Triboelectricity in capacitive biopotential measurements. *IEEE Trans. Biomed. Eng.* **2011**, *58*, 1268–1277. [CrossRef] [PubMed]

22. Giancoli, D.C. *Physics: Principles with Applications*; Prentice Hall: Upper Saddle River, NJ, USA, 1998.

23. Bard, A.J.; Faulkner, L.R.; Leddy, J.; Zoski, C.G. *Electrochemical Methods: Fundamentals and Applications*; Wiley: Hoboken, NJ, USA, 1980; Volume 2.

24. Merrill, D.R.; Bikson, M.; Jefferys, J.G. Electrical stimulation of excitable tissue: Design of efficacious and safe protocols. *J. Neurosci. Methods* **2005**, *141*, 171–198. [CrossRef] [PubMed]

25. Ludwig, K.A.; Miriani, R.M.; Langhals, N.B.; Joseph, M.D.; Anderson, D.J.; Kipke, D.R. Using a common average reference to improve cortical neuron recordings from microelectrode arrays. *J. Neurophysiol.* **2009**, *101*, 1679–1689. [CrossRef] [PubMed]

26. Du, Z.J.; Kolarcik, C.L.; Kozai, T.D.Y.; Luebben, S.D.; Sapp, S.A.; Zheng, X.S.; Nabity, J.A.; Cui, X.T. Ultrasoft microwire neural electrodes improve chronic tissue integration. *Acta Biomater.* **2017**, *53*, 46–58. [CrossRef] [PubMed]

27. Salatino, J.W.; Ludwig, K.A.; Kozai, T.D.Y.; Purcell, E.K. Glial responses to implanted electrodes in the brain. *Nat. Biomed. Eng.* **2017**, *1*, 862–877. [CrossRef]

28. Wellman, S.M.; Eles, J.R.; Ludwig, K.A.; Seymour, J.P.; Michelson, N.J.; McFadden, W.E.; Vazquez, A.L.; Kozai, T.D. A Materials Roadmap to Functional Neural Interface Design. *Adv. Funct. Mater.* **2017**, *28*, 1701269. [CrossRef] [PubMed]

29. Patel, P.R.; Zhang, H.; Robbins, M.T.; Nofar, J.B.; Marshall, S.P.; Kobylarek, M.J.; Kozai, T.D.Y.; Kotov, N.A.; Chestek, C.A. Chronic In Vivo Stability Assessment of Carbon Fiber Microelectrode Arrays. *J. Neural Eng.* **2016**, *13*, 066002. [CrossRef] [PubMed]

30. Kozai, T.D.; Jaquins-Gerstl, A.S.; Vazquez, A.L.; Michael, A.C.; Cui, X.T. Brain tissue responses to neural implants impact signal sensitivity and intervention strategies. *ACS Chem. Neurosci.* **2015**, *6*, 48–67. [CrossRef] [PubMed]

31. Kolarcik, C.L.; Luebben, S.D.; Sapp, S.A.; Hanner, J.; Snyder, N.; Kozai, T.D.Y.; Chang, E.; Nabity, J.A.; Nabity, S.T.; Lagenaur, C.F.; et al. Elastomeric and soft conducting microwires for implantable neural interfaces. *Soft Matter* **2015**, *11*, 4847–4861. [CrossRef] [PubMed]

32. Kozai, T.D.Y.; Li, X.; Bodily, L.M.; Caparosa, E.M.; Zenonos, G.A.; Carlisle, D.L.; Friedlander, R.M.; Cui, X.T. Effects of caspase-1 knockout on chronic neural recording quality and longevity: Insight into cellular and molecular mechanisms of the reactive tissue response. *Biomaterials* **2014**, *35*, 9620–9634. [CrossRef] [PubMed]

33. Kozai, T.D.Y.; Langhals, N.B.; Patel, P.R.; Deng, X.; Zhang, H.; Smith, K.L.; Lahann, J.; Kotov, N.A.; Kipke, D.R. Ultrasmall implantable composite microelectrodes with bioactive surfaces for chronic neural interfaces. *Nat. Mater.* **2012**, *11*, 1065–1073. [CrossRef] [PubMed]

34. Guitchounts, G.; Markowitz, J.E.; Liberti, W.A.; Gardner, T.J. A carbon-fiber electrode array for long-term neural recording. *J. Neural Eng.* **2013**, *10*, 046016. [CrossRef] [PubMed]

35. Sohal, H.S.; Clowry, G.J.; Jackson, A.; O'Neill, A.; Baker, S.N. Mechanical flexibility reduces the foreign body response to long-term implanted microelectrodes in rabbit cortex. *PLoS ONE* **2016**, *11*, e0165606. [CrossRef] [PubMed]

36. Sohal, H.S.; Jackson, A.; Jackson, R.; Clowry, G.J.; Vassilevski, K.; O'Neill, A.; Baker, S.N. The sinusoidal probe: A new approach to improve electrode longevity. *Front. Neuroeng.* **2014**, *7*, 10. [CrossRef] [PubMed]

37. Harris, J.P.; Capadona, J.R.; Miller, R.H.; Healy, B.C.; Shanmuganathan, K.; Rowan, S.J.; Weder, C.; Tyler, D.J. Mechanically adaptive intracortical implants improve the proximity of neuronal cell bodies. *J. Neural Eng.* **2011**, *8*, 066011. [CrossRef] [PubMed]

38. Canales, A.; Jia, X.; Froriep, U.P.; Koppes, R.A.; Tringides, C.M.; Selvidge, J.; Lu, C.; Hou, C.; Wei, L.; Fink, Y.; et al. Multifunctional fibers for simultaneous optical, electrical and chemical interrogation of neural circuits in vivo. *Nat. Biotechnol.* **2015**, *33*, 277–284. [CrossRef] [PubMed]

39. Xie, C.; Liu, J.; Fu, T.M.; Dai, X.; Zhou, W.; Lieber, C.M. Three-dimensional macroporous nanoelectronic networks as minimally invasive brain probes. *Nat. Mater.* **2015**, *14*, 1286–1292. [CrossRef] [PubMed]

40. Patel, P.R.; Na, K.; Zhang, H.; Kozai, T.D.; Kotov, N.A.; Yoon, E.; Chestek, C.A. Insertion of linear 8.4 μm diameter 16 channel carbon fiber electrode arrays for single unit recordings. *J. Neural Eng.* **2015**, *12*, 046009. [CrossRef] [PubMed]

41. Ware, T.; Simon, D.; Liu, C.; Musa, T.; Vasudevan, S.; Sloan, A.; Keefer, E.W.; Rennaker, R.L., 2nd; Voit, W. Thiol-ene/acrylate substrates for softening intracortical electrodes. *J. Biomed. Mater. Res. Part B Appl. Biomater.* **2014**, *102*, 1–11. [CrossRef] [PubMed]

42. Nguyen, J.K.; Park, D.J.; Skousen, J.L.; Hess-Dunning, A.E.; Tyler, D.J.; Rowan, S.J.; Weder, C.; Capadona, J.R. Mechanically-compliant intracortical implants reduce the neuroinflammatory response. *J. Neural Eng.* **2014**, *11*, 056014. [CrossRef] [PubMed]

43. Schluter, E.W.; Mitz, A.R.; Cheer, J.F.; Averbeck, B.B. Real-time dopamine measurement in awake monkeys. *PLoS ONE* **2014**, *9*, e98692. [CrossRef] [PubMed]

44. Clark, J.J.; Sandberg, S.G.; Wanat, M.J.; Gan, J.O.; Horne, E.A.; Hart, A.S.; Akers, C.A.; Parker, J.G.; Willuhn, I.; Martinez, V. Chronic microsensors for longitudinal, subsecond dopamine detection in behaving animals. *Nat. Methods* **2009**, *7*, 126–129. [CrossRef] [PubMed]

45. Seymour, J.P.; Kipke, D.R. Neural probe design for reduced tissue encapsulation in CNS. *Biomaterials* **2007**, *28*, 3594–3607. [CrossRef] [PubMed]

46. Kozai, T.D.; Catt, K.; Li, X.; Gugel, Z.V.; Olafsson, V.T.; Vazquez, A.L.; Cui, X.T. Mechanical failure modes of chronically implanted planar silicon-based neural probes for laminar recording. *Biomaterials* **2015**, *37*, 25–39. [CrossRef] [PubMed]

47. Kozai, T.D.Y.; Du, Z.; Gugel, Z.V.; Smith, M.A.; Chase, S.M.; Bodily, L.M.; Caparosa, E.M.; Friedlander, R.M.; Cui, X.T. Comprehensive chronic laminar single-unit, multi-unit, and local field potential recording performance with planar single shank electrode arrays. *J. Neurosci. Methods* **2015**, *242*, 15–40. [CrossRef] [PubMed]

48. Mechler, F.; Victor, J.D. Dipole characterization of single neurons from their extracellular action potentials. *J. Comput. Neurosci.* **2012**, *32*, 73–100. [CrossRef] [PubMed]

49. Henze, D.A.; Borhegyi, Z.; Csicsvari, J.; Mamiya, A.; Harris, K.D.; Buzsaki, G. Intracellular features predicted by extracellular recordings in the hippocampus in vivo. *J. Neurophysiol.* **2000**, *84*, 390–400. [CrossRef] [PubMed]

50. Kozai, T.D.Y.; Catt, K.; Du, Z.; Na, K.; Srivannavit, O.; Haque, R.-U.M.; Seymour, J.; Wise, K.D.; Yoon, E.; Cui, X.T. Chronic In Vivo Evaluation of PEDOT/CNT for Stable Neural Recordings. *IEEE Trans. Biomed. Eng.* **2016**, *63*, 111–119. [CrossRef] [PubMed]

51. De Gennaro, L.; Ferrara, M. Sleep spindles: An overview. *Sleep Med. Rev.* **2003**, *7*, 423–440. [CrossRef] [PubMed]

52. Shahriari, K. Safe and Effective Techniques for Surgically Inserting Flexible Microelectrode Arrays into the Cortex. Ph.D. Thesis, Arizona State University, Tempe, AZ, USA, 2001.

53. Ludwig, K.A.; Uram, J.D.; Yang, J.; Martin, D.C.; Kipke, D.R. Chronic neural recordings using silicon microelectrode arrays electrochemically deposited with a poly(3,4-ethylenedioxythiophene) (PEDOT) film. *J. Neural Eng.* **2006**, *3*, 59–70. [CrossRef] [PubMed]

54. Shon, Y.M.; Chang, S.Y.; Tye, S.J.; Kimble, C.J.; Bennet, K.E.; Blaha, C.D.; Lee, K.H. Comonitoring of adenosine and dopamine using the wireless instantaneous neurotransmitter concentration system: Proof of principle. *J. Neurosurg.* **2010**, *112*, 539–548. [CrossRef] [PubMed]

55. Swamy, B.K.; Venton, B.J. Subsecond detection of physiological adenosine concentrations using fast-scan cyclic voltammetry. *Anal. Chem.* **2007**, *79*, 744–750. [CrossRef] [PubMed]

56. Jackson, J.D. *Classical Electrodynamics*; John Wiley & Sons: New York, NY, USA, 1999.

57. Webster, J.G.; Eren, H. *Measurement, Instrumentation, and Sensors Handbook*, 2nd ed.; CRC Press: Boca Raton, FL, USA, 2014; p. 2.

58. Kahn, A. Motion artifacts and streaming potentials in relation to biological electrodes. In Proceedings of the Dig 6th International Conference Medical Electronics and Biological Engineering, Tokyo, Japan, 22–27 August 1965; Volume 112, pp. 562–563.

59. Abidian, M.R.; Ludwig, K.A.; Marzullo, T.C.; Martin, D.C.; Kipke, D.R. Interfacing conducting polymer nanotubes with the central nervous system: chronic neural recording using poly(3,4-ethylenedioxythiophene) nanotubes. *Adv. Mater.* **2009**, *21*, 3764–3770. [CrossRef] [PubMed]

60. Paralikar, K.; Rao, C.; Clement, R.S. Automated reduction of non-neuronal signals from intra-cortical microwire array recordings by use of correlation technique. In Proceedings of the 2008 30th Annual International Conference of the IEEE Engineering in Medicine and Biology Society, Vancouver, BC, Canada, 20–25 August 2008; pp. 46–49.

61. Ludwig, K.A.; Langhals, N.B.; Joseph, M.D.; Richardson-Burns, S.M.; Hendricks, J.L.; Kipke, D.R. Poly(3,4-ethylenedioxythiophene) (PEDOT) polymer coatings facilitate smaller neural recording electrodes. *J. Neural Eng.* **2011**, *8*, 014001. [CrossRef] [PubMed]

62. Purcell, E.K.; Thompson, D.E.; Ludwig, K.A.; Kipke, D.R. Flavopiridol reduces the impedance of neural prostheses in vivo without affecting recording quality. *J. Neurosci. Methods* **2009**, *183*, 149–157. [CrossRef] [PubMed]

63. Subbaroyan, J.; Martin, D.C.; Kipke, D.R. A finite-element model of the mechanical effects of implantable microelectrodes in the cerebral cortex. *J. Neural Eng.* **2005**, *2*, 103–113. [CrossRef] [PubMed]

64. Rolston, J.D.; Gross, R.E.; Potter, S.M. Common median referencing for improved action potential detection with multielectrode arrays. In Proceedings of the 2009 Annual International Conference of the IEEE Engineering in Medicine and Biology Society, Minneapolis, MN, USA, 3–6 September 2009; pp. 1604–1607.

65. Paralikar, K.J.; Rao, C.R.; Clement, R.S. New approaches to eliminating common-noise artifacts in recordings from intracortical microelectrode arrays: Inter-electrode correlation and virtual referencing. *J. Neurosci. Methods* **2009**, *181*, 27–35. [CrossRef] [PubMed]

66. Phillips, P.E.; Wightman, R.M. Critical guidelines for validation of the selectivity of in-vivo chemical microsensors. *TrAC Trends Anal. Chem.* **2003**, *22*, 509–514. [CrossRef]

67. Garris, P.A.; Ensman, R.; Poehlman, J.; Alexander, A.; Langley, P.E.; Sandberg, S.G.; Greco, P.G.; Wightman, R.M.; Rebec, G.V. Wireless transmission of fast-scan cyclic voltammetry at a carbon-fiber microelectrode: Proof of principle. *J. Neurosci. Methods* **2004**, *140*, 103–115. [CrossRef] [PubMed]

68. Johnson, J.A.; Hobbs, C.N.; Wightman, R.M. Removal of Differential Capacitive Interferences in Fast-Scan Cyclic Voltammetry. *Anal. Chem.* **2017**, *89*, 6166–6174. [CrossRef] [PubMed]

69. Simakov, A.B.; Webster, J.G. Motion Artifact from Electrodes and Cables. *Iran. J. Electr. Comput. Eng.* **2010**, *9*, 139–143.

70. Atcherley, C.W.; Laude, N.D.; Parent, K.L.; Heien, M.L. Fast-scan controlled-adsorption voltammetry for the quantification of absolute concentrations and adsorption dynamics. *Langmuir* **2013**, *29*, 14885–14892. [CrossRef] [PubMed]
71. Nicolai, E.N.; Trevathan, J.K.; Ross, E.K.; Lujan, J.L.; Blaha, C.D.; Bennet, K.E.; Lee, K.H.; Ludwig, K.A. Detection of norepinephrine in whole blood via fast scan cyclic voltammetry. In Proceedings of the 2017 IEEE International Symposium on Medical Measurements and Applications (MeMeA), Rochester, MN, USA, 7–10 May 2017; p. 111.
72. Schwerdt, H.N.; Shimazu, H.; Amemori, K.-I.; Amemori, S.; Tierney, P.L.; Gibson, D.J.; Hong, S.; Yoshida, T.; Langer, R.; Cima, M.J. Long-term dopamine neurochemical monitoring in primates. *Proc. Natl. Acad. Sci. USA* **2017**, *114*, 13260–13265. [CrossRef] [PubMed]
73. Singh, Y.S.; Sawarynski, L.E.; Dabiri, P.D.; Choi, W.R.; Andrews, A.M. Head-to-head comparisons of carbon fiber microelectrode coatings for sensitive and selective neurotransmitter detection by voltammetry. *Anal. Chem.* **2011**, *83*, 6658–6666. [CrossRef] [PubMed]
74. Cody, P.A.; Eles, J.R.; Lagenaur, C.F.; Kozai, T.D.; Cui, X.T. Unique electrophysiological and impedance signatures between encapsulation types: An analysis of biological Utah array failure and benefit of a biomimetic coating in a rat model. *Biomaterials* **2018**, *161*, 117–128. [CrossRef] [PubMed]

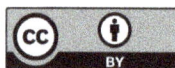

micromachines

MDPI

Article

Acquisition of Neural Action Potentials Using Rapid Multiplexing Directly at the Electrodes

Mohit Sharma [1],*, Avery Tye Gardner [1], Hunter J. Strathman [2], David J. Warren [2], Jason Silver [1] and Ross M. Walker [1],*

[1]   Department of Electrical and Computer Engineering, University of Utah, Salt Lake City, UT 84112, USA;
     tye.gardner@utah.edu (A.T.G.); jason.silver@utah.edu (J.S.)
[2]   Department of Biomedical Engineering, University of Utah, Salt Lake City, UT 84112, USA;
     h.strathman@utah.edu (H.J.S.); david.warren@utah.edu (D.J.W.)
*   Correspondence: mohit.sharma@utah.edu (M.S.); ross.walker@utah.edu (R.M.W.);
     Tel.: +1-801-585-1494 (M.S. & R.M.W.)

Received: 1 September 2018; Accepted: 17 September 2018; Published: 20 September 2018

Abstract: Neural recording systems that interface with implanted microelectrodes are used extensively in experimental neuroscience and neural engineering research. Interface electronics that are needed to amplify, filter, and digitize signals from multichannel electrode arrays are a critical bottleneck to scaling such systems. This paper presents the design and testing of an electronic architecture for intracortical neural recording that drastically reduces the size per channel by rapidly multiplexing many electrodes to a single circuit. The architecture utilizes mixed-signal feedback to cancel electrode offsets, windowed integration sampling to reduce aliased high-frequency noise, and a successive approximation analog-to-digital converter with small capacitance and asynchronous control. Results are presented from a 180 nm CMOS integrated circuit prototype verified using in vivo experiments with a tungsten microwire array implanted in rodent cortex. The integrated circuit prototype achieves <0.004 mm^2 area per channel, 7 μW power dissipation per channel, 5.6 μV$_{rms}$ input referred noise, 50 dB common mode rejection ratio, and generates 9-bit samples at 30 kHz per channel by multiplexing at 600 kHz. General considerations are discussed for rapid time domain multiplexing of high-impedance microelectrodes. Overall, this work describes a promising path forward for scaling neural recording systems to numbers of electrodes that are orders of magnitude larger.

Keywords: neural recording; neural amplifier; microelectrode array; intracortical; sensor interface; windowed integration sampling; mixed-signal feedback; multiplexing

1. Introduction

Penetrating microelectrodes that record neural signals currently achieve the highest temporal and spatial resolution available for measuring nervous system activity in vivo [1,2]. Multichannel electrode arrays can be implanted into regions of the central and peripheral nervous systems, and extracellular measurements of neuronal activity can be taken by interfacing the electrodes to signal acquisition electronics that are composed of amplifiers, filters, and analog-to-digital converters (ADCs). This general approach is frequently used in experimental neuroscience [3–5], as well as in research toward prosthetics and brain-computer interfaces that are directly controlled by neural activity [6–8]. Recently, neural interface technologies based on microelectrode arrays have seen dramatic growth and interest that has been supported by progress in materials, fabrication, electronics, and neuroscience [9].

A key goal for the future is to scale the number of implanted electrode sites up by orders of magnitude. In neuroscience, this goal is important for accessing larger populations of neurons to provide a more complete view of information processing in the brain. For medical applications of neural interfaces, scaling has great potential to provide more effective therapies and prosthetic devices. Regions of the human neocortex contain approximately 50,000 neurons/mm^3 [10], but neural interfaces used in human clinical trials [6–8] can only provide cellular-level signals from around 200 different neurons sampled in a roughly 10 mm^3 volume of tissue. Today, most microelectrode arrays have between 16 and 256 electrode sites, typically positioned at a few hundred micrometer spacing (<10 sites/mm^2) [1,2]. There are large ongoing efforts focused on scaling up to thousands of electrodes and beyond [11–15]. These projects often target orders of magnitude higher density of the electrode sites (>1000 sites/mm^2) [13–15]. Fully implantable acquisition electronics are needed to support this scaling, because passive wiring of each electrode site to external electronics incurs a number of surgical and reliability problems [1,16].

Massive system scaling requires reconsideration of the traditional approach to designing acquisition electronics. The conventional approach is to use individual amplifiers and filters dedicated to each electrode site (Figure 1a). While this approach offers simple solutions to many of the technical issues involved in acquiring neural signals, the resulting silicon chip area per channel is too large to support thousands of electrodes and beyond without dominating the size and form factor of a fully implantable microsystem. Progress has been made in reducing the size of traditional acquisition electronics (e.g., there are >2000 articles listed under "neural amplifier" in the Inspec database at the time of this writing), but state-of-the-art designs still typically result in 0.04–0.1 mm^2 of chip area per electrode channel (10–25 channels/mm^2) [17].

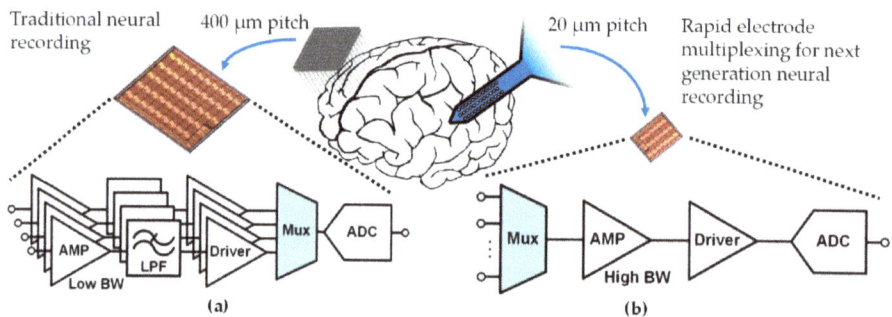

Figure 1. (**a**) Conventional neural recording electronics use individual amplifiers and filters dedicated to each electrode, and often employ back-end multiplexing to a smaller number of analog-to-digital converters. (**b**) Rapid multiplexing directly at the electrodes can be used to share amplifiers and filters across many electrodes, leading to a drastic reduction in the size of the electronics. Small channel area enables high-density arrays with active electronics closer to the electrode.

A promising approach for reducing the area of the acquisition electronics is to use time division multiplexing to rapidly sample multiple electrode sites with a single front-end circuit, without preamplification (Figure 1b). However, rapid multiplexing directly at the electrodes raises challenges related to electrode offsets and aliasing of high-frequency noise. These challenges have been shown to be tractable for non-penetrating microelectrode arrays used in electrocorticography (ECoG) [18,19], but these low-impedance arrays measure average neural activity from large groups of neurons and generally do not provide the spatial or temporal resolution needed to observe action potentials.

To the authors' best knowledge, this paper presents the first in vivo demonstration of a rapidly multiplexed neural recording system without preamplification, designed for high-impedance, penetrating microelectrode arrays that provide measurements of action potentials (APs). Time division multiplexing is often used after amplification to reduce ADC area [17,20–23] (Figure 1a), and has also been used for serialized analog communication in neural recording systems [24–26]. However, these prior works all use multiplexing after amplification, which does not reduce the area of the amplifiers and thus has limited benefit. In the work presented in this report, a 180 nm CMOS circuit was designed to address issues from electrode offsets and high-frequency noise aliasing that become problematic when rapidly multiplexing electrodes directly to a single front-end amplifier, without preamplification, in order to enable drastic area reductions.

The rest of this paper is organized as follows. Section 2 describes the fundamental theory of acquiring rapidly multiplexed signals from microelectrode arrays without preamplification, and presents informative electrode characterization measurements. Section 3 proposes a circuit architecture for rapid multiplexing directly at the electrodes, along with details of a fabricated prototype. Section 4 presents test results for the prototype, including in vivo experiments with signals recorded from the rodent cortex. Section 5 provides a discussion and implications for future research.

2. Rapidly Multiplexed Neural Recording: Theory and Practical Issues

Figure 2 illustrates the input signal that arises from rapidly multiplexing multiple electrode sites to a single front-end amplifier. This paradigm uses time domain multiplexing to switch between electrodes at a high enough rate (e.g., 600 kHz) such that each different electrode can be sampled at a frequency that is typically used when acquiring APs (e.g., $f_{ch} = 30$ kHz). Since each electrode is visited for only a short time (microseconds or less) within the overall sampling period, the total electrode voltage appears as a step input to the electronics, which confounds traditional filtering. As a result, the multiplexed signal amplitude is dominated by DC offsets arising from polarization potentials at the interfaces between electrodes and the tissue [27]. To accurately sample the smaller AP signals, the bandwidth of the recording electronics must be made large such that the step transients can settle fully. This large bandwidth creates challenges for achieving adequate signal-to-noise ratio (SNR) in the presence of high-frequency noise. Overall, rapid multiplexing without preamplification requires more careful consideration of electrode properties than the traditional approach. This section describes the fundamental challenges to rapid multiplexing, and offers high-level solutions.

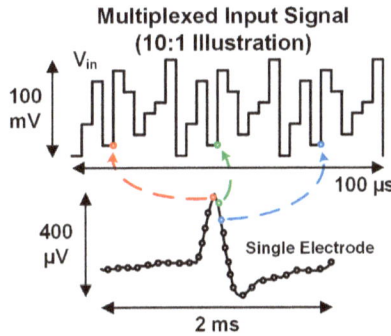

Figure 2. Illustration of the signal that arises from rapidly multiplexing multiple electrodes to the input of a single acquisition circuit. The amplitude of the signal is dominated by DC offsets from differences in polarization potentials between recording and reference electrodes. The goal is to acquire much smaller action potential signals, which are multiplexed in the time domain.

2.1. DC Offsets from the Electrodes

Electrochemical polarization naturally develops an equilibrium potential at the electrode-tissue interface [27]. Commonly, a single low impedance reference electrode is used when recording from a multichannel electrode array, e.g., a single platinum wire that is separate from the array itself [27]. The reference electrode develops its own equilibrium potential, which differs significantly from the equilibrium potentials of the recording electrodes. The difference between the potentials of a recording and reference electrode manifests as a DC offset signal when recording. These DC offset voltages are typically much larger than APs, and can be in the 1–50 mV range depending on the materials and geometries of the recording and reference electrodes (when performing "bipolar" recording between two identical electrodes, the DC offsets are usually smaller but still often within the millivolt range).

Unfortunately, quantitative studies of DC offsets seen during recording are generally lacking in the literature. Differences also exist between the equilibrium potentials of each recording electrode in a multichannel array, due to manufacturing tolerances that result in physical differences, as well as differences in the local chemistry around each implanted electrode [27]. The DC offsets observed during recording also depend on the input impedance of the acquisition electronics and any leakage currents from protection diodes or other devices [28].

Dedicating an individual amplifier to each electrode site (Figure 1a) [17,20,21,23,29–31] allows simple high-pass filtering to separate the electrode offsets from APs before amplification up to the full scale range of the ADC (~1 V). When rapidly multiplexing before amplification, a high-pass filter is not feasible, because the DC offsets and APs both appear as a step input and do not change appreciably during the time allotted for generating a sample (microseconds or less). Indeed, applying such a high-pass filter to the waveform illustrated in Figure 2 would simply remove its average value.

One solution is to limit the overall gain in the signal path and use a high-resolution ADC to digitize both the modulated offset signal as well as the much smaller APs. However, assuming that the DC offsets are 50× larger than the APs, this approach requires an additional 6 bits of resolution (~16 bits in total). While such resolution is achievable, the resulting ADC specifications are challenging to achieve with low power and low circuit area, since the ADC must also run at a high sample rate of $f_s = M \cdot f_{ch}$, where M is the number of multiplexed electrodes. The architecture presented in this report uses a mixed-signal DC offset rejection approach that greatly reduces the burden on the ADC by avoiding the need for increased resolution.

2.2. Noise from Acquisition Electronics

Whether employing rapid multiplexing (Figure 1b) or the traditional approach (Figure 1a), noise from the acquisition electronics must be made low enough to accurately acquire AP signals. The target noise specification depends on the intrinsic signal quality that can be achieved with particular microelectrodes. There is a great incentive to avoid overdesigning the electronics in terms of noise performance, because circuit power dissipation trades directly with thermal noise power [32]. The most common philosophy when targeting fully implantable electronics is to roughly match the circuit noise specification to the background noise level from the electrodes (5–10 μV_{rms}, as discussed in Section 2.3), so that there is a significant, yet non-dominating, contribution of noise from the electronics. In a traditional neural recording circuit design, the bandwidth of the signal path is generally chosen in the 5–10 kHz range [17], stemming from the spectral content of APs (0.5–5 kHz) [33]. This low bandwidth limits noise, and hence allows reduction of power dissipation.

Noise equivalent bandwidth (NEB) is a useful metric for comparing the traditional and rapidly multiplexed approaches to neural recording. The NEB of a filter response, $H(f)$, is defined as the bandwidth of a brick-wall filter that would pass the same amount of noise:

$$NEB \triangleq \int_0^\infty |H(f)|^2 \, df. \tag{1}$$

For example, a single pole response has a NEB equal to $\pi f_p/2$, where f_p is the pole frequency.

To acquire rapidly multiplexed APs, the bandwidth of the acquisition channel must be large enough to allow complete transient settling of the multiplexed waveform (Figure 2) in the time period allocated to each electrode (microseconds or less). The settling requirement necessitates a larger bandwidth than the traditional approach. Assuming instantaneous voltage sampling with a single pole low-pass filter response, transient settling necessitates a bandwidth of

$$f_{BW} = \frac{-\ln(\varepsilon_{dtol})}{2\pi T_s}, \tag{2}$$

where ε_{dtol} is the tolerable dynamic settling error (0.1% for 10-bit accuracy), and T_s is the amount of time available for settling. To achieve a per-channel sampling rate of f_{ch} (~30 kHz) across M

multiplexed electrodes, the ADC must sample at a rate of $f_s = M \cdot f_{ch}$, allowing a maximum settling time of $T_s = 1/f_s$ for each electrode. The NEB for multiplexed acquisition using instantaneous voltage sampling thus increases proportionally to M, in order to maintain f_{ch} for each electrode:

$$NEB_{vs} = \frac{\pi}{2} f_{BW} = -f_s \ln(\varepsilon_{dtol})/4 = -M f_{ch} \ln(\varepsilon_{dtol})/4. \tag{3}$$

This increased NEB necessitates a reduction in the acquisition circuit's noise power spectral density (PSD) to maintain the same total integrated noise specification as a traditional neural recording circuit, since noise at frequencies higher than $f_{ch}/2$ will alias and show up in the samples. Reducing the wideband noise PSD is achieved by investing more power in the amplifier (Amp in Figure 1b) to reduce its input-referred thermal noise. Assuming that f_{ch} is chosen to be 3× the AP bandwidth (a typical case), the NEB of a multiplexed acquisition circuit (Figure 1b) that uses instantaneous voltage sampling increases above the NEB of a traditional acquisition circuit (Figure 1a) according to

$$NEB_{vs} = -M \ln(\varepsilon_{dtol})(3/2\pi)NEB_{trad}, \tag{4}$$

where NEB_{trad} is the NEB of a traditional neural recording circuit (Figure 1a). Assuming $\varepsilon_{dtol} = 0.1\%$ to allow accurate detection of APs in the presence of large DC offsets, $NEB_{vs} \cong 3.5M \cdot NEB_{trad}$. Assuming a one-to-one tradeoff between the circuit's thermal noise PSD and its power dissipation (the typical case [32]), the NEB enlargement translates to 3.5× higher power per channel for a multiplexed acquisition circuit that uses instantaneous voltage sampling, compared to a traditional neural recording circuit with the same total integrated noise. This power penalty is quite large, but can be avoided by alternative sampling methods. In this work, windowed integration sampling (WIS) was used to reduce the NEB of the rapidly multiplexed acquisition circuit by ~3.5× versus instantaneous voltage sampling, restoring the power per channel back to the traditional range.

Windowed integration sampling (WIS) [31,34,35] is an alternative to instantaneous voltage sampling that breaks the tradeoff between settling accuracy and NEB. The fundamental idea is to integrate the signal over a finite window of time, and then sample the result. Integration reduces high-frequency noise according to a sinc characteristic in frequency, which can be understood by examining the Laplace transform of a continuous moving average function:

$$y(t) = \int_{t-T_s}^{t} v_{in}(t\prime)dt\prime \tag{5}$$

$$|\{y(t)\}| = \frac{|2\sin(\omega T_s/2)|}{\omega}|v_{in}(\omega)|, \tag{6}$$

where $\{\cdot\}$ is the Laplace transform and ω is frequency. The samples $y(nT_{ch})$ contain aliased high-frequency noise of $v_{in}(\omega)$, but the sinc magnitude response attenuates high frequencies with a NEB that depends on the duration of T_s, which is shown by analyzing Equation (6) with a normalized DC gain of 1:

$$NEB_{wis} = \int_0^\infty \frac{\sin^2(\pi f T_s)}{(\pi f T_s)^2} df = \frac{1}{\pi T_s}\int_0^\infty \text{sinc}^2(x)dx = \frac{1}{2T_s}. \tag{7}$$

The NEB of WIS can be written in terms of the NEB of the traditional neural recording approach as

$$NEB_{wis} = M(3/\pi)NEB_{trad}. \tag{8}$$

Thus, the power consumption per channel of a multiplexed system using WIS can be about the same as a traditional system, while the area per channel can be divided by M. Multiplexing with voltage sampling incurs an extra multiplicative penalty of $\ln(\varepsilon_{dtol})/2$ compared to WIS (see Equation (4)). For example, given $M = 10$, $f_{ch} = 30$ kHz ($T_s \cong 3.3$ μs), $\varepsilon_{dtol} = 0.1\%$, the NEB of instantaneous voltage sampling is 518 kHz while the NEB of WIS is only 150 kHz, a factor of 3.5× smaller.

Besides thermal noise, MOSFET devices display $1/f$ noise (also called "flicker" or "pink" noise), which originates from trapping and de-trapping of carriers in states close to the interface between the silicon and gate insulation material [36]. This noise source is substantial in the AP band, and motivates large transistor sizes to reduce its PSD. Interestingly, the $1/f$ noise requirements and tradeoffs are the same for both traditional and rapidly multiplexed acquisition circuits, which can be seen by considering that each channel is sampled at f_{ch} in both approaches, leading to a discrete time spectrum confined to $f_{ch}/2$ for both. This leads to similar transistor sizes for both approaches, although the area is amortized across channels when using rapid multiplexing.

With an equivalent power per channel that is neither worse nor better than a traditional neural recording circuit, the rapidly multiplexed approach can be seen as combining all the power consumption that would be spent in multichannel circuitry into one faster circuit that uses dynamic operation (speed) to reduce circuit area. This strategy generally leverages one of the main strengths of CMOS technology, i.e., high-speed operation, which is not utilized by the traditional approach.

2.3. Noise from the Electrodes

Excluding noise from the acquisition electronics, the noise floor for the traditional approach to AP recording (Figure 1a) is dominated by biological activity in the AP band [33], with a relatively minor contribution from thermal noise generated by the electrode, tissue, and their electrochemical interface. When rapidly multiplexing, however, this thermal noise becomes an increasing concern due to the larger bandwidth required. High-frequency noise from the electrode-tissue system will alias into the AP spectrum, and increase the variance of the acquired samples. WIS is effective in reducing the contribution of high-frequency noise, but residual aliased noise still presents a limit on the number of electrodes that can be multiplexed while achieving an acceptable noise floor and SNR.

Recently, we performed wideband spectral measurements of implanted electrodes [37–40] (Figure 3). These measurements characterize the noise at high frequency as thermal in origin, on the basis of impedance magnitude and phase measurements. The measured high-frequency noise PSD is generally <20 $nV_{rms}/\sqrt{Hz}$ for typical penetrating microelectrodes. Background biological noise is generally in the 5–10 μV_{rms} range in the AP band [17], which would correspond to 75–150 $nV_{rms}/\sqrt{Hz}$ white noise across 0.5–5 kHz. Our studies [38] have also shown that high-frequency electromagnetic interference can be eliminated through proper referencing, grounding, and shielding, and that biological noise is confined to low frequencies (<10 kHz) [37]. Overall, thermal noise is the dominant concern at high frequencies and can be accurately predicted by impedance magnitude and phase measurements [38].

The thermal noise originates from the real part of the impedance within the bioelectrochemical cell, and can be predicted using

$$v_n{}^2(f) = 4kT\mathrm{Re}[Z(f)], \tag{9}$$

where $v_n{}^2(f)$ is the voltage noise power spectral density, k is Boltzmann's constant, T is absolute temperature, and $\mathrm{Re}[Z(f)]$ is the real part of the impedance between the measurement point and ground [41]. This prediction is highly accurate for in vitro measurements, as well as in vivo for frequencies above typical biological bandwidths. Figure 3a,b shows in vitro and in vivo spectral measurements of a representative 16-channel tungsten microwire array (Tucker-Davis Technologies, Alachua, FL, USA) and a representative 16-channel silicon "Utah" microelectrode array [42] (Blackrock Microsystems, Salt Lake City, UT, USA), respectively. The in vivo measurements were performed under isoflurane anesthesia, which is known to suppress local cortical spiking activity [43], revealing the baseline noise floor. The real part of the measured impedance was used to predict the thermal noise (dashed lines), whereas the solid lines are direct spectral measurements [38]. For the in vitro measurements, the measured noise and predicted thermal noise match well across the spectrum. For in vivo measurements, there is excess low-frequency noise/activity attributed to biological sources other than local AP activity [37–39,44].

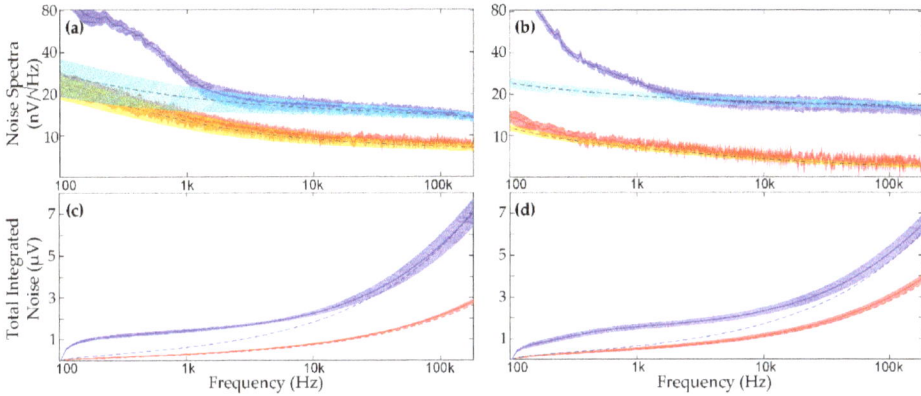

Figure 3. Noise characterizations for representative 16-channel microelectrode arrays. (**a**) Silicon microelectrodes (Blackrock Microsystems) and (**b**) microwire electrodes (Tucker-Davis Technologies) both in vitro (saline, bottom traces) and in vivo (rodent cortex, top traces). The dashed lines indicate the impedance predicted thermal noise spectrum, the solid lines show measured noise, and shading indicates the variance. (**c**) Total integrated noise (TIN) for the representative silicon microelectrode array and (**d**) microwire array, in vitro (bottom traces) and in vivo (top traces), with measured noise (solid) and impedance predicted thermal noise (dashed). Colored shadows show variance within each electrode array. The predicted thermal noise is shown to accurately reflect the measured TIN at high frequencies, indicating thermal noise is the dominant noise source for wideband applications like rapidly multiplexed recording.

Figure 3c,d shows the running integral of the measured PSDs in vitro and in vivo for silicon and microwire arrays, respectively. The total integrated noise (TIN), which quantifies the noise floor of the system, is thermally dominated as shown by the accuracy of the predicted and measured TIN. The accuracy of the predicted thermal TIN indicates that the real part of the impedance can be used as an accurate estimator of high-frequency noise from the electrode-tissue system.

Because the impedance is a good predictor of noise, it is useful to describe the electrode-tissue interface with an equivalent circuit that can be used for simulation and design. The overall impedance is frequently modeled using a Randles equivalent circuit [45,46], often using a constant phase element (CPE) for accurate representation of both magnitude and phase:

$$Z_{CPE} = \frac{1}{Y_0(j\omega)^{\alpha}},\tag{10}$$

where ω is radial frequency and Y_0 and α are fitting parameters. A simple model is shown in Figure 4 [27,47], where R_s is the access resistance, R_p represents faradaic reactions, the CPE models the interface's double-layer capacitance, and C_{in} is the input capacitance of measurement instrumentation or acquisition electronics. C_{in} can interact with the high impedance of the electrodes to create a high-frequency pole, and is therefore important to the model matching. Parameters were extracted using the Gamry E-chem Analyst software (v7.06) for fitting the Figure 4a model to typical electrode impedance measurements (example parameters are shown in the figure). Figure 4c,d shows an example in vivo impedance and phase measurement compared to the fitted model for the microwire and silicon arrays, respectively. There is a high degree of agreement in impedance and low frequency phase. The high frequency phase shows a roll off incongruent with the input capacitance, but can be modeled with a capacitor parallel to the electrode model (not shown since the physical mechanism is unclear). The accuracy of the model in conjunction with the accuracy of the thermal noise prediction using Equation (9) indicates that an accurately parameterized model is a good method for predicting total thermal noise when designing neural recording electronics in general. This prediction is shown in Figure 4e for both types of arrays, neglecting C_{in} so that the prediction is system independent.

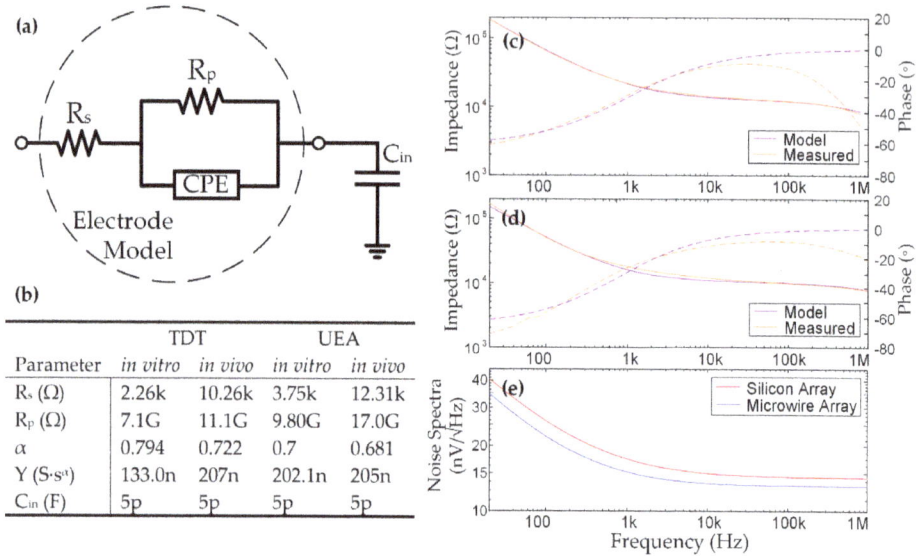

Figure 4. (**a**) Randles equivalent circuit electrode model. R_s represents the access resistance, which is the summation of several factors including electrode material, tissue encapsulation, protein binding, and cellular morphology between the recording and reference electrodes [47]. Faradaic reactions are represented by R_p, which is also called the charge-transfer resistance and is representative of electrode surface oxidation and reduction reactions [27]. (**b**) Calculated model parameters in vitro and in vivo. (**c**) Measured and modeled in vivo impedance magnitude and phase for the representative silicon microelectrode array. (**d**) Measured and modeled in vivo impedance magnitude and phase for the representative microwire array. (**e**) Model predicted thermal noise neglecting the effect of C_{in}.

Parameter	TDT in vitro	TDT in vivo	UEA in vitro	UEA in vivo
R_s (Ω)	2.26k	10.26k	3.75k	12.31k
R_p (Ω)	7.1G	11.1G	9.80G	17.0G
α	0.794	0.722	0.7	0.681
Y (S·s$^\alpha$)	133.0n	207n	202.1n	205n
C_{in} (F)	5p	5p	5p	5p

This model can be used to assess the impact of high-frequency noise on rapidly multiplexed recording. Figure 5 shows how the overall thermal TIN is affected by the multiplexing factor (M), with a comparison between voltage sampling and WIS (see Section 2.2). The curves were generated using Equations (3) and (7), and the model parameters in Figure 4. Figure 5 shows that WIS provides a roughly 3× decrease in the thermal TIN root-mean-square (rms) amplitude compared to voltage sampling. Since the dominant noise source at high frequencies is R_s, the total integrated noise can be linearly extrapolated to higher frequencies to assess higher multiplexing factors. It can be seen that rapid multiplexing using voltage sampling becomes impractical for M values as low as 4 when budgeting for a <10 μV_{rms} thermal noise contribution, while WIS allows ~7 μV_{rms} for $M = 20$.

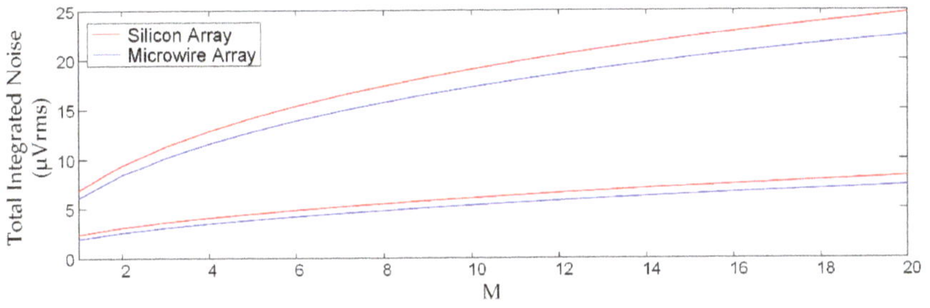

Figure 5. Comparison of voltage sampling (VS, top pair) and windowed integration sampling (WIS, bottom pair) for the representative silicon and microwire arrays using the Figure 4 model with a per channel sampling rate set to f_{ch} = 30 kHz. Voltage sampling results in prohibitively large noise even for M = 4, whereas WIS allows for M = 20 with acceptable noise performance. A design should ideally account for the thermal noise along with expected biological noise and signal amplitudes in order to optimize for in vivo signal detection.

3. Rapidly Multiplexed Neural Recording Circuit Architecture

The architecture shown in Figure 6 was developed to address the acquisition issues discussed in Section 2. The first stage is a capacitive feedback low noise amplifier (LNA) based on an operational transconductance amplifier (OTA), which is followed by an open-loop transconductance amplifier (G_M) that forms a windowed integration sampler in combination with the input capacitance ($C_{IN,adc}$) of a successive approximation (SAR) ADC. The prototype system supports up to 32 multiplexed electrodes (M = 1–32), and is designed to generate samples of each electrode at f_{ch} = 30 kHz by rapidly multiplexing the electrodes at $f_s = M \cdot f_{ch}$, which is 300 kHz to 1 MHz depending on M.

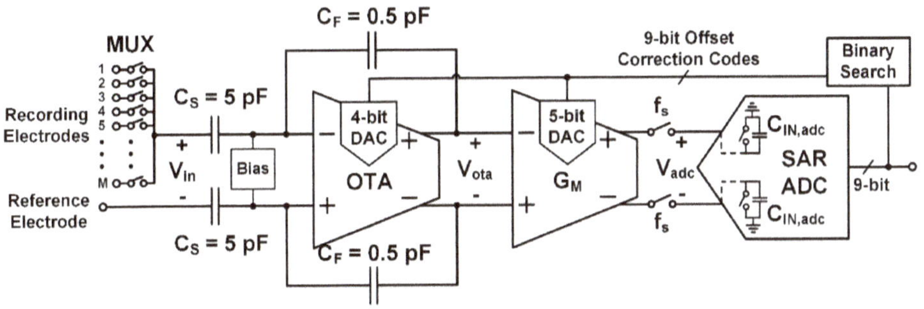

Figure 6. Diagram of the proposed rapidly multiplexed neural recording architecture. A capacitive feedback amplifier is used for pre-amplification with a gain of 10. Windowed integration sampling (WIS) is implemented with an open-loop transconductor (G_M) driving the input capacitance ($C_{IN,adc}$) of a successive approximation ADC. Mixed-signal feedback is used to reject DC offsets between the recording and reference electrodes by injecting correction signals through digital-to-analog converters (DACs) in the analog signal path.

When each electrode is selected, the DACs in the OTA and G_M amplifiers are updated to cancel DC offsets. The offset correction DAC codes are calculated using a binary search algorithm that processes the acquired data from the ADC. Since the electrode DC offsets do not change rapidly, the DAC codes can be recalculated every second (1 Hz). The LNA implements a closed-loop gain of 10 given by C_S/C_F, which relaxes noise requirements on the subsequent stages. Since the LNA gain is fairly low, it allows residual uncorrected offset from the electrodes and the OTA itself to pass without causing clipping at V_{ota} (Figure 6). The WIS operation provides additional voltage gain given by $G_M T_s/C_{IN,adc}$, which is designed at 100 with $M = 20$ ($T_s = 1.5$ µs). Thus, an overall 60 dB passband gain is used for amplifying APs. The transconductor (G_M) uses a 5-bit DAC to remove residual offset at the LNA output, in order to maximize the useful dynamic range of the circuit and relax the ADC resolution requirement. Integration of the signal current onto $C_{IN,adc}$ reduces the high-frequency noise from the LNA and the electrodes ($NEB_{wis} \cong 333$ kHz for $T_s = 1.5$ µs, $M = 20$). This WIS operation attenuates high-frequency noise before it aliases as a result of forming a discrete time sample (see Equations (6) and (7) in Section 2.2).

The multiplexer itself (MUX in Figure 6) contributes thermal noise due to the on-resistance of the switches, but this noise can be made negligible without requiring large switch sizes (e.g., 12×0.18 µm^2 switches were used in this design, corresponding to 160 Ω resistance and 0.94 µV$_{rms}$ noise). With small switches, charge injection and clock feedthrough are not significant given the 5 pF C_S capacitance and typical electrode double layer capacitances (~1 nF). Simulation and measurements of the fabricated prototype confirmed that charge injection and clock feedthrough do not significantly affect offset, noise, or linearity in this design.

Figure 7 shows a timing diagram of the circuit operation, with an illustration of the LNA output (V_{ota}). When an electrode is selected, a brief period of time (T_{conv}) is reserved to allow the electrode signal to settle through the LNA before the G_M amplifier is connected and WIS begins. During the T_{conv} phase the sample from the last electrode selected is also being digitized by the ADC, which uses an asynchronous, self-timed controller that does not require a clock [48]. $C_{IN,adc}$ is reset subsequently before the T_s phase begins. For the current prototype implementation, $T_{conv} > 110$ ns is required for ADC conversion, allowing the WIS integration time (T_s) to be ≥ 930 ns for $M = 1$–32. In general, the NEB reduction from WIS depends on the timing overhead that T_{conv} takes away from the maximum possible T_s. However, even at M = 32, T_{conv} only takes up 11% of the total available period ($T_{conv} + T_s$) and hence does not severely degrade the NEB reduction (~3× versus voltage sampling). The LNA provides fast voltage settling, since the bias current required to reduce circuit noise results in a large bandwidth (7.5 MHz translating to $\varepsilon_{dtol} = 0.1\%$ at the end of T_{conv}).

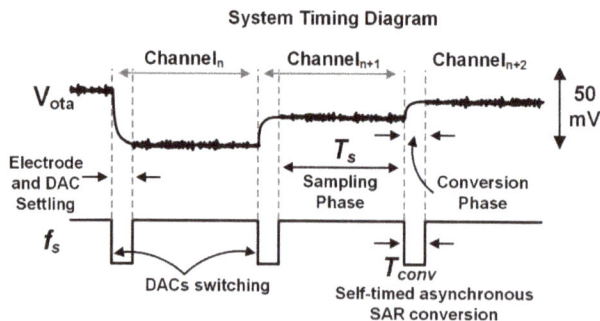

Figure 7. Illustration of the multiplexed recording circuit operation showing the OTA output (top) along with timing information. The OTA DAC provides coarse cancellation of the electrode DC offsets. After a short period of time (T_{conv}) reserved for settling of the electrode, LNA, and DACs, the electrode signal is integrated onto the input capacitance of the ADC ($C_{IN,adc}$).

3.1. LNA Design

A closed loop capacitive feedback topology was chosen for the LNA, since it provides good linearity, well controlled gain, and ease of input biasing. The transistor level implementation of the OTA amplifier, shown in Figure 8, is optimized for noise and power efficiency. The topology consists of a cascoded NMOS differential pair, and resistor-degenerated active loads split into parallel branches to implement a 4-bit offset correction DAC. The output voltage (V_{ota} in Figures 6 and 7) does not experience high signal swing, because APs typically produce amplitudes <1 mV peak on extracellular electrodes, and electrode DC offsets are suppressed by the LNA's offset correction DAC (+/−5 mV residual input referred offset). Thus, an efficient single stage OTA topology can be used, which is power efficient and easy to stabilize (load compensated).

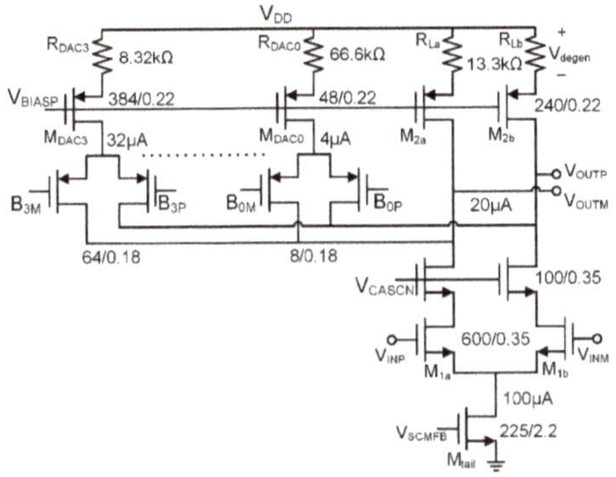

Figure 8. Transistor level design of the OTA in Figure 6. The topology leverages the low output signal swing requirements by using an efficient single stage structure. Coarse offset correction is achieved with a 4-bit digital-to-analog converter (DAC) implemented with binary weighted active load slices that steer current between the differential outputs.

The differential pair transistors ($M_{1a,b}$) operate in weak inversion and were sized in order to optimize the tradeoff between thermal noise and flicker noise. This tradeoff is essentially the same as with traditional capacitive feedback amplifiers used in neural recording (see Section 2.2), and has been studied extensively [17]. The degenerated active loads have a $g_m R$ product of 6, to suppress flicker noise from the PMOS devices as much as possible given the available headroom ($V_{degen} \approx 260$ mV). The LNA was designed for an input referred noise of 5 μV_{rms} within a NEB of 333 kHz ($M = 20$), which translates to a 8.7 nV/$\sqrt{Hz}$ spectral density. Therefore, each branch of the differential pair was biased at a drain current of 50 μA, resulting in a unity gain bandwidth of ~7.5 MHz, which is sufficient for 0.1% settling in 166 ns (T_{conv}). Since electrode offsets imbalance the differential pair, the noise of M_{tail} is not entirely canceled. Therefore, its g_m/I_D was made relatively low (16 V^{-1}).

A 4-bit current source DAC topology was chosen here for offset correction, which allows high switching speed (~166 ns settling in this design). One can derive a relation between the input offset and the compensating current imbalance that the DAC must inject:

$$V_{os,in} = V_{INP} - V_{INM} = \frac{C_F + C_S + C_P}{C_S} n U_T \ln(I_{D1b}/I_{D1a}), \tag{11}$$

where $V_{INP,M}$ are the input voltages of the OTA, C_F and C_S are the feedback network capacitances shown in Figure 6, C_P is the parasitic input capacitance of the OTA, n is subthreshold slope factor, U_T is the thermal voltage, and I_{D1a} and I_{D1b} are the drain currents in the differential pair. The 4-bit offset correction DAC can compensate ±65 mV of electrode offset, using a least significant bit (LSB) size of 4 μA that translates to 10 mV input referred offset. This DAC can also correct for the offset of the amplifier itself, although the OTA's offset is far below the LSB size ($\sigma = 400$ μV input referred based on Monte Carlo simulation). Residual electrode offset and the OTA's offset are corrected by the fine correction DAC in the G_M amplifier, described below. The low gain of the LNA (10) ensures that residual offset does not saturate its output, and the fine correction DAC in the G_M amplifier ensures that the final signal chain output is not saturated by offset despite the 60 dB overall passband gain.

The input node biasing circuit of the LNA (Bias in Figure 6) consists of reset switches, which periodically (>1 s) connect the input nodes to a reference voltage. The OTA also uses a switched capacitor common mode feedback circuit (not shown) connected to M$_{tail}$, which is split with a 20% fixed bias segment to facilitate startup.

3.2. Transconductance Amplifier Design

The output of the transconductance amplifier (G$_M$ in Figure 6) swings across the full scale range of the ADC (+/−0.9 V differential). A folded cascode topology (Figure 9) was chosen to satisfy this swing requirement while achieving high output resistance to avoid gain error in the WIS operation [34]. Given the relaxed 1/f noise requirements provided by the LNA's gain, the input differential pair devices (M$_{1a,b}$ in Figure 9) do not need to be sized large. This led to the choice of implementing the 5-bit fine offset correction DAC by changing the size of the input pair [28], resulting in low area overhead and fast settling (<166 ns). An alternative would be a capacitive DAC at the G$_M$ input nodes [18], but this approach would require capacitive coupling between the LNA and G$_M$ amplifiers, and the input pair DAC is a simpler implementation.

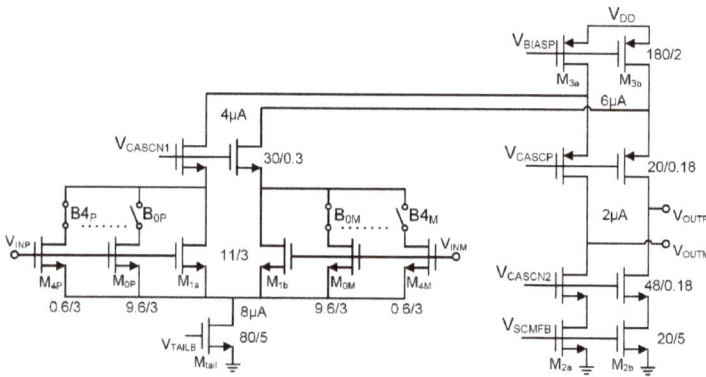

Figure 9. Transistor level design of the transconductance amplifier used in the windowed integration sampler (G$_M$ in Figure 6). A folded cascode architecture was selected for high output resistance and moderate output swing. A 5-bit fine offset correction digital-to-analog converter was implemented through an array of differential pair devices.

For an approximate understanding, the weak inversion current equation can be used to derive the offset referred to the G$_M$ input nodes, which leads to [28]:

$$V_{os} = nU_T \ln(W_{1a}/W_{1b}),$$

(12)

where $W_{1a,b}$ are the total widths of the input pair devices, which change as a function of the DAC codes. The LNA passes a worst case residual offset of approximately 50 mV at its output. The G$_M$ DAC's offset correction range was designed for ±57 mV to leave some margin for mismatch effects and for ease of DAC sizing.

A switched capacitor common mode feedback circuit (not shown) was connected to the output active load transistors (M$_{2a,b}$), which were split with a 25% fixed bias segment to facilitate startup.

3.3. SAR ADC Design

A successive approximation register (SAR) ADC was chosen for low power dissipation, adequate conversion speed, and for streamlined integration with the WIS operation. Moderate resolution (8–10 bits) is acceptable given the offset correction DACs, which preserve useful dynamic range for AP signals. Small CDAC unit capacitors (2.4 fF) [49] and asynchronous digital control [48] were used to reduce power and area in the ADC. The 9-bit design uses top-plate sampling on an 8-bit CDAC, with a monotonic switching procedure [48]. A fully dynamic latch based comparator was used for low power consumption. The CDAC consists of split capacitor elements to maintain a constant common mode voltage at the comparator inputs [50]. The total CDAC capacitance is approximately 600 fF ($C_{IN,adc}$ in Figure 6), and is constructed with custom metal-oxide-metal (MOM) capacitors in three metal layers. The asynchronous, self-timed SAR controller simplifies clocking by only requiring a master sample clock, and can achieve sample rates up to 9 MHz in this design.

4. Experimental Results

4.1. Bench Testing of the CMOS Prototype

The rapidly multiplexed circuit described in Section 3 was implemented in the ON Semiconductor 180 nm CMOS process with 6 metal layers. The micrograph of the fabricated test chip is shown in Figure 10. The chip contains a 32:1 input multiplexer, the core circuits described in Section 3, and programmable bias generator blocks. A master clock is generated externally and used for multiplexer control, DAC updating, and common mode feedback circuit clocking. Reference voltages for the LNA input bias, common-mode feedback circuits, and ADC were generated off-chip. The design has a core circuit area of 245 μm × 315 μm, while the overall test chip itself is pad-limited and is 1.7 mm × 2.3 mm. The chip was mostly tested for a multiplexing factor of $M = 20$, with a multiplexing clock rate of 600 kHz. The power supply voltage is 1 V and the total power consumption is 140 μW, which translates to 7 μW per channel for $M = 20$. The test chip was packaged in an 80 pin, 12 mm × 12 mm thin quad frame package (TQFP). Test PCBs consist of a motherboard for various functions and connections, and a daughterboard to hold the test chip.

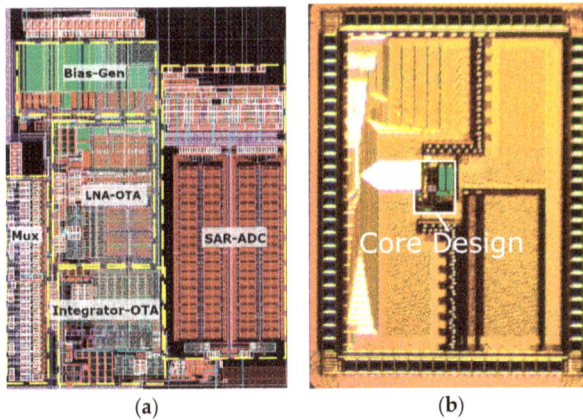

Figure 10. (a) Layout of the core circuitry of the fabricated CMOS design; (b) micrograph of the fabricated test chip, with core circuitry highlighted in the center.

The digital and analog inputs to the chip as well as the ADC outputs were all processed through a National Instruments (NI; Austin, TX, USA) platform consisting of a multifunction data acquisition card (DAQ, PXIe-6368) and a high-performance arbitrary waveform generator (AWG, PXIe-5451). The test system was controlled with the NI DAQmx API through Python 2.7. The binary search algorithm for finding offset correction codes (Figure 6) was also implemented in Python for flexibility when prototyping. Data processing was performed in Python and MATLAB.

Gain was measured using an attenuated sinusoidal input from the AWG, and reading of the ADC output codes. Gain was measured at 59.1 dB, and is flat up to the 15 kHz channel Nyquist frequency. Bandwidth limiting for AP detection is accomplished with software digital filters (see Section 4.2 below). The total harmonic distortion (THD) was measured using an input signal from the AWG and a fast Fourier transform (FFT) of the ADC output codes. Simulations showed a worst case THD at the

LNA output to be 1.5%, while measurements of the full chain THD (including integrator and ADC) indicated 2%. The common mode rejection ratio (CMRR) was simulated at the LNA output with an input offset of 63 mV and the maximum offset correction DAC settings, indicating a worst case CMRR of 65 dB. The measured worst case CMRR was 50 dB for the full chain, which is likely due to mismatch in the circuitry.

The input referred noise of the overall circuitry was measured from the ADC output codes with a grounded input (Figure 11), resulting in 5.6 μV_{rms}. With a total chip current of 140 μA, bandwidth of 15 kHz (set by the ADC Nyquist frequency), and $M = 20$, the noise efficiency factor (NEF) [51] is 4.74 when considered on a per channel basis, which is within the range of traditional neural recording circuitry [17]. The ADC was measured by itself for signal to noise plus distortion ratio (SNDR) with a 1 kHz sinusoidal input delivered through auxiliary test pads, resulting in 53.8 dB (ENOB of 8.3 bits) as shown in Figure 12a. The power consumption of the ADC is 6.5 μW at 600 kHz (325 nW per channel for $M = 20$), corresponding to 37 fJ per conversion step. The DNL and INL were measured using the histogram method, indicating a DNL of 0.86/−0.89 and INL of 1/−0.91 as shown in Figure 12b. Parasitic extraction simulations of the OTA demonstrate a gain bandwidth product (GBW) of 7.84 MHz and phase margin of 90°, compared to 7.67 MHz and 90° from nominal simulations. The higher GBW after layout extraction is due to differences in device fingering. Monte Carlo simulations indicate $\sigma = 400\ \mu V$ input referred offset for the OTA (200 runs), which is consistent with measurement results across three chips. Parasitic extraction of the overall test chip indicates 270 fF of capacitive loading from wiring, pads, ESD, and device parasitics, while the 5 pF C_S capacitance of the LNA presents 6.7 MΩ impedance when periodically connected to a given electrode at $f_{ch} = 30$ kHz. This input loading is commensurate with traditional neural recording circuitry [17], and can be reduced if needed for particular microelectrodes through feedback strategies typically used in chopper amplifiers [52,53].

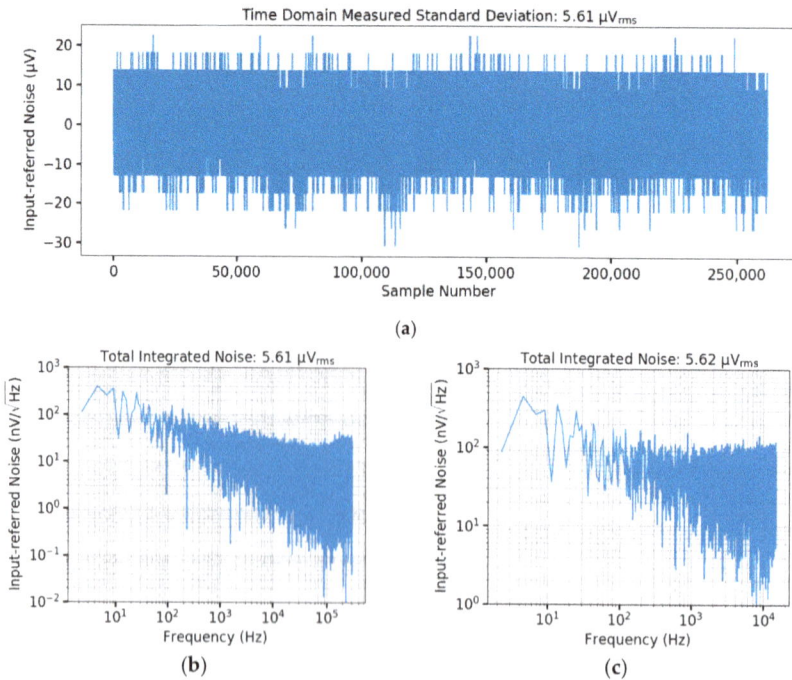

(a)

(b)   (c)

Figure 11. Full system input-referred noise measured from the ADC output codes. (a) Time domain plot of 262,144 ADC samples (400 ms time record); (b) Single channel FFT spectrum with sampling frequency of 600 kHz; (c) Spectrum of demultiplexed samples with 30 kHz sampling per channel.

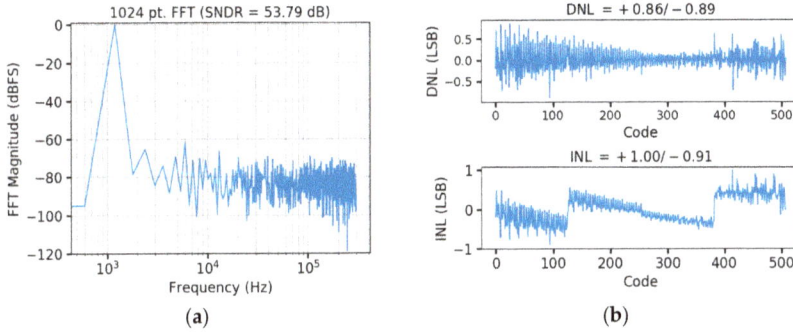

Figure 12. ADC test results. (**a**) FFT with 1 kHz input sinusoid showing 53.8 dB SNDR; (**b**) Linearity measurements showing DNL of +0.86/−0.89 and INL of +1.00/−0.91.

Table 1 shows the power and area of the individual circuit blocks shown in Figures 6 and 10a. The power is dominated by the LNA, since it dominates the input referred noise of the design. The area contributions of the LNA, G_M block, and the ADC are similar, with the ADC being the largest because of its CDAC. It should be noted that the ADC area in particular would be reduced greatly if implemented in a smaller CMOS process node. Table 2 summarizes the bench measurements of the design for $M = 20$ and compares the performance to state-of-the-art traditional AP recording circuits. This design achieves the lowest area per channel for AP recording, while being competitive in the rest of the specifications. This was achieved in an older CMOS process node and with a conventional capacitive feedback LNA design, demonstrating the efficacy of the rapidly multiplexed approach. Of particular note is that the power per channel and NEF per channel metrics are in the same range as traditional neural recording circuits, demonstrating that there is no fundamental advantage or disadvantage to the approach in terms of power dissipation. For offset correction, this work used dynamic offset correction DACs, similarly to the single channel design presented in [28]. The work in [54] pursues analog-to-time conversion, with extensive use of digital blocks that benefit from CMOS process scaling. However, that work needs to be extended to a multi-channel architecture and should deal with electrode offsets that are modulated by the chopping technique. Finally, this work achieves over an order of magnitude reduction in the area per channel compared to state-of-the art multichannel designs [55–57]. The technique of rapidly multiplexed AP acquisition is unique to this work, and the proof of concept demonstration should be viewed as the starting point for further circuit innovation and optimization.

Table 1. Area and power of distribution among design blocks.

Block	Power	Area
MUX	0.6 μW	0.0059 mm^2
LNA	110 μW	0.011 mm^2
G_M	12 μW	0.009 mm^2
SAR ADC	6.5 μW	0.025 mm^2
Bias-Gen	10 μW	0.0087 mm^2

Table 2. Measured performance of the rapidly multiplexed CMOS design ($M = 20$) and comparison to state-of-the-art neural recording circuits.

Parameter	[28]	[54]	[55]	[56]	[57]	This Work
Process	65 nm	65 nm	180 nm	180 nm	65 nm	180 nm
Supply Voltage	0.5 V	0.5 V	0.45 V	0.5–1.8 V	1 V	1 V
Supply Current per Channel	10.08 μA	2.55 μA	1.6 μA	18 μA	3.28 μA	7 μA (140 μA total)
Gain [V/V]	N/A	N/A	52	N/A	52.1	59.1
Bandwidth	10 kHz	11 kHz	10 kHz	9.2 kHz	8.2 kHz	15 kHz
Input-Referred Noise [μV$_{rms}$]	4.9	3.8	3.2	3.37	4.13	5.6
Noise Efficiency Factor	5.99	2.2	1.57	2.61	3.19	4.74
THD	2%	0.1%	N/A	N/A	1%	2%
CMRR	75 dB	60 dB	73 dB	60 dB	80 dB	50 dB
Circuit Area per Channel [mm^2]	0.013	0.006	N/A	0.098	0.042	0.0039 (0.077 total)

4.2. In Vivo Testing of the CMOS Prototype

One 16-channel (2×8) tungsten microwire array (Tucker-Davis Technologies) was implanted into the cortex of a male Sprague Dawley rat (500 g). The array was customized to have varying shaft lengths from 1 to 3.8 mm in length, and was positioned perpendicular to the midline to allow for recording from the more lateral barrel cortex as well as the motor cortex. All studies were conducted with the approval of the Institutional Animal Care and Use Committee at the University of Utah. The surgical procedure was similar to that outlined in [38]. Anesthesia was induced using 5% vaporized isoflurane in a specialized induction chamber and maintained at 1.5–3%. Two incisions (approximately 2.5 mm apart) were made along the midline of the skull. Two more incisions were made to connect the tops and bottoms and create a rectangular opening. Blunt dissection was used to separate the skin from the underlying fascia. Four bone screws were inserted into the skull: one in each corner of the exposed skull surface along the medial face of the temporal ridge. An approximately 3.5 mm diameter craniotomy was performed over the insertion site using a hand drill. The underlying dura was then incised and manipulated using a 26 G needle to expose the cortex. The array was slowly inserted into the tissue using a stereotaxic arm with the longer 3.8-mm shanks most lateral and the 1-mm shanks most medial from the midline. After the desired depth was reached, the craniotomy was filled with Kwik-Cast silicone elastomer (World Precision Instruments, Sarasota, FL, USA) and the skull was covered with UV cure epoxy to protect and stabilize the array.

All recordings were performed in the same experimental session (two days after surgery) on a single rat implanted with one microwire array as described above. During the recording session, the animal was anesthetized using a ketamine (70 mg/kg)/xylazine (10 mg/kg) cocktail. To better assess the multiplexed measurements, additional recordings were made using the well-established Cerebus Neural Recording system (v.6.04.02, Blackrock Microsystems). Each of the 16 recording channels used in the Cerebus system produced a dual output: a continuous time data stream with an analog bandpass filter from 0.3 Hz to 7.5 kHz, and a second channel with a digital filter from 750 Hz to 7.5 kHz used for action potential (AP) detection. Both channels used a 30 kHz sampling frequency.

Figure 13 shows continuous recordings from two different electrodes selected for their robust threshold crossing activity, each recorded from the rapidly multiplexed CMOS test chip and the Cerebus system (not simultaneously). In Figure 13a,c, data are shown from the two electrodes when multiplexed and sampled at 600 kHz, corresponding to an effective multiplexing factor of $M = 16$. The 300 kHz data streams were then demultiplexed and downsampled to 37.5 kHz by throwing away samples, using custom MATLAB software. The same two electrodes recorded from the Cerebus system were sampled from two different channels at a rate of 30 kHz, and data are shown in Figure 13b,d. All four traces show periodic bouts of high-amplitude bursts strongly correlated with threshold crossing events. Figure 14 shows the preservation of similar wave shapes and peak-to-peak amplitudes across the two recording systems. All events come from the same 4-s recordings shown in Figure 13, which displays the Figure 14 threshold crossing events with the raster plot at the bottom of each panel. Spike sorting was performed using custom MATLAB software with time-amplitude window thresholds similar to the "hoops" described in [58]. Some variations in the averaged threshold crossing waveforms appear as patterns in the pre- and post-crossing segments. These minor patterns result from averaging a limited number of threshold crossing events (the number of events is shown in each panel of Figure 14), and are similar between the two recording systems.

The signal-to-noise-ratio was calculated as the peak-to-peak amplitude of the mean waveform divided by the standard deviation of noise in the waveform [59]:

$$SNR = \frac{max(\overline{W}) - min(\overline{W})}{SD_\varepsilon}, \tag{13}$$

where $\overline{W}$ is the mean waveform and ε is a matrix containing the difference of each point of individual waveforms from the mean. The two electrodes recorded with the test chip (Figure 13a,b) were found to have SNRs of 2.1 and 2.2, respectively. The same two electrodes when recorded from with the Cerebus system had SNRs of 2.4 and 2.2, respectively, showing good agreement between the two recording systems. The similarity of the acquired data between the CMOS test chip and the Cerebus system provides confidence in the ability to acquire APs using the rapidly multiplexed approach. The test chip results in a slightly higher background noise level of 9.9 μV_{rms} for Figure 13a and 10.1 μV_{rms} for Figure 13c, compared to the Cerebus recordings corresponding to 6.6 μV_{rms} for Figure 13a and 7.8 μV_{rms} for Figure 13b (computed by removing threshold crossing events from the overall waveform). This modest increase in the background noise is expected given the additional circuit noise and electrode thermal noise (5.6 μV_{rms} and roughly 6 μV_{rms} across the 18.75 kHz Nyquist zone, respectively).

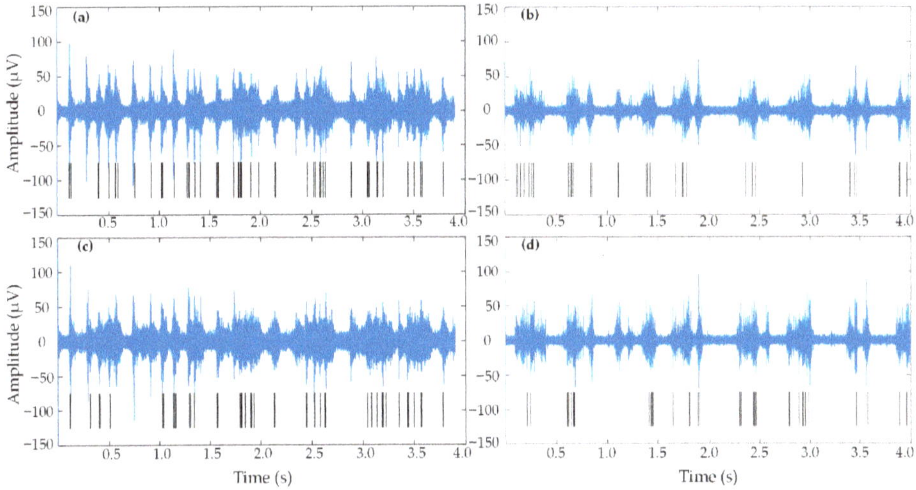

Figure 13. Continuous data from the rapidly multiplexed CMOS test chip (left column) and the Cerebus system (right column). All data were filtered from 800 Hz to 4 kHz using a digital bandpass filter implemented in MATLAB. Black lines under each plot indicate threshold crossing events. The top row contains data from the same electrode recorded from the test chip (**a**) and Cerebus (**b**). The second row contains data from a second electrode recorded from the test chip (**c**) and Cerebus (**d**).

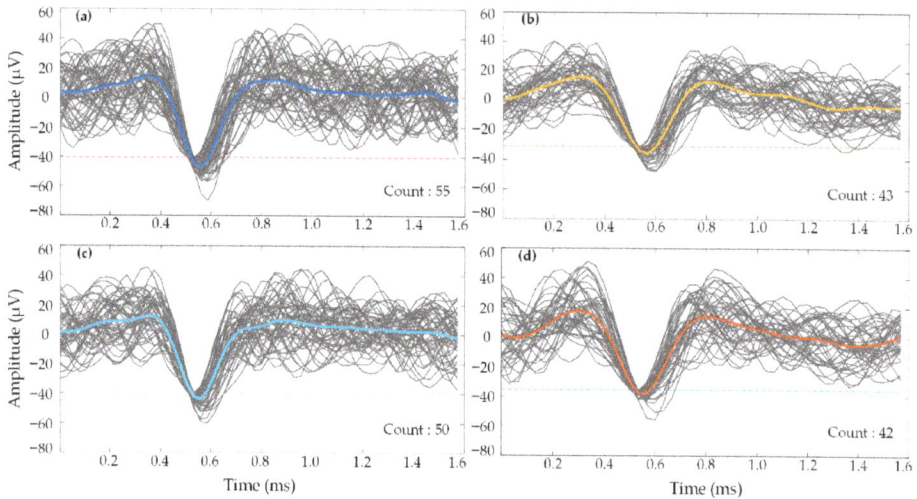

Figure 14. Waveforms of threshold crossing events recorded from the rapidly multiplexed chip (left column) and Cerebus (right column) extracted from the data shown in Figure 14. (**a,b**) show waveforms from one electrode, (**c,d**) are taken from a second electrode. Bold, colored traces represent the mean of each electrode's threshold crossing waveforms. Dotted lines indicate the threshold.

5. Discussion

This report describes a new approach to acquiring neuronal action potentials from multichannel electrode arrays, based on time domain multiplexing of multiple electrode sites to a single integrated circuit. The implications of electrode DC offsets and high-frequency noise were discussed. Windowed integrator sampling was presented as an approach to mitigate high-frequency noise from the electrodes as well as electronics, enabling far higher multiplexing ratios than traditional voltage sampling. A CMOS integrated circuit architecture was proposed, which incorporates the windowed integrator sampling technique as well as mixed-signal DC offset cancellation. Transistor level design details of a proof-of-concept implementation were also presented. Finally, experimental results were reported from bench testing of the CMOS circuitry as well as acquisition of putative action potentials (possibly multi-unit) from a standard microwire electrode array implanted in rodent cortex.

The proposed approach replaces traditional multichannel neural recording circuitry with a single circuit that acquires signals from multiple electrodes. Sophisticated circuit techniques were required to maintain noise and power performance at levels that are commensurate with traditional neural recording circuitry, while achieving a dramatic reduction in circuit area. This approach can be viewed as combining the power dissipation of many traditional neural recording channels into a single circuit with higher bandwidth, leveraging high-speed operation. The reduction in circuit area, and the potential for further reduction, is critical for scaling neural recording systems to higher channel counts by enabling fully implantable electronics that are better matched to the size and density of emerging electrode arrays technologies [13–15]. Limitations on the multiplexing ratio imposed by high-frequency electrode noise still dictate that a number of copies of the circuitry be used to support electrode arrays with hundreds of channels and beyond, but the approach is compelling in terms of reduced area per channel as well as reduced complexity at the system level.

The rapidly multiplexed acquisition approach is particularly well suited for high channel count microelectrode arrays, where active circuitry is integrated with the device through homogenous fabrication [15,19,25] or advanced heterogeneous approaches [29,60,61]. The technique in itself does not address interconnect limitations that arise when adopting headstage recording architectures where active circuits (chips) are connected to electrode arrays through standard printed circuit boards and connectors (i.e., not fully implantable) [3–5]. Standard CMOS I/O bondpad dimensions often result in "pad-limited" implementations, such as the test chip shown in Figure 10b. However, the rapidly multiplexed approach does improve those architectures as well, since it allows for more chip area that can be used for signal processing, data compression, and communication circuits, which are increasingly important. The main goal of this report is to provide proof-of-concept evidence that rapid multiplexing, directly at the electrodes, without preamplification, is feasible for acquiring action potentials from multichannel electrode arrays. Future work should address fully implantable integration with arrays, and assessment of long term reliability. Issues must be investigated such as thermal considerations, dissolution of electrode materials, stability of packaging and encapsulation, and long term tissue response. These considerations are critical for any fully implantable active array, and rapid multiplexing does not fundamentally present new barriers (e.g., the power dissipation and electrode loading are commensurate with traditional neural recording circuitry [17]). Nevertheless, thorough studies of electrode behavior in the context of rapid multiplexing should be explored, and is part of our own ongoing work. In vivo characterization of a wider range of electrode array technologies should also be pursued, with rapid multiplexing in mind.

It is expected that many further improvements can be made. This report is intended to highlight new avenues of research in integrated circuits, microelectrode array design, and signal processing methods. Co-design of rapidly multiplexed systems across these three dimensions is a particularly interesting goal. Directions for future work in CMOS circuit design include offset cancellation techniques as well as noise mitigation techniques. Windowed integrator sampling and mixed-signal feedback were shown to be effective approaches, but there are likely others as well. There is also significant room for improvement in the core amplifier and ADC circuits beyond the prototype presented in this work, e.g., leveraging more advanced IC process technologies.

The results indicate that rapidly multiplexed action potential acquisition without preamplification is possible, which to our best knowledge has not been shown before. Overall, this report demonstrates a compelling candidate approach for scaling up neural recoding systems.

Author Contributions: Conceptualization, M.S. and R.M.W.; Methodology, M.S., A.T.G., H.J.S., D.J.W., J.S. and R.M.W.; Validation, D.J.W. and R.M.W.; Formal analysis, M.S., A.T.G., H.J.S., J.S. and R.M.W.; Investigation, M.S., A.T.G., H.J.S., D.J.W, J.S. and R.M.W.; Resources, D.J.W.; Data Curation, A.T.G. and H.J.S.; Writing—Original Draft Preparation, M.S., A.T.G., H.J.S. and R.M.W.; Writing—Review & Editing, D.J.W.; Supervision, D.J.W. and R.M.W.; Project Administration, R.M.W.; Funding Acquisition, J.S. and R.M.W.

Funding: This research was funded in part by a National Science Foundation Graduate Research Fellowship under Grant 1256065 and in part by the National Institutes of Health under Grant R21EY027618.

Acknowledgments: The authors would like to thank John Rolston, Loren Reith, Stuart Cogan, and Ryan Caldwell for useful discussions; John Mize for implantation assistance and training; and Analog Devices and Linear Technology (now also Analog Devices) for parts. Special thanks are given to ON Semiconductor for providing test chip fabrication.

Conflicts of Interest: D.J.W. has a potential financial interest related to sales of the Utah Electrode Array by Blackrock Microsystems if certain intellectual property aspects are optionally included in its design. The funders had no role in the design of the study; in the collection, analyses, or interpretation of data; in the writing of the manuscript, and in the decision to publish the results.

References

1. Gunasekera, B.; Saxena, T.; Bellamkonda, R.; Karumbaiah, L. Intracortical Recording Interfaces: Current Challenges to Chronic Recording Function. *ACS Chem. Neurosci.* **2015**, *6*, 68–83. [CrossRef] [PubMed]
2. Marblestone, A.H.; Zamft, B.M.; Maguire, Y.G.; Shapiro, M.G.; Cybulski, T.R.; Glaser, J.I.; Amodei, D.; Stranges, P.B.; Kalhor, R.; Dalrymple, D.A.; et al. Physical Principles for Scalable Neural Recording. *Front. Comput. Neurosci.* **2013**, *7*, 1–34. [CrossRef] [PubMed]
3. Schwarz, D.A.; Lebedev, M.A.; Hanson, T.L.; Dimitrov, D.F.; Lehew, G.; Meloy, J.; Rajangam, S.; Subramanian, V.; Ifft, P.J.; Li, Z.; et al. Chronic, Wireless Recordings of Large-Scale Brain Activity in Freely Moving Rhesus Monkeys. *Nat. Methods* **2014**, *11*, 670–676. [CrossRef] [PubMed]

4.   Yin, M.; Borton, D.A.; Komar, J.; Agha, N.; Lu, Y.; Li, H.; Laurens, J.; Lang, Y.; Li, Q.; Bull, C.; et al. Wireless Neurosensor for Full-Spectrum Electrophysiology Recordings during Free Behavior. *Neuron* **2014**, *84*, 1170–1182. [CrossRef] [PubMed]

5.   Foster, J.D.; Nuyujukian, P.; Freifeld, O.; Gao, H.; Walker, R.; Ryu, S.I.; Meng, T.H.; Murmann, B.; Black, M.J.; Shenoy, K.V. A Freely-Moving Monkey Treadmill Model. *J. Neural Eng.* **2014**, *11*, 046020. [CrossRef] [PubMed]

6.   Hochberg, L.R.; Serruya, M.D.; Friehs, G.M.; Mukand, J.A.; Saleh, M.; Caplan, A.H.; Branner, A.; Chen, D.; Penn, R.D.; Donoghue, J.P. Neuronal Ensemble Control of Prosthetic Devices by a Human with Tetraplegia. *Nature* **2006**, *442*, 164–171. [CrossRef] [PubMed]

7.   Collinger, J.L.; Wodlinger, B.; Downey, J.E.; Wang, W.; Tyler-Kabara, E.C.; Weber, D.J.; McMorland, A.J.C.; Velliste, M.; Boninger, M.L.; Schwartz, A.B. High-Performance Neuroprosthetic Control by an Individual with Tetraplegia. *Lancet* **2013**, *381*, 557–564. [CrossRef]

8.   Gilja, V.; Pandarinath, C.; Blabe, C.H.; Nuyujukian, P.; Simeral, J.D.; Sarma, A.A.; Sorice, B.L.; Perge, J.A.; Jarosiewicz, B.; Hochberg, L.R.; et al. Clinical Translation of a High-Performance Neural Prosthesis. *Nat. Med.* **2015**, *21*, 1142–1145. [CrossRef] [PubMed]

9.   Stevenson, I.H.; Kording, K.P. How Advances in Neural Recording Affect Data Analysis. *Nat. Neurosci.* **2011**, *14*, 139–142. [CrossRef] [PubMed]

10.   Rajkowska, G.; Halaris, A.; Selemon, L.D. Reductions in Neuronal and Glial Density Characterize the DL PFC Cortex in Bipolar Disorder. *Biol. Psychiatry* **2001**, *49*, 741–752. [CrossRef]

11.   Khodagholy, D.; Gelinas, J.N.; Thesen, T.; Doyle, W.; Devinsky, O.; Malliaras, G.G.; Buzsáki, G. NeuroGrid: Recording Action Potentials from the Surface of the Brain. *Nat. Neurosci.* **2015**, *18*, 310–315. [CrossRef] [PubMed]

12.   Rios, G.; Lubenov, E.V.; Chi, D.; Roukes, M.L.; Siapas, A.G. Nanofabricated Neural Probes for Dense 3-D Recordings of Brain Activity. *Nano Lett.* **2016**, *16*, 6857–6862. [CrossRef] [PubMed]

13.   Berenyi, A.; Somogyvari, Z.; Nagy, A.J.; Roux, L.; Long, J.D.; Fujisawa, S.; Stark, E.; Leonardo, A.; Harris, T.D.; Buzsaki, G. Large-Scale, High-Density (up to 512 Channels) Recording of Local Circuits in Behaving Animals. *J. Neurophysiol.* **2014**, *111*, 1132–1149. [CrossRef] [PubMed]

14.   Chung, J.E.; Joo, H.R.; Fan, J.L.; Liu, D.F.; Barnett, A.H.; Chen, S.; Geaghan-Breiner, C.; Karlsson, M.P.; Karlsson, M.; Lee, K.Y.; et al. High-Density, Long-Lasting, and Multi-Region Electrophysiological Recordings Using Polymer Electrode Arrays. *bioRxiv* **2018**. [CrossRef]

15.   Jun, J.J.; Steinmetz, N.A.; Siegle, J.H.; Denman, D.J.; Bauza, M.; Barbarits, B.; Lee, A.K.; Anastassiou, C.A.; Andrei, A.; Aydin, Ç.; et al. Fully Integrated Silicon Probes for High-Density Recording of Neural Activity. *Nature* **2017**, *551*, 232–236. [CrossRef] [PubMed]

16.   Barrese, J.C.; Rao, N.; Paroo, K.; Triebwasser, C.; Vargas-Irwin, C.; Franquemont, L.; Donoghue, J.P. Failure Mode Analysis of Silicon-Based Intracortical Microelectrode Arrays in Non-Human Primates. *J. Neural Eng.* **2013**, *10*, 66014. [CrossRef] [PubMed]

17.   Bharucha, E.; Sepehrian, H.; Gosselin, B. A Survey of Neural Front End Amplifiers and Their Requirements toward Practical Neural Interfaces. *J. Low Power Electron. Appl.* **2014**, *4*, 268–291. [CrossRef]

18.   Smith, W.A.; Uehlin, J.P.; Perlmutter, S.I.; Rudell, J.C.; Sathe, V.S. A Scalable, Highly-Multiplexed Delta-Encoded Digital Feedback ECoG Recording Amplifier with Common and Differential-Mode Artifact Suppression. In *2017 Symposium on VLSI Circuits, Proceedings of the 2017 Symposium on VLSI Circuits, Kyoto, Japan, 5–8 June 2017*; IEEE: Piscataway, NJ, USA, 2017; pp. C172–C173.

19.   Viventi, J.; Kim, D.-H.; Vigeland, L.; Frechette, E.S.; Blanco, J.A.; Kim, Y.-S.; Avrin, A.E.; Tiruvadi, V.R.; Hwang, S.-W.; Vanleer, A.C.; et al. Flexible, Foldable, Actively Multiplexed, High-Density Electrode Array for Mapping Brain Activity In Vivo. *Nat. Neurosci.* **2011**, *14*, 1599–1605. [CrossRef] [PubMed]

20.   Guo, J.; Ng, W.; Yuan, J.; Li, S.; Chan, M. A 200-Channel Area-Power-Efficient Chemical and Electrical Dual-Mode Acquisition IC for the Study of Neurodegenerative Diseases. *IEEE Trans. Biomed. Circuits Syst.* **2016**, *10*, 567–578. [CrossRef] [PubMed]

21.   Zou, X.; Liu, L.; Cheong, J.H.; Yao, L.; Li, P.; Cheng, M.; Goh, W.L.; Rajkumar, R.; Dawe, G.S.; Cheng, K.-W.; et al. A 100-Channel 1-mW Implantable Neural Recording IC. *IEEE Trans. Biomed. Circuits Syst. I* **2013**, *60*, 2584–2596. [CrossRef]

22.   Lee, J.; Rhew, H.G.; Kipke, D.R.; Flynn, M.P. A 64 Channel Programmable Closed-Loop Neurostimulator with 8 Channel Neural Amplifier and Logarithmic ADC. *IEEE J. Solid State Circuits* **2010**, *45*, 1935–1945. [CrossRef]

23. Chae, M.S.; Yang, Z.; Yuce, M.R.; Hoang, L.; Liu, W. A 128-Channel 6 mW Wireless Neural Recording IC with Spike Feature Extraction and UWB Transmitter. *IEEE Trans. Neural Syst. Rehabil. Eng.* **2009**, *17*, 312–321. [CrossRef] [PubMed]

24. Mohseni, P.; Najafi, K.; Eliades, S.J.; Wang, X. Wireless Multichannel Biopotential Recording Using an Integrated FM Telemetry Circuit. *IEEE Trans. Neural Syst. Rehabil. Eng.* **2005**, *13*, 263–271. [CrossRef] [PubMed]

25. Wise, K.D.; Anderson, D.J.; Hetke, J.F.; Kipke, D.R.; Najafi, K. Wireless Implantable Microsystems: High-Density Electronic Interfaces to the Nervous System. *Proc. IEEE* **2004**, *92*, 76–97. [CrossRef]

26. Bai, Q.; Wise, K.D. Single-Unit Neural Recording with Active Microelectrode Arrays. *IEEE Trans. Biomed. Eng.* **2001**, *48*, 911–920. [CrossRef] [PubMed]

27. Cogan, S.F. Neural Stimulation and Recording Electrodes. *Annu. Rev. Biomed. Eng.* **2008**, *10*, 275–309. [CrossRef] [PubMed]

28. Muller, R.; Gambini, S.; Rabaey, J.M. A 0.013 mm^2, 5 mW, DC-Coupled Neural Signal Acquisition IC with 0.5 V Supply. *IEEE J. Solid State Circuits* **2012**, *47*, 232–243. [CrossRef]

29. Shulyzki, R.; Abdelhalim, K.; Bagheri, A.; Salam, M.T.; Florez, C.M.; Velazquez, J.L.P.; Carlen, P.L.; Genov, R. 320-Channel Active Probe for High-Resolution Neuromonitoring and Responsive Neurostimulation. *IEEE Trans. Biomed. Circuits Syst.* **2015**, *9*, 34–49. [CrossRef] [PubMed]

30. Harrison, R.R.; Watkins, P.T.; Lovejoy, R.; Kier, R.; Black, D.J.; Greger, B.; Solzbacher, F. A Low-Power Integrated Circuit for a Wireless 100- Electrode Neural Recording System. *IEEE J. Solid State Circuits* **2007**, *42*, 123–133. [CrossRef]

31. Gao, H.; Walker, R.M.; Nuyujukian, P.; Makinwa, K.A.A.; Shenoy, K.V.; Murmann, B.; Meng, T.H. HermesE: A 96-Channel Full Data Rate Direct Neural Interface in 0.13 μm CMOS. *IEEE J. Solid State Circuits* **2012**, *47*, 1043–1055. [CrossRef]

32. Vittoz, E.A. Weak Inversion for Ultra Low-Power and Very Low-Voltage Circuits. In Proceedings of the 2009 IEEE Asian Solid State Circuits Conference, Taipei, Taiwan, 16–18 November 2009; IEEE: Piscataway, NJ, USA, 2009. [CrossRef]

33. Fee, M.S.; Mitra, P.P.; Kleinfeld, D. Variability of Extracellular Spike Waveforms of Cortical Neurons. *J. Neurophysiol.* **1996**, *76*, 3823–3833. [CrossRef] [PubMed]

34. Mirzaei, A.; Chehrazi, S.; Bagheri, R.; Abidi, A.A. Analysis of First-Order Anti-Aliasing Integration Sampler. *IEEE Trans. Circuits Syst. I* **2008**, *55*, 2994–3005. [CrossRef]

35. Poberezhskiy, Y.; Poberezhskiy, G. Sampling with Weighted Integration for Digital Receivers. In Proceedings of the 1999 IEEE MTT-S International Topical Symposium on Technologies for Wireless Applications, Vancouver, BC, Canada, 21–24 February 1999; IEEE: Piscataway, NJ, USA. [CrossRef]

36. Chang, J.; Abidi, A.A.; Viswanathan, C.R. Flicker Noise in CMOS Transistors from Subthreshold to Strong Inversion at Various Temperatures. *IEEE Trans. Electron. Devices* **1994**, *41*, 1965–1971. [CrossRef]

37. Gardner, A.T.; Strathman, H.J.; Warren, D.J.; Walker, R.M. Signal and Noise Sources from TDT Microwire Arrays Implanted in Rodent Cortex. *IEEE Life Sci. Conf.* **2018**. accepted.

38. Gardner, A.T.; Strathman, H.J.; Warren, D.J.; Walker, R.M. Impedance and Noise Characterizations of Utah and Microwire Electrode Arrays. *IEEE J. Electromagn. RF Microwaves Med. Biol.* **2018**, *2*, 1–8.

39. Gardner, A.T.; Mize, J.; Warren, D.J.; Walker, R.M. Comparative Characterization of in vivo and in vitro Noise of the SIROF Utah Electrode Array. In Proceedings of the 2017 IEEE SENSORS, Glasgow, UK, 29 October–1 November 2017; IEEE: Piscataway, NJ, USA, 2007. [CrossRef]

40. Sharma, M.; Gardner, A.T.; Silver, J.; Walker, R.M. Noise and Impedance of the SIROF Utah Electrode Array. In Proceedings of the 2016 IEEE SENSORS, Orlando, FL, USA, 30 October–3 November 2016; IEEE: Piscataway, NJ, USA, 2016. [CrossRef]

41. Nyquist, H. Thermal Agitation of Electric Charge in Conductors. *Phys. Rev.* **1928**, *32*, 110. [CrossRef]

42. Maynard, E.M.; Nordhausen, C.T.; Normann, R.A. The Utah Intracortical Electrode Array: A Recording Structure for Potential Brain-Computer Interfaces. *Electroencephalogr. Clin. Neurophysiol.* **1997**, *102*, 228–239. [CrossRef]

43. Venkatraman, S.; Hendricks, J.; Richardson-Burns, S.; Jan, E.; Martin, D.; Carmena, J.M. PEDOT Coated Microelectrode Arrays for Chronic Neural Recording and Stimulation. In Proceedings of the 2009 4th International IEEE/EMBS Conference on Neural Engineering, Antalya, Turkey, 29 April–2 May 2009; IEEE: Piscataway, NJ, USA, 2009. [CrossRef]

44. Buzsáki, G.; Anastassiou, C.A.; Koch, C. The Origin of Extracellular Fields and Currents-EEG, ECoG, LFP and Spikes. *Nat. Rev. Neurosci.* **2012**, *13*, 407–420. [CrossRef] [PubMed]

45. Randles, J.E.B. Kinetics of Rapid Electrode Reactions. *R. Soc. Chem.* **1947**, *1*, 11–19. [CrossRef]

46. Sankar, V.; Patrick, E.; Dieme, R.; Sanchez, J.C.; Prasad, A.; Nishida, T. Electrode Impedance Analysis of Chronic Tungsten Microwire Neural Implants: Understanding Abiotic vs. Biotic Contributions. *Front. Neuroeng.* **2014**, *7*, 1–12. [CrossRef] [PubMed]

47. Williams, J.C.; Hippensteel, J.A.; Dilgen, J.; Shain, W.; Kipke, D.R. Complex Impedance Spectroscopy for Monitoring Tissue Responses to Inserted Neural Implants. *J. Neural Eng.* **2007**, *4*, 410–423. [CrossRef] [PubMed]

48. Liu, C.C.; Chang, S.J.; Huang, G.Y.; Lin, Y.Z. A 10-bit 50-MS/s SAR ADC with a Monotonic Capacitor Switching Procedure. *IEEE J. Solid State Circuits* **2010**, *45*, 731–740. [CrossRef]

49. Harpe, P.J.A.; Zhou, C.; Bi, Y.; van der Meijs, N.P.; Wang, X.; Philips, K.; Dolmans, G.; de Groot, H. 26 mW 8 bit 10 MSPS Asynchronous SAR ADC for Low Energy Radios. *IEEE J. Solid State Circuits* **2011**, *46*, 1585–1595. [CrossRef]

50. Tripathi, V.; Murmann, B. An 8-bit 450-MS/s Single-Bit/Cycle SAR ADC in 65-nm CMOS. In Proceedings of the 2013 Proceedings of the ESSCIRC (ESSCIRC), Bucharest, Romania, 16–20 September 2013; IEEE: Piscataway, NJ, USA, 2013. [CrossRef]

51. Steyaert, M.S.J.; Sansen, W.M.C.; Zhongyuan, C. A Micropower Low-Noise Monolithic Instrumentation Amplifier for Medical Purposes. *IEEE J. Solid State Circuits* **1987**, *22*, 1163–1168. [CrossRef]

52. Lee, J.; Lee, G.H.; Kim, H.; Cho, S.H. An Ultra-High Input Impedance Analog Front End Using Self-Calibrated Positive Feedback. *IEEE J. Solid State Circuits* **2018**, *53*, 2252–2262. [CrossRef]

53. Fan, Q.; Sebastiano, F.; Huijsing, J.H.; Makinwa, K.A.A. A 1.8 mW 60 nV/$\sqrt{Hz}$ Capacitively-Coupled Chopper Instrumentation Amplifier in 65 nm CMOS for Wireless Sensor Nodes. *IEEE J. Solid State Circuits* **2011**, *46*, 1534–1543. [CrossRef]

54. Leene, L.B.; Constandinou, T.G. A 0.006 mm^2 1.2 µW Analog-to-Time Converter for Asynchronous Bio-Sensors. *IEEE J. Solid State Circuits* **2018**, *53*, 2604–2613. [CrossRef]

55. Han, D.; Zheng, Y.; Rajkumar, R.; Dawe, G.S.; Je, M. A 0.45 V 100-Channel Neural-Recording IC with Sub-µW/Channel Consumption in 0.18 µm CMOS. *IEEE Trans. Biomed. Circuits Syst.* **2013**, *7*, 735–746. [CrossRef] [PubMed]

56. Park, S.Y.; Cho, J.; Lee, K.; Yoon, E. Dynamic Power Reduction in Scalable Neural Recording Interface Using Spatiotemporal Correlation and Temporal Sparsity of Neural Signals. *IEEE J. Solid State Circuits* **2018**, *53*, 1102–1114. [CrossRef]

57. Ng, K.A.; Xu, Y.P. A Low-Power, High CMRR Neural Amplifier System Employing CMOS Inverter-Based OTAs with CMFB through Supply Rails. *IEEE J. Solid State Circuits* **2016**, *51*, 724–737. [CrossRef]

58. Santhanam, G.; Sahani, M.; Ryu, S.I.; Shenoy, K.V. An Extensible Infrastructure for Fully Automated Spike Sorting during Online Experiments. In Proceedings of the The 26th Annual International Conference of the IEEE Engineering in Medicine and Biology Society, San Francisco, CA, USA, 1–5 September 2004; IEEE: Piscataway, NJ, USA, 2004. [CrossRef]

59. Kelly, R.C.; Smith, M.A.; Samonds, J.M.; Kohn, A.; Bonds, A.B.; Movshon, J.A.; Lee, T.S. Comparison of Recordings from Microelectrode Arrays and Single Electrodes in the Visual Cortex. *J. Neurosci. Off. J. Soc. Neurosci.* **2007**, *27*, 261–264. [CrossRef] [PubMed]

60. Walker, R.M.; Subramanian, I.S.; Bajwa, A.A.; Rieth, L.; Silver, J.; Ahmed, T.; Tasneem, N.; Sharma, M.; Gardner, A.T. Integrated Neural Interfaces. In Proceedings of the 2017 IEEE 60th International Midwest Symposium on Circuits and Systems (MWSCAS), Boston, MA, USA, 6–9 August 2017; IEEE: Piscataway, NJ, USA, 2017. [CrossRef]

61. Park, S.-Y.; Cho, J.; Na, K.; Yoon, E. Modular 128-Channel Δ - ΔΣ Analog Front-End Architecture Using Spectrum Equalization Scheme for 1024-Channel 3-D Neural Recording Microsystems. *IEEE J. Solid State Circuits* **2018**, *53*, 501–514. [CrossRef]

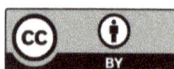

micromachines

MDPI

Review

A Bidirectional Neuromodulation Technology for Nerve Recording and Stimulation

Jian Xu [1], Hongsun Guo [1], Anh Tuan Nguyen [1], Hubert Lim [1,2,3] and Zhi Yang [1,*]

[1] Department of Biomedical Engineering, University of Minnesota, 312 Church Street SE, Minneapolis, MN 55455, USA; xuxx1268@umn.edu (J.X.); guoxx691@umn.edu (H.G.); nguy2833@umn.edu (A.T.N.); hlim@umn.edu (H.L.)
[2] Department of Otolaryngology, Head and Neck Surgery, University of Minnesota, 516 Delaware Street SE, Minneapolis, MN 55455, USA
[3] Institute for Translational Neuroscience, University of Minnesota, 2101 6th Street SE, Minneapolis, MN 55455, USA
* Correspondence: yang5029@umn.edu; Tel.: +1-612-626-1114

Received: 17 September 2018; Accepted: 19 October 2018; Published: 23 October 2018

Abstract: Electrical nerve recording and stimulation technologies are critically needed to monitor and modulate nerve activity to treat a variety of neurological diseases. However, current neuromodulation technologies presented in the literature or commercially available products cannot support simultaneous recording and stimulation on the same nerve. To solve this problem, a new bidirectional neuromodulation system-on-chip (SoC) is proposed in this paper, which includes a frequency-shaping neural recorder and a fully integrated neural stimulator with charge balancing capability. In addition, auxiliary circuits consisting of power management and data transmission circuits are designed to provide the necessary power supply for the SoC and the bidirectional data communication between the SoC and an external computer via a universal serial bus (USB) interface, respectively. To achieve sufficient low input noise for sensing nerve activity at a sub-10 μV range, several noise reduction techniques are developed in the neural recorder. The designed SoC was fabricated in a 0.18 μm high-voltage Bipolar CMOS DMOS (BCD) process technology that was described in a previous publication and it has been recently tested in animal experiments that demonstrate the proposed SoC is capable of achieving reliable and simultaneous electrical stimulation and recording on the same nerve.

Keywords: system-on-chip; neuromodulation; bidirectional; closed-loop; sciatic nerve; vagus nerve; precision medicine

1. Introduction

Electroceuticals is a new research area in bioelectronics that aims to create implants, including chips that are as small as a grain of rice, and the implants are expected to simultaneously monitor and modulate nerve activity to treat diseases and augment or replace drugs [1–4]. With these implants, electrical stimulation is combined with low-noise and artifact-free recording, enabling closed-loop neuromodulation therapies for a variety of chronic disorders including hypertension, heart failure, gastrointestinal disorders, type II diabetes, and inflammatory disorders [5,6]. The effectiveness of electroceutical therapy can be monitored and optimized for each patient by applying controlled amounts of charge into the nerve while monitoring the neural responses from the treated organ or system at the same time. For example, vagus nerve stimulation is emerging as an alternative method for treating multiple health disorders, such as seizures, depression, rheumatoid arthritis and tinnitus. To minimize side effects and optimize treatment, the stimulation levels could be titrated to the lowest levels required to elicit the desired spiking activity along the ascending and/or descending vagus nerve and also to elicit specific firing patterns in the nerve relevant for treatment. Another example is in providing better neural prosthetics to amputees for controlling robotic hands by monitoring motor and sensory neural activity from ulnar and median nerves to control the hand movements as well as electrically stimulate the nerves to restore sensory sensations and feedback based on the recorded signals.

Highly effective electroceuticals are not in currently use because state-of-the-art bioelectronics do not have three critical features [7–10]. First, existing neural recording technologies have sufficient noise characteristics for sensing action potentials in brain recordings, but this is inadequate for resolving small neural signals from noise sources in cuff electrode interfaces on nerves [11]. Second, penetrating electrodes can improve the signal quality by recording closer to the nerve fiber, but the signals typically decay over time due to the foreign body response caused by electrode penetration and damage of the nerve as well as the micro-motion of the tethered electrodes relative to the soft nerve tissue [12]. Third, electrical stimulation produced by adjacent electrodes generates large noise and recording artifacts on the same nerve that can be multiple orders of magnitude larger than the spontaneous or evoked nerve activity, making it extremely challenging to perform simultaneous recording and stimulation on the same nerve [13].

In this paper, a neuromodulation system-on-chip (SoC) is proposed for nerve recording and stimulation. We have recently pioneered a new neural recorder architecture that does not need built-in analog filters, thus avoiding the filter noise that is a major noise source in nerve recordings [14–18]. We also propose new techniques that can significantly reduce activity-dependent noise (shot noise) in the electrode interface, which is another primary noise source. The combination of "filterless" amplification and shot noise suppression permits an entirely different approach to improve signal quality at a sub-10 µV range. Thus, we aim to develop an ultra-low-noise recording chip for sensing nerve activity at a sub-10 µV range, even with electrical stimulation on the same nerve. We will test and use the SoC in animal experiments to monitor nerve activity in the presence of stimulation artifacts.

The paper is organized as follows. The research background and limitations in the nerve recording technology field are discussed in Section 2. Section 3 presents the design of the proposed bidirectional neuromodulation system that was described in detail in the previous publications [16,18,19] and reviewed in this paper. New animal experimental results obtained with a prototype of our neuromodulation system are presented in Section 4. Section 5 summarizes this paper.

2. Background and Limitations

It is well known that the ability to simultaneously stimulate and record nerve activity is currently limited and that new technologies are required to provide high-fidelity chronic recording and stimulation in animals for basic science studies and, eventually, for human clinical applications. In particular, there are three limitations that prevent chronically stable nerve recording and stimulation.

Limitation 1: There is poor signal-to-noise ratio (*SNR*) of recorded signals on nerves. Epineural electrodes such as cuff electrodes provide a robust and stable interface for recording whole nerve activity, but the electrical isolation caused by the epineurium/perineurium reduces the magnitude of detected signals, which translates into low *SNR* [20,21]. The main reasons for low *SNR* are given as follows. (1) The biological noise in epineural electrodes can significantly distort recordings and require heavy filtering. Due to insufficient recording precision and the difficulty of resolving nonstationary signals and noise through filtering, residual biological noise can be intermixed with the desired nerve signals. (2) Part of the electrode-tissue interface noise is ohmic that in principle cannot be separated from signals. However, several models and more recent measurement data [22–24] suggest that a large portion of electrode noise is non-ohmic. For example, [25] compared an electrode with 100-fold increased surface area that should have reduced the ohmic noise by ten-fold, but the measured total electrode noise was only reduced by 40%. (3) The amount of electronic noise in nerve recording can be quite large due to elevated filter noise. When recording from a nerve in the abdomen, for example, the constant motion of viscera guarantees large amplitude motion artifacts. To sufficiently attenuate motion artifacts to avoid saturating electronics, a built-in analog high-pass filter with a corner frequency of at least ten times higher than the artifact frequency is required. This requirement increases the analog filter noise over the neural signal band to tens of μV and beyond. In some other cases, circuits and devices that have low-noise characteristics in benchtop testing do not work well in actual experiments. For example, [26–28] have reported a neural interface based on epineural electrodes and low-noise neural amplifiers [11,29], where the measured *SNR* on a sciatic nerve preparation is only 1–3 dB, which is not high enough to isolate the small nerve signals.

Limitation 2: There is an inability to record microvolt-level nerve activity in the presence of stimulation pulses applied to the same nerve. The stimulation artifacts often produce a shift in the differential mode signal and the common mode signal, both of which need to be properly rejected. The subtraction of stimulation artifacts requires compensating for the frequency-dependent amplitude and phase of the transfer function [8]. This subtraction cannot be routinely done because it requires a high precision amplifier buffer to store superimposed artifacts and neural signals, and a fast recovery from stimulation artifacts. We did a survey on recent recording electronics and found that every extra bit of increased precision requires a four-fold increase in the supply power [30–35]. In other words, an 8-bit increase in precision translates into a >60,000 times increase in power. Thus, it is not possible to implant a 10 W nerve recorder into the body. Furthermore, fast recovery from stimulation artifacts is another challenge. Electrical stimulation saturates the recorder and increases the noise floor in addition to creating "ringing" in the signals that only slowly stabilizes towards zero. The closer the stimulation and recording electrodes, the more artifacts and noise appear in the recorded signals. As a result, a typical nerve experimental setup requires direct electrical stimulation of a portion of the nerve and recording of the nerve at another distant location. Therefore, current technologies described in the literature cannot yet support simultaneous recording and stimulation on the same nerve.

Limitation 3: There is an inability to extract signals of individual fascicles with current noninvasive electrodes. Considerable research effort has been devoted to developing and improving neural interfaces using a variety of designs and materials. Noninvasive nerve interface approaches provide small signals from a highly limited number of electrodes. Current technologies have demonstrated successful recording from the sciatic nerve, where the recorded compound action potentials (CAPs) are sufficiently greater than the background noise activity [36,37]. However, when using a noninvasive wire or cuff electrode, it is still not readily possible to acquire more resolved neural activity from the sciatic nerve or other peripheral nerves (i.e., representing nerve fibers or small groups of fibers that is possible with penetrating electrodes) using current commercial devices.

In this paper, a bidirectional neuromodulation SoC is proposed for simultaneous nerve recording and stimulation. With several new techniques that will be presented in Section 3, the proposed SoC is supposed to be able to overcome many of the limitations described above.

3. Bidirectional Closed-Loop Neuromodulation System Design

Figure 1 shows an exemplary bidirectional neuromodulation system for supporting simultaneous recording and stimulation without one impeding the other. The neuromodulation system includes a SoC and auxiliary circuits, where the SoC consists of a fully integrated neural recorder and a electrical neural stimulator that are implemented in a high-voltage Bipolar CMOS DMOS (BCD) process technology, and the auxiliary circuits that comprise power management and data transmission circuits are implemented using consumable components. The operation of the SoC is facilitated by the customized auxiliary circuits. In this design, the function of the power management circuits is to provide the required power supply and voltage references for the SoC. The function of the data transmission circuits is to provide the bidirectional data communication between the SoC and an external computer via a customized universal serial bus (USB) interface, which is developed for adjusting system parameters, such as total loop gain, data acquisition bandwidth, stimulation waveforms & patterns, stimulation rate, stimulation current/voltage, etc. In order to perform simultaneous nerve recording and stimulation experiments, both the neural recorder and neural stimulator are connected to the same sciatic nerve of a guinea pig.

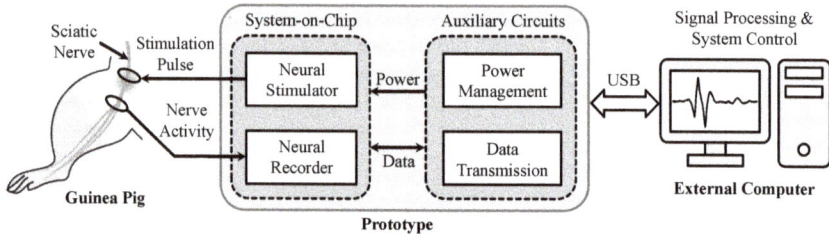

Figure 1. An illustration of the proposed bidirectional neuromodulation system for nerve recording and stimulation experiments.

3.1. Neural Recorder Design

For the neural recorder design, we have previously presented a frequency-shaping (FS) technique [17] that can remove electrode offset without requiring a sub-Hz high-pass filter, increase input impedance by 5–10-fold, compress neural data dynamic range, and support full bandwidth recording up to several kHz [14,16]. Figure 2 gives the detailed block diagrams of the proposed recorder that is developed for nerve recording experiments, which includes a frequency-shaping amplifier (FSA) stage with noise optimization techniques, a programmable low-pass filter stage, an M-bit analog-to-digital converter (ADC), and a digital signal processor (DSP). The FSA stage has a frequency dependent gain characteristic such that artifacts appearing at low frequencies are attenuated and nerve activity at high frequencies is amplified, and the low-pass filter is used to remove high-frequency noise outside the signal bandwidth. After the recorded signals are digitized by the ADC, a matched digital filter is then applied to reconstruct data supposedly observed at the electrode and the reconstruction data are passed to the DSP for information decoding.

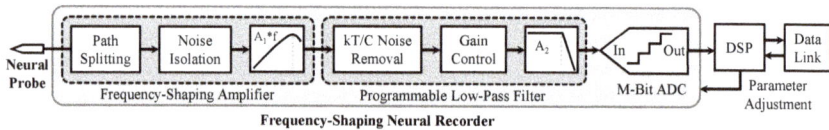

Figure 2. Block diagrams of the proposed neural recorder.

To substantially reduce input noise floor at low frequencies, one noise reduction technique of path splitting is developed in the FSA stage to generate two separate amplification pathways for low-frequency (1–300 Hz) and high-frequency (300–5000 Hz) signal acquisition. Also, a noise isolation method is added in the FSA stage to avoid charge transfer from parasitic capacitor C_p to the feedback capacitor C_f for further noise optimization. To reduce parasitic capacitors, all the switches and amplifier input-pair transistors are designed with small size, and the amplifier input-pair transistors are biased in the sub-threshold region. In addition, it is well known that switched-capacitor circuits usually bring in kT/C noise caused from switch-on resistance. In the proposed neural recorder, to achieve high input impedance, the value of C_f is set to be tens of fF, thus large kT/C noise will appear on C_f after the reset switch is turned off. Fortunately, the kT/C noise on C_f is generated during resetting phase and remains constant during amplification phase. Given the noise generation is not directly correlated with the signal transfer, an auto-zero kT/C noise cancellation scheme is proposed to reduce the noise on C_f with three steps: reset the charge, sample the kT/C noise, and remove the kT/C noise.

To extend the signal application range of the designed recorder, the recording bandwidth, bias current, and sampling frequency are designed to be adjustable from 1–625 Hz to 1–5000 Hz,

25 nA to 200 nA, and 5 kHz to 40 kHz, respectively. More details about circuit implementation of the proposed recorder are presented in [16,18].

3.2. Neural Stimulator Design

In our device design, we propose an integrated, current-mode microstimulator that can support high voltage compliance and high output impedance, where the output waveform, current, timing, and pattern are fully programmable for each channel in real time [19]. Both passive and active charge-balancing schemes are implemented to reduce the residual voltage and its accumulation over time, which are important safety features, especially for chronic applications.

Figure 3a shows the simplified diagrams of one stimulator channel that consists of three major functional blocks: current drivers, digital circuits, and charge-balancing circuits. Each current driver includes two matched sub-drivers, namely (S_{A1}, S_{A2}) and (S_{C1}, S_{C2}), which can be independently controlled to deliver flexible stimulation waveforms. Two charge-balancing schemes are integrated into the stimulator to remove residual charge on the electrode. In the passive scheme, the output is connected to the ground electrode through a switch. In the active scheme, a comparator is used to monitor the electrode voltage after each stimulus and digital circuits are then employed to adjust stimulation parameters accordingly, including relative anodic/cathodic timing (t_A, t_C) and current (S_{A0}, S_{C0}). Figure 3b also shows examples of stimulation waveforms and patterns used in the experiments, which demonstrate the capabilities of the proposed stimulator for producing a broad range of current waveforms. The stimulator is programmed through a single-wire customized communication protocol. Additionlly, the controller utilizes a 32-bit data frame at 1 Mbit/s, where the first 16-bit encodes the channel identification and the second 16-bit is the instruction set. Thus, the controller can support 2^{16} independent channels and 2^{16} distinct commands. Stimulation parameters are loaded when the device is powered on. The stimulation waveforms and patterns are then automatically generated by the internal clock generator. During normal operation, individual parameters can be reprogrammed in real time with a 32 µs latency by sending the appropriate commands to the device.

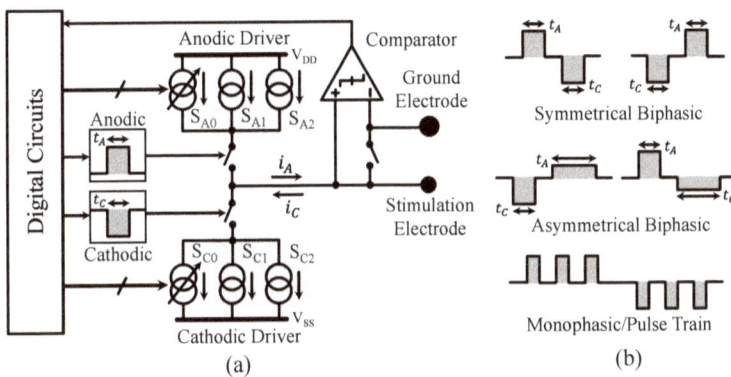

Figure 3. (a) Simplified functional block diagrams of one stimulator channel; (b) Examples of stimulation waveforms and patterns used in the experiments. Reproduced with permission from Anh Tuan Nguyen, A Programmable Fully Integrated Microstimulator for Neural Implants and Instrumentation; published by IEEE Biomedical Circuits and Systems Conference (BioCAS), 2016.

3.3. Auxiliary Circuits Design

Figure 4 presents the detailed block diagrams of the auxiliary circuits that include a nano low power flash field-programmable gate array (FPGA) (AGLN250-CS81, Microsemi Corporation, Aliso Viejo, CA, USA), a USB chip (FT245R, Future Technology Devices International Ltd., Glasgow, UK), ultra-low noise voltage reference circuits (ADR445, Analog Devices, Norwood, MA, USA;

ADA4896-2, Analog Devices), and several low noise voltage regulators (ADP222, Analog Devices; LTC3260, Linear Technologies, Milpitas, CA, USA). The digital output data of the designed SoC are sent to the nano FPGA for signal processing and information encoding. Afterwards, the FPGA output data are transferred to the external computer using a USB to parallel first-in first-out (FIFO) interface. Meanwhile, control signals from the external computer can be sent back to the SoC for adjusting the system parameters through the same data transmission protocol. Thus, the designed data interface can provide bidirectional communication between the SoC and the external computer. Note that the prototype as shown in Figure 1 is also powered by the external computer through the USB cable. In the power management circuits, the voltage regulators are used to generate different power supplies (1.8 V, 3.3 V, and ±5 V) for both the SoC and auxiliary circuits, and the voltage reference circuits are designed to provide ultra-low noise voltage references (0 V, 0.9 V, and 1.8 V) for the SoC.

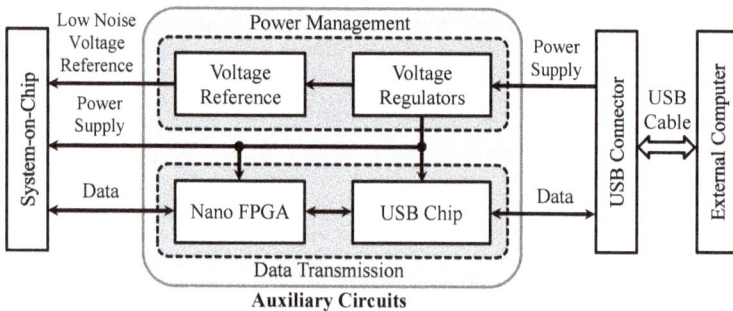

Figure 4. Block diagrams of the auxiliary circuits, which include a nano flash field-programmable gate array (FPGA) , a universal serial bus (USB) interface chip, a voltage reference chip, and several voltage regulators.

4. Experimental Prototype and Animal Experimental Results

4.1. Experimental Prototype

A prototype SoC including both neural recorder and stimulator was fabricated in a one-poly six-metal (1P6M) high-voltage (HV) 0.18 μm BCD process, and the chip micrograph is given in Figure 5. The core area of the designed two-channel neural recorder is 2.2 mm × 1.2 mm, where the analog frontend circuits consisting of an FSA stage and a programmable low-pass filter stage occupy a circuit area of 500 μm × 600 μm per channel, ADC occupies a circuit area of 1300 μm × 350 μm per channel, digital circuits occupy a circuit area of 1300 μm × 500 μm, and clock generator occupies a circuit area of 250 μm × 720 μm. The core area of the designed two-channel neural stimulator is 1.4 mm × 0.65 mm, where the backend current drivers utilize high-voltage (5 V and 20 V) transistors, digital circuits adopt low-voltage (1.8 V) transistors, and level shifters are added between the stimulator current drivers and digital circuits.

Figure 6a gives the printed circuit board (PCB) layout illustration of the designed neuromodulation system prototype with four layers, where the SoC chip and auxiliary circuits are connected with two flexible layers (analog and digital wires). The power management circuits and designed SoC chip are placed on the bottom side while the data transmission circuits, a micro USB connector, and several passive components are designed on the top side. Figure 6b shows the physical photograph of the designed neuromodulation system prototype. In this design, the miniaturized prototype is developed for nerve recording and stimulation experiments in a small animal model.

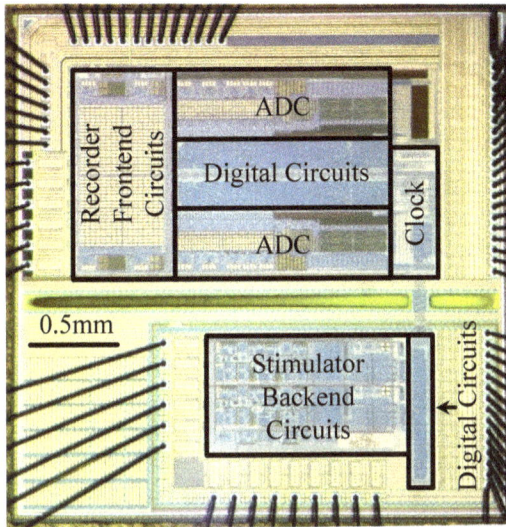

Figure 5. Chip microphoto of the designed neural recorder and neural stimulator in a high-voltage 0.18 μm Bipolar CMOS DMOS (BCD) process.

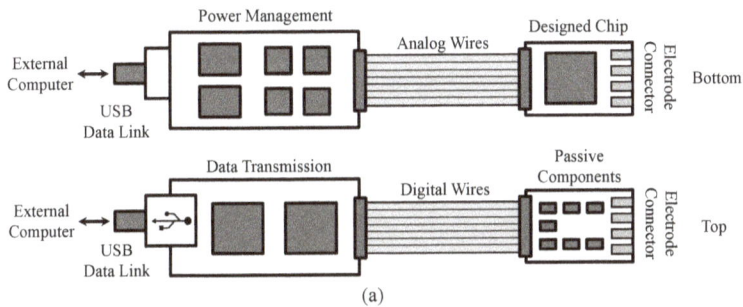

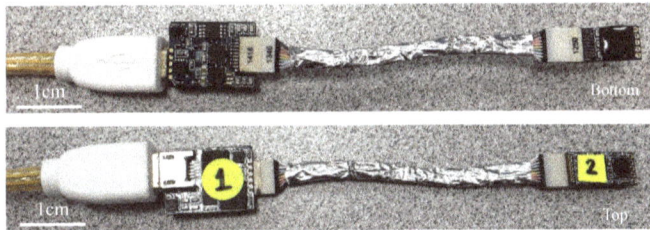

Figure 6. (**a**) Layout illustration (bottom and top side) of the designed neuromodulation system prototype; (**b**) Physical photograph (bottom and top side) of the designed neuromodulation system prototype.

4.2. Animal Surgery and Experimental Preparation

Animal experiments were performed in a sound attenuating, electrically shielded booth, and guinea pigs (450 ± 50 g; Elm Hill, Chelmsford, MA, USA) were used in accordance with the policies of University of Minnesota Institutional Animal Care and Use Committee. The animals were anesthetized with an intramuscular injection of ketamine (40 mg/kg) and xylazine (10 mg/kg) with 0.1 mL supplements every 45–60 min to maintain an areflexive state. Heart rate and blood oxygenation were continuously monitored via a pulse oximeter and body temperature was maintained at $38.0 \pm 0.5\ °C$ using a heating blanket and rectal thermometer.

In the nerve preparation as shown in Figure 7, the left sciatic nerve was exposed and separated from surrounding tissue. Two platinum wires (AS 770-36, Cooner Wire, Chatsworth, CA, USA) were wrapped around the exposed nerve distal to the spine for delivering constant current pulses (0.5 mA, biphasic, 500 µs pulse duration) to the nerve. Five silver wires (AS 766-36, Cooner Wire, Chatsworth, CA, USA) were used to wrap around the sciatic nerve proximal to the spine for recording. The middle silver wire was used as reference while the other four wires were used as two pairs of recording sites.

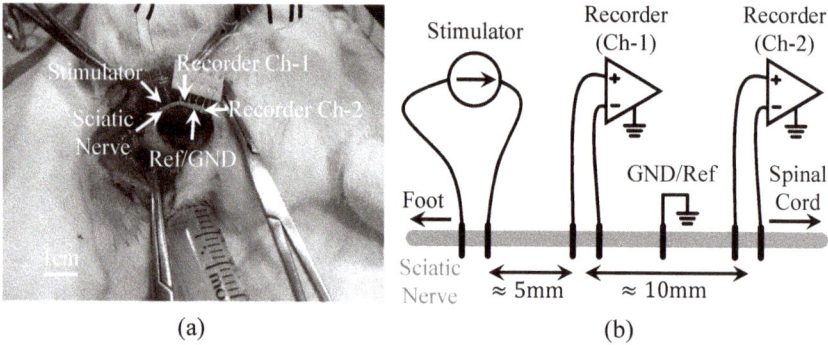

Figure 7. Nerve activity recording from a guinea pig's sciatic nerve, where a two-channel fully differential nerve recording is performanced on the same nerve with current stimulation in a bipolar configuration. (**a**) Physical photograph and (**b**) illustration of experimental setup for simultaneous stimulation and recording.

4.3. Animal Experimental Results from the Proposed Prototype

To demonstrate the proposed prototype is capable of acquiring CAPs, Figure 8 presents the recorded signals from a guinea pig's sciatic nerve, where 2 mA, biphasic, 500 µs current pulses were presented to the guinea pig's left foot to trigger nerve activity along the sciatic nerve. A single-channel fully differential nerve recording acquired the activity along the guinea pig's sciatic nerve. The recorded nerve activity was filtered at 300–5000 Hz, and the peak-to-peak amplitude of the stimulation artifacts and CAPs is approximately 2.1 mVpp and 250 µVpp, respectively.

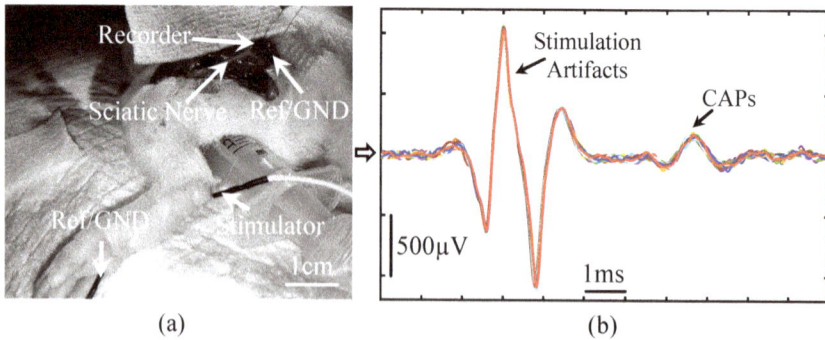

Figure 8. Compound action potentials (CAPs) recordings from a guinea pig's sciatic nerve, where the stimulation current is presented to the guinea pig's left foot and a one-channel fully differential nerve recording is performed on the sciatic nerve. (**a**) Illustration of experimental setup; (**b**) Recorded compound action potentials in response to foot stimulation with 2 mA, biphasic, 500 µs pulse duration current. In total, 30 trials are plotted, where each colored curve represents a single trial.

Figure 7a,b show the physical photograph and illustration, respectively, of the experimental setup for recording and stimulating on the same sciatic nerve. The nerve is exposed and in contact with platinum and silver wire electrodes. From left (foot) to right (spinal cord), we placed one stimulation channel and two recording channels, and the spacing between the two recording channels is about 10 mm. One way to verify whether the data consist of actual nerve activity (instead of muscle responses or other surrounding biological or artifact signals) is to confirm that the signals are propagating along the nerve, which is a challenging task. Figure 9a shows ten trials of the recorded waveforms in response to electrical stimulation on the same nerve, where 0.5 mA, biphasic, 500 μs current pulses were presented to the guinea pig's sciatic nerve to trigger nerve activity. The signals include stimulation artifacts, nerve activity, motion artifacts, and electromyography (EMG) signals. The data were filtered at 300–5000 Hz. Figure 9b–d show the zoom-in of the recorded stimulation artifacts, nerve activity, motion artifacts/EMG, respectively. As shown in Figure 9, electrical stimulation can evoke neural responses. However, the stimulation artifacts can be quite large that are likely masking neural activity immediately evoked after stimulation onset. Note that there is no apparent delay in recorded stimulation artifacts across the recording channels, which is expected since the current flow spreads nearly instantaneously from the stimulation electrodes to both sets of recording electrodes. Interestingly, we observed nerve activity at about 8–20 ms after stimulation onset in which the recording channel closest to the spinal cord (channel-2, red) exhibited activity before channel-1 (blue; Figure 9a,c). This suggests that electrical stimulation may activate the sciatic nerve, which initially propagates towards the spinal cord. We may not have been able to detect those ascending signals because they were masked by the electrical artifacts. However, there are feedback signals from the spinal cord that propagate back from the spinal cord to the foot along the sciatic nerve, which would correspond to the spike activity shown in Figure 9a,c. There is about a 200–300 μs phase delay between the recorded spike activity from the two channel recordings, which is consistent with the conduction velocity expected for the sciatic nerve in rodents [38,39]. The EMG or muscle responses are likely elicited by the initial electrical stimulus activating the sciatic nerve down to the muscles rather than those feedback signals since the muscle activity exists even when there were no noticeable feedback signals. There does not appear to be any systematic delay between recording channels for the muscle activity, which is consistent with the two channels recording far-field muscle signals that reach both sets of electrodes nearly simultaneously. There also exists additional spike activity with longer delays after stimulation onset, which predominantly appears to originate from the spinal cord down the sciatic nerve since the activity appears more frequently on channel-2 before channel-1. Overall, these data demonstrate the powerful capabilities of our stimulation and recording system in sensing low amplitude neural signals and conduction delays in sub-populations of nerve fibers using simple non-invasive wire electrodes around the sciatic nerve, which is enabled by the low noise properties of our device. Further improvements are being pursued by our collaborative research group to better reduce and quickly suppress the electrical artifacts to detect any spike activity that may have been masked immediately after stimulation onset.

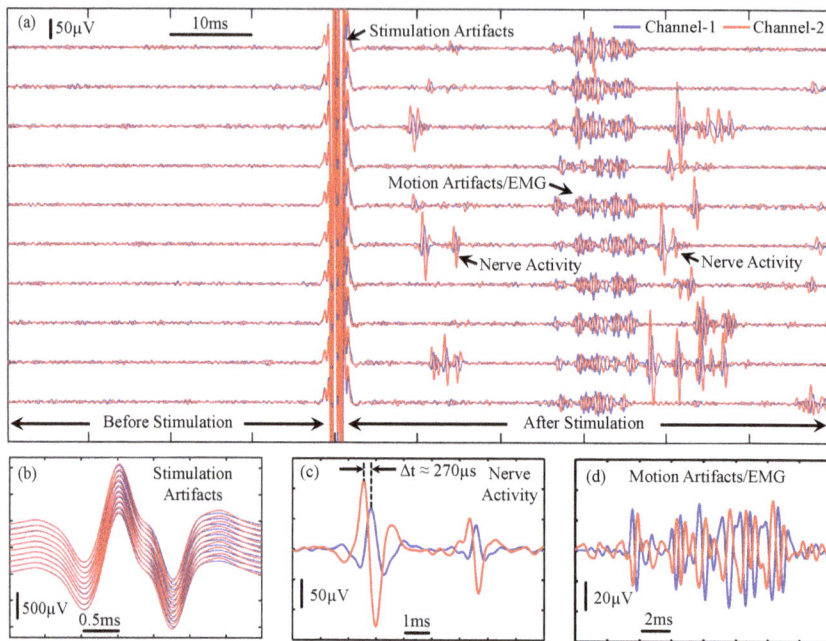

Figure 9. Measurement results of nerve recording and stimulating on the same sciatic nerve. (**a**) Ten trials of the recorded nerve activity showing the recorded waveforms in response to electrical stimulation of the sciatic nerve; (**b**–**d**) Zoom-in of the recorded stimulation artifacts, nerve activity, and motion artifacts/electromyography (EMG), respectively.

4.4. Animal Experimental Results from Commercial System

To demonstrate the performance of the proposed neuromodulation prototype, we also compare the measurement results with one commercial system (Tucker–Davis Technologies (TDT), Alachua, FL, USA; PZ2-64 (Amplifier) and RZ2 (BioAmp Processor)). Figure 10 shows the measured nerve activity at 1.6–7500 Hz with the TDT system when using the same experimental setup as shown in Figure 7, where the stimulator is connected to the foot and the recorder is interfaced with the left sciatic nerve of a guinea pig, and the stimulation electrode delivers current pulses to the nerve. The measured noise floor without (Figure 10a) and with (Figure 10b) the electrical stimuli is similar, and its peak-to-peak value is ~40 µVpp. Thus, the stimulation on the foot does not noticeably increase the noise floor of nerve recording. Figure 11 shows the measured nerve activity at 1.6–7500 Hz with the TDT system when using the same experimental setup as shown in Figure 8, where both the stimulator and recorder are connected to the left sciatic nerve of a guinea pig, and the stimulation electrode delivers current pulses to the nerve. Measurement results show the peak-to-peak value of the recorded noise floor without (Figure 11a) and with (Figure 11b) the electrical stimuli. The ordinate signal amplitudes and scale bars are drastically larger when the electrical stimuli are presented versus when no stimuli are presented (i.e., ~1800 µVpp and ~60 µVpp, respectively). It is clearly shown that presenting stimuli on the same nerve can increase the noise floor by 30-fold, even with high-end standard commercial physiology devices. Therefore, it has been very difficult for current neuromodulaiton technologies to simultaneously support electrical recording and stimulation on the same nerve, a challenge that we have begun to overcome with our neuromodulation system.

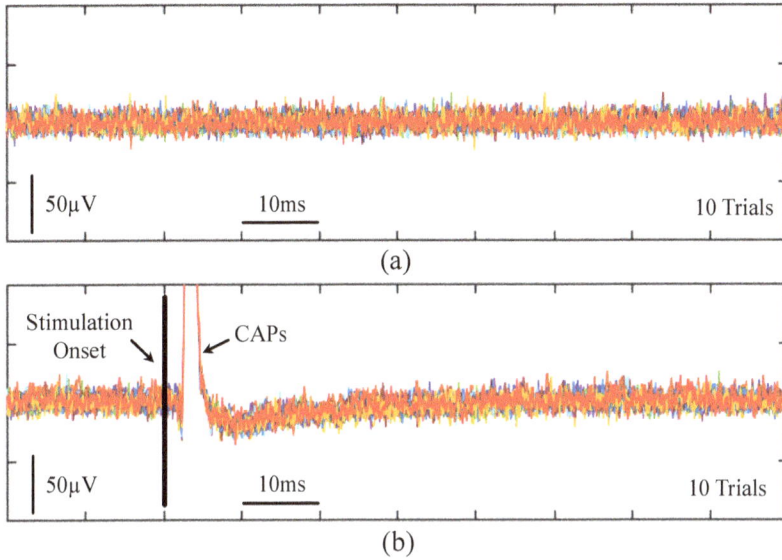

Figure 10. Measured nerve activity with a commercial system (Tucker–Davis Technologies (TDT), Alachua, FL, USA; PZ2-64 (Amplifier) and RZ2 (BioAmp Processor)) when the stimulation electrode is connected to the foot and the recording electrode is interfaced with the left sciatic nerve of a guinea pig. (**a**) Ten trials of the measured nerve activity when the stimulation electrode does not deliver current. (**b**) Ten trials of the measured nerve activity when the stimulation electrode delivers 2.82 mA, biphasic, 205 µs current pulses.

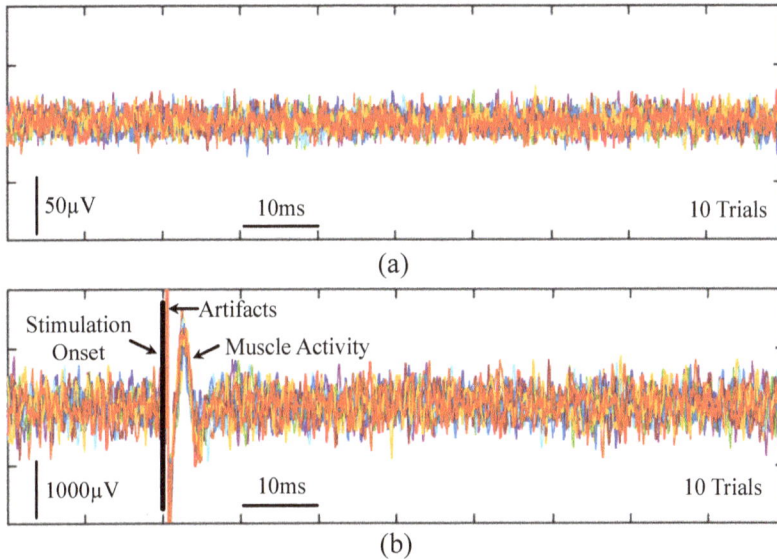

Figure 11. Measured nerve activity with the TDT system when both the stimulation electrode and recording electrode are connected to the left sciatic nerve of a guinea pig. (**a**) Ten trials of the measured nerve activity when the stimulation electrode does not deliver current; (**b**) Ten trials of the measured nerve activity when the stimulation electrode delivers 14.13 µA, biphasic, 205 µs current pulses. Note the drastic change in signal amplitudes and ordinate scale bars in (**b**) compared to (**a**).

5. Conclusions

A bidirectional neuromodulation SoC has been proposed for simultaneous nerve recording and stimulation. Several methods have been proposed in our device design to reduce both electronic noise and electrode noise. First, we have pioneered a new switched-capacitor neural recorder architecture based on the frequency-shaping technique, which does not require any analog high-pass filter in the frontend circuits. As a result, the filter-related noise, artifacts, and distortions can be avoided through the frequency-shaping filterless neural amplification. Second, several noise optimization presented in Section 3.1 have been developed in the frontend circuits to reduce transistor thermal noise and switched-capacitor noise. Third, to reduce activity-dependent noise (shot noise) in the electrode interface, high input impedance is designed in the recorder to reduce current passing through the electrode interface. Fourth, because the recorder is implemented with switched-capacitor circuits, the electrode shot noise becomes zero when the recorder is disconnected from the electrode. Thus, the electrode noise can be minimized by adjusting the "electrode-on" duty cycle. These improvements in the design have enabled the proposed SoC to potentially detect nerve activity at a sub-10 μV range, even with electrical stimulation on the same nerve.

For verification, the designed SoC has been tested with two sets of animal experiments, in which the results demonstrate the SoC is capable of acquiring high-fidelity nerve activity along with stimulation artifacts, CAPs, and motion artifacts/EMG. Further improvements are being pursued to better suppress the electrical artifact during stimulation to enable more immediate recordings after stimulation onsent. The successful development of simultaneous recording and stimulation technologies for nerve interfacing applications with low-noise recording capability will open up new opportunities to study the function and interactions of nerves and organs, as well as advance clinical opportunities for precise treatment of various diseases and health conditions.

In the future, wireless and wearable transcutaneous power delivery and data telemetry will be required to enable the neural devices to be implanted and the subjects to move freely in their daily activities. To miniaturize the SoC as small as a grain of rice when incorporating all the circuits, the wireless power deliver and data telemetry would be also designed with custom VLSI circuits. In addition, new calibration algorithms and shielding methods are required to reduce wireless interferences. These technical challenges are currently being investigated by our research group.

Funding: This research was funded in part by the DARPA under Grant HR0011-17-2-0060, in part by the NIH under Grant R01-MH111413-01, in part by a startup package provided by the College of Science and Engineering and MnDRIVE Program at the University of Minnesota, in part by the Institute for Engineering in Medicine Fund at the University of Minnesota, and in part by the MnDRIVE Fellowships in Neuromodulation at the University of Minnesota. The APC was funded by the startup package provided by the College of Science and Engineering and MnDRIVE Program at the University of Minnesota.

Conflicts of Interest: The authors declare no conflict of interest.

References

1. Burns, J.; Hsieh, Y.H.; Mueller, A.; Chevallier, J.; Sriram, T.S.; Lewis, S.J.; Chew, D.; Achyuta, A.; Fiering, J. High density penetrating electrode arrays for autonomic nerves. In Proceedings of the 38th Annual International of the IEEE EMBS Conference, Orlando, FL, USA, 17–20 August 2016; pp. 2802–2805.
2. Boretius, T.; Badia, J.; Pascual-Font, A.; Schuettler, M.; Navarro, X.; Yoshida, K.; Stieglitz, T. A transverse intrafascicular multichannel electrode (time) to interface with the peripheral nerve. *Biosens. Bioelectron.* **2010**, *26*, 62–69. [CrossRef] [PubMed]
3. Abdelhalim, K.; Kokarovtseva, L.; Velazquez, J.; Genov, R. 915-MHz FSK/OOK Wireless Neural Recording SoC With 64 Mixed-Signal FIR Filters. *IEEE J. Solid-State Circuits* **2013**, *48*, 2478–2493. [CrossRef]
4. Biederman, W.; Yeager, D.; Narevsky, N.; Koralek, A.; Carmena, J.; Alon, E.; Rabaey, J. A Fully Integrated, Miniaturized (0.125 mm²) 10.5 μW Wireless Neural Sensor. *IEEE J. Solid-State Circuits* **2013**, *48*, 960–970. [CrossRef]
5. Reardon, S. Electroceuticals spark interest. *Nature* **2014**, *511*, 18. [CrossRef] [PubMed]

6. Famm, K.; Litt, B.; Tracey, K.J.; Boyden, E.S.; Slaoui, M. Drug discovery: A jump-start for electroceuticals. *Nature* **2013**, *496*, 159–161. [CrossRef] [PubMed]

7. Bensmaia, S.J.; Miller, L.E. Restoring sensorimotor function through intracortical interfaces: Progress and looming challenges. *Nat. Rev. Neuronsci.* **2014**, *15*, 313–325. [CrossRef] [PubMed]

8. Chernyy, N.; Schiff, S.J.; Gluckman, B.J. Time dependence of stimulation/recording-artifact transfer function estimates for neural interface systems. In Proceedings of the 31th Annual International Conference of the IEEE Engineering in Medicine and Biology Society (EMBS 2009), Minneapolis, MN, USA, 3–6 September 2009; pp. 1380–1383.

9. Clark, G.A.; Ledbetter, N.M.; Warren, D.J.; Harrison, R.R. Recording sensory and motor information from peripheral nerves with utah slanted electrode arrays. In Proceedings of the 33th Annual International Conference of the IEEE Engineering in Medicine and Biology Society (EMBS 2011), Boston, MA, USA, 30 August–3 September 2011; pp. 4641–4644.

10. Yang, Z.; Xu, J.; Nguyen, A.T.; Wu, T.; Zhao, W.; Tam, W.K. Neuronix enables continuous, simultaneous neural recording and electrical microstimulation. In Proceedings of the 38th Annual International Conference of the IEEE Engineering in Medicine and Biology Society (EMBS 2016), Orlando, FL, USA, 16–20 August 2016; pp. 4451–4454.

11. Rieger, R.; Taylor, J.; Demosthenous, A.; Donaldson, N.; Langlois, P.J. Design of a low noise preamplifier for nerve cuff electrode recording. *IEEE J. Solid-State Circuits* **2003**, *38*, 1373–1379. [CrossRef]

12. Lotti, F.; Ranieri, F.; Vadala, G.; Zollo, L.; Di Pino, G. Invasive intraneural interfaces: Foreign body reaction issues. *Front. Neurosci.* **2017**, *11*, 00497. [CrossRef] [PubMed]

13. Loi, D.; Carboni, C.; Angius, G.; Angotzi, G.N.; Barbaro, M.; Raffo, L.; Raspopovic, S.; Navarro, X. Peripheral neural activity recording and stimulation system. *IEEE Trans. Biomed. Circuits Syst.* **2011**, *5*, 368–379. [CrossRef] [PubMed]

14. Xu, J.; Yang, Z. A 50 μW/Ch Artifacts-Insensitive Neural Recorder Using Frequency-Shaping Technique. In Proceedings of the IEEE Custom Integrated Circuits Conference (CICC), San Jose, CA, USA, 22–25 September 2013; pp. 1–4.

15. Xu, J.; Wu, T.; Yang, Z. A power efficient frequency shaping neural recorder with automatic bandwidth adjustment. In Proceedings of the 2014 IEEE International Asian Solid-State Circuit Conference (A-SSCC), Kaohsiung, Taiwan, 10–12 November 2014; pp. 197–200.

16. Xu, J.; Wu, T.; Liu, W.; Yang, Z. A Frequency Shaping Neural Recorder With 3 pF Input Capacitance and 11 Plus 4.5 Bits Dynamic Range. *IEEE Trans. Biomed. Circuits Syst.* **2014**, *8*, 510–527. [CrossRef] [PubMed]

17. Xu, J.; Wu, T.; Yang, Z. A New System Architecture for Future Long-Term High-Density Neural Recording. *IEEE Trans. Circuits Syst. II Express Briefs* **2013**, *60*, 402–406. [CrossRef]

18. Xu, J.; Nguyen, A.T.; Zhao, W.; Guo, H.; Wu, T.; Wiggins, H.; Keefer, E.W.; Lim, H.; Yang, Z. A Low-Noise, Wireless, Frequency-Shaping Neural Recorder. *IEEE J. Emerg. Sel. Top. Circuits Syst.* **2018**, *8*, 187–200. [CrossRef]

19. Nguyen, A.; Xu, J.; Tam, W.; Zhao, W.; Wu, T.; Yang, Z. A Programmable Fully Integrated Microstimulator for Neural Implants and Instrumentation. In Proceedings of the IEEE Biomedical Circuits and Systems Conference, Shanghai, China, 17–19 October 2016; pp. 472–475.

20. Navarro, X.; Krueger, T.B.; Lago, N.; Micera, S.; Stieglitz, T.; Dario, P. A critical review of interfaces with the peripheral nervous system for the control of neuroprostheses and hybrid bionic systems. *J. Peripher. Nerv. Syst.* **2005**, *10*, 229–258. [CrossRef] [PubMed]

21. FitzGerald, J.J.; Lacour, S.P.; McMahon, S.B.; Fawcett, J.W. Microchannels as axonal amplifiers. *IEEE Trans. Biomed. Eng.* **2008**, *55*, 1136–1146. [CrossRef] [PubMed]

22. Cogan, S.F. Neural stimulation and recording electrodes. *Annu. Rev. Biomed. Eng.* **2008**, *10*, 275–309. [CrossRef] [PubMed]

23. Lempka, S.; Johnson, M.; Moffitt, M.; Otto, K.; Kipke, D.; McIntyre, C. Theoretical analysis of intracortical microelectrode recordings. *J. Neural Eng.* **2011**, *8*, 045006. [CrossRef] [PubMed]

24. Yang, Z.; Zhao, Q.; Keefer, E.; Liu, W. Noise characterization, modeling, and reduction for in-*vivo* neural recording. In Proceedings of the Advances in Neural Information Processing Systems, Vancouver, BC, Canada, 7–10 December 2009; pp. 2160–2168.

25. Scholvin, J.; Kinney, J.P.; Bernstein, J.G.; Moore-Kochlacs, C.; Kopell, N.; Fonstad, C.G.; Boyden, E.S. Close-packed silicon microelectrodes for scalable spatially oversampled neural recording. *IEEE Trans. Biomed. Eng.* **2016**, *63*, 120–130. [CrossRef] [PubMed]

26. Garde, K.; Keefer, E.; Botterman, B.; Galvan, P.; Romero-Ortega, M.I. Early interfaced neural activity from chronic amputated nerves. *Front. Neuroeng.* **2009**, *2*, 1–11. [CrossRef] [PubMed]

27. Seo, D.; Neely, R.M.; Shen, K.; Singhal, U.; Alon, E.; Rabaey, J.M.; Carmena, J.M.; Maharbiz, M.M. Wireless recording in the peripheral nervous system with ultrasonic neural dust. *Neuron* **2016**, *91*, 529–539. [CrossRef] [PubMed]

28. Micera, S.; Carpaneto, J.; Raspopovic, S. Control of hand prostheses using peripheral information. *IEEE Rev. Biomed. Eng.* **2010**, *3*, 48–68. [CrossRef] [PubMed]

29. Dweiri, Y.M.; Eggers, T.; McCallum, G.; Durand, D.M. Ultra-low noise miniaturized neural amplifier with hardware averaging. *J. Neural Eng.* **2015**, *12*, 046024. [CrossRef] [PubMed]

30. Gao, H.; Walker, R.; Nuyujukian, P.; Makinwa, K.; Shenoy, K.; Murmannn, B.; Meng, T. HermesE: A 96-Channel Full Data Rate Direct Neural Interface in 0.13 μm CMOS. *IEEE J. Solid-State Circuits* **2012**, *47*, 1043–1055. [CrossRef]

31. Muller, R.; Gambini, S.; Rabaey, J. A 0.013 mm^2, 5μW, DC-Coupled Neural Signal Acquisition IC With 0.5 V Supply. *IEEE J. Solid-State Circuits* **2012**, *47*, 232–243. [CrossRef]

32. Harrison, R.; Watkins, P.; Kier, R.; Lovejoy, R.; Black, D.; Greger, B.; Solzbacher, F. A Low-Power Integrated Circuit for a Wireless 100-Electrode Neural Recording System. *IEEE J. Solid-State Circuits* **2007**, *42*, 123–133. [CrossRef]

33. Harrison, R.; Charles, C. A Low-Power Low-Noise CMOS Amplifier for Neural Recording Applications. *IEEE J. Solid-State Circuits* **2003**, *38*, 958–965. [CrossRef]

34. Wattanapanitch, W.; Fee, M.; Sarpeshkar, R. An Energy-Efficient Micropower Neural Recording Amplifier. *IEEE Trans. Biomed. Circuits Syst.* **2007**, *1*, 136–147. [CrossRef] [PubMed]

35. Lee, S.; Lee, H.; Kiani, M.; Jow, U.; Ghovanloo, M. An Inductively Powered Scalable 32-Channel Wireless Neural Recording System-on-a-Chip for Neuroscience Applications. *IEEE Trans. Biomed. Circuits Syst.* **2010**, *4*, 360–371.

36. Patel, Y.A.; Butera, R.J. Differential fiber-specific block of nerve conduction in mammalian peripheral nerves using kilohertz electrical stimulation. *J. Neurophysiol.* **2015**, *113*, 3923–3929. [CrossRef] [PubMed]

37. Patel, Y.A.; Willsie, A.; Clements, I.P.; Aguilar, R.; Rajaraman, S.; Butera, R.J. Microneedle cuff electrodes for extrafascicular peripheral nerve interfacing. In Proceedings of the 38th Annual International Conference of the IEEE Engineering in Medicine and Biology Society (EMBC), Orlando, FL, USA, 16–20 August 2016; pp. 1741–1744.

38. Wenk, H.N.; Brederson, J.D.; Honda, C.N. Morphine Directly Inhibits Nociceptors in Inflamed Skin. *J. Neurophysiol.* **2006**, *95*, 2083–2097. [CrossRef] [PubMed]

39. Waxman, S.G. Determinants of conduction velocity in myelinated nerve fibers. *Muscle Nerve* **1980**, *3*, 141–150. [CrossRef] [PubMed]

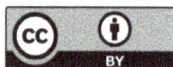

micromachines

MDPI

Article

LED Optrode with Integrated Temperature Sensing for Optogenetics

S. Beatriz Goncalves [1,2], José M. Palha [2], Helena C. Fernandes [2], Márcio R. Souto [2], Sara Pimenta [2], Tao Dong [1,3], Zhaochu Yang [1], João F. Ribeiro [2] and José H. Correia [1,2,*]

[1] Institute of Applied Micro-Nano Science and Technology—IAMNST, Chongqing Key Laboratory of Colleges and Universities on Micro-Nano Systems Technology and Smart Transducing, Chongqing Engineering Laboratory for Detection, Control and Integrated System, National Research Base of Intelligent Manufacturing Service, Chongqing Technology and Business University, Nan'an District, Chongqing 400067, China; sgoncalves@dei.uminho.pt (S.B.G.); Tao.Dong@usn.no (T.D.); Zhaochu.Yang@usn.no (Z.Y.)

[2] CMEMS-UMinho, Department of Industrial Electronics, University of Minho, Guimaraes 4800-058, Portugal; jose.palha@dei.uminho.pt (J.M.P.); a65352@alunos.uminho.pt (H.C.F.); a68554@alunos.uminho.pt (M.R.S.); sara.pimenta@dei.uminho.pt (S.P.); jribeiro@dei.uminho.pt (J.F.R.)

[3] Institute for Microsystems-IMS, Faculty of Technology, Natural Sciences and Maritime Sciences, University of South-Eastern Norway (USN), Postboks 235, 3603 Kongsberg, Norway

* Correspondence: higino.correia@dei.uminho.pt

Received: 23 July 2018; Accepted: 4 September 2018; Published: 17 September 2018

Abstract: In optogenetic studies, the brain is exposed to high-power light sources and inadequate power density or exposure time can cause cell damage from overheating (typically temperature increasing of 2 °C). In order to overcome overheating issues in optogenetics, this paper presents a neural tool capable of assessing tissue temperature over time, combined with the capability of electrical recording and optical stimulation. A silicon-based 8 mm long probe was manufactured to reach deep neural structures. The final proof-of-concept device comprises a double-sided function: on one side, an optrode with LED-based stimulation and platinum (Pt) recording points; and, on the opposite side, a Pt-based thin-film thermoresistance (RTD) for temperature assessing in the photostimulation site surroundings. Pt thin-films for tissue interface were chosen due to its biocompatibility and thermal linearity. A single-shaft probe is demonstrated for integration in a 3D probe array. A 3D probe array will reduce the distance between the thermal sensor and the heating source. Results show good recording and optical features, with average impedance magnitude of 371 kΩ, at 1 kHz, and optical power of 1.2 mW·mm^{-2} (at 470 nm), respectively. The manufactured RTD showed resolution of 0.2 °C at 37 °C (normal body temperature). Overall, the results show a device capable of meeting the requirements of a neural interface for recording/stimulating of neural activity and monitoring temperature profile of the photostimulation site surroundings, which suggests a promising tool for neuroscience research filed.

Keywords: silicon neural probes; LED chip; thermoresistance; temperature monitoring; optogenetics

1. Introduction

The central nervous system is the part of the human body that is least understood, and there is a constant effort to develop novel and useful tools and techniques to increase knowledge about it. Advances in microtechnologies allowed the development of micrometer-size devices that promote the interface between biological neural tissue and physical and electronic components. These instruments, known as neural probes, are usually invasive and with multiple recording sites [1].

Optogenetics is a recent technology that combines genetics and optics to promote stimulation or inhibition in specific photosensitive cells of brain tissue when exposed to light [2]. Combined with optogenetics, neural probes are now capable of simultaneously performing electrophysiology studies and stimulation based on light pulses, with increased cell-type selectivity and millisecond-scale temporal precision [3]. An optogenetic implantable tool is known as optrode.

Optrode designs can be categorized based on its approach to deliver light to the tissue, i.e., as devices integrating customized optical fibers, waveguide systems or LEDs. Commercial optogenetics-compatible neural probes, like those available by Neuronexus or Cambridge Neurotech, integrate exclusively optical fibers as light sources. These approaches present various drawbacks discussed in a recent review [4], where LED probes stand out by overcoming coupling light losses and maximizing delivered light power due to the proximity to target cells. Nowadays, there are various LED-based penetrating optrodes reported in the literature [5–10]. In our work, the LED optrode distinguishes from those designs due to integration of a temperature monitoring system.

Design requirements to manufacture a relevant optrode have been reported [4,11]. One of these challenges consists of preventing cell damage from overheating processes in the stimulation focus area. Thus, it becomes crucial to assess thermal properties of optical sites under various conditions, avoiding inadequate light-power density or exposure time, which can cause overheating. Probes providing in situ heat monitoring can be particularly important in academic scenarios, where photostimulation protocols are frequently customized to each experiment and application.

The core body temperature maintains a near constant (37 °C) over a broad range of environment temperatures. However, the human brain is quite sensitive to fluctuations in temperature [12]. The knowledge on brain temperature fluctuations is limited, and, therefore, there is no established threshold above which irreversible heat-induced brain injury occurs [13]. Haveman et al. reported microscopic damage in many brain areas (striatum, cortex, hippocampus and thalamus) when subjected to temperatures of 39 °C [14]. Rises in temperature of approximately 2 °C have been used as a threshold to prevent brain damage [15], corresponding nowadays to the regulatory limit recommended by the American Association of Medical Instrumentation (AAMI). Nevertheless, this temperature reference may vary based on different species, animal age and brain activity state [13,15].

By directly exposing light sources to tissue, LED-based optrodes could be easily affected by overheating, as a light emitter converts energy into heat. Although previous studies using LED-optrodes have measured rises of temperature in vivo below 1 °C (using thermal cameras) [16,17], monitoring device temperature is crucial, since the lack of monitoring could cause damage of neural cells and greatly disturb brain functions. In this regard, McAlinden et al. [17] and, more recently, Dong et al. [18] measured the heating profile of LEDs using thermal cameras. In this paper, an approach to manufacture a thin-film thermoresistance (RTD) sensor on an LED-optrode body is presented, capable of monitoring the temperature on the stimulation surroundings, preventing temperature rises over 2 °C.

An RTD is a temperature sensor that operates on the measurement principle that a material's electrical resistance changes with temperature. RTDs have been used to add functionality in biodevices for blood flow [19], heart [20], and superficial [21] and deep [22–25] brain measurement applications. For high-performance thermal sensing coupled to an optrode, the proposed thermal sensor needs to meet the following main requirements: (1) Micrometer-size dimensions, so it can be integrated in the probe body. For this application, thin-film RTDs, which enable smaller dimensions, were used. Thin-film RTDs allow good time responses, vibration resistance, and are relatively inexpensive and stable [26]; (2) Good resolution. RTD must be capable of monitoring temperature fluctuations in the medium that are inferior to the maximum increase in temperature before cell damage (2 °C); (3) Temperature range of 0 °C to 60 °C. The wide temperature range was chosen for future applications, e.g., low temperatures required in neurosurgery procedures [27].

In this paper, a Pt RTD was fabricated using microfabrication lithographic methods. Pt RTDs were previously reported in gas [28] and heat [29] flow devices. Pt was chosen due to its biocompatibility and linear behavior with temperature variations within the proposed temperature range [30]. Moreover,

Pt is the material also used for manufacturing the optrode recording sites, which avoids increasing fabrication complexity of the device.

In summary, the focus in this paper is to demonstrate a simple and robust manufacturing approach to produce a multifunction single-shaft probe for rodents' applications, combining optogenetics with electrophysiology and temperature sensing, avoiding overheating processes. An 8 mm deep and 600 μm wide optrode coupled with a 300 μm long Pt RTD was successfully manufactured, capable of spanning nearly any mice brain structure. Electrochemical, optical and thermal characterization of the device is also presented and discussed, which validated the proposed device as a valuable tool in neuroscience.

2. Probe Design

As a device capable of delivering light to neurons and electrically recording them, the proposed optrode comprises 10 recording points (50 × 50 μm^2) around a single LED chip (ELC-470-37, Roithner LaserTechnik GmbH, Wien, Austria) with dimensions of 280 × 310 × 85 μm^3. The recording points are metallic Pt thin-films responsible to convert ionic into electronic currents, and therefore record electrical activity of neurons. The LED chip is the light source, which delivers light to photosensitive engineered brain cells, so they can express the intended biological effect.

The proposed device also includes a Pt RTD for temperature sensing, aiming to prevent tissue overheating around the implant (>2 °C). RTD is positioned in the shaft on the opposite site of the LED and recording sites, which would allow the temperature sensor to be positioned even closer to the stimulation focus of a neighbor shaft. Thus, this design becomes interesting for a close-packed 3D array by assembled individual shafts on top of each other, as illustrated in Figure 1. The goal of this study is to demonstrate a multifunctional probe, thus just the fabrication of a single shaft is demonstrated. The single-shaft configuration could be assembled into an array by the stacking method reported by Chang et al. [31].

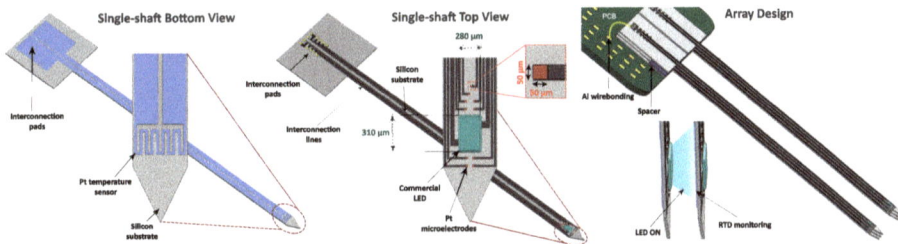

Figure 1. Design of the 3D silicon neural array concept. Pt thermoresistance (RTD) patterning on a single shaft (**bottom view**), and on the opposite side 10 recording sites and an LED chip (**top view**).

RTD design must meet the dimension requirements of the proposed device. Therefore, its geometry was dimensioned based on Pouillet law—Equation (1)—that computes resistance (R) from input resistivity (ρ), length (L) and cross-sectional area (t, thickness and W, width) of the resistive material. To increase RTD's length, a serpentine geometry (Figure 2) and the following parameters were chosen: t = 50 nm; W = 20 μm; theoretical ρ_{Pt} = 1.05 × 10^{-4} Ω·mm; L = 3.27 mm, which resulted in an RTD area of 300 × 520 μm^2, and a theoretical resistance of 343.35 Ω. The higher the length, the higher RTD resistance. Higher resistance can improve accuracy in one side but can also increase device noise. Thus, a sensible trade-off between those factors must be achieved. Top RTD geometry included a large area to promote a better electrical contact between the serpentine and its pads via interconnection lines. Pad resistance represents less than 2% of the RTD resistance:

$$R = \rho \frac{L}{t\,W}. \tag{1}$$

The Si probe outline is 8 mm long and 600 µm wide with a sharp tip that facilitates probe implantation. Probe geometry is accomplished by conventional blade cutting technology, using a diamond blade (NBC-ZB 2050, Disco, Tokyo, Japan) suitable for Si wafer dicing [32].

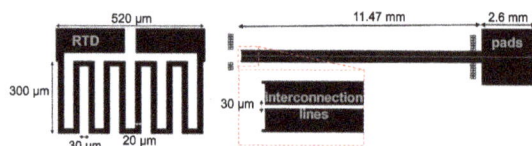

Figure 2. Design and geometrical dimensions of RTD patterned on the optrode.

3. Methods

This section includes the fabrication methodology and electrochemical, optical and thermal characterization processes used to manufacture and validate single-shaft optrodes.

3.1. Microfabrication

Figure 3 summarizes the manufacturing process of the proposed single-shaft device. This process begins with the fabrication of the Pt RTD (Figure 1 Bottom view) followed by the manufacturing of the recording sites and the pads for the LED (Figure 1 Top view). This order aims to start with the simpler fabrication steps first.

In this paper, n-type [100] 525 µm thick Si wafers (with 1 µm of SiO_2 at wafer surface) were selected for producing neural shafts. Si wafers were chosen due to the legacy of microfabrication technologies used for micromachining Si devices, their compatibility to complementary metal-oxide-semiconductor (CMOS) processes, and good mechanical proprieties [33]. The chosen Si doping and crystal orientation ensures the maximum shaft robustness after the dicing step. Initially, Si samples were cleaned with acetone on a 20 min ultrasonic bath, rinsed with deionized (DI) water and heated at 110 °C during 20 min for dehydration. The cleaning step promotes a better adhesion of the substrate surface in the further fabrication steps.

RTD is patterned by photolithography. Firstly, 10 nm of TiO_2 as electrical insulation layer is deposited over the entire wafer to enhance adhesion between SiO_2 surface of wafers and RTD and pad's material [34]. Thin-film deposition parameters are shown in Table 1. Then, spin-coating of a 7 µm thick layer of negative photoresist (AZ nLOF 2070, MicroChemicals GmbH, Ulm, Germany) that is an image reversal resist. The samples are exposed to ultraviolet (UV) light (Figure 3a), using the lithographic mask in Figure 4b, and immersed in developer (AZ 726 MIF, MicroChemicals GmbH) to dissolve the unexposed photoresist (Figure 3b). Next, it is performed a metalization step (50 nm Pt) over the samples (Figure 3(c1)), to create RTD geometry—see Table 1. Then, the negative photoresist layer is lifted by its immersion in stripper (TechniStrip NI555, MicroChemicals GmbH), so that only the thin metal films remain in the substrate (Figure 3(d1)). After RTD patterning, steps (a) to (d) are repeated for interconnection lines and pads fabrication of the RTD using chromium and aluminum (30 nm Cr/600 nm Al) metallic layers (Figure 3(c2,d2))—see Table 1. For these steps, it used the mask in Figure 4a. Finally, an 800 nm Si_3N_4 passivation layer is deposited, thick enough to protect RTD and its pads (Figure 3e).

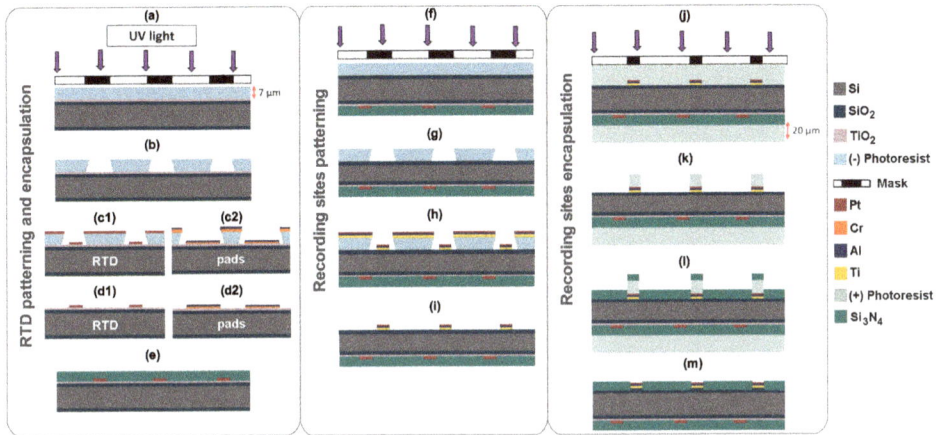

Figure 3. Cross-section view of the neural device fabrication process flow (not to scale).

Table 1. Parameters of the thin-films deposition to manufacture the optrode with RTD.

Material	Technology	Thickness (nm)	Pressure (mbar)	Gas injection (sccm)	Power (W)	Rate (Å/s)
TiO_2	RF sputtering	10	2×10^{-3}	10 (Ar); 2 (O_2)	200	0.1
Pt	DC sputtering	50 and 60	6×10^{-3}	40 (Ar)	100	3.4
Cr	e-beam	30	6.3×10^{-6}	–	140	1
Al	e-beam	600 and 200	5.3×10^{-6}	–	700	23
Ti	e-beam	15	4.3×10^{-6}	–	350	0.8
Si_3N_4	RF sputtering	800 and 400	6×10^{-3}	7 (Ar); 13 (N_2)	150	0.3

After RTD manufacturing, samples undergo lithographic steps (Figure 3f,g), using the lithographic mask shown in Figure 4c, with the same negative photoresist for the interconnection lines, pads and recording sites patterning. Then, Ti/Al/Pt (15 nm/200 nm/60 nm) metalization layers (Figure 3h) are deposited. Deposition parameters are shown in Table 1. Next, samples are again immersed in stripper (TechniStrip NI555, MicroChemicals GmbH), removing photoresist from the wafer (Figure 3i).

Another photolithographic process is performed to protect the samples against silicon dust during the dicing phase, sequentially on top and then on the bottom surface (Figure 3j). In this stage, a layer of 20 µm thick positive photoresist (AZ 4562, MicroChemicals GmbH) is deposited by spin-coating. Then, samples are exposed to UV light, using the mask shown in Figure 4d. Before the developer step in the pattering process, the cutting phase is performed in order to get the desired probe geometry, carried on a DAD-2H/6T dicing machine (Disco, Tokyo, Japan) performing cuts 150 µm thick. The cutting step is performed before passivation step because mechanical cutting of wafers introduces Si dust over the samples. Thus, the resist layer serves as a debris protective layer. Probe outline is set as 8 mm long, 600 µm wide with a sharp tip. A detailed dicing step for probe shaping is reported elsewhere [35], and the tip sharpening process is accomplished by using an automatic cutting program of the dicing machine, which allows the user to set a target cut angle (in this case, 45°).

The samples are then cleaned with DI water, and the photoresist removed with developer (AZ 351B, MicroChemicals GmbH), exposing only passivation area (Figure 3k). A deposition of 400 nm thick layer of Si_3N_4 as the insulation material was performed (Figure 3l), followed by the removal of the resist layer with acetone (top and bottom), exposing the recording sites and LED pads (Figure 3m). Finally, the blue-light LED chip is welded with solder paste (EM907, Kester) on the probe. LED's contact pads are coated with a thin layer of a biocompatible transparent glue (PERMABOND 102), in order to protect LED against wet conditions.

After manufacturing, the optrode is fixed to a Printed Circuit Board (PCB) using cyanoacrylate, and its contact pads are packaged by Al wire-bonding. The PCB provides connection for external hardware for the LED chip and the RTD pads, and it is also coupled to an 18-pin connector (A79014-001, Omnetics, Minneapolis, MN, USA) to ensure external connectivity for recording sites.

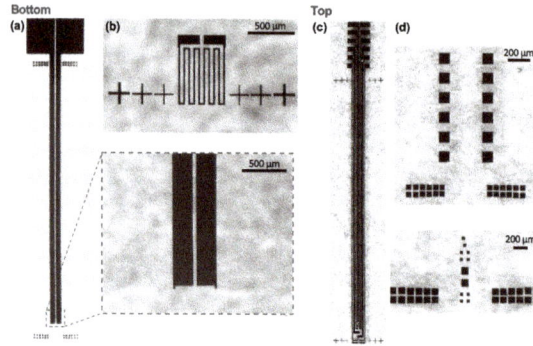

Figure 4. Lithographic masks used during fabrication process of the optrode. (**a**) RTD's interconnection lines and pads; (**b**) RTD; (**c**) interconnection lines, recording sites, and pads for LED and recording points; (**d**) connection pads to external electronics (top) and exposure of recording sites and pads for the LED (bottom).

3.2. Characterization

The characterization process of the proposed device aimed to validate its threefold goal: record electrical neural activity; stimulate engineered target cells sensitive to blue light; and monitor temperature profile around the probe. For this purpose, electrochemical, optical and thermal measurements were performed in vitro.

Electrochemical impedance spectroscopy (EIS) is a valuable technique in assessing the recording capabilities of recording sites and, because the voltage excursions at the electrode are small, may also be a useful and benign method for the in vivo assessment of an electrode [36]. The impedance measurements were performed in a Gamry system (Reference 600, Gamry Instruments, Warminster, PA, USA), using a standard three-electrode configuration: $40 \times 40 \times 0.25$ mm^3 Pt foil as counter electrode, Ag/AgCl as reference electrode, and 0.9% NaCl solution as electrolyte at room temperature. Impedance (Z) was measured for frequencies from 100 Hz to 1 MHz at a constant 10 mV rms alternating current (AC) voltage.

Photostimulation is validated by measuring power intensity of the light source. Reported minimum light intensity to promote a biological effect in engineered cells is 1 mW·mm^{-2} [3]. LED light power was measured using a photodiode sensor (FDS100-CAL, Thorlabs, Newton, NJ, USA), coupled to a 1 mm diameter pinhole. Power (*P*) can be obtained by Equation (2), where I is the current produced by the photodiode and $\Re$ is the photodiode's responsivity at a wavelength (λ):

$$P_\lambda = \frac{I}{\Re_\lambda}. \tag{2}$$

The fabricated RTD was validated by measuring its resistance (*R*) with a four-wire setup. Temperature measurements were carried out inside a temperature-controlled furnace (0 °C to 100 °C and 5 °C steps) coupled to an acquisition system (DT800, dataTaker, Scoresby, Australia) and software interface (DeLogger, dataTaker). A commercial RTD sensor, hereafter refereed as Pt100 (DM-510, Thorlabs), is used as comparative tool for the temperature measurements with a 600 μm long RTD. All measurements were carried out with a current of 0.1 mA. RTD's temperature in °C (*T*) can be obtained with its resistance (R), temperature coefficient of resistance (TCR) and resistance at 0 °C (R_0), as shows Equation (3) [29]. TCR is given by R_0 and R_{100} (resistance at 100 °C)—Equation (4) [37]:

$$T = (\frac{R}{R_0} - 1)TCR, \tag{3}$$

$$TCR = \frac{R_{100} - R_0}{100 \times R_0}. \tag{4}$$

RTD's resistivity (ρ_{exp}) was obtained with van der Pauw method [38]. ρ_{exp} can be obtained with Equations (5)–(7). Moreover, the sensitivity of the RTDs can be obtained as the slope of the second-order polynomial fit [39]:

$$R_A = \frac{V_{12}}{2I_{43}} + \frac{V_{43}}{2I_{12}} \quad \text{and} \quad R_B = \frac{V_{14}}{2I_{23}} + \frac{V_{23}}{2I_{14}}, \tag{5}$$

$$e^{\frac{-\pi R_A}{R_S}} + e^{\frac{-\pi R_B}{R_S}} = 1, \tag{6}$$

$$\rho_{exp} = R_s t. \tag{7}$$

4. Results and Discussion

The fabrication methodology based on lithography, thin-film depositions and blade dicing successfully accomplished an optrode design with the proposed features: 10 recording sites for electrical recording of neural activity; integration of one commercial LED chip for optical stimulation; and, finally, an RTD for temperature sensing of photostimulation site surroundings.

Microfabrication results are shown in Figure 5. Geometrical features of Si optrodes resulted in 8 mm long, 600 µm wide and 525 µm thick shafts. Maximize length of penetrating interfaces is important so the device is capable of reaching deeper neural structures than current designs [5]. For rodents' applications, the probe cross-section must still be optimized. Here, it was demonstrated a single LED-based probe concept, whose dimensions are mainly limited by the dimensions of the commercial LED chip.

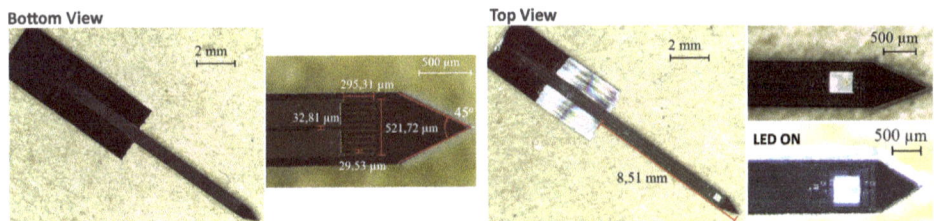

Figure 5. Results of the fabricated optrode integrating 10 Pt recording sites and commercial LED chip, and also a Pt RTD on its backside.

Traditionally, µ-LEDs are either (1) monolithical manufactured onto the device structure by deposition of gallium nitride (GaN) layers on a substrate [5,6]; or (2) integrated in the probe by LED transfer techniques [7–10]. Here, the latter approach due to employment of a commercial LED chip was used. While the first approach has the disadvantage of offering limited substrate choices, manual assembly of LED to substrate represents a harder task and might yield challenges. Further developments to our probe could include monolithically manufacture LEDs onto the probe, as demonstrated by other studies [5,40], ultimately leading to probe cross-section reduction. An interesting approach to address high-footprint commercial LED chips is reported by Ayub et al. [41].

In that study, LED chips are mounted on a thin polyimide-based substrate, stiffened using a micromachined ladder-like silicon structure. This approach avoids thicker probes by transfer LED chip to the surface of a stiff and thick substrate. Although minimizing probes cross-section is a preferable feature, with our approach, wider probes are necessary to accommodate wide LED chips and recording sites.

Light intensity tests for the LED chip, performed with the previously mentioned photodiode and pinhole, measured an average photodiode current of 168.5 μA when a current of 20 mA is applied to the LED. Considering the LED's peak emission wavelength (approximately 470 nm—Figure 6) and the photodiode responsivity of 0.14 A/W (at 470 nm), extracted from its datasheet, LED optical power measured was 1.2 mW·mm^{-2}—Equation (2). This result is superior to the reported minimum light intensity (1 mW·mm^{-2}) to effectively promote photomodulation in brain tissue [3].

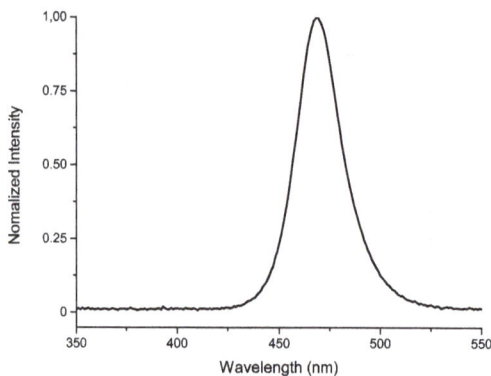

Figure 6. Experimental LED's normalized light intensity as a function of the wavelength. LED peak intensity is at approximately 470 nm.

By using a thermal camera, McAlinden et al. [17] measured the temperature rise profile of 40 μm-diameter GaN LEDS. They reported a maximum temperature rise of 1.5 °C over 100 ms light pulse. More recently, Dong et al. [18] demonstrated temperature variation over pulsed and continuous illumination regime, using the same forward current (20 mA) and a similar area (240 × 320 μm^2) LEDs as the emitter proposed in this paper (250 × 280 μm^2). Their results show a maximum temperature rise of 2 °C for 350 ms pulse light train and 3 °C for continuous irradiance over 15 min. Moreover, this study measured a 400 μm penetration depth (depth that can be attained while still presenting the optical power of 1 mW·mm^{-2}) for a Lambertian emitter.

Another important geometrical characteristic of the probe is its tip shape. Here, Si shafts present sharpened tips (opening angle 45°). Sharp tips on these devices have been reported to result in lower implantation forces, and thus lower tissue damage [42–44].

Currently, a high-density probe includes more than 1000 channels [45–47], which advantageously span wider tissue areas and allow unprecedented opportunities for extracellular electrophysiology studies. On the other hand, they suffer higher signal attenuations by noise and crosstalk wiring. Conversely to these high-density designs, the proposed approach includes more functionalities (optical stimulation and temperature monitoring), not only recording capability as those reports. In fact, Kim et al. demonstrated a multi-functional operation that includes only a single 400 μm^2 Pt recording site [22].

Figure 7 shows EIS average result for the fabricated 50 × 50 μm^2 recording sites. At 1 kHz (neurons firing rate), they show an average of 371 kΩ suitable for electrophysiology studies [48].

RTD was also successfully manufactured on one surface of the device. RTD design includes its location on the opposite side of the LED, which still makes it possible to monitor vicinity of the stimulation focus. In contrast to our approach, RTD could be fabricated next to the LED chip [24]. The downside of this approach is that it takes additional surface space in the shafts and overall complexity of fabrication to integrate an additional sensor. In this sense, Dehkhoda et al. reported an interesting study by presenting a temperature monitoring system that uses the LED both as emitter and its own sensor, taking advantage of the LED reverse current to measure the generated heat at the surface of the device.

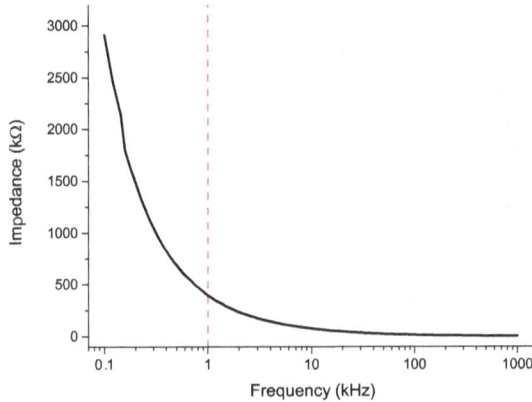

Figure 7. Impedance results for the Pt 50 × 50 µm^2 recording sites.

Experimental Pt resistivity over the temperature range defined in the requirements (0 °C to 60 °C) is shown in Figure 8, where higher temperatures result in higher values of resistivity, as expected. Average RTD resistivity was 2.33 × 10^{-4} Ω·mm, similar to theoretical value (1.05 × 10^{-4} Ω·mm). RTD's resistance at 0 °C and 100 °C, R_0 and R_{100}, respectively, were also measured to obtain the *TCR* coefficient of the fabricated RTD (Equation (4)). Table 2 shows the resistance values for RTD and Pt100. Pt100 *TCR* magnitude is consistent with the theoretical value of bulk pure platinum (0.0039 °C^{-1}) [49]. RTD's sensitivity is 2.4 Ω·°C^{-1} in the temperature range of 35 °C to 40 °C. This value is in accordance with Pt RTDs reported by Fiedler et al., where Pt1000 and Pt5000 sensitivities were 1.7 Ω·°C^{-1} and 8.8 Ω·°C^{-1}, respectively [50]. Table 3 compares the sensitivity and *TCR* values of the RTD in this work and previously reported studies.

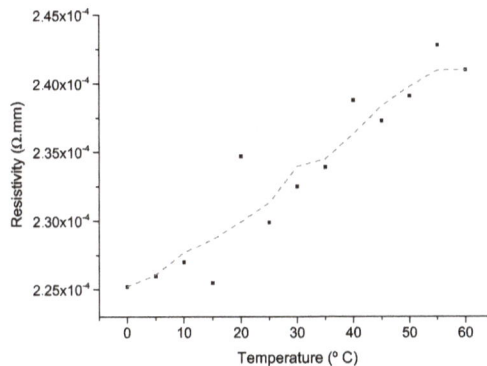

Figure 8. RTD's resistivity vs. temperature. The dashed line results from a processing data five-point adjacent-averaging smoothing method, which replaces a point using the average of its five closest points.

Table 2. Resistance values at 0 °C (R_0) and 100 °C (R_{100}) for RTD and commercial Pt100. The calculated *TCR* value is also included.

Sample	R_0	R_{100}	TCR
Pt100	100.23 Ω	137.71 Ω	0.0037 °C^{-1}
RTD	1548.58 Ω	1787.55 Ω	0.0015 °C^{-1}

Table 3. Comparison of RTD developed in this work and previous studies.

Ref.	Material	Sensitivity (Ω·°C^{-1})	TCR (°C^{-1})	Resolution (°C)
[19]	Au	-	-	0.03
[20]	Poly-Si	-	-	0.9
[49]	Pt	0.781	0.0028	-
[50]	Pt	8.8	-	0.5
[51]	Pt	-	0.0015	1
[52]	Au	-	0.0032	0.25
[53]	Pt	1.485	0.0035	-
This work	Pt	2.4	0.0015	0.19

Figure 9 presents temperature measurements with Pt100 and RTD over a wide range of temperatures (0 °C to 100 °C), and at an approximately normal body temperature (35 °C)—Figure 10. These results show RTD's accurate temperature measurements in the entire range of temperatures. In addition, it is noticeable that RTD measurements show higher noise amplitudes relative to the Pt100 results, which might be related with higher thermal mass of the Pt100. In particular, at 37 °C (normal body temperature), RTD has an average and maximum error of 0.19 °C and 0.64 °C, respectively. This means that temperature recording with the fabricated RTD might provide on average an estimated difference of 0.19 °C from real tissue temperature. These results are suitable for monitoring temperature variations below 2 °C required in this application. In Table 3, it is possible to see the final resolution is better than most RTD reported. In fact, even the RTD maximum error (0.64 °C) presented is lower than most approaches reported to monitor brain thermal variation. Therefore, we believe a average error of 0.19 °C is a promising result for this kind of devices.

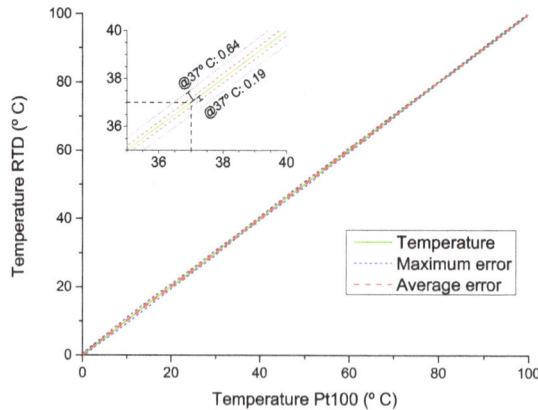

Figure 9. Comparative temperature measurements using Pt100 vs. RTD (green line). Measurement accuracy is given by error lines: maximum error (blue dashed line) and average error (red dashed line).

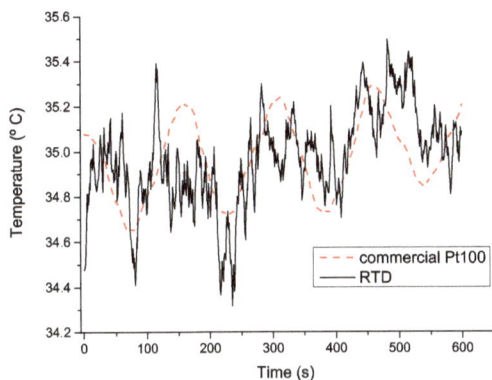

Figure 10. Measurements temperature results with a commercial Pt100 and the proposed RTD when medium is set to 35 °C.

Passivation layer on RTD is a required step with a twofold goal: (1) electrical insulation, and (2) avoiding electrical stimulation of neurons in its vicinity. Current as low as 10 µA has been reported to promote microstimulation of neurons as far as four millimeters away [54]. One possible limiting factor in RTD performance (response time) is the use of Si_3N_4 as a passivation layer due to low thermal conductivity. Fekete et al. demonstrated, however, a good thermal monitoring in mice tissue using a thin-film Pt sensor insulated with a Si_3N_4 layer [24].

Future work for this optrode-RTD combination design will include initially in vitro measurements of the environment thermal profile with the LED on, followed by in vivo validation of thermal brain monitoring in the vicinity of LED-based stimulation and electrophysiology studies.

5. Conclusions

The fabrication and in vitro validation of a single LED optrode was demonstrated in this paper. Its design accommodates optical stimulation, electrophysiological recording sites and temperature sensing with an RTD thin-film integrated in a silicon probe. The proposed multi-functional device is envisioned to help validated neural probes with optical stimulation capability, avoiding overheating processes. The manufacturing methodology relied on standard microfabrication technologies: lithography, thin-film depositions and low-cost traditional mechanical blade dicing technology. Fabrication results suggest a robust probe design, with 8 mm long single-shaft with a sharp tip. The 2D dicing methodology, applied to silicon wafers, facilitates the integration with patterning process, frequently used in MEMS and CMOS industry. Low impedance values of recording sites and sufficient light power results show great potential for this design to modulate neural activity in both cortical and deeper brain regions. RTD's average accuracy of 0.2 °C suggests that this is a promising tool for thermal mapping of brain tissue in the vicinity of the stimulation focus.

Author Contributions: The work presented in this paper was a collaboration of all authors. J.M.P., H.C.F., M.R.S., S.P. and J.F.R. conceived and designed the experiments; J.M.P., H.C.F. and S.P. performed the experiments; S.B.G., S.P., J.F.R. and J.H.C. analysed the data; T.D. and Z.Y. contributed with analysis tools; S.B.G. wrote the paper.

Acknowledgments: This work is supported by the Innovation Team for Chongqing Higher Education Construction Plan on "Smart Micro/Nano-Systems Technology and Applications" with project number CXTDX201601025. S. B. Goncalves is supported by the Portuguese Foundation for Science and Technology (FCT) under grant PD/BD/105931/2014, MIT Portugal Program. This work is also supported by FCT with the reference project UID/EEA/04436/2013, by FEDER funds through the COMPETE 2020—Programa Operacional Competitividade e Internacionalizacão (POCI) with the reference project POCI-01-0145-FEDER-006941 and project PTDC/CTM-REF/28406/2017 (02/SAICT/2017). ANI also supports this work through the Brain-Lighting project by FEDER funds through Portugal 2020, COMPETE 2020 with the reference POCI-01-0247-FEDER-003416.

Conflicts of Interest: The authors declare no conflict of interest.

Micromachines **2018**, *9*, 473

Abbreviations

The following abbreviations are used in this manuscript:

RTD   Resistance Temperature Detector
e-beam   Electron-Beam
EIS   Electrochemical Impedance Spectroscopy
UV   Ultraviolet
DI   Deionized
TCR   Temperature Coefficient of Resistance
CMOS   Complementary Metal-Oxide-Semiconductor
RF   Radio-Frequency
DC   Direct Current
AC   Alternating Current

References

1. Maharbiz, M.M.; Muller, R.; Alon, E.; Rabaey, J.M.; Carmena, J.M. Reliable Next-Generation Cortical Interfaces for Chronic Brain–Machine Interfaces and Neuroscience. *Proc. IEEE* **2017**, *105*, 73–82. [CrossRef]
2. Deisseroth, K. Optogenetics: 10 years of microbial opsins in neuroscience. *Nat. Neurosci.* **2015**, *18*, 1213–1225. [CrossRef] [PubMed]
3. Boyden, E.S.; Zhang, F.; Bamberg, E.; Nagel, G.; Deisseroth, K. Millisecond-timescale, genetically targeted optical control of neural activity. *Nat. Neurosci.* **2005**, *8*, 1263–1268. [CrossRef] [PubMed]
4. Goncalves, S.B.; Ribeiro, J.F.; Silva, A.F.; Costa, R.M.; Correia, J.H. Design and Manufacturing Challenges of Optogenetic Neural Interfaces: A Review. *J. Neural Eng.* **2017**, *14*, 041001. [CrossRef] [PubMed]
5. Wu, F.; Stark, E.; Ku, P.; Wise, K.D.; Buzsáki, G.; Yoon, E. Monolithically Integrated μLEDs on Silicon Neural Probes for High-Resolution Optogenetic Studies in Behaving Animals. *Neuron* **2015**, *88*, 1136–1148. [CrossRef] [PubMed]
6. Scharf, R.; Tsunematsu, T.; McAlinden, N.; Dawson, M.D.; Sakata, S.; Mathieson, K. Depth-specific optogenetic control in vivo with a scalable, high-density μLED neural probe. *Nat. Sci. Rep.* **2016**, *8*, 28381. [CrossRef] [PubMed]
7. Kwon, K.Y.; Sirowatka, B.; Weber, A.; Li, W. Opto-μEcoG Array: A Hybrid Neural Interface With Transparent μEcoG Electrode Array and Integrated LEDs for Optogenetics. *IEEE Trans. Biomed. Circuits Syst.* **2013**, *7*, 593–600. [CrossRef] [PubMed]
8. Cao, H.; Gu, L.; Mohanty, S.K.; Chiao, J.C. An Integrated μ-LED Optrode for Optogenetic Stimulation and Electrical Recording. *IEEE Trans. Biomed. Eng.* **2013**, *60*, 225–229. [CrossRef] [PubMed]
9. Ayub, S.; Gossler, C.; Schwaerzle, M.; Klein, E.; Paul, O.; Schwarz, U.T.; Ruther, P. High-Density Probe with Integrated Thin-Film Micro Light Emitting Diodes (μ-LEDs) For Optogenetic Applications. In Proceedings of the 2016 IEEE 29th International Conference on Micro Electro Mechanical Systems (MEMS), Shanghai, China, 24–28 January 2016; pp. 379–382.
10. Goßler, C.; Bierbrauer, C.; Moser, R.; Kunzer, M.; Holc, K.; Pletschen, W.; Köhler, K.; Wagner, J.; Schwaerzle, M.; Ruther, P.; et al. GaN-based micro-LED arrays on flexible substrates for optical cochlear implants. *J. Phys. D Appl. Phys.* **2014**, *47*, 205401. [CrossRef]
11. Alt, M.T.; Fiedler, E.; Rudmann, L.; Ordonez, J.S.; Ruther, P.; Stieglitz, T. Let There Be Light—Optoprobes for Neural Implants. *Proc. IEEE* **2017**, *105*, 101–138. [CrossRef]
12. Wang, H.; Wang, B.; Normoyle, K.P.; Jackson, K.; Spitler, K.; Sharrock, M.F.; Miller, C.M.; Best, C.; Llano, D.; Du, R. Brain temperature and its fundamental properties: A review for clinical neuroscientists. *Front. Neurosci.* **2014**, *8*, 307. [CrossRef] [PubMed]
13. Kiyatkin, E.A. Brain Hyperthermia During Physiological and Pathological Conditions: Causes, Mechanisms, and Functional Implications. *Curr. Neurovasc. Res.* **2004**, *1*, 77-90. [CrossRef]
14. Haveman, J.; Sminia, P.; Wondergem, J.; van der Zee, J.; Hulshof, M.C. Effects of hyperthermia on the central nervous system: What was learnt from animal studies? *Int. J. Hyperth.* **2005**, *21*, 473-487. [CrossRef] [PubMed]
15. Childs, C. Human brain temperature: Regulation, measurement and relationship with cerebral trauma: Part 1. *Br. J. Neurosurg.* **2008**, *22*, 486–496. [CrossRef] [PubMed]

16. Kim, S.; Tathireddy, P.; Normann, R.A.; Solzbacher, F. In vitro and in vivo study of temperature increases in the brain due to a neural implant. In Proceedings of the 2007 3rd International IEEE/EMBS Conference on Neural Engineering, Kohala Coast, HI, USA, 2–5 May 2007; pp. 163–166.

17. McAlinden, N.; Massoubre, D.; Richardson, E.; Gu, E.; Sakata, S.; Dawson, M.D.; Mathieson, K. Thermal and optical characterization of micro-LED probes for in vivo optogenetic neural stimulation. *Opt. Lett.* **2013**, *38*, 992–994. [CrossRef] [PubMed]

18. Dong, N.; Berlinguer-Palmini, R.; Soltan, A.; Ponon, N.; O'Neil, A.; Travelyan, A.; Maaskant, P.; Degenaar, P.; Sun, X. Opto-electro-thermal optimization of photonic probes for optogenetic neural stimulation. *J. Biophotonics* **2018**, *30*, e201700358. [CrossRef] [PubMed]

19. Li, C.; Wu, P.M.; Hartings, J.A.; Wu, Z.; Cheyuo, C.; Wang, P.; LeDoux, D.; Shutter, L.A.; Ramaswamy, B.R.; Ahn, C.H.; et al. Micromachined lab-on-a-tube sensors for simultaneous brain temperature and cerebral blood flow measurements. *Biomed. Microdevices* **2012**, *14*, 759–768. [CrossRef] [PubMed]

20. Li, K.S.; Chao, T.Y.; Cheng, Y.T.; Chen, J.K.; Chen, Y.S. Temperature sensing probe integrated with an SU-8 flexible ribbon cable for heart surgery application. In Proceedings of the 2011 16th International Solid-State Sensors, Actuators and Microsystems Conference, Beijing, China , 5–9 June 2011; pp. 2180–2183.

21. Wu, Z.; Li, C.; Hartings, J.; Narayan, R.K.; Ahn, C. Polysilicon-based flexible temperature sensor for brain monitoring with high spatial resolution. *J. Micromech. Microeng.* **2016**, *27*, 025001. [CrossRef]

22. Kim, T.I.; McCall, J.G.; Jung, Y.H.; Huang, X.; Siuda, E.R.; Li, Y.; Song, J.; Song, Y.M.; Pao, H.A.; Kim, R.H.; et al. Injectable, Cellular- Scale Optoelectronics with Applications for Wireless Optogenetics. *Science* **2013**, *340*, 211–216. [CrossRef] [PubMed]

23. Lee, B.C.; Lim, Y.G.; Kim, K.H.; Lee, S.; Moon, S. Microfabricated neural thermocouple arrays probe for brain research. In Proceedings of the 2009 International Solid-State Sensors, Actuators and Microsystems Conference, Denver, CO, USA, 21–25 June 2009; pp. 338–341.

24. Fekete, Z.; Csernai, M.; Kocsis, K.; Horváth, A.C.; Pongrácz, A.; Barthó, P. Simultaneous in vivo recording of local brain temperature and electrophysiological signals with a novel neural probe. *J. Neural Eng.* **2017**, *14*, 34001. [CrossRef] [PubMed]

25. Billard, M.W.; Basantani, H.A.; Horn, M.W.; Gluckman, B.J.A. Flexible Vanadium Oxide Thermistor Array for Localized Temperature Field Measurements in Brain. *IEEE Sens. J.* **2016**, *16*, 2211–2212. [CrossRef]

26. Innovative Sensor Technology, I.S.T.A.G.; Temperature Sensors. Available online: https://wwwist-agcom/en/products-services/temperature-sensors (accessed on 22 March 2018).

27. Galvin, I.M.; Levy, R.; Boyd, J.G.; Day, A.G.; Wallace, M.C. Cooling for cerebral protection during brain surgery. *Cochrane Database Syst. Rev.* **2015**, *1*, CD006638. [CrossRef] [PubMed]

28. Mailly, F.; Giani, A.; Bonnot, R.; Delannoy, F.; Foucaran, A.; Boyer, A. Anemometer with hot platinum thin film. *Sens. Actuators A Phys.* **2001**, *94*, 32–38. [CrossRef]

29. Zribi, A.; Barthès, M.; Bègot, S.; Lanzetta, F.; Rauch, J.Y.; Moutarlier, V. Design, fabrication and characterization of thin film resistances for heat flux sensing application. *Sens. Actuators A Phys.* **2016**, *245*, 26–39. [CrossRef]

30. Aslam, M.; Hatfield, J.V. Fabrication of thin film microheater for gas sensors on polyimide membrane. *Proc. IEEE Sens.* **2003**, *1*, 389–392. [CrossRef]

31. Chang, C.; Chiou, J. Development of a Three Dimensional Neural Sensing Device by a Stacking Method. *Sensors* **2010**, *10*, 4238–4252. [CrossRef]

32. Disco Electroformed Bond Blades: NBC-Zseries. Available online: https://www.disco.co.jp/eg/products/catalog/pdf/nbcz.pdf (accessed on 7 August 2018).

33. Dean, R.N.; Luque, A. Applications of Microelectromechanical Systems in Industrial Processes and Services. *IEEE Trans. Ind. Electron.* **2009**, *56*, 913–925. [CrossRef]

34. Vieira, E.M.F.; Ribeiro, J.F.; Sousa, R.; Silva, M.M.; Dupont, L.; Goncalves, L.M. Titanium Oxide Adhesion Layer for High Temperature Annealed $Si/Si_3N_4/TiO_x/Pt/LiCoO_2$ Battery Structures. *J. Electron. Mater.* **2016**, *45*, 910–916. [CrossRef]

35. Goncalves, S.B.; Ribeiro, J.F.; Silva, A.F.; Correia, J.H. High Aspect Ratio Neural Probe using conventional Blade Dicing. *J. Phys. Conf. Ser.* **2016**, *757*, 012011. [CrossRef]

36. Chang, B.Y.; Park, S.M. Electrochemical Impedance Spectroscopy. *Annu. Rev. Anal. Chem.* **2010**, *3*, 207–229. [CrossRef] [PubMed]

37. Iles, G.S.; Tindall, R.F. A Thick Film Platinum Resistance Thermometer. *Platin. Met. Rev.* **1975**, *19*, 42–47.

38. Van der Pauw, L.J. A Method of Measuring the Resistivity Hall Coefficient on Lamellae of Arbitrary Shape. *Philips Tech. Rev.* **1958**, *20*, 220–224. [CrossRef]
39. Moser, E.; Mathiesen, I.; Andersen, P. Association between brain temperature and dentate field potentials in exploring and swimming rats. *Science* **1993**, *259*, 1324–1326. [CrossRef] [PubMed]
40. Mcalinden, N.; Gu, E.; Dawson, M.D.; Sakata, S.; Mathieson, K. Optogenetic activation of neocortical neurons in vivo with a sapphire-based micro-scale LED probe. *Front. Neural Circuits* **2015**, *9*, 25. [CrossRef] [PubMed]
41. Ayub, S.; Gentet, L.J.; Fiaáth, R.; Schwaerzle, M.; Borel, M.; David, F.; Barthó, P.; Ulbert, I.; Paul, O.; Ruther, P. Hybrid intracerebral probe with integrated bare LED chips for optogenetic studies. *Biomed. Microdevices* **2017**, *19*, 49. [CrossRef] [PubMed]
42. Jensen, W.; Yoshida, K.; Hofmann, U.G. In-Vivo Implant Mechanics of Flexible, Silicon-Based ACREO Microelectrode Arrays in Rat Cerebral Cortex. *IEEE Trans. Biomed. Eng.* **2006**, *53*, 934–940. [CrossRef] [PubMed]
43. Han, M.; Manoonkitiwongsa, P.S.; Wang, C.X.; McCreery, D.B. In Vivo Validation of Custom-Designed Silicon-Based Microelectrode Arrays for Long-Term Neural Recording and Stimulation. *IEEE Trans. Biomed. Eng.* **2012**, *59*, 346–354. [CrossRef] [PubMed]
44. Sharp, A.A.; Ortega, A.M.; Restrepo, D.; Curran-Everett, D.; Gall, K. In Vivo Penetration Mechanics and Mechanical Properties of Mouse Brain Tissue at Micrometer Scales. *IEEE Trans. Biomed. Eng.* **2009**, *56*, 45–53. [CrossRef] [PubMed]
45. Lopez, C.M.; Putzeys, J.; Raducanu, B.C.; Ballini, M.; Wang, S.; Andrei, A.; Rochus, V.; Vandebriel, R.; Severi, S.; Hoof, C.; et al. A Neural Probe With Up to 966 Electrodes and Up to 384 Configurable Channels in 0.13 µm SOI CMOS. *IEEE Trans. Biomed. Eng.* **2017**, *11*, 510–522. [CrossRef]
46. Scholvin, J.; Kinney, J.P.; Bernstein, J.G.; Moore-Kochlacs, C.; Kopell, N.; Fonstad, C.G.; Boyden, E.S. Close-Packed Silicon Microelectrodes for Scalable Spatially Oversampled Neural Recording. *IEEE Trans. Biomed. Eng.* **2016**, *63*, 120–130. [CrossRef] [PubMed]
47. Raducanu, B.C.; Yazicioglu, R.F.; Lopez, C.M.; Ballini, M.; Putzeys, J.; Wang, S.; Andrei, A.; Rochus, V.; Welkenhuysen, M.; Helleputte, N.V.; et al. Time Multiplexed Active Neural Probe with 1356 Parallel Recording Sites. *Sensors* **2017**, *17*, 2388. [CrossRef] [PubMed]
48. Negi, S.; Bhandari, R.; Rieth, L.; Solzbacher, F. In vitro comparison of sputtered iridium oxide and platinum-coated neural implantable microelectrode arrays. *Biomed. Mater.* **2010**, *5*, 015007. [CrossRef] [PubMed]
49. Xiao, S.Y.; Che, L.F.; Li, X.X.; Wang, Y.L. A novel fabrication process of MEMS devices on polyimide flexible substrates. *Microelectron. Eng.* **2008**, *85*, 452–457. [CrossRef]
50. Fiedler, E.; Cruz, M.F.; Monjara, O.F.; Stieglitz, T.; Member, S. Evaluation of Thin-film Temperature Sensors for Integration in Neural Probes. In Proceedings of the 2015 7th International IEEE/EMBS Conference on Neural Engineering (NER), Montpellier, France, 22–24 April 2015; pp. 22–24.
51. Moser, Y.; Gijs, M.A.M. Miniaturized Flexible Temperature Sensor. *J. Microelectromech. Syst.* **2007**, *16*, 1349–1354. [CrossRef]
52. Wang, J.; Xie, H.; Chung, T.; Chan, L.L.H.; Pang, S.W. Neural Probes with Integrated Temperature Sensors for Monitoring Retina and Brain Implantation and Stimulation. *IEEE Trans. Neural Syst. Rehabil. Eng.* **2017**, *25*, 1663–1673. [CrossRef] [PubMed]
53. Yang, Z.; Zhang, Y.; Itoh, T.; Maeda, R. Flexible Implantable Microtemperature Sensor Fabricated on Polymer Capillary by Programmable UV Lithography With Multilayer Alignment for Biomedical Applications. *J. Microelectromech. Syst.* **2014**, *23*, 21–29. [CrossRef]
54. Tehovnik, E.J. Electrical stimulation of neural tissue to evoke behavioral responses. *J. Neurosci. Methods* **1996**, *65*, 1–17. [CrossRef]

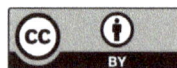

micromachines

MDPI

Article

Scalable, Modular Three-Dimensional Silicon Microelectrode Assembly via Electroless Plating

Jörg Scholvin [1], Anthony Zorzos [1], Justin Kinney [1], Jacob Bernstein [1], Caroline Moore-Kochlacs [1,2], Nancy Kopell [2], Clifton Fonstad [1] and Edward S. Boyden [1,*]

[1] Massachusetts Institute of Technology, Cambridge, MA 02139, USA; scholvin@MIT.EDU (J.S.); anthonyzorzos@gmail.com (A.Z.); jkinney@mit.edu (J.K.); jgbernstein@gmail.com (J.B.); caromk@gmail.com (C.M.-K.); fonstad@mit.edu (C.F.)

[2] Department of Mathematics, Boston University, Boston, MA 02215, USA; nk@math.bu.edu

[*] Correspondence: esb@media.mit.edu

Received: 31 July 2018; Accepted: 24 August 2018; Published: 30 August 2018

Abstract: We devised a scalable, modular strategy for microfabricated 3-D neural probe synthesis. We constructed a 3-D probe out of individual 2-D components (arrays of shanks bearing close-packed electrodes) using mechanical self-locking and self-aligning techniques, followed by electroless nickel plating to establish electrical contact between the individual parts. We detail the fabrication and assembly process and demonstrate different 3-D probe designs bearing thousands of electrode sites. We find typical self-alignment accuracy between shanks of <0.2° and demonstrate orthogonal electrical connections of 40 µm pitch, with thousands of connections formed electrochemically in parallel. The fabrication methods introduced allow the design of scalable, modular electrodes for high-density 3-D neural recording. The combination of scalable 3-D design and close-packed recording sites may support a variety of large-scale neural recording strategies for the mammalian brain.

Keywords: electrode array; microelectrodes; neural recording; silicon probe; three-dimensional; electroless plating

1. Introduction

Silicon microfabricated neural probes [1–10] offer the capability of scalable neural recording in acute and chronic neuroscience experiments [8–11], since hundreds of, or more, electrode recording sites can be created on an implantable 1-D or 2-D shank using scalable microfabrication techniques. Recently we designed, implemented and used 2-D silicon microelectrode arrays bearing close-packed recording sites, designed with small enough spacing to enable spatial oversampling of extracellular action potentials—and thus, scalable, tetrode-style analysis to be performed on the data obtained [12]. Here we explore another key aspect of scalability, namely how to fabricate silicon microfabricated neural probes with electrode pads distributed in 3-D, not just 2-D, patterns. 1-D and 2-D microfabricated silicon probes primarily record in a small part of the brain and by design cover a one- or two-dimensional subset of the brain. Most silicon based probe technologies have the ability to record in 2-D, either in a vertical plane ("Michigan probes" [2]) with recording sites along each shank using in-plane microfabrication, or a horizontal plane ("Utah array" [13]) with recording sites at the shank tips, using bulk micromachining techniques.

1.1. Overview of 3-D Approaches

To record from an entire region of the brain, or across multiple regions simultaneously, the neural recording sites need to cover a 3-D volume. Therefore, a 3-D probe needs to consist of many shanks, each bearing multiple electrode recording sites that record at many points along its length. But, because microfabricated devices are currently inherently two-dimensional, combining them into a 3-D structure presents engineering challenges, such as the question of how to create mechanical and electrical connectivity between individual 2-D parts, in a scalable, modular way. Since the introduction of the first 3-D neural probes comprised out of individual 2-D parts [14], different technologies for assembling arrays have been explored: ultrasonic bonding [15–17], pressed contacts [18–20], solder reflow [21] (also used in early explorations for 3-D integrated circuits (ICs) [22]), conductive silver paste [23], post-packaging nickel or gold electrolytic plating [24,25], folding parts [26,27], self-assembly [28], electrostatic- [29] or magnetic-field [30] assisted assembly, die stacking with wirebonding [31] and different types of packaged stacking [10,32–35]. These solutions all share the principle of combining (or, in the case of [26–30], folding) individual 2-D probes in order to create 3-D arrays and are summarized in Table 1. The above studies primarily focus on pioneering new modalities of 3-D assembly. Our primary focus is to explore the scalability of 3-D assembly of modular microfabricated neural probes, aiming to develop robust, powerful methods for assembling probes bearing many thousands of electrode recording sites and beyond. We approach this by introducing electroless plating as a way of forming, in a simple single step, all of the electrical connections at the same time—thereby enabling a new efficient and scalable fabrication method.

Our methods can subsequently be combined with heterogeneous integration of amplifier circuits [36] to reduce the total number of actual wires leaving the device, for example, through wirebonds to a circuit board, because the external package size determines which in vivo recording scenarios the probe can be used in and can additionally govern the scale that is meaningfully achievable with a given probe design.

Table 1. 3-D Probe Fabrication Technologies.

Reference	Method [a]	Design [b]	Total Sites	Connection [k] Count	Pitch
Nordhausen 1996 [9]	Monolithic	10 × 10 × 1	100	n/a	n/a
Hoogerwerf 1991 [14]	Electrolytic	4 × 4 × 16	256	16 [g]	-
Hoogerwerf 1994 [24]	Electrolytic	4 × 4 × 8	128	16 [g]	-
Barz 2013 [25]	Electrolytic	4 × 4 × 4	64	64	70 μm
Herwik 2009 [18]	Pressed	4 × 4 × 5	80	80	70 μm
Kisban 2010 [20]	Pressed	2 × 4 × 5	80	80	35 μm [d]
Aarts 2011 [19]	Pressed	4 × 4 × 5	80	80	70 μm [e]
Bai 2000 [16]	Ultrasonic	4 × 4 × 4	32	32 [g]	-
Yao 2007 [17]	Ultrasonic	4 × 8 × 32	1024	32 [g]	-
Perlin 2008 [15]	Ultrasonic	4 × 4 × 4	64	64	40 μm
Malhi 1987 [c] [22]	Solder	9 × 1 × 22	198	198	-
Cheng 2014 [21]	Solder	5 × 4 × 5	100	100	150 μm
Lee 2009 [23]	Silver Paste	4 × 4 × 1	16	16	800 μm [e]
Takeuchi 2004 [30]	Folding	2 × 3 × 3	18	n/a	n/a
Wang 2010 [28]	Folding	2 × 2 × 4	32	n/a	n/a
John 2011 [26]	Folding	3 × 3 × 2	18	n/a	n/a
Chen 2011 [29]	Folding	2 × 2 × 2	8	n/a	n/a
Merriam 2011 [a] [27]	Folding	4 × 4 × 4	64	n/a	n/a
Chiou 2010 [31]	Die Stacking	4 × 4 × 4	64	n/a	n/a
Rios 2016 [37]	Die Stacking	4 × 4 × 64	1024	256	200 μm
Du 2009 [33]	Package	4 × 2 × 8 [h]	64	n/a	n/a
Langhals 2009 [35]	Package	4 × 4 × 4	64	n/a	n/a
Merriam 2011 [b] [32]	Package	5 × 4 × 8	160	n/a	n/a
Barz 2014 [34]	Package	2 × 2 × 8	32	n/a	n/a
Barz 2017 [34]	Package	2 × 2 × 8	32	n/a	n/a
Shobe 2015 [10]	Package	4 × 4 × 64 [f]	1024	n/a	n/a
Michon 2016 [38]	Micro-Drive	16 × 2 × 8	256	n/a	n/a

[a] Abbreviated methods, we define as "Package" assembly a method that uses non-microfabricated parts to combine 2-D probes. [b] Inserts/probe × Shanks/insert × Sites/shank. [c] Not used in a neural probe but relevant 3-D IC exploration. [d] Design conditions had a very strong impact on connection yield. [e] Not specified in the paper but inferred from images and drawings or previous work. [f] Design varies slightly from a uniform 4 × 4 × 64 configuration

to accommodate brain region under study. ^g Active probe that uses multiplexing to reduce the connection count. ^h Double sided shanks. ^k The need for fine-pitched connection will vary, depending on the total number of recording sites, the target animal model and recording volume (which sets the space in which the connections must be made).

1.2. Creating a Scalable 3-D Probe Design

Virtual reality awake head-fixed setups [39], for example, for mouse behavior, have become widespread in neuroscience because they enable neural recording and imaging during animal behavior experiments, without the weight and size constraints of freely moving animal behavior experiments [40]. A design example of a 3-D scalable probe appropriate for such an experiment is shown in Figure 1. The need for scalability is particularly important for 3-D probe arrays, because to tile a 3-D volume, one needs a far greater number of recording sites than required to tile a 2-D section.

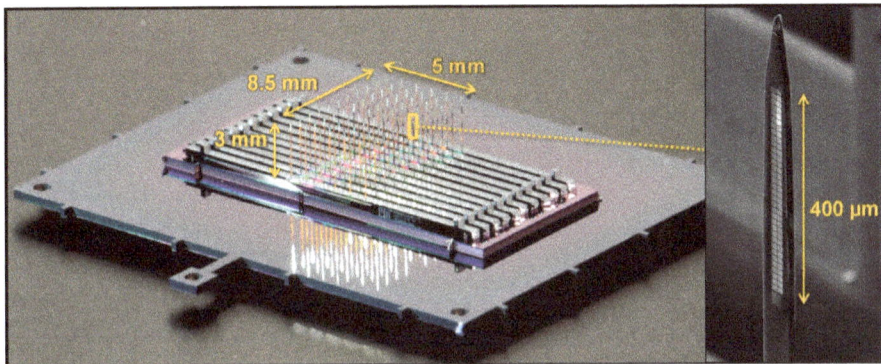

Figure 1. Photograph of a high-density 3-D probe, consisting of a 6 × 11 grid of shanks. Each shank contains a set of 2 × 34 close packed recording sites (as seen in the scanning electron microscope (SEM) inset), for a total number of 4488 sites across a volume of 5 × 8.5 × 0.4 mm.

We describe new principles for scalable, modular mechanical and electrical assembly of 3-D structures, using self-locking mechanical components that allow easy by-hand assembly and we introduce the use of electroless nickel (EN) plating to form orthogonal electrical connections between individual parts in a scalable way. The electrical connections are formed without the need for electrical access to the sites, relieving potential constraints on future monolithic or heterogeneously integrated neural amplifier circuits (as outlined in [36]). Our method therefore supports equally well passive and active probes (i.e., probes without and with integrated amplifiers or other circuitry, respectively) and is carried out prior to probe packaging, relieving constraints on the final packaging steps.

We utilize our close-packed 2-D probe technology of [12] as the unit building block for our 3-D arrays. With probe designs scaling possibly into the thousands of recording sites and beyond [41], the close-packed recording sites can be of benefit in automating the large-scale data analysis that will be necessary when recording from a large number of sites across many brain regions.

1.3. Scope of the Design

We focus this paper only on the design and fabrication challenges of probe arrays but not on the downstream packaging and in vivo testing—which will partly depend on the final application; such testing may then require refinement or alteration of the design depending on how well the probe performance matches the goal. For example, awake headfixed extracellular recordings in rodents can utilize probe arrays attached to printed circuit boards with conventional methods such as wirebonding or flip-chip assembly. In contrast, chronic applications may require flexible cables to be used (e.g., as described in [20,42–45]), although this may dictate a lower channel count due to packaging restrictions. Our goal is to demonstrate methods of creating highly scalable Si based electrode arrays and we accordingly uncouple their design from the packaging choice. But for highly-scaled 3-D probes aimed at in vivo headfixed recordings, we can draw on existing solutions used in the semiconductor probe card industry, where systems face even more complex packaging constraints and designs connect and route over 10,000 high-speed wires out from a small space to sophisticated test equipment [46]. The semiconductor industry roadmap also sets out to increase the maximum number of pins to around 50,000 by 2028 [47], with each connection supporting significantly higher bandwidth than a passive probe or active neural amplifier requires. Probe-card packaging technologies can inform us about the current technological limits relevant for awake headfixed experiments, where the size and weight of the setup is not a determining factor.

2. Materials and Methods

2.1. Fabrication and Assembly Overview

The process for fabricating the silicon parts for the 3-D probes described in this paper is nearly identical to that for the 2-D probes previously reported [12]. We will refer to that work for detailed fabrication methods, while noting the differences here. The key innovation reported here involves the mechanical and electrical assembly of individual 2-D probes into a 3-D structure and the necessary layout changes required for accomplishing this. The overall principle of the mechanical assembly is shown in Figure 2.

We build a 3-D array from four types of components: individual 2-D probe inserts (point A in Figure 2a,b) which are placed into a slotted holder plate (point B in Figure 2a,b), similar in principle to [14,48]. The 2-D inserts as well as the holder plate contain electrical wiring and exposed pads for electroplating, packaging and neural recording. The electroplating pads (point J in Figure 2a) are later connected with electroless nickel plating. We identify the two sides of the holder plate according to how the array is shown in Figure 1, with the probe shanks pointing up. Thus, the top side of the holder plate is on the same side as the probe shanks, while the bottom side of the holder plate contains the pads and wiring. The choice for placing the pads on the bottom side of the holder plate is not critical but it helps to increase the space available to redistribute wires from the shank to the contact pads (point J in Figure 2a) within each 2-D insert. We can also imagine a holder plate with metal pads on both sides, in an effort to double the wiring density (or, for active 2-D probes, to assist in spatially isolating different signal types).

The 2-D inserts are placed into the opening slots from the top side. In contrast to our previous work on 3-D waveguide arrays [48], we introduce a self-locking hook (point C in Figure 2a,b) that locks the 2-D inserts into place. This hook is inserted on the bottom side of the holder plate, through a set of openings etched into the 2-D inserts (point H in Figure 2a). The hook is a simple deep reactive ion etched (DRIE) silicon structure. Finally, on the top side of the holder plate, a pair of self-locking tapered comb structures (point D in Figure 2a,b) is inserted to help with self-aligning the 2-D inserts to all point in the same direction.

The different components and their respective cross sections are shown in Figure 3, along with a comparison of the process steps in Table 2. Once the parts are fabricated and mechanically assembled into a 3-D structure, electroless nickel deposition forms the electrical connections and prepares the probe for wirebonding or other packaging steps. To wirebond these probes, a dedicated wirebond chuck will need to be prepared, so that after attaching the probe to a printed circuit board (PCB), the shanks are protected. We used a similar approach when carrying out the electrical measurements on an assembled probe (using an aluminum block with a recessed area for the shanks). The cross section and side-view of an assembled probe is shown in Figure 4. The next two sections explain the design and process choices made for the mechanical and electrical assembly.

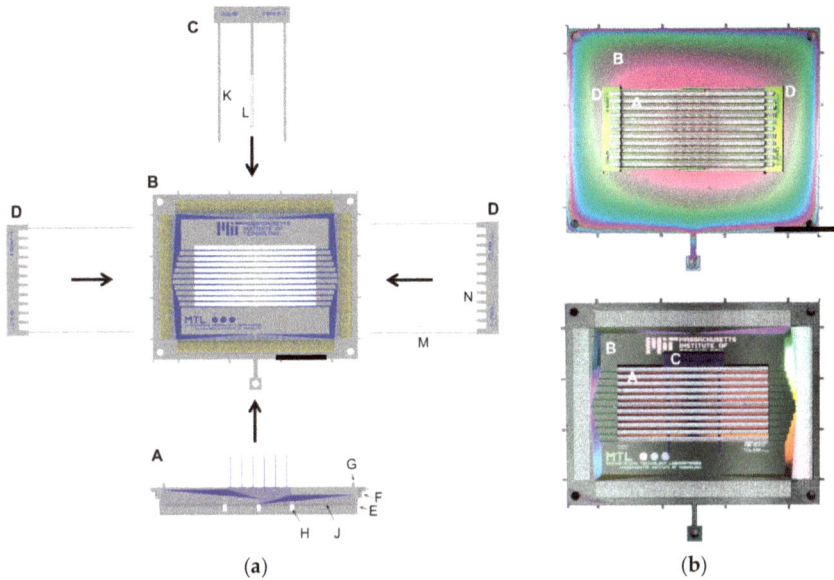

(a)   (b)

Figure 2. (**a**) Principle of the mechanical assembly for the probe shown in Figure 1. The 2-D inserts (A) are slid into the openings in the holder plate (B). A slight taper (E) on the 2-D insert facilitates the hand-assembly and a small bump (G) protects the shanks when pushing the 2-D inserts down with tweezers. On the bottom, a self-locking hook (C) with two guide beams (K) and locking beams (L) is then pushed through the openings in the 2-D inserts (H). A pair of self-locking alignment structures (D) is inserted on the top. Its tapered combs (N) push the 2-D inserts (A) into alignment and lock themselves into place: vertically confined by an indent (F) and horizontally by interlocking beams (M). The recording sites on the 2-D insert are wired down to the contact pads (J) and are described in the electrical assembly section. The fabrication steps for the individual parts are shown in Figures 3 and 4. (**b**) The top and bottom photographs show an assembled device from above and below, respectively, with the individual components labeled. Scale bars are 10 mm. A typical step-by-step assembly sequence is: (step 1) lay out the individual components for assembly, (step 2) grip holder plate (B) with reverse tension tweezers, (step 3) sequentially pick up the inserts (A) with fine tweezers and insert through the slots in (B), (step 4) inspect and tap down with tweezers onto the inserts to make sure they are fully inserted into the holder plate, (step 5) pick up the self-locking hook (C) with fine tweezers and insert the guide beams (K) through the openings of the inserts (H). It can help to lift the reverse tension tweezers with the probe to better see, or place a mirror below the probe for visual guidance. (step 6) once the guide beams are inserted, use either tweezers or your finger to gently push the hook through completely. As the guide beams pass through each insert, a small resistance can be felt when pushing, due to the hooks (L) going through the openings (H) of each insert. (step 7) using tweezers, pick up the two alignment structures (D) and place on the top side of the probe body (B), roughly aligning them. (step 8) using two sets of tweezers, one in each hand, push the two structures (D) closer until they slide into position. The tweezers should be open in this step, allowing both pushing and rotating of the two parts (D) as they approach and lock. Avoid pushing both parts forward at the same time but alternate between them. Use your dominant hand for the last fine push that locks the beams of (D) together and aligns the probe.

(A) 2-D Inserts

(B) Holder Plate

(C) Assembly Supports

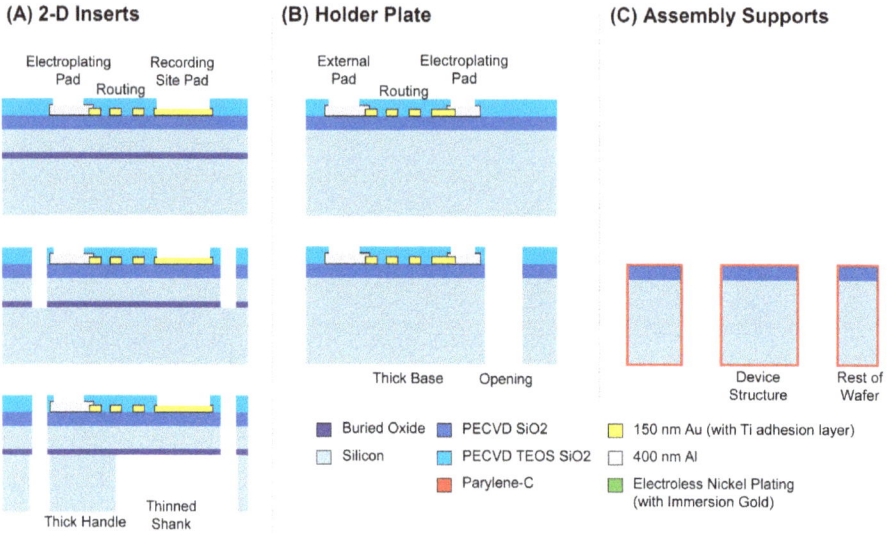

Electroplating Pad · Routing · Recording Site Pad

External Pad · Routing · Electroplating Pad

Thick Base · Opening

Device Structure · Rest of Wafer

Thick Handle · Thinned Shank

■ Buried Oxide ■ PECVD SiO2 □ 150 nm Au (with Ti adhesion layer)
□ Silicon ■ PECVD TEOS SiO2 □ 400 nm Al
■ Parylene-C ■ Electroless Nickel Plating (with Immersion Gold)

Figure 3. The three different design components, with photographs of the finished 150 mm diameter wafers (top) and process cross-sections (bottom). The cross sections are not to scale. Parts (**A**), the 2-D inserts, are fabricated identically to our 2-D probe components reported in [12] with the exception of using 400 nm Al as the optical lithography metal (instead of 250 nm Au). Part (**B**) is the holder plate and identical to A except that the DRIE etch consists of a single through-etch from the front-side, instead of a front- followed by a back-side etch in A. Finally, part (**C**) is a single silicon deep reactive ion etch (DRIE) step to create the self-locking hooks and the alignment comb structures.

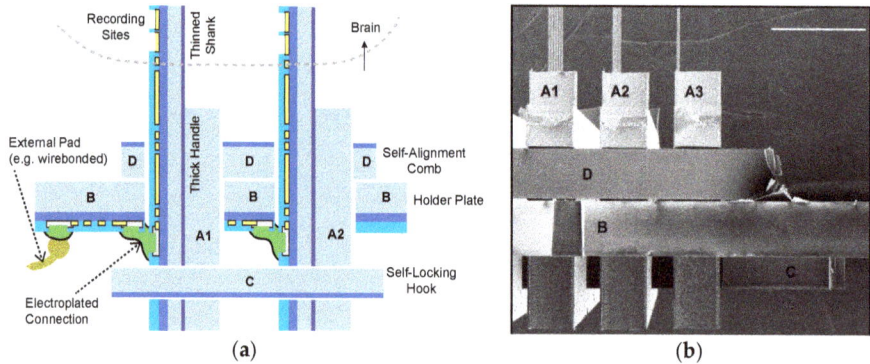

(a)

(b)

Figure 4. (**a**) Cross-section schematic of the assembled probe, with the different parts from Figure 3 labeled (drawing not to scale). (**b**) SEM image showing a close-up side-view of the probe in Figure 1, with the corresponding parts labelled. The scale bar is 1 mm. After completed assembly, the probe can subsequently be encapsulated in epoxy (not shown here), protecting the electroplated and external connections, while leaving the thinned shanks free from encapsulation (similar to how we epoxy-encapsulate our 2-D probes in [12]).

Table 2. Overview of Processing Steps. Summary of the process steps to fabricate the components of Figure 3. The process is adopted from and uses the same tools as our 2-D probes in [12].

Step	2-D Inserts (A)	Holder Plate (B)	Mechanical Supports (C,D)
Starting material	150 mm SOI wafer, thicknesses: 15 μm device layer, 0.8 μm buried oxide, 510 μm handle	150 mm wafer, 525 μm thick, double-sided polished	150 mm wafer, 525 μm thick, double-sided polished
Clean wafers and insulation	Piranha clean 1 μm of PECVD SiO_2	Piranha clean 1 μm of PECVD SiO_2	Omitted
Electron beam lithography metallization (liftoff)	10 nm Ti/150 nm Au/5 nm Ti, mask is 400 nm of PMMA 495A8	10 nm Ti/150 nm Au/5 nm Ti mask is 400 nm of PMMA 495A8	Omitted
Optical lithography metallization (liftoff)	50 nm Ti/400 nm Al, mask is 1.5 μm of AZ5214E	50 nm Ti/400 nm Al mask is 1.5 μm of AZ5214E	Omitted
Upper insulation	1 μm of PECVD TEOS	1 μm of PECVD TEOS	Omitted
Electron beam lithography small recording site etch	CF_4/CHF_3 based SiO_2 etch, mask is 800 nm of PMMA 495A11	CF_4/CHF_3 based SiO_2 etch, mask is 800 nm of PMMA 495A11	Omitted
Optical lithography large pad etch	CF_4/CHF_3 based SiO_2 etch, mask is 1 μm of SPR-700	CF_4/CHF_3 based SiO_2 etch, mask is 1 μm of SPR-700	Omitted
Frontside DRIE etch [a]	CF_4/CHF_3 based etch of frontside SiO_2, then 15 μm etch of Si device layer to buried oxide. Mask is 8 μm of AZ4620.	CF_4/CHF_3 based etch of frontside SiO_2, then 15 μm etch of Si device layer to buried oxide. Mask is 8 μm of AZ4620.	Etch 525 μm through wafer, mask is 8 μm of AZ4620
SOI wafer buried oxide etch	CF_4/CHF_3 based etch of 0.8 μm of buried oxide.	Omitted	Omitted
Backside DRIE etch	Etch 510 μm through wafer from the backside, mask is 8 μm of AZ4620	Omitted	Omitted
Clean wafers	Barrel ash in oxygen plasma	Barrel ash in oxygen plasma	Barrel ash in oxygen plasma
Insulation on full wafer	Omitted	Omitted	0.1 μm [c] of PECVD SiO_2 1 μm of Parylene-C
Remove parts	Break out devices	Break out devices	Break out devices
Insulation on individual parts	(optional) Place dies facing down onto a Si wafer and deposit 100 nm PECVD Si_3N_4 to insulate backside [b]	Place dies facing down onto a Si wafer and deposit 100 nm PECVD Si_3N_4 to insulate backside [b]	Omitted

[a] For the 15 μm frontside SOI etch, because the etch depth is sufficiently shallow we now use 1 μm of SPR-700 resist for improved alignment accuracy. [b] This step needs to be carefully tested, to avoid any deposition on the front side where the recording sites or metal pads could be impaired by a film of dielectric. Only a thin film should be used, sufficient to provide insulation but not thick enough to risk accidental covering of the front-side. If necessary, a dilute HF dip can be performed to remove any accidental, thin, front-side deposition. [c] Optional deposition, used to color-code different wafers.

2.2. Mechanical Assembly Procedures

2.2.1. Inserts and Holder Plate

The mechanical assembly is designed to be simple and done by hand using mechanical tweezers, without a need for robotic assembly. The holder plate (point B in Figure 2a,b) can be fixed in space using forceps or by using a customized holder. The individual 2-D inserts (point A in Figure 2a,b) are placed into the holder plate slots, which is an easy task as long as these openings are wider by about 5 to 10 μm. The inserts have tapered sides (point E in Figure 2a) to allow initial misalignment when inserting them into the openings. Once inserted, we tap down on the inserts with tweezers and ensure they are placed all the way into the holder plate.

2.2.2. Self-Locking Hook

Once all of the 2-D inserts are in place, a self-locking hook is inserted on the underside of the holder plate, locking all of the 2-D inserts into position (point C in Figure 2a,b). We use a design with at least three beams. The pair of outer beams is longer and solid and they function as guide beams (point K in Figure 2a). The inner beam(s) each contain a pair of locking beams (point L in Figure 2a), which will self-lock once inserted through the 2-D probe openings (point H in Figure 2a). The purpose of the guide beams is to enter first and align the insertion. Without the guide beams, it is very difficult to insert the hook by hand, because any off-angle insertion will easily break the fragile center hook pair. Any initial misalignment is self-corrected by the guide beams and they are strong enough to not break during this process. Once the guide beams are inserted, the self-locking hook can be pushed through, either using tweezers or the tip of a finger (this has the benefit of feeling the changes in mechanical resistance when the locking beams pass each insert—helpful at least initially when practicing the assembly).

The geometry of the locking beams was initially chosen using a simple cantilever beam formula (to get the necessary displacement of the tips yet stay well below the stress limits of silicon) and then experimentally optimized using a range of different designs. In our current designs, the locking beam's length is always identical—with an aspect ratio of $L/W = 4500 \ \mu m/95 \ \mu m = 47$. During insertion, the hook tip is displaced by as much as 50 μm, resulting in a maximum simulated stress of 0.07 GPa (calculated using finite element methods), well below the silicon fracture strength of around 1.5 to 2.0 GPa [49].

2.2.3. Self-Alignment Combs

The final step in the mechanical assembly is to insert a pair of self-aligning and self-locking tapered combs on the top side of the holder plate (point D in Figure 2a,b). We introduced these structures in [48] but show important improvements in their design here.

Because the openings in the holder plate must be slightly larger than the 2-D inserts placed through them, it is possible for each insert to point in a slightly different direction. The purpose of the tapered combs is to prevent misaligned shanks because they can result in excessive tissue damage. The opening will be larger than the insert for three reasons: First, there can be variations in the 2-D insert's thickness caused by wafer thickness variations. But these are small and can be adjusted for in the design, thus posing no major concern. Second, variations can be by design. The dimensions of the opening in the holder plate are lithographically defined and thus set precisely. However, to facilitate insertion, some tolerance is necessary (e.g., on the order of 10 μm for hand-assembly). Third, variations can be due to non-vertical sidewalls of the etched openings, which is harder to control. The sidewall angles of the DRIE depend on the tool and recipe optimization and can add significant uncertainty. When etching through 525 μm thick wafers, the bottom of the trench is wider than the top; we observed around 30 μm of widening (or a 3.3° tilt from the vertical). The precise value can vary with tool condition and etch recipe parameters. While recipe optimization could reduce the trench widening, an effective solution is to etch half-way through the wafer from each side with the trenches meeting up in the middle (e.g., as done in [15]). This adds another lithography step and some front-to-back alignment uncertainty (up to a few μm) can remain. Even with robotic assembly and near-perfect etch precision, small non-vertical DRIE sidewalls or process misalignments can still allow probes to rotate. Consequently, the alignment structures remain beneficial even when assembly and process conditions are improving and their presence allows us to avoid challenging optimization and monitoring of processing tolerances and instead build in a 5 to 10 μm gap that greatly facilitates assembly.

2.2.4. Improvements to the Self-Alignment Combs

Our initial use of the self-alignment combs in [48] was a single design of alignment beams, where two identical structures self-interlocked. Rather than having many hook pairs between each insert (as done in [48]), we found two interlocking hooks located at the ends of the structure were sufficient to provide mechanical stability (point M in Figures 2a and 5). Placing the interlocking hooks only at the ends allows us to reduce the pitch between the 2-D inserts.

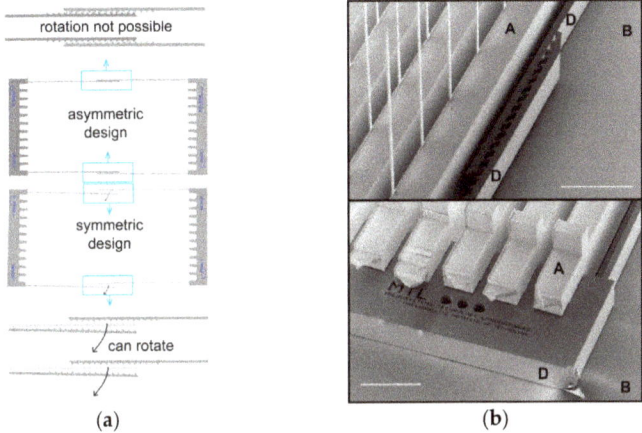

Figure 5. (a) Different locking designs for the self-alignment combs. For narrow distances, the symmetric design is acceptable but as the two combs are spaced further apart, rotations can cause problems and an asymmetric design instead is preferred. (b) The SEM on the right shows detailed views of the tapered comb (D) locked between the 2-D inserts (A) and holder plate (B) in the bottom image and its beams (D) locked onto itself in the top image. The scale bar is 1 mm.

The symmetric interlocking hook design is suitable for smaller inserts (e.g., inserts of 5 mm size). However, for larger inserts such as the ones we are presenting here (the base of the insert in Figure 1 is 1.9 cm wide), a problem arises: when sliding the structures into place, the symmetry of the interlocking structures means that small rotations in one direction can result in a lack of self-locking (bottom of Figure 5a). We adjusted the design to use asymmetric structures: one with the locking beams on the outside and another with the beams on the inside (top of Figure 5a). This removes the freedom to rotate and ensures that the structures will stay interlocked in place since small rotations will be counteracted in either direction.

A further improvement made relates to the contact between the self-alignment combs and the 2-D insert. The comb structure has a slightly tapered shape, so that the comb gradually presses against the 2-D inserts. If the surfaces touching are both silicon, they cannot be pressed well into each other and their points of contact will be minimal. We decided to coat the combs with a 1 μm layer of Parylene-C, to provide a thin, soft coating on the alignment combs. When pressed against the silicon 2-D inserts, the soft Parylene-C provides a press-fit type mechanism. Pushing in the alignment combs becomes easier and adds stability as the point of contact between the combs and the inserts is now larger. We chose Parylene-C because it is easy to deposit uniformly on finished wafers with DRIE through-etched patterns. We use Parylene-C only to provide a press-fit coating for the assembly and do not deposit it on the shanks, or any other neural recording related parts of the probe.

2.2.5. Alternative Assembly Methods

The assembly described above is done by hand but a robotic or micromanipulator based assembly could be developed in the future and would allow reduction of tolerances, useful for more aggressively scaled electrical connections. Our initial 2-D insert design had additional features, which we eventually omitted from the final design. However, we describe these initial design features briefly here, because they may become relevant in the future if robotic assembly is used.

In our initial design, the 2-D probe inserts were not locked into place until the bottom hook was inserted. If, however, the inserts needed to be held in place temporarily, a small set of hooks could be included, as shown in Figure 6. These smaller side-hooks snap into place when the 2-D insert is inserted through the holder plate. The single large opening shown in Figure 2 can also be interrupted with a number of bridges, to utilize more than two side-hooks. These bridges can also help give mechanical strength to the holder plate if the pitch between inserts is very small, although we did not notice that to be a problem. However, we discovered that the main problem with the side-hooks is their fragility (being very thin yet stiff beams). During manual assembly, the natural shaking of the hand resulted in an estimated two-thirds of the side-hooks breaking. By itself, this may not be problematic but the side-hook length is much larger than the wafer thickness and broken side-hooks therefore create a significant challenge: with the hook broken, the 2-D insert now has substantial space to move around, easily creating a horizontal misalignment between the electrical pads on the holder plate and those on the 2-D insert. This can make the electrical assembly impossible. Thus, we decided not to use the bridges or side-hook concepts and instead went with a simpler, tapered insert design. A robotic assembly method may however find the side-hooks beneficial, because robotic precision may avoid breaking them.

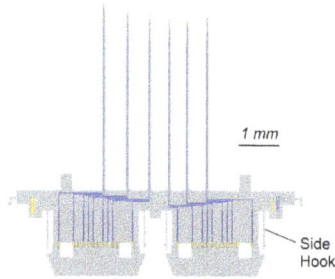

Figure 6. Design drawing of a 2-D insert with side-hooks.

2.3. Electrical Assembly Procedures

To electrically connect the 2-D probe inserts with the holder plate, a connection across a gap and between pads on two orthogonal surfaces (the holder plate and the 2-D insert) must be made. Our goal was to create a scalable approach that could easily form thousands of connections. The mechanical constraints (because the points of connection are in a "canyon" which does not allow easy mechanical access) rule out ultrasonic bonding as a practical method. We also decided against solder based methods, because we thought that connections at a pitch at tens of microns would be extremely challenging and because sample preparation with solder would require additional process steps prior to DRIE. Instead, we focused on different ways of electroplating to form connections (e.g., similar to [24]). The layout for each method is shown in Figure 7 and we compare their merits in Table 3.

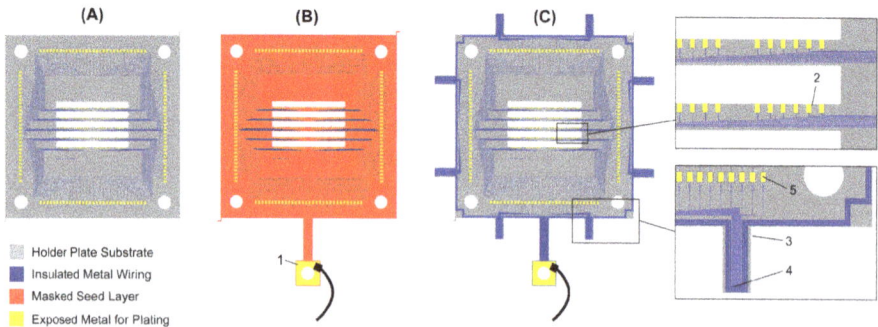

Figure 7. Layout illustrations for the different electroplating methods: (**A**) packaged and electroless plating, (**B**) seed and masked plating and (**C**) design with short-circuit beams. All cases aim to electroplate

the small pads near the opening in the holder plate, shown as (2) but differ in how plating current is supplied to these pads. The larger external contact pads (5) can be plated as well, facilitating final packaging. The design in (A) has the lowest complexity. In (B), a seed is masked with exposed pads only at the desired plating sites. Plating current is then supplied at the contact (1), for example, by attaching a temporary clip. For short-circuit beam plating (C), no seed layer is used but instead all sites are routed and connected to a wiring frame (4), which consists of several wiring rings, resulting in a tree-like structure to balance the voltage drop for each pad. After plating, the shorts are disconnected by breaking off the external short circuit beams at (3).

Table 3. Comparison of Electroplating Approaches.

Detail	Packaged Plating	Short-Circuited Breakout Beams	Seed and Mask	Electroless
Method	Electrolytic	Electrolytic	Electrolytic	Electroless
Common metal choices	Au, Ni, Cu	Au, Ni, Cu	Au, Ni, Cu	Ni, Cu
Holder plate design type (see Figure 7)	"A"	"C"	"B"	"A"
Can be plated before packaging	No	Yes	Yes	Yes
Requires further processing after plating	No	Yes	Yes	No
Minimum pitch [a]	$W_{pad} + 2\,W_{gap}$	$W_{pad} + 2\,W_{gap}$	$W_{pad} + 2\,W_{gap}$	$W_{pad} + W_{gap}$
Requires direct wiring access to plating pads	Yes	Yes	No	No
Advantages	• Pads can be plated individually • Ability to electrically detect plating endpoint, especially if pads are individually plated	• No seed layer or plating mask needed	• Controlled plating of all pads in parallel • Most common plating method in microfabrication	• Tightest pad pitch • Aluminum pad compatible • Zincate and brief Ni plating can be done on full wafer before assembly
Disadvantages	• Devices must be fully packaged before plating • Package must be compatible with plating chemicals	• Temporary short circuit wiring requires extra space • Breaking the short-circuit beams can be difficult • Careful resistance balancing needed	• Requires chemical etching of mask and seed • Mask and seed must be DRIE and O2 plasma ashing compatible	• Pad cleanliness is very important, to avoid uneven plating

[a] W_{pad} is the width of the contact pad and W_{gap} is the distance between the 2-D insert and the contact pad on the holder plate. The minimum pitch is the width of the pad and the spacing. For electrolytic plating, a distance of W_{gap} needs to be covered, so that the minimum spacing to avoid short-circuiting pads is $2\,W_{gap}$. For electroless plating, the gap is bridged from both sides and thus only $W_{gap}/2$ is plated per side, with a minimum spacing of W_{gap}.

2.3.1. Post-Package Electrolytic Plating

In packaged plating (e.g., [24,25]), the probe is first assembled and packaged (e.g., to a PCB), so that individual sites on the holder plate can be electrically accessed through the package connector. This allows flexibility in the plating: each pad can be individually plated, or pads can be plated in parallel. Individual plating can allow end-point detection of the plating but this approach does not scale well with the number of pads. Because the probe must first be completely packaged, any electroplating yield problems will not be identified until after packaging, increasing the time and cost caused by non-yielding devices. The package also needs to be compatible with the electroplating chemicals.

2.3.2. Electrolytic Plating with Seed Layer and Mask

A common approach for electroplating in microfabrication is to use a masked seed layer to plate from, shown in Figure 7B. The seed blankets the entire device (in our case the holder plate) and is selectively covered by an insulating mask with only the desired plating sites exposed. Photoresist is often used as a convenient mask material. By plating with a seed and mask, a single point of contact to the seed can supply the plating current for all sites in parallel, independent of what devices or wiring is implemented in the actual silicon below the seed. After plating, the mask and seed are chemically removed. In our process, the mask and seed must be fabricated prior to the DRIE etch. Therefore, it is not possible to use photoresist as a plating mask. This restriction complicates the choice of mask material. We initially implemented this approach with electrolytic Cu plating using a thin evaporated Cu seed (e.g., 100 nm), masked by a thin film (e.g., 150 nm) of plasma-enhanced chemical vapor deposition (PECVD) SiN_x or SiO_2. The Cu seed required either Ti or Cr to be used as an adhesion layer (e.g., 10 to 20 nm). However, our choice of Cu was not ideal, because of metal adhesion and removal issues (caused by the presence of difficult to remove Cu/Cr or Cu/Ti intermetallics). The mask layer removal in diluted HF was also not ideal, because it attacked the probe insulating dielectric films. Thus, switching from Cu to Ni or Au as the seed and plating metal could help to reduce some of these problems. But the requirement for chemical etching to remove the mask would remain.

2.3.3. Seedless Plating with Temporary Short Circuits

We also investigated an intermediate step between packaged plating and plating with a seed and mask (Figures 7C and 8). In this approach, we modify the wiring layout on the holder plate and short-circuit all of the pads together, so that they can be plated in parallel. This method removes the need for a seed or mask layer and also the need to first package the device. The short-circuits must be temporary and we route the wiring to the outside of the holder plate, where they are short-circuited together and connected to a single plating access site. This approach requires balancing of the line resistance and we implemented a tree-like structure along the short circuit ring's perimeter. If a simple short circuit ring is used, distant plating sites will fail to plate due to significant potential drops along the way. After plating, short-circuits are removed by physically cleaving the beams with side-cutting pliers. The disadvantage we found with this method is a lack of scalability and added design complexity. The space on the short circuit beams is fixed, requiring either a larger number of wider beams, or finer metal traces as we scale up the pad count. We also found that breaking off the short circuit beams poorly can sometimes result in broken metal wires short-circuiting because of the ductility of the metal. An alternative may thus be to use laser-cutting rather than cleaving.

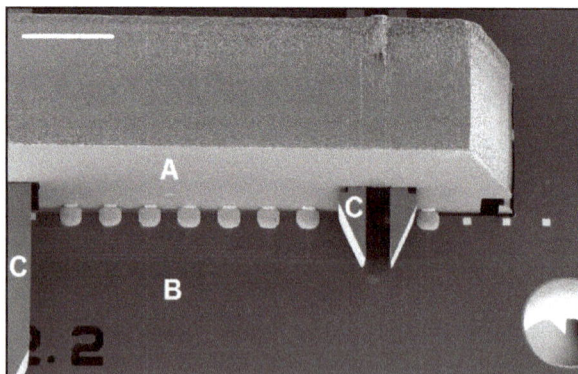

Figure 8. SEM image of an earlier electrolytic plating design, showing 2-D insert (A), holder plate (B) and self-locking hook (C). The scale bar is 400 μm.

2.3.4. Electroless Plating

The previous methods all relied on electrolytic plating, where plating current is supplied externally. In contrast, electroless (or autocatalytic) plating is able to deposit metal without the need for an external current supply. This method is ideal for our designs, because it minimized the process complexity and avoids the handling complexities to make a temporary single electrical contact on the assembled 3-D probe. The design of the holder plate is shown in Figure 7A. We decided to use electroless nickel (EN) plating, because it provides a well-established plating protocol compatible with plating on Al pads. We use a standard phosphorous nickel solution (Fidelity 9012, OMGroup Inc., Piscataway, NJ, USA). The process starts with a pre-treatment for Al substrates: 5 min in OMG 3152 soak cleaner, 15 seconds in OMG 3133 acid etch, 30 s de-smut in 50% v/v nitric acid and 25% v/v sulfuric acid, 60 s in OMG 3116M zincate, 30 seconds de-smut in 50% v/v nitric acid, 60 seconds OMG 3116M zincate—with deionized (DI) water rinsing between steps. All solutions are mixed and operated according to the manufacturer's specifications. The pre-treatment prepares the Al pads with a seed layer of zinc and is followed by EN plating. The plating time depends on the gap that needs to be bridged but will typically be between 30 and 60 min.

To hold the probe during plating, we use a Teflon carrier, custom-made by the Massachusetts Institute of Technology (MIT) Central Machine Shop (Figure 9). The carrier allows easy handling while protecting the probe and accommodates different inserts, one for each holder-plate design. In the carrier, the probe is held at a 45° angle to facilitate H_2 gas evolution during plating and to avoid getting evolving gas trapped on or under a horizontal surface.

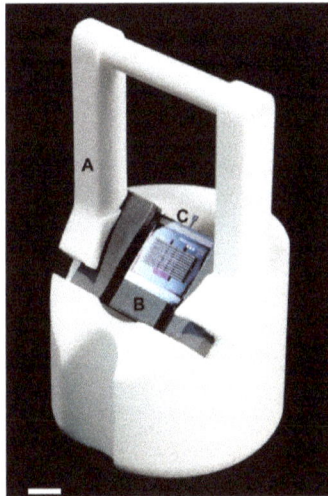

Figure 9. Teflon-based holder (A) for electroless plating. The darker insert (B) is specific to the probe (C) and holds the assembled probe at a 45-degree angle, to facilitate the removal of evolving gas from the plating sites to avoid gas getting trapped under a horizontal surface. The insert (B) can also be used to hold the probe during mechanical assembly steps (see section). The scale bar is 1 cm.

While the main purpose of the plating is to form the connections between the holder plate and the 2-D probe inserts, the external wiring pads also are plated (see Figure 7). Once the EN plating is complete, we follow with an immersion-gold step (Bright Electroless Gold, Transene, Danvers, MA, USA) to protect the Ni from corrosion and to make the external pads packaging compatible (e.g., for wirebonding).

Electroless nickel does not catalyze on the materials present on the probe shanks (Au recording sites, SiO$_2$ insulator, Si shank). It is nonetheless a good idea to protect the probe shanks during plating with photoresist and removing the resist with acetone when plating is complete (as also suggested by [24]). Otherwise, stray Ni deposits may occasionally form especially on rough surfaces—for example, the DRIE sidewall or indented Au pad may trap contaminants in the plating bath that can then act as plating seeds.

2.3.5. Comparison

The above electroplating methods are summarized in Table 3. Based on our experience with the different methods, we find that electroless plating can enable scalable probe fabrication, by minimizing microfabrication process complexity and because plating can occur before packaging all in a single step regardless of the number of connections to be made. EN plating is also compatible with integration or attachment of complementary metal–oxide–semiconductor (CMOS) integrated circuits (e.g., similar to [7,17]) to the holder plate, because no electrical access to the plating sites is needed. However, the plating process is sensitive to substrate cleanliness. Organic contamination (e.g., from photoresist residues or the DRIE handle-mounting) must be properly cleaned, otherwise some pads may not plate. Regardless of the plating method used, the finest connection pitch that can be achieved depends on the gap that has to be bridged. The minimum pitch depends on the width of the pad and the spacing. Electrolytic plating needs to grow metal for a distance of W$_{gap}$ (see Figure 8) and the minimum spacing to avoid short-circuiting neighboring pads is 2W$_{gap}$. In contrast, electroless plating bridges the gap from both sides (Figure 10) and only W$_{gap}$/2 is plated per side, giving a minimum spacing of W$_{gap}$. These dependencies are summarized in Table 3.

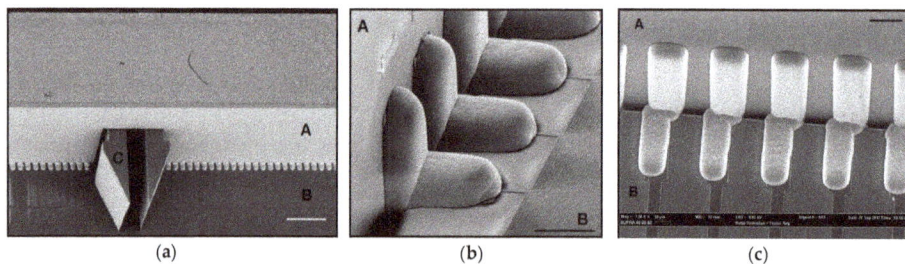

Figure 10. (**a**) SEM image of the 40 μm pitch connections of a 4480 recording site probe (design 3b in Table 4), with the 2-D insert (A), the holder plate (B) and the self-locking hook (C). (**b**) Electrical connections and shown with more detail. (**c**) An earlier test-design, also using a 40 μm connection pitch, with a narrow gap indicates the potential for a much narrower connection pitch. Scale bars are 200 μm (a) and 20 μm (b,c) respectively.

We currently first assemble the 3-D probe before plating any of the parts. If a larger number of probes are required, it may become more time-efficient to initiate plating on the entire wafer—cleaning, zincate pre-treatments and a thin (e.g., 1 μm) initial EN plating—before breaking out the structures and assembling them into individual 3-D probes. After assembling the pre-plated structures, the probe can then be immediately placed into EN plating to form the final connections, simplifying the post-assembly processing.

We found that the protrusions at the end of the holder plate in Figure 7C make handling the device much easier and we introduced smaller protrusion on the edges of all our holder-plate designs. Similarly, the long bridge for seed/mask plating (Figure 7B) provides an easy way to pick up the device with tweezers. Our final designs use EN plating and while functionally equivalent to Figure 7A, have the physical outline of the holder plate in Figure 7C.

Table 4. Design summary of example designs in this paper.

ID	Design (Part Names)	Recording Site Configuration [a]	3-D Array Configuration [b]	Connections per 2-D Insert[c]	Total Connections	Connection Pitch	Device Purpose
1a	B160–F160	2×20 @ 13.0 μm	9×4	160	1440	60 μm	Conservative design
1b	B160–F20	2×2 @ 9.5/14 μm	9×40	160	1440	60 μm	Large shank count, tetrode tips
2	B160–F30	1×9 @ 250.0 μm	9×17	160	1440	60 μm	Optical-only lithography
3a	B408–F408	2×34 @ 13.0 μm	11×6	408	4488	40 μm	Standard design
3b	B409–F408	2×34 @ 13.0 μm	11×6	408	4488	40 μm	Compact holder plate
4	B1000–F1006	4×42 @ 13.0 μm	10×6	1008	10,080	26 μm	Aggressive design
5	B1000–F1010	2×50 @ 13.0 μm	10×10	1008	10,080	26 μm	Aggressive design
6	B10–F10	1×1	8×80	149	1192	16.5 to 113.7 μm	Pitch and DRIE etch testing

[a] Rows/shank × Columns/shank @ Site pitch in μm (identical for columns and rows except 1b). [b] Inserts/probe × Shanks/insert. [c] For more connections than recording sites per insert (e.g., design 5 and 6), the layout code leaves some connections open, yet the connections are still formed in the electrical assembly. Configurations of the different probes fabricated in this paper. Part names begin with B for the holder plates and F for the 2-D probe inserts. Electrical characteristics are shown in Table 5.

Table 5. Electrical Characterization of Probe Components. Measurement accuracy is ±5%, driven by the quality of the contact to the metal pad during measurement, rather than the measurement equipment itself. One measurement was taken per point.

Design	Wire Length (mm)	Wire Aspect Ratio (n_{sq} = L/W)	Resistance (kΩ)	Capacitance (pF)
Holder B10	5.6	1900	1.02	0.56
Insert F10 [a]	1.9	1050	n/a	0.08
Holder B160	11.3	7200	8.53	1.39
Insert F30	2.1	950	0.29	0.09
Insert F160	4.0	7700	9.30	0.28
Holder B408	13.0	14,200	21.7	1.82
Holder B409	13.9	34,750	55.1	1.28
Insert F408	5.3	8700	9.45	0.48
Holder B1000	15.8	39,400	66.1	1.88
Insert F1006	8.2	14,100	18.1	0.71
Insert F1010	5.4	11,300	12.8	0.63

[a] No resistance measurement for F10 because only 1 site/shank. Design names correspond to the details shown in Table 4.

3. Results

3.1. Example Designs

We have built a number of different sample designs, summarized in Table 4. Each shank has close-packed recording sites (except for designs B160-F30 and B10-F10). The connection pitch ranges from a conservative 60 μm (B160-F160) to an aggressive 26 μm pitch (B1000-F1006, B1000-F1010). Testing was carried out on design 6, with was created with the goal of testing the minimum electroplating pitch and to demonstrate an aggressive number of very narrow shanks to test the DRIE etch capabilities. The following sections show the mechanical and electrical characteristics of these designs.

3.2. Mechanical Characterization

To measure the alignment accuracy of the probe shanks, we mapped out the probe tip locations under an optical microscope with a digital stage. This allowed us to track the actual versus expected locations of the shank tips, with results shown in Figure 11. For these measurements, we placed a 3-D probe under the microscope and moved the stage in well-defined steps. At each step, we took microscope images focused on the shank tips and processed the results by measuring the actual versus expected pixel location of the tip, with a resulting measurement accuracy of around 3 μm. After mapping all of the probe's inserts, we moved the stage back to the first position to verify that the probe had not shifted relative to the first image. Based on the characterization of six probes of three different designs, we find that the self-alignment method is effective with less than 0.2° misalignment. However, we noticed several probe inserts where the position was significantly different from its expected value (seen as the tail-end in Figure 11). Closer inspection of these probes revealed that they were using 2-D inserts from two wafers that had very different dielectric film stress (caused by a temporary tool problem that resulted in high stress instead of zero-stress in the final 1 μm tetraethoxysilane (TEOS) film deposited). While the inserts were well aligned, the probe shanks had different radii of curvature depending on the wafer they came from. Therefore, either all of the inserts should come from the same wafer or batch, or the shank bending should be characterized with an optical profilerometer before the devices are broken out of the wafer. Ideally, though, the dielectrics should be properly stress-balanced with minimal bending, thus avoiding the mismatch we encountered.

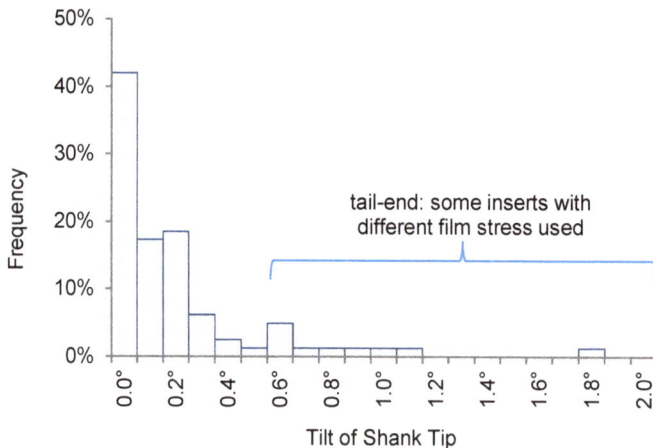

Figure 11. Measurements of the alignment accuracy based on six assembled 3-D probes. The strongly tilted shank tips were due to probe parts from wafers with different film stresses, resulting in an increased misalignment due to shank bending. For inserts with identical film stress, the shank tips are pointing within ±0.2° of their mean, equivalent to the tip of a 5 mm long shank being within 20 μm of the intended position.

3.3. Electrical Characterization

Because the electrode recording sites are identical to that of our previously published 2-D designs [12], we here focus on the electrical and mechanical connectivity from 2-D to 3-D. Electrical measurements of line resistance and parasitic capacitance for the individual 2-D components, using a microprobe station and an impedance meter (HP4284A), are shown in Table 5. Measurements of the line resistances were done by connecting some of the ends of adjacent wires together on each component.

We tested electrically assembled 3-D probes by measuring the resistance of wire pairs running from the holder plate and connected together on the 2-D insert. The electroplated contacts showed a resistance of 43 Ω. Wire pairs not connected were confirmed to be open circuits.

To characterize the smallest electroplating pitch, we used a test design where each insert had a graduation of pitch values ranging from 16.5 µm to 113.7 µm (partially shown in Figure 12). We found that a pitch of 35 to 40 µm was easily achieved. The 26 µm pitch of the aggressive design turned out to be slightly too aggressive to allow successful contact formation with the 10 µm tolerance gap used. An SEM of the electrical connections of our standard design (design 3b in Table 4 and shown in Figure 1) with a 40 µm pitch is shown in Figure 9. We believe that by reducing the width of the pads and reducing the opening gap, a connection pitch down to 25 µm should be feasible (e.g., based on using an 8 µm wide pad and an 8 µm gap, which allows for a good overplating tolerance). Further increases in the number of connections may also be achieved by widening the base of the 2-D inserts (rather than reducing the pitch between connections).

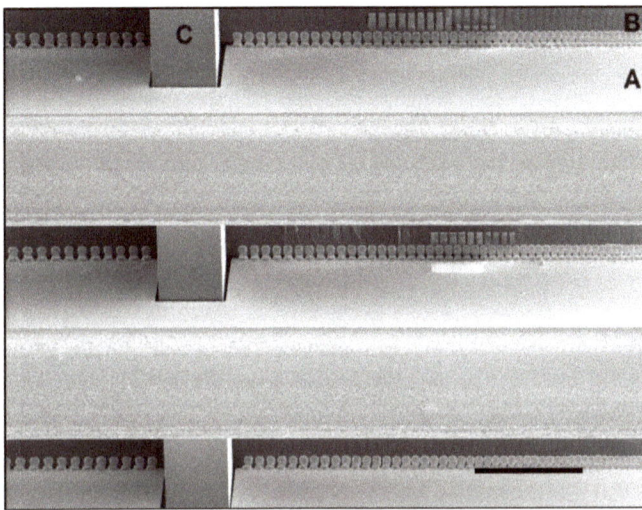

Figure 12. Example of a plating pitch test, showing several 2-D inserts (A) after electrical connections were formed to the holder plate (B). The self-locking hook (C) is visible. Each insert has a very fine pitch on the right and then relaxes the pitch towards the left. The finest pitch pads are visibly merged and overplated. Pads towards the left are clearly separated. The transition in this example occurred at around 35–40 µm but depends on the amount of plating necessary to bridge the gap (see Table 3). Scale bar is 500 µm.

4. Discussion

In this paper, we have focused on creating a scalable architecture for 3-D microelectrodes for neural recording. Scalability was demonstrated for both for the number of shanks and the number of recording sites per shank. Increases in the number of recording sites per shank are generally achieved through innovating the microfabrication process (the focus of our previous work [12]), while increases in the number of shanks requires a simultaneous innovation of scalable mechanical and electrical assembly methods, which has been the focus of this paper.

Increasing the number of shanks on an individual 2-D insert is relatively simple, because only adjustments in the layout need to be made. Increasing the number of 2-D inserts is possible as well, yet requires a tighter pitch between inserts. This can be achieved by using thinner 2-D inserts. The inserts can be entirely thinned back by the second DRIE etch step, similar to how the shanks themselves are thinned in our existing process—resulting in an identical thickness (here, 15 μm) of both the shanks and the 2-D insert's base. However, this introduces conflicting requirements between the desire for thin shanks and a thicker base to simplify handling and avoid thin-film stress-induced bending of the base. But, these requirements can be uncoupled: by inserting a back-thinning step prior to the second DRIE, one can allow the base portion of the 2-D insert to be thinned back independently from the shanks and thus achieve an optimal thickness for both the shank and the base. For example, a base thickness of 50 to 100 μm may provide a suitable tradeoff between an array with tight pitch (e.g., 150 μm) and the mechanical stability to handle the inserts in assembly process (e.g., the waveguide arrays built in [48] used inserts of 50 μm thickness).

With automated layout generation (see [12]), many different probe geometries can be included on the same wafer (see Figure 3). This will enable us to readily create many designs that are targeted to different specific applications. Each 3-D probe can also consist of a set of unique 2-D inserts to span a more complex, or behavior-specific brain region (e.g., as demonstrated by [10]). The placement of recording sites can be individualized for each shank and the location and length of each shank can be tuned to perfectly suit a specific neuroscience goal.

The mechanical properties of Si shanks allow further scaling of the cross-sectional geometries [50], enabling a larger number of shanks for a constant tissue displacement of, for example, under 1%. Previous multielectrode designs have successfully used tissue displacement ratios of 2% for 100 Si shanks [13] and 2.8% for 30 microwires [51] in vivo and designs as low as 0.1% were suggested in [14]. Rapid insertion has been used for 100-shank designs with cone-shaped tips [52]. However, both the shape of the tip and the diameter of the shank have a strong impact on the optimal insertion speed and thus the chisel-tip geometries of the shanks presented in this paper may enable a slow and gradual insertion, similar to the design and analysis described in [53].

5. Conclusions

We have demonstrated fabrication and assembly technologies for 3-D probes and showed new methods to build scalable and close packed electrode recording sites, focusing on scalability of both the number of shanks as well as the number of recording sites per shank. Advanced packaging technologies in the semiconductor industry can enable these probes to be connected to and used for awake headfixed recordings in the future. The use of scaled 3-D probes in vivo will benefit from recent advances in surgery and experimental design (e.g., [39,54]) that will allow scaling up the number of recording sites without the constraints that chronic implant systems require.

The designs we introduced may help with explorations of the scalability of 3-D microelectrodes and the possibilities of wafer thinning and amplifier/multiplexer integration (either monolithic or heterogeneous) points towards a continued ability to scale in the future. A combination of these methods with our 3-D array assembly can significantly increase the number of recording sites beyond what we introduce here, we envision by two orders of magnitude or more, for the same number of external wires. Such scaling will bring along new engineering design challenges in packaging, thermal and power management and experimental design and data analysis. But the promise of extreme scalability is the capability to record a significant portion of the neurons in the mouse brain, obtaining and analyzing orders of magnitudes more information than currently possible.

Author Contributions: Conceptualization, J.S., A.Z., J.K., J.B., C.M.-K., N.K., C.F. and E.S.B.; Investigation, J.S.; Writing—Original Draft Preparation, J.S., J.K., C.F., E.S.B.; Supervision, E.S.B., C.F., N.K.

Funding: This work was supported by John Doerr, the HHMI-Simons Faculty Scholars Program, the Simons Center for the Social Brain at MIT, the Paul Allen Family Foundation, NIH Director's Pioneer Award DP1NS087724, NIH grants R01NS067199, 2R44NS070453-03A1, 1R01NS102727, 1R43MH101943, 1R43MH109332, 1R24MH106075 and R01DA029639, Cognitive Rhythms Collaborative NSF DMS 1042134, IET Harvey Prize, Google, New York Stem Cell Foundation, NSF CBET 1053233 and DARPA HR0011-14-2-0004.

Acknowledgments: Devices were fabricated at MIT's Microsystems Technology Laboratories (MTL). DRIE etching was carried out at the Harvard Center for Nanoscale Systems, a Member of the National Nanotechnology Infrastructure Network. We thank the MIT Central Machine Ship for fabricating the plating carriers and Andrew Gallant at MIT for preparing the CAD drawings of the carriers. We thank OMGroup Inc. for the electroless nickel plating chemicals and Doug Richard for valuable plating advice and suggesting the customized plating carrier design.

Conflicts of Interest: The authors declare no conflict of interest. The funding sponsors had no role in the design of the study; in the collection, analyses, or interpretation of data; in the writing of the manuscript and in the decision to publish the results.

References

1. Wise, K.D.; Angell, J.B.; Starr, A. An integrated-circuit approach to extracellular microelectrodes. *IEEE Trans. Biomed. Eng.* **1970**, *3*, 238–247. [CrossRef]
2. Najafi, K.; Wise, K.D.; Mochizuki, T. A high-yield IC-compatible multichannel recording array. *IEEE Trans. Electron Devices* **1985**, *32*, 1206–1211. [CrossRef]
3. Norlin, P.; Kindlundh, M.; Mouroux, A.; Yoshida, K.; Jensen, W.; Hofmann, U.G. A 32-Site Neural Recording Probe Fabricated by Double-Sided Deep Reactive Ion Etching of Silicon-on-Insulator Substrates. In Proceedings of the 12th Micromechanics Europe Workshop (MME-2001), Cork, Ireland, 16–18 September 2001.
4. Du, J.; Blanche, T.J.; Harrison, R.R.; Lester, H.A.; Masmanidis, S.C. Multiplexed, high density electrophysiology with nanofabricated neural probes. *PLoS ONE* **2011**, *6*, e26204. [CrossRef] [PubMed]
5. Blanche, T.J.; Spacek, M.A.; Hetke, J.F.; Swindale, N.V. Polytrodes: High-density silicon electrode arrays for large-scale multiunit recording. *J. Neurophysiol.* **2005**, *93*, 2987–3000. [CrossRef] [PubMed]
6. Herbawi, A.S.; Larramendy, F.; Galchev, T.; Holzhammer, T.; Mildenberger, B.; Paul, O.; Ruther, P. CMOS-Based Neural Probe with Enhanced Electronic Depth Control. In Proceedings of the 18th International Conference on Solid-State Sensors, Actuators and Microsystems (Transducers), Anchorage, AK, USA, 21–25 June 2015.
7. Lopez, C.M.; Andrei, A.; Mitra, S.; Welkenhuysen, M.; Eberle, W.; Bartic, C.; Puers, R.; Yazicioglu, R.F.; Gielen, G.G.E. An implantable 455-active-electrode 52-channel CMOS neural probe. *IEEE J. Solid-State Circuit.* **2014**, *49*, 248–261. [CrossRef]
8. Berényi, A.; Somogyvári, Z.; Nagy, A.J.; Roux, L.; Long, J.D.; Fujisawa, S.; Stark, E.; Leonardo, A.; Harris, T.D.; Buzsáki, G. Large-scale, high-density (up to 512 channels) recording of local circuits in behaving animals. *J. Neurophysiol.* **2014**, *111*, 1132–1149. [CrossRef] [PubMed]
9. Nordhausen, C.T.; Maynard, E.M.; Normann, R.A. Single unit recording capabilities of a 100 microelectrode array. *Brain Res.* **1996**, *726*, 129–140. [CrossRef]
10. Shobe, J.L.; Claar, L.D.; Parhami, S.; Bakhurin, K.I.; Masmanidis, S.C. Brain activity mapping at multiple scales with silicon microprobes containing 1024 electrodes. *J. Neurophysiol.* **2015**, *114*, 2043–2052. [CrossRef] [PubMed]
11. Drake, K.L.; Wise, K.D.; Farraye, J.; Anderson, D.J.; BeMent, S.L. Performance of planar multisite microprobes in recording extracellular single-unit intracortical activity. *IEEE Trans. Biomed. Eng.* **1988**, *35*, 719–732. [CrossRef] [PubMed]
12. Scholvin, J.; Kinney, J.P.; Bernstein, J.G.; Moore-Kochlacs, C.; Kopell, N.; Fonstad, C.G.; Boyden, E.S. Close-packed silicon microelectrodes for scalable spatially oversampled neural recording. *IEEE Trans. Biomed. Eng.* **2016**, *63*, 120–130. [CrossRef] [PubMed]
13. Campbell, P.K.; Jones, K.E.; Huber, R.J.; Horch, K.W.; Normann, R.A. A silicon-based, three-dimensional neural interface: Manufacturing processes for an intracortical electrode array. *IEEE Trans. Biomed. Eng.* **1991**, *38*, 758–768. [CrossRef] [PubMed]
14. Hoogerwerf, A.C.; Wise, K.D. A Three-Dimensional Neural Recording Array. In Proceedings of the International Conference on Solid-State Sensors and Actuators. Digest of Technical Papers, San Francisco, CA, USA, 24–27 June 1991.
15. Perlin, G.E.; Wise, K.D. A Compact Architecture for Three-Dimensional Neural Microelectrode Arrays. In Proceedings of the 30th Annual International Conference of the IEEE Engineering in Medicine and Biology Society, Vancouver, BC, Canada, 20–25 August 2008.

16. Bai, Q.; Wise, K.D.; Anderson, D.J. A high-yield microassembly structure for three-dimensional microelectrode arrays. *IEEE Trans. Biomed. Eng.* **2000**, *47*, 281–289. [PubMed]

17. Yao, Y.; Gulari, M.N.; Wiler, J.A.; Wise, K.D. A microassembled low-profile three-dimensional microelectrode array for neural prosthesis applications. *J. Microelectromech. Syst.* **2007**, *16*, 977–988. [CrossRef]

18. Herwik, S.; Kisban, S.; Aarts, A.A.A.; Seidl, K.; Girardeau, G.; Benchenane, K.; Zugaro, M.B.; Wiener, S.I.; Paul, O.; Neves, H.P.; et al. Fabrication technology for silicon-based microprobe arrays used in acute and sub-chronic neural recording. *J. Micromech. Microeng.* **2009**, *19*, 074008. [CrossRef]

19. Aarts, A.A.A.; Srivannavit, O.; Wise, K.D.; Yoon, E.; Puers, R.; Van Hoof, C.; Neves, H.P. Fabrication technique of a compressible biocompatible interconnect using a thin film transfer process. *J. Micromech. Microeng.* **2011**, *21*, 074012. [CrossRef]

20. Kisban, S.; Holzhammer, T.; Herwik, S.; Paul, O.; Ruther, P. Novel method for the assembly and electrical contacting of out-of-plane microstructures. In Proceedings of the 23rd International Conference on Micro Electro Mechanical Systems (MEMS), Hong Kong, China, 24–28 January 2010.

21. Cheng, M.Y.; Yao, L.; Tan, K.L.; Lim, R.; Li, P.; Chen, W. 3D probe array integrated with a front-end 100-channel neural recording ASIC. *J. Micromech. Microeng.* **2014**, *24*, 125010. [CrossRef]

22. Malhi, S.D.S.; Davis, H.E.; Stierman, R.J.; Bean, K.E.; Driscoll, C.C.; Chatterjee, P.K. Orthogonal Chip Mount—A 3D Hybrid Wafer Scale Integration Technology. In Proceedings of the International Electron Devices Meeting, Washington, DC, USA, 6–9 December 1987.

23. Lee, Y.T.; Lin, C.W.; Lin, C.M.; Yeh, S.R.; Chang, Y.C.; Fu, C.C.; Fang, W. A 3D Glass Microprobe Array with Embedded Silicon for Alignment and Electrical Connection. In Proceedings of the International Solid-State Sensors, Actuators and Microsystems Conference, Denver, CO, USA, 21–25 June 2009.

24. Hoogerwerf, A.C.; Wise, K.D. A three-dimensional microelectrode array for chronic neural recording. *IEEE Trans. Biomed. Eng.* **1994**, *41*, 1136–1146. [CrossRef] [PubMed]

25. Barz, F.; Holzhammer, T.; Paul, O.; Ruther, P. Novel Technology for the In-plane to Out-of-plane Transfor of Multiple Interconnection Lines in 3D Neural Probes. In Proceedings of the 17th International Conference on Solid-State Sensors, Actuators and Microsystems (Transducers & Eurosensors XXVII), Barcelona, Spain, 16–20 June 2013.

26. John, J.; Li, Y.; Zhang, J.; Loeb, J.A.; Xu, Y. Microfabrication of 3D neural probes with combined electrical and chemical interfaces. *J. Micromech. Microeng.* **2011**, *21*, 105011. [CrossRef]

27. Merriam, S.M.E.; Srivannavit, O.; Gulari, M.N.; Wise, K.D. A three-dimensional 64-site folded electrode array using planar fabrication. *J. Microelectromech. Syst.* **2011**, *20*, 594–600. [CrossRef]

28. Wang, M.F.; Maleki, T.; Ziaie, B. A self-assembled 3D microelectrode array. *J. Micromech. Microeng.* **2010**, *20*, 035013. [CrossRef]

29. Chen, C.H.; Chuang, S.C.; Su, H.C.; Hsu, W.L.; Yew, T.R.; Chang, Y.C.; Yeh, S.R.; Yao, D.J. A three-dimensional flexible microprobe array for neural recording assembled through electrostatic actuation. *Lab Chip* **2011**, *11*, 1647–1655. [CrossRef] [PubMed]

30. Takeuchi, S.; Suzuki, T.; Mabuchi, K.; Fujita, H. 3D flexible multichannel probe array. *J. Micromech. Microeng.* **2004**, *14*, 104–107. [CrossRef]

31. Chiou, J.C.; Chang, C.W. Development of Three Dimensional Neural Sensing Device by Stacking Method. In Proceedings of the IEEE Sensors 2010 Conference, Kona, HI, USA, 1–4 November 2010.

32. Merriam, M.E.; Dehmel, S.; Srivannavit, O.; Shore, S.E.; Wise, K.D. A 3-D 160-Site Microelectrode Array for Cochlear Nucleus Mapping. *IEEE Trans. Biomed. Eng.* **2011**, *58*, 397–403. [CrossRef] [PubMed]

33. Du, J.; Riedel-Kruse, I.H.; Nawroth, J.C.; Roukes, M.L.; Laurent, G.; Masmanidis, S.C. High-Resolution three-dimensional extracellular recording of neuronal activity with microfabricated electrode arrays. *J. Neurophysiol.* **2009**, *101*, 1671–1678. [CrossRef] [PubMed]

34. Barz, F.; Paul, O.; Ruther, P. Modular Assembly Concept for 3D Neural Probe Prototypes Offering High Freedom of Design and Alignment Precision. In Proceedings of the 36th Annual International Conference of the IEEE Engineering in Medicine and Biology Society, Chicago, IL, USA, 26–30 August 2014.

35. Langhals, N.B.; Kipke, D.R. Validation of a Novel Three-Dimensional Electrode Array Within Auditory Cortex. In Proceedings of the Annual International Conference of the IEEE Engineering in Medicine and Biology Society, Minneapolis, MN, USA, 3–6 September 2009.

36. Scholvin, J.; Kinney, J.P.; Bernstein, J.G.; Moore-Kochlacs, C.; Kopell, N.J.; Fonstad, C.G.; Boyden, E.S. Heterogeneous neural amplifier integration for scalable extracellular microelectrodes. In Proceedings of the 38th Annual International Conference of the IEEE Engineering in Medicine and Biology Society (EMBC), Orlando, FL, USA, 16–20 August 2016.

37. Rios, G.; Lubenov, E.V.; Chi, D.; Roukes, M.L.; Siapas, A.G. Nanofabricated neural probes for dense 3-D recordings of brain activity. *Nano Lett.* **2016**, *16*, 6857–6862. [CrossRef] [PubMed]

38. Michon, F.; Aarts, A.; Borghs, G.; Bruce, M.; Fabian, K. Integration of silicon-based probes and micro-drive array for chronic recordings of large populations of neurons in behaving animals. *J. Neural Eng.* **2016**, *13*, 1–11. [CrossRef] [PubMed]

39. Dombeck, D.A.; Khabbaz, A.N.; Collman, F.; Adelman, T.L.; Tank, D.W. Imaging Large-Scale Neural Activity with Cellular Resolution in Awake, Mobile Mice. *Neuron* **2007**, *56*, 43–57. [CrossRef] [PubMed]

40. Harvey, C.D.; Collman, F.; Dombeck, D.A.; Tank, D.W. Intracellular dynamics of hippocampal place cells during virtual navigation. *Nature* **2009**, *461*, 941–946. [CrossRef] [PubMed]

41. Scholvin, J.; Fonstad, C.G.; Boyden, E.S. Scaling models for microfabricated in vivo neural recording technologies. In Proceedings of the 8th International IEEE/EMBS Conference on Neural Engineering (NER), Shanghai, China, 25–28 May 2017.

42. Hetke, J.F.; Lund, J.L.; Najafi, K.; Wise, K.D.; Anderson, D.J. Silicon ribbon cables for chronically implantable microelectrode arrays. *IEEE Trans. Biomed. Eng.* **1994**, *41*, 314–321. [CrossRef] [PubMed]

43. Ledochowitsch, P.; Tiefenauer, R.F.; Pepin, B.; Maharbiz, M.M.; Blanche, T.J. Nanoflex for Neural Nanoprobes. In Proceedings of the The 17th International Conference on Solid-State Sensors, Actuators and Microsystems (Transducers & Eurosensors XXVII), Barcelona, Spain, 16–20 June 2013.

44. Sun, T.; Park, W.T.; Cheng, M.Y.; An, J.Z.; Xue, R.F.; Tan, K.L.; Je, M. Implantable polyimide cable for multichannel high-data-rate neural recording microsystems. *IEEE Trans. Biomed. Eng.* **2012**, *59*, 390–399. [CrossRef] [PubMed]

45. Hetke, J.F.; Najafi, K.; Wise, K.D. Flexible miniature ribbon cables for long-term connection to implantable sensors. *Sensor Actuators A-Phys.* **1990**, *23*, 999–1002. [CrossRef]

46. Thacker, H.D.; Bottoms, W.R. Wafer-Level testing of gigascale integrated circuits. In *Integrated Interconnect Technologies for 3D Nanoelectronic Systems*; Artech House: Norwood, MA, USA, 2009.

47. International Technology Roadmap for Semiconductors. Available online: https://www.semiconductors.org/clientuploads/Research_Technology/ITRS/2015/0_2015%20ITRS%202.0%20Executive%20Report%20(1).pdf (accessed on 24 August 2018).

48. Zorzos, A.N.; Scholvin, J.; Boyden, E.S.; Fonstad, C.G. Three-dimensional multiwaveguide probe array for light delivery to distributed brain circuits. *Opt. Lett.* **2012**, *37*, 4841–4843. [CrossRef] [PubMed]

49. Gaither, M.S.; Gates, R.S.; Kirkpatrick, R.; Cook, R.F.; DelRio, F.W. Etching process effects on surface structure, fracture strength and reliability of single-crystal silicon theta-like specimens. *J. Microelectromech. Syst.* **2013**, *22*, 589–602. [CrossRef]

50. Najafi, K.; Ji, J.; Wise, K.D. Scaling limitations of silicon multichannel recording probes. *IEEE Trans. Biomed. Eng.* **1990**, *37*, 1–11. [CrossRef] [PubMed]

51. Kruger, J.; Aiple, F. Multimicroelectrode investigation of monkey striate cortex: Spike train correlations in the infragranular layers. *J. Neurophysiol.* **1988**, *60*, 798–828. [CrossRef] [PubMed]

52. Rousche, P.J.; Normann, R.A. A method for pneumatically inserting an array of penetrating electrodes into cortical tissue. *Ann. Biomed. Eng.* **1992**, *20*, 413–422. [CrossRef] [PubMed]

53. Edell, D.J.; Toi, V.V.; McNeil, V.M.; Clark, L.D. Factors influencing the biocompatibility of insertable silicon microshafts in cerebral cortex. *IEEE Trans. Biomed. Eng.* **1992**, *39*, 635–643. [CrossRef] [PubMed]

54. Pak, N.; Siegle, J.H.; Kinney, J.P.; Denman, D.J.; Blanche, T.J.; Boyden, E.S. Closed-loop, ultraprecise, automated craniotomies. *J. Neurophysiol.* **2015**, *113*, 3943–3953. [CrossRef] [PubMed]

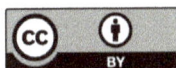

micromachines

MDPI

Article

Development, Modeling, Fabrication, and Characterization of a Magnetic, Micro-Spring-Suspended System for the Safe Electrical Interconnection of Neural Implants

Katharina Hoch [1], Frederick Pothof [1], Felix Becker [1], Oliver Paul [1,2] and Patrick Ruther [1,2,*]

[1] Department of Microsystems Engineering (IMTEK), University of Freiburg, 79110 Freiburg, Germany; katharina.hoch@imtek.uni-freiburg.de (K.H.); frederick.pothof@imtek.uni-freiburg.de (F.P.); felix.becker@imtek.uni-freiburg.de (F.B.); paul@imtek.de (O.P.)

[2] BrainLinks-BrainTools Cluster of Excellence, University of Freiburg, 79110 Freiburg, Germany

* Correspondence: ruther@imtek.de; Tel.: +49-761-203-7197

Received: 31 July 2018; Accepted: 21 August 2018; Published: 23 August 2018

Abstract: The development of innovative tools for neuroscientific research is based on in vivo tests typically applied to small animals. Most often, the interfacing of neural probes relies on commercially available connector systems which are difficult to handle during connection, particularly when freely behaving animals are involved. Furthermore, the connectors often exert high mechanical forces during plugging and unplugging, potentially damaging the fragile bone structure. In order to facilitate connector usage and increase the safety of laboratory animals, we developed a new magnetic connector system circumventing the drawbacks of existing tools. The connector system uses multiple magnet pairs and spring-suspended electrical contact pads realized using micro-electromechanical systems (MEMS) technologies. While the contact pad suspension increases the system tolerance in view of geometrical variations, we achieved a reliable self-alignment of the connector parts at ±50 µm provided by the specifically oriented magnet pairs and without the need of alignment pins. While connection forces are negligible, we can adjust the forces during connector release by modifying the magnet distance. With the connector test structures developed here, we achieved an electrical connection yield of 100%. Based on these findings, we expect that in vivo experiments with freely behaving animals will be facilitated with improved animal safety.

Keywords: neural interfacing; micro-electromechanical systems (MEMS) technologies; microelectromechanical systems; neuroscientific research; magnetic coupling; freely-behaving

1. Introduction

The goal of neuroscientific research is to analyze brain functionality, and to understand and treat neuronal disorders. For this, neuroscientists and physicians use neural implants to record or trigger neural activity on the brain surface as well as directly within the brain tissue. During the past decades, extensive research in the field of neurotechnology targeting the continuous development and improvement of neural implants has helped to establish appropriate diagnostic methods and clinical treatments for a broad variety of neural diseases. Exemplary disorders such as Parkinson's disease, epilepsy and dystonia, for which drug treatment might become ineffective over time, can nowadays be successfully targeted by deep brain stimulation or diagnosed by neural implants followed by a subsequent surgical resection of the affected brain areas [1–4], respectively. Furthermore, auditory and visual prostheses such as the well-established cochlear implants or innovative retina implants are based on the ongoing improvement in recording and stimulation techniques [5–8].

Basic neuroscientific research is most often performed on small animals such as rodents [9]. In the case of translational efforts towards clinical applications, neuroscientific tools and procedures need to be further approved in larger animals such as non-human primates (NHP) [10–12], sheep [13] or pigs [14]. Depending on the complexity and duration of these experiments, probes to be implanted and validated are interfaced either by transcutaneous connectors [15] or via fully implantable, wireless recording systems [16].

Figure 1a illustrates a recording experiment using a silicon-based neural probe implanted into the cortex of a rat. As sketched, the neural probe is attached to a printed circuit board (PCB) carrying a small strip connector, e.g., of the Omnetics Nano Series (Omnetics, Minneapolis, MN, USA) [17,18] or MOLC/FOLC (Samtec, New Albany, IN, USA) type [19]. Following probe implantation, the probe and PCB are permanently anchored to the skull using dental cement, which at the same time seals the craniotomy that exposed the brain surface prior to probe implantation. Obviously, the skulls of mice and rats require careful handling during surgery. In particular, when connecting and disconnecting the external instrumentation either directly or via a longer tether cable (Figure 1a) using the aforementioned connectors, excessive force may easily damage the fragile bone structure.

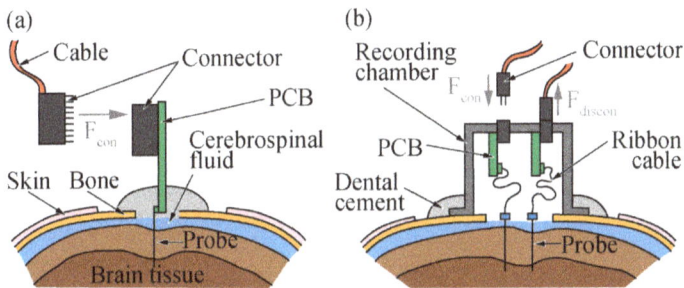

Figure 1. Silicon-based probes (**a**) directly interfacing a printed circuit board (PCB) fixed to the skull using dental cement, and (**b**) floating with the brain interfacing a PCB fixed to a recording chamber. The electrical interface between probe and an external instrumentation is accomplished via small strip connectors providing a tethered connection (F_{con} and F_{discon} represent forces exerted during connection and disconnection, respectively).

The example of a recording chamber, as often used in the case of NHP experiments to mechanically protect the surgical area as well as the connectors between the various recording sessions, is shown in Figure 1b. In this case, the neural implant is interfaced to a small connector fixed in the recording chamber via a highly flexible ribbon cable connected to an intermediate PCB [10,20]. When the connector is being plugged in, connecting forces F_{con} are effectively distributed across the chamber sidewalls avoiding local mechanical stress peaks on the skull surface. In contrast, unintended forces pulling the cable in different directions relative to the connector orientation might induce torque on the connector, eventually damaging the cable or the connector itself.

The interconnections formed in the case of these specific animal experiments are often quite rigid and need comparably large connection forces. As an example, Omnetics Nano Series connectors require connection and disconnection forces up to 2 N per contact [21]. Forces exerted during connection and disconnection potentially harm the fragile skull of small animals while unintended forces applied during experimental use might damage the connectors or interfacing cables, or harm the bone structure by large mechanical torque. In addition to issues related to excessive or unintended forces and torque, some connector variants are often not intended for repeated connection and disconnection. Wear may result in unreliable electrical connection. Thus, innovative connector systems circumventing the aforementioned issues are required. They need to be laid out for experiments on small animals such as mice and rats, require minimal connection and disconnection forces, and also enable simple and fast handling in the case of experiments with freely behaving animals. Furthermore, the connector needs to be compatible with a broad variety of different devices such as silicon-based probes [20,22], flexible polymer-based electrode arrays [23,24], and other devices. Even the above-mentioned wireless recording systems may benefit from an enhanced connector system, as any headstage—may it be wireless or not—has to be connected to the neural probe in some way.

One technical solution to reduce connecting/disconnecting forces implies magnetic coupling of the two connector parts. Such a magnetic break-away connection was initially introduced for a deep fryer equipped with a magnetic power cord [25]. This connector variant was spread to a broader audience when Apple applied it in its laptops as the magnetically attached power supply MagSafe® (Apple, Cupertino, CA, USA). The connection is designed such that unintended forces acting on the power cord immediately unclasp the connection, therefore preventing the laptop from being pulled and damaged unintentionally. The connector unit applies a ferromagnetic material and five gold-plated, spring-mounted contacts on one side. The counterpart contains five concave contact pads surrounded by a permanent magnet which provides the force needed to fix both connector parts and at the same time shields the electrical pins. This connector is approximately 17 mm wide and 5 mm tall. *MagSafe* was granted a patent in 2007 [26].

To the best of our knowledge, there are only a few magnetically-coupled connector systems available for neural implants. One example, a magnetic fiber stub for optogenetic stimulation experiments has been developed by Plexon (Dallas, TX, USA) [27]. It is intended to be combined with either a magnetic head-mounted light-emitting diode (LED) or an optical patch cable which contains a magnetic ferrule. The interface comprises a stainless steel tubing and a ring magnet enabling free rotation while being connected to the external component. This effectively reduces the torque on the implant which is highly beneficial for experiments with freely behaving animals.

A percutaneous connector with up to 128 channels using spring-loaded pin contacts has been introduced by Smith and Guillory [28]. The magnetic coupling system comprises a ferrous ring on one connector part and several magnets in the respective counterpart. The precise alignment of both connector halves is achieved by an alignment pin. The magnetic connector system presented by Shah et al. [29] features up to 64 channels. It consists of several magnets circularly mounted around the connector center with alternating magnetization directions of the individual magnets. This design includes an additional anisotropic conductive film (ACF) placed between the two connector halves acting as an interconnect sheet to guarantee a good electrical contact. The alignment of the connector parts is again achieved by means of passive alignment features. Both percutaneous connector variants fulfill the above-mentioned requirements to some extent. Connection and disconnection seem to work without the need of large forces while providing a stable electric transmission. However, the connector dimension renders these devices impractical for experiments with small animals. The alignment pins reduce the ease of operation and prevent disconnection by lateral forces in experiments with freely behaving animals, thus reducing the safety of the animals.

In the present work, we propose a new magnetic connector system offering minimal connection and disconnection forces, a secure disconnection when unintended lateral forces are applied, and fast and easy device handling during connection. The latter advantage is achieved by the omission of alignment pins. Although the connection is less rigid, and thus, the risk of animal harm or device failure is reduced to a minimum, the mechanical system is strong enough to ensure a stable electrical connection. The initial idea of implementing spring-suspended contact pads in a MEMS-based connector and its fabrication were previously presented in [30]. Here we provide a comprehensive description of the novel connector system and the underlying fabrication process, an in-detail mechanical and electrical characterization, as well as an analytical model of the spring-suspended contact pads. The insights gained from this model in conjunction with the experimental system characterization enable the definition of an optimal connector design for future modules to be applied in neuroscientific experiments.

2. Materials and Methods

2.1. Module Design

The aim of this work is to develop a novel connector system for neural implants. In contrast to most of the existing interconnection technologies, the system is designed to work with low connection and disconnection forces, and thus, to be suitable for experiments with small rodents, among other applications. As illustrated in Figure 2, the connector system comprises two connector parts. They are pulled together by small magnets enabling a reliable signal transmission between adjacent electrical contact pads. While the lower part interfacing the neural probe is permanently fixed to the skull of the animal, the counterpart is equipped with a tether cable giving access to the external instrumentation. As magnets are used, connection forces are negligible while the disconnection force is defined by the strength and number of magnets applied. By installing the magnets in different directions of magnetization, the two connector parts self-align once in close proximity. As no alignment features are needed, the connection is easily released as soon as external forces parallel to the plane of connection exceed a threshold value. This magnetic break-away connection prevents animal harm and device failure.

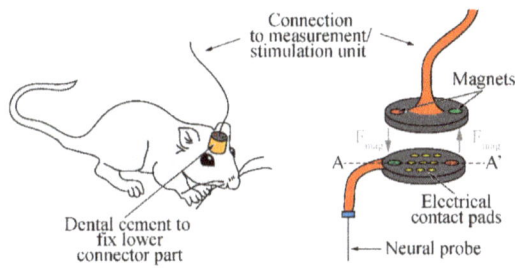

Figure 2. Schematic of basic connector concept applying small magnets to magnetically pull the connector parts together. Different magnet orientations are exploited to self-align the parts when being brought in contact.

In addition to the magnetic break-away connection, the study compared different contact pad compliances, as illustrated in Figure 3. Protruding gold (Au) bumps realized, e.g., by electroplating were used as electrical contacts. In the case of the stiff connector variant (Figure 3b1), both parts comprise silicon (Si) chips of the same thickness. In contrast to this approach, the connector variant shown in Figure 3b2 applies spring-suspended pads on the upper connector part to account for possible module bow and warp, and for differences in the electroplated pad heights.

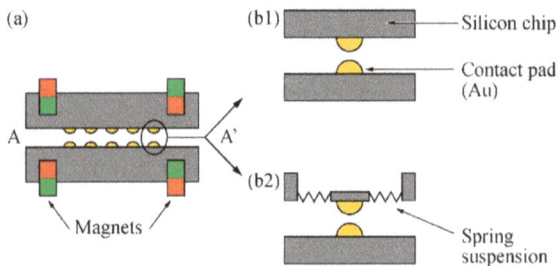

Figure 3. (**a**) Cross-section of connector parts illustrating the adjacent contact pads and (**b**) respective pad compliances using either (**b1**) a stiff pad contact or (**b2**) spring-suspended pads on the upper connector part.

Connector test modules, as schematically shown in Figure 4, were designed and fabricated in order to investigate the relevant connection forces, contact resistance and interconnection yield. They comprise a module carrier that can be interfaced via zero-insertion force (ZIF) [31] connectors enabling a time-efficient electrical validation of the connector system. A circular module cover (diameter 10 mm, thickness 380 µm) constitutes the upper connector part shown in Figure 2. Depending on the connector variant, as shown in Figure 3b, 32 rigid or spring-suspended contact pads are integrated in the module cover at a center-to-center distance of 1250 µm while the same number of rigid pads are used in the module carrier. In a real connector system used for animal experiments, the module carrier and cover are interfaced to the implantable probe and a tether cable, respectively, as indicated in Figure 2.

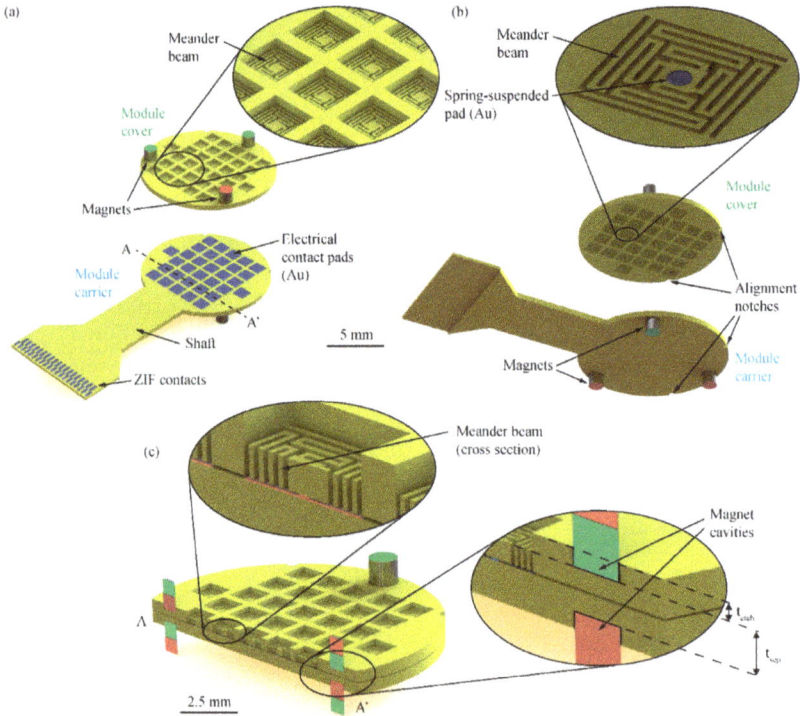

Figure 4. Connector modules seen from (**a**) above and (**b**) below. The module cover comprises spring-suspended pads and three magnets integrated on its top side. The module carrier contains quadratic contact pads connected to a zero insertion force (ZIF) interface and magnets on its bottom side. Cover and carrier comprise additional alignment notches for inspection purposes; magnet orientation is indicated by the red and green color. (**c**) Cross-section of connected modules along line A-A in (**a**). Magnet distance is denoted t_{sep}. Adapted from [30].

The module carrier and cover each comprise three circular cavities (diameter 1 or 1.2 mm, depth $\geq$ 180 µm) for cylindrical magnets. The cavities are implemented in the module face opposite to the contact pads. As illustrated by the different colors in Figure 4, one of the three magnet pairs is mounted with opposite direction of magnetization. This guarantees that the two halves of the connector can only be mated in a unique orientation.

In order to enhance the compliance of the contact pads and to increase the system tolerance towards deviations in the contact pad heights, as well as the potential bow and warp of the connector modules, one variant of the module cover is equipped with spring-suspended contact pads. The metallized contact pads with a diameter of 150 µm are integrated on quadratic structures with a side length of 250 µm. As shown in Figure 4b, each pad is symmetrically suspended on four meander-shaped beams (total length 2455 µm, width 40 µm, thickness t_b) within a rigid, quadratic frame (side length 970 µm). The number of meander beam sections and their respective lengths were determined with the help of an analytical model and finite element (FE) simulations. All corners of the meander structure are rounded in order to avoid mechanical stress concentrations. While the rigid frame has a thickness of 380 µm equivalent to the wafer thickness t_{wafer}, beams and contact support structures are thinned down to $t_b = t_{wafer} - t_{etch}$, where t_{etch} represents the etch depth of the magnet cavities. The beam thickness corresponds to half of the magnet distance t_{sep}, as indicated in Figure 4c.

While the rigid contact pads on the module carrier are of quadratic shape (length 930 µm), circular pads (diameter 150 µm) are implemented on the module cover. The relatively large size difference of the pads allows to compensate for in-plane misalignments of both connector parts of up to 840 µm. For test purposes, the electroplated pad heights on the carrier and cover were varied between 1 and 8 µm. Metal lines on the carrier base connecting the pads with the ZIF section along the 4-mm-wide shaft are made of chromium (Cr) and Au.

To facilitate and accelerate the electrical characterization, the test modules were designed in a way that contact pads on the module cover are short-circuited in pairs. In this way, mated connector parts can be efficiently interfaced via the ZIF interface on the module carrier enabling the extraction of connection yield and contact resistance. The lateral alignment of the module cover and carrier relative to each other is validated by optical inspection under a microscope using two semi-circular alignment notches (diameter 500 µm) implemented in the rim of carrier and cover (see Figure 4b).

Cylindrical, nickel-plated neodymium magnets (Supermagnete, Gottmadingen, Germany; height and diameter of 1 ± 0.1 mm) were used for the test modules. They weigh 6 mg and have a maximum energy product of 342–358 kJ/m^3.

2.2. Module Fabrication

The test structures are designed so that module carrier and cover can be fabricated on a common Si substrate using a single process flow. Both module variants presented in Figure 3b were fabricated simultaneously in the same process. Figure 5 summarizes the main clean room fabrication steps for these Si test structure modules. As substrates, 380-µm-thick Si wafers covered by a 1-µm-thick thermal silicon oxide (SiO$_2$) layer on both sides were used.

Following the initial cleaning of the wafers in acetone, isopropanol and Piranha solution, a lift-off process was used to pattern the metallization. This applies hexamethyldisilazane (HMDS) as an adhesion promoter, and spin-coating and hard-baking of the 700-nm-thick photo-insensitive resist LOR5A (MicroChem Corp., Westborough, MA, USA) and the 1.8-µm-thick positive photoresist AZ1518 (Microchemicals GmbH, Ulm, Germany). During ultra-violet (UV) light exposure, only the AZ1518 resist is modified, which results in a locally increased solubility. During the subsequent development using tetramethylammonium hydroxide (TMAH), the AZ1518 is dissolved in areas exposed to UV light. In contrast, LOR5A is dissolved isotropically where the structure of the AZ resist gives access to the TMAH solution. Due to this isotropic behavior and a strictly time-controlled development, an undercut of about 1 µm was obtained (see Figure 5a), which facilitated the subsequent lift-off of the metal layer. The metallization, i.e., 50 nm chromium (Cr) and 200 nm Au were sputter-deposited (Figure 5b) with the Cr layer used as an adhesion promoter between the SiO$_2$ and Au layers. The resist strip lifts the metal on top of the patterned AZ1518, resulting in well-defined contact pads and conducting leads on the Si substrate.

Patterning the metallization was followed by the plasma enhanced chemical vapor deposition (PECVD) of a 1-µm-thin passivation layer (Figure 5c). Similar to an established fabrication process of Si-based neural probes [32], the passivation comprises a stack of multiple silicon oxide (SiO$_x$) and silicon nitride (Si$_x$N$_y$) layers providing an optimal stress compensation. This passivation also serves as a protection layer for the metal structures during the subsequent process steps carried out on the wafer rear, which brings the wafer front into contact to wafer chucks.

The photolithography on the wafer rear applied another dehydration bake and the adhesion promoter HMDS. Next, a 10-µm-thick layer of the positive photoresist AZ9260 (Microchemicals GmbH) was spin-coated and structured using UV lithography. This serves as the etch mask for the rear SiO_2 layer patterned using reactive ion etching (RIE). This was followed by deep reactive ion etching (DRIE) of Si (see Figure 5d) to define the magnet cavities, the areas under the ZIF pads on the carrier modules, and the areas where the spring-suspended contact pads will be realized in the module covers. To obtain test structures with different suspension beam thicknesses, the etch depth was varied between 200 µm and 330 µm. In addition, the outer rear shape of the individual components was defined in this step.

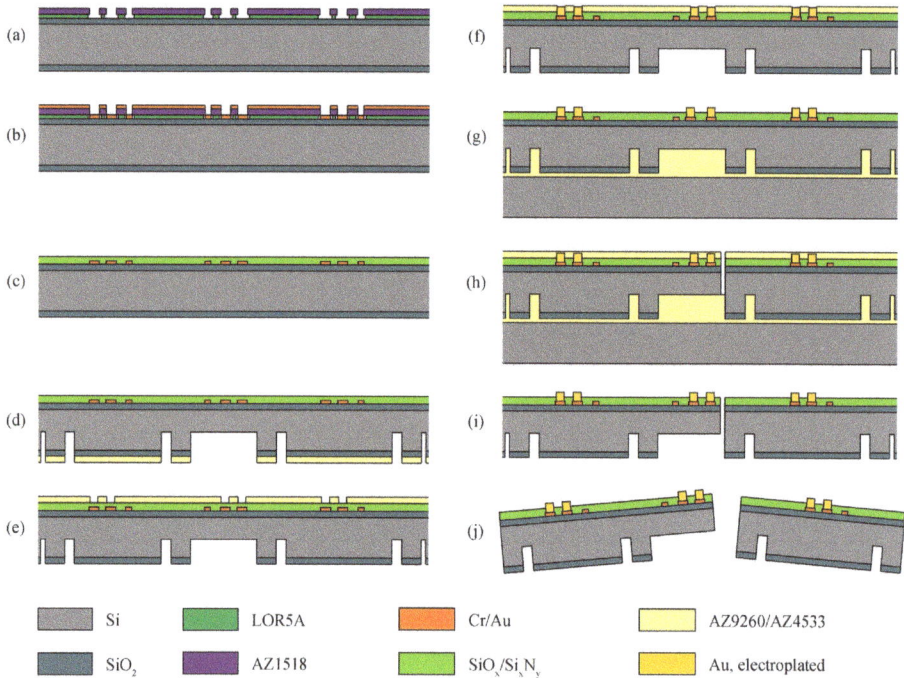

Figure 5. Fabrication process to realize the connector modules by means of microsystems processes performed on the wafer front (**a–c,h**) and rear (**d–g**), followed by the separation of the individual parts (**i,j**). Adapted from [30].

Stripping the photoresist in acetone and isopropanol, the wafer processing continued with a further photolithography step on the front to open the passivation at the contact pads that will be thickened by electroplating. Again, a 10-µm-thick layer of AZ9260 was spin-coated and structured by UV lithography (Figure 5e) followed by RIE to open the passivation. Subsequently, the contact pads were electroplated at a current density of 0.75 mA/cm^2 resulting in a deposition rate of approximately 0.0475 µm/min according to Faraday's law of electrolysis. Using the AZ9260 resist as a masking layer, wafers of different contact pad heights were realized. Following electroplating, the AZ9260 resist was stripped and the wafer was transferred onto a handle wafer fixed using the resist AZ4533 (Microchemicals GmbH) (see Figure 5g). The handle wafer is needed for stability reasons, especially for the final front etching, where the Si parts are separated from each other.

The next photolithography step was carried out on the wafer front, again using a dehydration bake, HMDS-based adhesion promotion as well as spin-coating and patterning of a 10-µm-thick layer of AZ9260. The resist was used as a mask in the RIE process to open the passivation layer. This was followed by a wet etch to remove the electroplating feed lines of the individual connector parts. The Au was etched with a potassium iodide (KI)-iodine(I_2)-solution (100 g KI and 25 g I_2 plus deionized (DI) water for 1 L of etch solution), whereas the Cr was removed with a ceric ammonium nitride (($NH4)_2Ce(NO_3)_6$)-nitric acid (HNO_3) solution (165 g ($NH_4)_2Ce(NO_3)_6$ and 90 mL HNO_3(69%) plus DI water for 1 L of etch solution). By means of DRIE, the wafer was then etched through to a depth ≤ 180 µm to achieve the trenches defining the geometry of the individual parts, which have already been pre-etched from the wafer rear (Figure 5h). The struts used to suspend the connector parts in the fabrication wafer were not etched from the wafer front.

After a final resist strip and release of the handle wafer, the Si components were suspended inside the fabrication wafer by the struts (Figure 5i). Individual parts were separated by applying torsional forces with the aid of a pair of tweezers (Figure 5j). This was then followed by the assembly and the fixation of the magnets in their cavities.

2.3. Modeling of Spring-Suspended Contact Pads

2.3.1. Analytical Model

An analytical model was derived to describe the mechanical behavior of the meander-shaped contact pad suspension. It considers both bending and torsion of the individual sections of the suspension beam and is based on the schematic shown in Figure 6a. As the suspension system with its four identical suspension beams is symmetric, only one of the beams is modeled, as illustrated in Figure 6b.

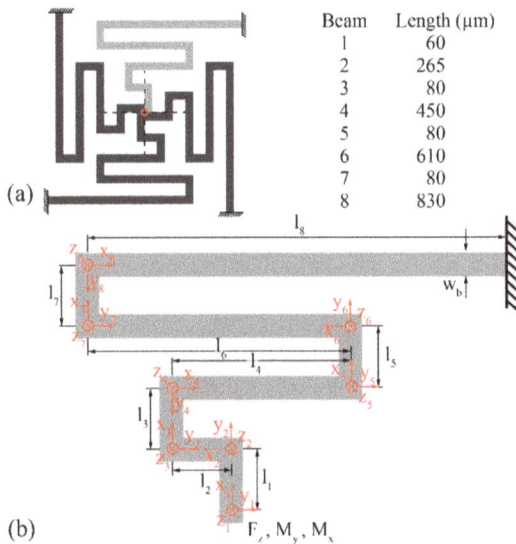

Beam	Length (µm)
1	60
2	265
3	80
4	450
5	80
6	610
7	80
8	830

Figure 6. (**a**) Symmetric suspension beam system comprised of four identical meander beams fixed to the rigid frame and lengths of the individual beam sections. (**b**) Mechanical model of one meander beam consisting of eight beams sections (lengths l_i ($i = 1, \ldots, 8$)) of width w_b and thickness t_b. The model applies the Young's modulus E_{Si}, area moment of inertia I, shear modulus G_{Si} and torsional moment of inertia I_t. The force F_{pad} applied to the complete suspension system is translated into the force $F_z = 0.25 F_{pad}$ and the moments M_x and M_y acting on a single meander beam (F_z, M_x and M_y are defined in the global *x-y-z*-coordinate system).

Each of the meander-shaped beams has one fixed support where the eighth beam section is connected to the Si frame which is assumed to be perfectly rigid. The other end is connected to the quadratic contact pad support onto which the force F_{pad} acts in the positive z-direction when the connector modules are brought into contact. Each beam section i ($i = 1, \ldots, 8$) is described by its respective length l_i, the area moment of inertia $I = w_b t_b^3/12$ where w_b and t_b denote the beam width and height, respectively, the torsional moment of inertia $I_t = t_b w_b^3/3(1 - 0.630 w_b/t_b + 0.052 w_b^5/t_b^5)$ [33], as well as the Young's modulus E_{Si}, Poisson's ratio v_{Si}, and the shear modulus $G_{Si} = E_{Si}/2(1 + v_{Si})$ of Si. Local coordinate systems x_i-y_i-z_i ($i = 1, \ldots, 8$) are used in each beam section i to define local internal forces and moments.

As indicated in Figure 6a, the pad suspension comprises four identical meander-shaped beams connected to a quadratic structure supporting the contact pad. In order to analyze the mechanical behavior of this beam system when a vertical force F_{pad} is applied in its center (see red dot in Figure 6a), the model evaluates one quarter only, obtained by cutting the pad suspension along the dashed lines shown in Figure 6a. The external force F_{pad} acting on the entire suspension is translated in forces F_j and moments M_j with $j = x, y, z$ acting on each individual meander beam. For symmetry reasons and because beam deflections were kept small, the model assumes that $F_x = F_y = 0$ and $M_z = 0$. This leaves the two moments M_x and M_y, shown in Figure 6b, as unknowns while the force F_z in z-direction equals $F_{pad}/4$. The moments together with the mating force F_z can now be transferred through the meandering suspension beam to calculate the internal forces and moments along the influence line resulting in the bending and torsional moments M_{y_i} and M_{x_i} as functions of x_i ($i = 1, \ldots, 8$), respectively. They are listed in Table 1.

Table 1. Bending and torsional moments M_{y_i} and M_{x_i}, respectively, of the individual beam sections i ($i = 1, \ldots, 8$) used in the analytical model shown in Figure 6 assuming that the force F_z and the moments M_x and M_y are applied on a single, meander-shaped suspension beam.

i	$M_{y_i}(x_i)$	$M_{x_i}(x_i)$
1	$-F_z x_1 - M_y$	$-M_x$
2	$-F_z x_2 - M_x$	$F_z l_1 + M_y$
3	$-F_z(l_1 + x_3) - M_y$	$-F_z l_2 - M_x$
4	$-F_z(-l_2 + x_4) + M_x$	$-F_z(l_1 + l_3) - M_y$
5	$-F_z(l_1 + l_3 + x_5) - M_y$	$F_z(l_2 - l_4) - M_x$
6	$-F_z(l_2 - l_4 + x_6) - M_x$	$F_z(l_1 + l_3 + l_5) + M_y$
7	$-F_z(l_1 + l_3 + l_5 + x_7) - M_y$	$-F_z(l_6 - l_4 + l_2) - M_x$
8	$-F_z(-l_6 + l_4 - l_2 + x_8) + M_x$	$-F_z(l_1 + l_3 + l_5 + l_7) - M_y$

Equation (1) in Table 1 can be summarized for $k > 0$ to

$$M_{y_k}(x_k) = -F_z x_k - (-1)^{\frac{k(k+1)}{2}} M_{x_{k-1}} \tag{1}$$

$$M_{x_k}(x_k) = (-1)^{\frac{k(k+1)}{2}} M_{y_{k-1}}(l_{k-1}) \tag{2}$$

with $M_{y_0}(l_0) = M_x$ and $M_{x_0} = -M_y$ as used in Table 1. The term $(-1)^{k(k+1)/2}$ generates the sequence $(-1, -1, 1, 1, -1, -1, 1, 1, \ldots)$ for all natural numbers $k > 0$.

In order to calculate the deflection of the pad suspension shown in Figure 6, the analytical model applies the energy theorem of mechanics that states that the work W done by external loads on a deformed body equals the stored elastic energy Π [34]. All further formulas in this section are taken from [35]. Consequently, the work carried out on the beam system by applying a force F_{pad} during connector mating is entirely transformed into elastic energy.

The specific strain energies $\prod_{b,i}^*$ and $\prod_{t,i}^*$ of bent and twisted beams, respectively, are given by

$$\prod_{b,i}^* = \frac{1}{2}\frac{M_{y_i}^2}{E_{\mathrm{Si}}I} \tag{3}$$

$$\prod_{t,i}^* = \frac{1}{2}\frac{M_{x_i}^2}{G_{\mathrm{Si}}I_t} \tag{4}$$

where M_{y_i} and M_{x_i} denote the bending and torsional moments acting on the i-th beam section, as given in Equation (1). The specific strain energies, which are given per unit length, are integrated over the total beam length $l_b = \sum_i l_i$ to achieve the total strain energy $\prod_{\mathrm{tot}}$ of the spring-suspension given by

$$\prod_{\mathrm{tot}} = \int_0^{l_b}\left(\prod_b^* + \prod_t^*\right)\mathrm{d}x \tag{5}$$

With the bending and torsional moments from Equation (1), one separately calculates the respective contributions of the individual beam sections i to the bending and torsional energies $\prod_{b,i}$ and $\prod_{t,i}$. They are listed in Table 2, normalized by $(2E_{\mathrm{Si}}I)^{-1}$ and $(2G_{\mathrm{Si}}I_t)^{-1}$, respectively.

Table 2. Specific strain energies $\prod_{b,i}^*$ and $\prod_{t,i}^*$ of bent and twisted beam sections i normalized by $(2E_{\mathrm{Si}}I)^{-1}$ and $(2G_{\mathrm{Si}}I_t)^{-1}$, respectively.

i	$2E_{\mathrm{Si}}I\prod_{b,i}$	$2G_{\mathrm{Si}}I_t\prod_{t,i}$
1	$l_1\left(l_1^2F_z^2/3 + l_1F_zM_y + M_y^2\right)$	$l_1M_x^2$
2	$l_2(l_2^2F_z^2/3 + l_2F_zM_x + M_x^2)$	$l_2\left(l_1^2F_z^2 + 2l_1F_zM_y + M_y^2\right)$
3	$l_3((3l_2^2 + 3l_1l_3 + l_3^2)F_z^2/3(2l_1 + l_3)F_zM_y + M_y^2)$	$l_3\left(l_2^2F_z^2 + 2l_2F_zM_x + M_x^2\right)$
4	$l_4((3l_2^2 + 3l_2l_4 + l_4^2)F_z^2/3 + (2l_2 + l_4)F_zM_x + M_x^2)$	$l_4((l_1^2 + 2l_1l_3 + l_3^2)F_z^2 2((l_1 + l_3)F_zM_y + M_y^2)$
5	$l_5((3l_1^2 + 6l_1l_3 + 3l_1l_5 + 3l_3^2 + 3l_3l_5 + l_5^2)F_z^2/3 + (2l_1 + 2l_3 + l_5)F_zM_y + M_y^2)$	$l_5((l_2^2 - 2l_2l_4 + l_4^2)F_z^2 2((l_4 - l_2)F_zM_x + M_x^2)$
6	$l_6((3l_2^2 - 6l_2l_4 + 3l_4^2 - 3l_4l_6 + 3l_2l_6 + l_6^2)F_z^2/3 + (2l_4 - 2l_2 - l_6)F_zM_x + M_x^2)$	$l_6((l_1^2 + 2l_1l_3 + 2l_1l_5 + l_3^2 + l_3l_5 + l_5^2)F_z^2 2((l_1 + l_3 + l_5)F_zM_y + M_y^2)$
7	$l_7((3l_1^2 + 6l_1l_3 + 3l_3^2 + 6l_1l_5 + 6l_3l_5 + 3l_5^2 + 3l_1l_7 + 3l_3l_7 + 3l_5l_7 + l_7^2)F_z^2/3 + (2l_1 + 2l_3 + 2l_5 + l_6)F_zM_y + M_y^2)$	$l_7((l_2^2 - 2l_2l_4 + 2l_2l_6 + l_4^2 - l_4l_6 + l_6^2)F_z^2 2(l_2 - l_4 + l_6)F_zM_x + M_x^2)$
8	$l_8((3l_4^2 - 6l_4l_6 + 3l_6^2 + 6l_2l_6 - 3l_2l_4 + 3l_2^2 - 3l_6l_8 + 3l_4l_8 - 3l_2l_8 + l_8^2)F_z^2/3 + (2l_6 - 2l_4 + 2l_2 - l_8)F_zM_x + M_x^2)$	$l_8((l_1^2 + 2l_1l_3 + 2l_1l_5 + 2l_1l_7 + l_3^2 + 2l_3l_5 + 2l_3l_7 + l_5^2 + 2l_5l_7 + l_7^2)F_z^2 + (l_1 + l_3 + l_5 + l_7)F_zM_y + M_y^2)$

Summarizing over all beam sections, the total strain energy $\prod_{\mathrm{tot}}$ is given by

$$\begin{aligned}\prod_{\mathrm{tot}} = {} & \frac{1}{E_{\mathrm{Si}}I}\left(A_1F_z^2 + A_2F_zM_y + A_3M_y^2 + A_4F_zM_x + A_5M_x^2\right) \\ & + \frac{1}{G_{\mathrm{Si}}I_t}\left(B_1F_z^2 + B_2F_zM_y + B_3M_y^2 + B_4F_zM_x + B_5M_x^2\right)\end{aligned} \tag{6}$$

with A_m and B_m being functions of the beam lengths l_i ($i = 1, \ldots, 8$), i.e., $A_m = f_m(l_1, \ldots, l_8)$ and $B_m = g_m(l_1, \ldots, l_8)$ for $m = 1, \ldots, 5$.

The result is an expression of the total strain energy $\prod_{\mathrm{tot}}$ with three unknowns acting on the central pad support, i.e., the force F_z, the bending moment M_y and the torsional moment M_x.

Castigliano's first theorem calculates the displacement or the angular rotation at the point of application of a force and moment in the direction of the force line of the causative force and the rotation axis of the causative moment, respectively. For this purpose, the derivatives of the total strain energy $\prod_{tot}(F_i, M_i)$ as a function of the applied external forces and moments are taken with respect to the relevant forces or moments. Here these are the vertical displacement,

$$\Delta_z = \frac{\partial \prod_{tot}}{\partial F_z} \tag{7}$$

and the two rotation angles φ_n, with $n = x, y$, given by

$$\varphi_n = \frac{\partial \prod_{tot}}{\partial M_n} \tag{8}$$

Due to symmetry considerations at the contact pad support, torsion around the x_1- and y_1-axis is zero at the transition from the meander beam to the contact pad. Castigliano's first theorem can therefore be used to calculate M_y and M_x as a function of F_z to fulfill this request. In other terms one has to solve

$$\frac{\partial \prod_{tot}(F_z, M_y, M_x)}{\partial M_y} = 0 \tag{9}$$

and

$$\frac{\partial \prod_{tot}(F_z, M_y, M_x)}{\partial M_x} = 0 \tag{10}$$

It can be shown that M_x and M_y are linear functions of F_z through the origin, i.e., $M_x = C_1 F_z$ and $M_y = C_2 F_z$ with $C_p = h_p(l_1, \ldots, l_8)$ for $p = 1, 2$.

As a consequence, one obtains an expression for the total strain energy $\prod_{tot}$ which only depends on F_z^2. By taking the derivative of this expression with respect to F_z, one obtains the displacement of the contact pad support in the z-direction given by

$$\Delta z = \frac{\partial \prod_{tot}}{\partial F_z} \tag{11}$$

Following Equations (6) and (11) with a quadratic dependence of $\prod_{tot}$ on F_z, one obtains a linear relation between Δz and the applied force F_z.

2.3.2. Finite Element Simulations

To validate the analytic results and for a fast estimation of the influence of certain parameters, a FE analysis was carried out using COMSOL (Version 5.2a, Burlington, MA, USA). The spring-suspension of an individual contact pad with four symmetrically positioned meander beams was simulated. With a beam width of w_b = 40 μm, a beam thickness of t_b = 200 μm, and the lengths of the individual beam sections as specified in Figure 6a, the geometrical dimensions were chosen in accordance with the fabricated test structures. As boundary conditions, fixed ends of the meander beams were assumed at the rigid Si frame. A vertical force of F_{pad} = 200 mN corresponding to the total strength of three magnet pairs was applied to the center of the contact pad. The whole structure was defined to be made of Si with a Young's modulus of 170 GPa and a Poisson's ratio of 0.28. Passivation layers and metal lines were neglected. The FE simulation was carried out with a free tetrahedral mesh with minimum and maximum element sizes of 0.1 and 10 μm, respectively, a maximum element growth rate of 1.3, a curvature factor of 0.2, and a resolution of narrow regions of 1.

2.4. Module Characterization

2.4.1. Mechanical Tests

The mechanical force F_{mag}, which is needed to overcome the attractive force of the magnets and to separate the two connector halves was measured using a tensile test setup (Z2.5 zwicki-Line,

Zwick/Roell, Ulm, Germany). In order to fix the connector module components in the test setup using pneumatic clamps, plastic cylinder supports were glued onto the rear sides of individual parts comprising three magnets each (Figure 7a). The magnetic force F_{mag} was recorded as a function of displacement Δz while separating the two connector parts in the vertical direction at a speed of 0.1 mm/min.

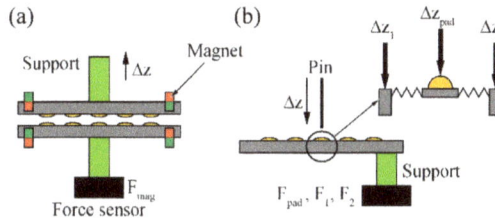

Figure 7. Schematic representation of mechanical testing using a tensile test device; characterization of (a) magnetic disconnection force F_{mag} and (b) mechanical yield of beam suspension.

In order to characterize the mechanical behavior and strength of the spring-suspended contact pads, the same tensile test setup was used as well. In this case, we mounted the plastic cylinders used for device clamping off-center on the connector modules comprising the spring-suspensions. With this arrangement we prevented any adhesive entering the trenches between the suspension beams during the assembly process. While the connector module is mounted on the lower clamp, a metal pin (500 μm diameter with sharp tip) is fixed to the movable clamp. The positioning of the pin with respect to the spring suspension is optically controlled using a video microscope. By moving this pin vertically onto the pad, the displacement-force curve $F_{pad}\left(\Delta z_{pad}\right)$ is recorded. It serves to extract the range of forces that can act perpendicularly on the connector plane without breaking the meander beams. As the fixation pin is glued off-center, we compensated for the compliance of the experimental setup by recording displacement-force curves $F_q\left(\Delta z_q\right)$ with $q = 1$, 2 when loading the connector module at two positions on the Si substrate next to the suspension frame, as indicated in Figure 7b. Beam suspension and frame compliance were tested at a speed of 0.1 mm/min of the pin for different meander beam thicknesses.

2.4.2. Electrical Tests

The electrical connection yield was determined by a two-wire resistance measurement. As described in Section 2.1, the contacts on the module cover are short-circuited in pairs. Hence, a two-wire resistance measurement on the ZIF section of the module carrier can determine whether two pairs of Au pads have electrical contact. Should any one of them fail, the measurement will reveal an open loop. A measured resistance below 15 kΩ was rated as a stable electrical connection. This comparably high resistance is explained by the only 6-μm-wide electrical leads between the ZIF section and the contact pads. Different combinations of contact-pad heights on the module carrier and module cover were tested.

In order to characterize the contact resistance between two pads, we used three corresponding pads P1 to P3 on the module carrier and cover each. While the three pads on the cover are short circuited with pad P2 being positioned in the middle, pads P1 and P3 on the carrier are interfaced to ZIF pads Z1 and Z4, respectively. In contrast, pad P2 of the module carrier is connected to ZIF pads Z2 and Z3. This enables a four-contact resistance measurement at the mating pads P2 using a wafer prober. A constant current $I_{1,3}$ was applied between the ZIF pads Z1 and Z3 while the voltage drop $\Delta V_{2,4}$ across the corresponding pads P2 on the module carrier and cover was determined via the ZIF pads Z2 and Z4. This allows the calculation of the contact resistance omitting the line resistances on both connector parts.

3. Results

3.1. Module Fabrication

The test structures for the novel connector system were successfully fabricated, as shown in Figure 8. The scanning electron micrograph in Figure 9a shows in detail the spring suspension of a contact pad. By varying the etch depth during rear DRIE, we obtained test modules with meander beam thicknesses of 200 µm, 100 µm, and 50 µm. Consequently, the vertical distance t_{sep} between two magnets in the mated connector state (Figure 4c) was set to 400 µm, 200 µm, and 100 µm.

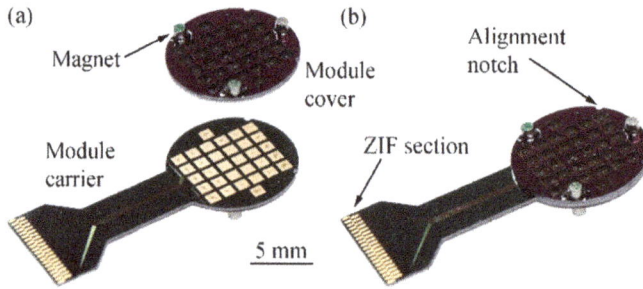

Figure 8. Fully assembled 32-channel Si test structure in the (**a**) separated and (**b**) connected state. Adapted from [30].

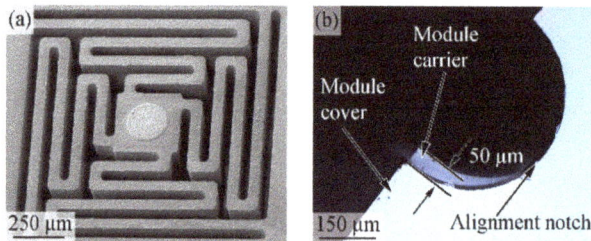

Figure 9. (**a**) Scanning electron micrograph of a spring-suspended contact pad. (**b**) Optical inspection of the self-alignment accuracy of two connector parts using respective alignment notches.

Using the notches implemented in the rim of the connector parts, the alignment accuracy was optically inspected during repeated connector mating. Following the system idea of magnetic self-alignment described in Section 2.1., no particular care was taken for a precise pre-alignment of the connector halves during the manual connection procedure. The optical inspection of mated connectors revealed a lateral alignment accuracy of better than 50 µm for each of the individual tests (cf. Figure 9b). It has to be kept in mind that the misalignment originates from a combination of relative translation and rotation of the two connector halves. As the misalignment is measured at the connector rim, the observed value represents the worst case, in particular for a pure rotational misalignment.

3.2. Modeling

The analytical model demonstrated that the displacement Δz of a spring-suspended contact pad depends linearly on the mating force F_{pad}. With the geometrical beam dimensions given in Figure 6a and the material properties of Si, i.e., E_{Si} = 170 GPa, ν_{Si} = 0.28 and G_{Si} = 66.4 GPa, the spring constant c_{model} of the meander beam system is extracted on the basis of Equations (6) and (11) as

$$c_{model} = 4\frac{F_z}{\Delta z(F_z)} = 31.5\frac{mN}{\mu m} \tag{12}$$

Using realistic magnetic forces of the three magnet pairs of 264 mN and the fact that 32 contact pads are implemented, the force F_{pad} per contact is 8.25 mN equivalent to a displacement of only Δz = 0.26 µm. This displacement might not be sufficient to overcome device bow, warp, and potential differences in the electroplating pad height, to form a stable electrical connection. To compensate for a certain under-dimensioning of the magnets used in this study we added an additional force of 460 mN by means of an additional weight placed on top of a connector cover. This results in a force of approximately 23 mN per contact and a theoretical pad displacement of 0.72 µm using the modelled spring constant.

Figure 10 shows the results of the COMSOL finite element simulations for a contact force of 200 mN acting on a single spring-suspended pad. As indicated in Figure 10a, a vertical displacement of 5.67 µm is obtained. This corresponds to a spring constant of c_{sim} = 35 mN/µm, slightly higher than c_{model} above. For this contact force, a maximum von Mises stress of 339 MPa is obtained in the surface of the beam suspension using the FE simulations (Figure 10b). This stress level is below the mechanical yield strength of Si reported to be in the range of 1 GPa [36] up to 7 GPa [37], depending on surface quality. Taking into account that the force used in the FE simulations is well above the applicable force using the chosen magnets, we expect that the mechanical strength of the suspension beams is more than sufficient.

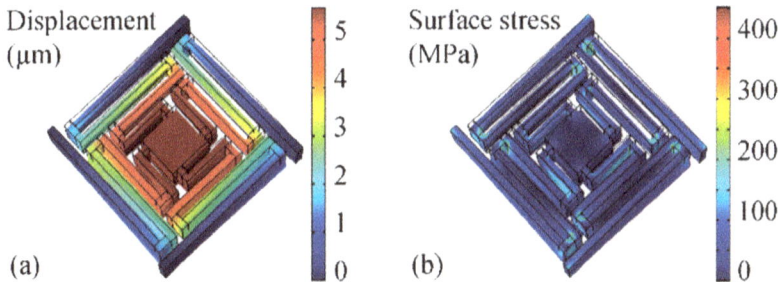

Figure 10. COMSOL FEA of a spring-suspended contact pad (vertical load 200 mN). (a) Displacement of the meander beam system. (b) Von Mises surface stress due to bending and torsion.

3.3. Module Characterization

Figure 11 shows the vertical disconnection force F_{mag} of the realized test structures as a function of the vertical displacement Δz for different magnet distances t_{sep}. For t_{sep} = 200 µm and 400 µm, maximum forces of 227 mN and 106 mN have been extracted, respectively. The fact that the two curves do not match exactly is explained by an unknown amount of epoxy inside the magnet cavities increasing the distance between the two magnets in the mated connector state.

Figure 12 shows the deflection of three representative spring-suspended contact pads under a vertical load F_{pad} (symbols). It is compared to the modeled and simulated data, indicated by the solid and dashed lines, respectively. The meander structures typically collapsed at vertical deflections between 11.9 µm and 13.6 µm and a respective force in the range of 300 mN. Following the FE simulations, the maximum force can be translated into a maximum von Mises stress in the beam structure of ca. 500 MPa. The fact that this value is below the data in the literature data [36,37] can be explained by the increased surface roughness of the DRIE processed beam sidewalls.

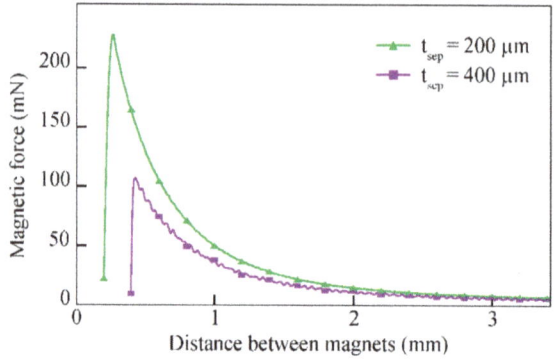

Figure 11. Magnetic disconnection force for two values of t_{sep} as a function of the vertical distance between the magnets. Adapted from [30].

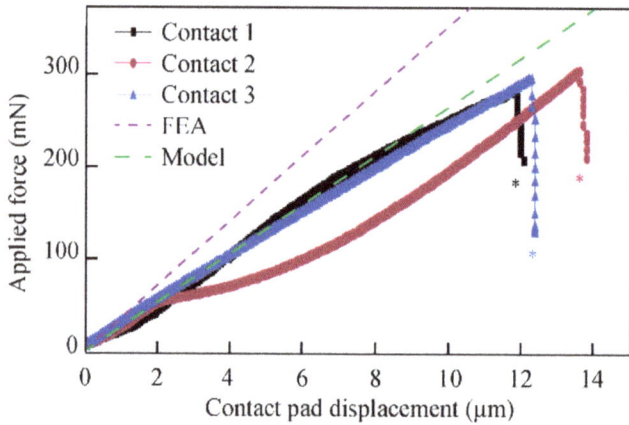

Figure 12. Vertical deflection of suspended contact pads vs applied force comparing experiment (three different pads), analytical model and FE simulations. Beam fracture is indicated by asterisks. Adapted from [30].

The electrical characterization of connector modules with different contact heights h_{cover} and $h_{carrier}$ on the module cover and carrier, respectively, is summarized in Table 3. It provides the connection yield as the percentage of successful electrical interconnection of 16 pairs of dual pad connections for the cover modules with spring-suspended (bold) and stiff contact pads (Figure 3b). It should be noted that the actual yield might be higher than the given numbers as a successful contact requests two pads to be effectively interfaced (see Section 2.1) In addition to the connection force exerted by the integrated magnets, an additional force of approximately 460 mN had to be applied to achieve a stable connection in the case of the spring-suspended contact pads. Depending on the pad height combination and thickness of the meander beam, an electrical connection yield of up to 100% was achieved for the spring-suspended variant. In the case of the stiff contact pads, despite the additional force weight applied, we could not achieve adequate percentages of stable electrical contacts.

Each connector configuration, i.e., combination of pad heights h_{cover} and $h_{carrier}$ and beam thickness t_b, was tested with one module comprising 32 channels, equivalent to 16 pairs of dual pad connections. As the statistical significance of our data is low, only certain trends in view of promising pad height combinations can be extracted. The contact resistance extracted using the 4-point-measurements, as described above, is in the range of 11 to 20 mΩ.

Table 3. Connection yield in % for different combinations of pad thicknesses h_1 and h_2, and beam heights t_b for spring-suspended (bold) and stiff contact pad variants. Due to the limited magnetic force of the magnets applied, an additional load of 460 mN was exerted on top of the modules. The heights of the circular and quadratic pads on the module cover and carrier are labeled as h_{cover} and $h_{carrier}$, respectively. Meander beam systems are thinned to $t_b = 200$ μm except (*) with $t_b = 50$ μm and (**) with $t_b = 100$ μm.

h_{cover} (μm)	$h_{carrier}$ (μm)			
	1	2	4	8
1	NA/7	NA/13	NA/0	NA/50
1 *	**90**/NA	**53**/NA	**40**/NA	**0**/NA
1 **	**35**/NA	**83**/NA	**100**/NA	**0**/NA
2	**94**/0	**100**/17	**94**/13	**0**/73
4	**100**/0	**100**/6	**100**/13	**0**/38
8	**84**/20	**92**/25	**92**/13	**16**/53

4. Discussion

The analytical model and the FE simulation provided slightly different spring constants c_{model} and c_{sim} (see also curves in Figure 12) of 31.5 and 35 mN/μm, respectively. A reason for this difference is certainly that the area moment of inertia used in the analytical model is assumed to be constant along the entire meander length. However, the beam corners have a considerably larger area moment of inertia than the beams. This likely explains the larger stiffness extracted from the FE simulation compared to the analytical model.

The discrepancy between FE simulations and the experimental tests of the beam suspension (Figure 12) can be explained by geometrical variations in the test structure dimensions due to the DRIE fabrication process, e.g., slightly tapered sidewalls, and the fact that the passivation layer and metal leads have not been included in the FE model. In the current design, the pad suspensions are somewhat stiff and this will be addressed in a future design optimization, where modified design parameters as well as alternative suspension geometries will be considered. Such alternative design may be based on helical designs with a reduced number of beams, ultimately enabling a size reduction with potentially smaller pad distances.

In view of system applicability, one has to consider the mechanical strength of the beam suspension, the forces exerted by the integrated magnets, the resulting connection yield and the alignment accuracy of both connector parts. For the given system dimensions, we extracted maximum vertical pad deflections between 11.9 and 13.6 μm at forces of ca. 300 mN per contact pad, i.e., a total force of 9.6 N for an entire connector comprising 32 pads. In that sense, the total pad height $h_1 + h_2$ of the module cover and carrier pads has to be limited to approximately 12 μm assuming that the magnetic force per pad can reach values of 300 mN. However, implementing the given small cylindrical magnets and a separation distance of 400 μm between the magnets, a maximum connection force of 264 mN for 32 pads, i.e., 8.25 mN per pad, cause beam deflections of only 0.26 μm. These deflections are well below the experimentally determined yield strength. Assuming a separation distance of $t_{sep} = 0$ μm achievable for $t_{etch} = t_{wafer}$, the connection force is increased to 1029 mN, still far below the maximum applicable deflections. Consequently, stronger, yet similarly compact magnets are required and have to be chosen such that the system dimensions are not increased too much.

The higher electrical connection yield of the spring-suspended connector variant in comparison to the stiff version successfully demonstrated the chosen connector concept. A connection yield of 100% for certain pad height combinations was, however, only achievable by applying an additional load of 460 mN on the entire connector. This clearly indicates that either more or stronger magnets need to be implemented in a redesign of the connector. The data summarized in Table 3 indicates that thicker pads on the module carrier, i.e., up to 8 μm, are not suitable for a stable electrical connection between the connector halves. Instead, using slightly protruding pad metallization on the cover module with h_{cover} = 4 μm provides the best results for $h_{carrier}$ between 1 and 4 μm. As discussed in Section 3.3, these findings need to be further validated by a statistically more significant number of test devices.

The lateral self-alignment accuracy of 50 μm is far better than needed for the applied pad sizes of 970 × 970 μm^2. A pronounced reduction in the pad size is thus possible. However, the current bottleneck in size reduction is the area occupied by the pad suspension relying on the proposed meander beam design.

The disconnection forces, in the range of several hundred mN per connector, are much smaller than those reported for other state-of-the-art magnetic connector systems. As an example, Shah et al. reported a normal disconnection force of 4.9 N for their connector system [29]. Hence, the implementation of stronger magnets as indicated by the applied models and the connection yield tests is still feasible without affecting animal safety.

5. Conclusions

A novel connector system for the safe electrical interconnection of neural implants based on a magnetic break-away mechanism was designed, fabricated, and extensively characterized. The system comprises spring-suspended contact pads compensating for the potential bow and warp of the connector components and differences on electroplated pad heights. The disconnection forces of the connector system are clearly reduced compared to other state-of-the-art devices. Therefore, the proposed design offers increased safety for future in vivo applications with freely moving animals. In addition, excessive lateral forces are inherently prevented, thus avoiding the action of mechanical torque on the connectors. Such undesired mechanical loads potentially harm the bone structure of the animal to which the connector is fixed. Safety is further increased by the omission of alignment pins, which is a unique feature of the new connector system.

The high self-alignment accuracy of better than 50 μm during connector mating clearly facilitates system handling when preparing the animals for a recording session. The correct positioning of the connector parts is inherently achieved by the specific arrangement of three magnet pairs. No manual pressure or any mechanical alignment features are needed. Compared to compact connectors as typically used in neuroscientific research, the connection procedure is straightforward and requires no specific training of the end-user.

Our study successfully demonstrated that the spring-suspension provides a high connection yield compared to a stiff connector variant. We identified pad height combinations on the two connector halves that showed the best performance regarding height compliance and thus electrical connection yield. As the high yield was only achieved by applying additional load exceeding the mating forces provided by the integrated magnets, future design optimizations of the connector need to implement more or stronger magnets.

So far, our magnetic, micro-spring-suspended system meets every demand of neuroscientific in-vivo experiments. Still, this has to be verified under real conditions.

The experimental findings regarding the mechanical suspension beam behavior were supported by a simplified analytical model derived in this study to describe the meander-like beams and by finite element simulations. Both the model and simulation predict similar spring constants. This knowledge will be used to define an optimal, application-specific design and respective fabrication parameters for future connector modules directly applicable in neuroscientific research.

Author Contributions: Conceptualization, K.H., F.P., F.B. and P.R.; Methodology, K.H., F.P. and P.R.; Project administration, P.R.; Supervision, F.P. and P.R.; Validation, K.H.; Writing—original draft, K.H.; Writing—review & editing, K.H., F.P., O.P. and P.R.

Funding: This research was funded by the European Union's Seventh Framework Program (FP7/2007-2013) under grant agreement No. 600 925 (NeuroSeeker). The article processing charge was funded by the German Research Foundation (DFG) and the University of Freiburg in the funding programme Open Access Publishing.

Acknowledgments: The authors gratefully acknowledge the support from IMTEK's Clean Room Service Center staff.

Conflicts of Interest: The authors declare no conflict of interest. The funders had no role in the design of the study; in the collection, analyses, or interpretation of data; in the writing of the manuscript, and in the decision to publish the results.

References

1. Limousin, P.; Krack, P.; Pollak, P.; Benazzouz, A.; Ardouin, C.; Hoffmann, D.; Benabid, A.-L. Electrical stimulation of the subthalamic nucleus in advanced Parkinson's disease. *N. Engl. J. Med.* **1998**, *339*, 1105–1111. [CrossRef] [PubMed]
2. Duncan, J.S. Epilepsy surgery. *Clin. Med.* **2007**, *7*, 137–142. [CrossRef]
3. Schulze-Bonhage, A.; Zentner, J. The preoperative evaluation and surgical treatment of epilepsy. *Dtsch. Arztebl. Int.* **2014**, *111*, 313–319. [CrossRef] [PubMed]
4. Bittar, R.G.; Yianni, J.; Wang, S.; Liu, X.; Nandi, D.; Joint, C.; Scott, R.; Bain, P.G.; Gregory, R.; Stein, J.; et al. Deep brain stimulation for generalised dystonia and spasmodic torticollis. *J. Clin. Neurosci.* **2005**, *12*, 12–16. [CrossRef] [PubMed]
5. Roche, J.P.; Hansen, M.R. On the horizon: Cochlear implant technology. *Otolaryngol. Clin. N. Am.* **2015**, *48*, 1097–1116. [CrossRef] [PubMed]
6. Zierhofer, C.M.; Hochmair-Desoyer, I.J.; Hochmair, E.S. Electronic design of a cochlear implant for multichannel high-rate pulsatile stimulation strategies. *IEEE Trans. Rehabil. Eng.* **1995**, *3*, 112–116. [CrossRef]
7. Da Cruz, L.; Coley, B.F.; Dorn, J.; Merlini, F.; Filley, E.; Christopher, P.; Chen, F.K.; Wuyyuru, V.; Sahel, J.; Stanga, P.; et al. The Argus II epiretinal prosthesis system allows letter and word reading and long-term function in patients with profound vision loss. *Br. J. Ophthalmol.* **2013**, *97*, 632–636. [CrossRef] [PubMed]
8. Rathbun, D.L.; Jalligampala, A.; Stingl, K.; Zrenner, E. To what extent can retinal prostheses restore vision? In Proceedings of the 7th International IEEE/EMBS Conference on Neural Engineering (NER), Montpellier, France, 22–24 April 2015; pp. 244–247. [CrossRef]
9. Berényi, A.; Somogyvári, Z.; Nagy, A.J.; Roux, L.; Long, J.D.; Fujisawa, S.; Stark, E.; Leonardo, A.; Harris, T.D.; Buzsáki, G. Large-scale, high-density (up to 512 channels) recording of local circuits in behaving animals. *J. Neurophysiol.* **2014**, *111*, 1132–1149. [CrossRef]
10. Pothof, F.; Bonini, L.; Lanzilotto, M.; Livi, A.; Fogassi, L.; Orban, G.A.; Paul, O.; Ruther, P. Chronic neural probe for simultaneous recording of single-unit, multi-unit, and local field potential activity from multiple brain sites. *J. Neural. Eng.* **2016**, *13*, 046006. [CrossRef] [PubMed]
11. Donoghue, J.P.; Nurmikko, A.; Black, M.; Hochberg, L.R. Assistive technology and robotic control using motor cortex ensemble-based neural interface systems in humans with tetraplegia. *J. Physiol.* **2007**, *579*, 603–611. [CrossRef] [PubMed]
12. Bonini, L.; Maranesi, M.; Livi, A.; Fogassi, L.; Rizzolatti, G. Space-dependent representation of objects and other's action in monkey ventral premotor grasping neurons. *J. Neurosci.* **2014**, *34*, 4108–4119. [CrossRef] [PubMed]
13. Gierthmuehlen, M.; Wang, X.; Gkogkidis, A.; Henle, C.; Fischer, J.; Fehrenbacher, T.; Kohler, F.; Raab, M.; Mader, I.; Kuehn, C.; et al. Mapping of sheep sensory cortex with a novel microelectrocorticography grid. *J. Comp. Neurol.* **2014**, *522*, 3590–3608. [CrossRef] [PubMed]
14. Ulyanova, A.V.; Koch, P.F.; Grovola, M.R.; Browne, K.D.; Russo, R.J.; Adam, C.D.; Smith, D.H.; Chen, H.I.; Johnson, V.E.; Cullen, D.K.; et al. Electrophysiological signature reveals laminar structure of the porcine hippocampus. *bioRxiv* **2017**, *1*, 201285. [CrossRef]
15. Brochier, T.; Zehl, L.; Hao, Y.; Duret, M.; Sprenger, J.; Denker, M.; Grün, S.; Riehle, A. Massively parallel recordings in macaque motor cortex during an instructed delayed reach-to-grasp task. *Sci. Data* **2018**, *5*, 180055. [CrossRef] [PubMed]

16. Kohler, F.; Gkogkidis, C.A.; Bentler, C.; Wang, X.; Gierthmuehlen, M.; Fischer, J.; Stolle, C.; Reindl, L.M.; Rickert, J.; Stieglitz, T.; et al. Closed-loop interaction with the cerebral cortex: A review of wireless implant technology. *Brain Comput. Interface* **2017**, *4*, 146–154. [CrossRef]

17. Fiedler, E.; Ordonez, J.; Stieglitz, T. Modular assembly of flexible thin-film electrode arrays enabled by a laser-structured ceramic adapter. In Proceedings of the 6th International IEEE/EMBS Conference on Neural Engineering (NER), San Diego, CA, USA, 6–8 November 2013; pp. 657–660. [CrossRef]

18. Rubehn, B.; Bosman, C.; Oostenveld, R.; Fries, P.; Stieglitz, T. A MEMS-based flexible multichannel ECoG-electrode array. *J. Neural Eng.* **2009**, *6*, 036003. [CrossRef] [PubMed]

19. Bernstein, J.G.; Allen, B.D.; Guerra, A.A.; Boyden, E.S. Processes for design, construction and utilisation of arrays of light-emitting diodes and light-emitting diode-coupled optical fibres for multi-site brain light delivery. *J. Eng.* **2015**, *2015*. [CrossRef] [PubMed]

20. Barz, F.; Livi, A.; Lanzilotto, M.; Maranesi, M.; Bonini, L.; Paul, O.; Ruther, P. Versatile, modular 3D microelectrode arrays for neuronal ensemble recordings: From design to fabrication, assembly, and functional validation in non-human primates. *J. Neural Eng.* **2017**, *14*, 036010. [CrossRef] [PubMed]

21. Data Sheet Omnetics Nano Series. Available online: http://www.omnetics.com/products/micro-and-nano-strips/nano-nps-npd-series#1852-tab4 (accessed on 4 June 2018).

22. Wise, K.D.; Sodagar, A.M.; Yao, Y.; Gulari, M.N.; Perlin, G.E.; Najafi, K. Microelectrodes, microelectronics, and implantable neural microsystems. *Proc. IEEE* **2008**, *96*, 1184–1202. [CrossRef]

23. Ordonez, J.; Schuettler, M.; Boehler, C.; Boretius, T.; Stieglitz, T. Thin films and microelectrode arrays for neuroprosthetics. *MRS Bull.* **2012**, *37*, 590–598. [CrossRef]

24. Luan, L.; Wei, X.; Zhao, Z.; Siegel, J.J.; Potnis, O.; Tuppen, C.A.; Lin, S.; Kazmi, S.; Fowler, R.A.; Holloway, S.; et al. Ultraflexible nanoelectronic probes form reliable, glial scar-free neural integration. *Sci. Adv.* **2017**, *3*, 1601966. [CrossRef] [PubMed]

25. News for "Break Away" Power Cords on Electric Deep Fryers. Available online: http://www.dowell.com.hk/breakawaycord_news.htm (accessed on 6 May 2017).

26. Rohrbach, M.D.; Doutt, M.E.; Andre, B.K.; Lim, K.; DiFonzo, J.C.; Gery, J.-M. Magnetic Connector for Electronic Device. U.S. Patent 7,311,526, 25 December 2007.

27. Kwon, K.Y.; Gnade, A.G.; Rush, A.D.; Patten, C.D. Head-mounted LED for optogenetic experiments of freely-behaving animal. In Proceedings of the SPIE BiOS, San Francisco, CA, USA, 13–18 February 2016; pp. 1–9. [CrossRef]

28. Smith, C.F.; Guillory, K.S. High-Density, Low-mating-force, magnetically-coupled, percutaneous connector for implanted electrode arrays. In Proceedings of the 3rd International IEEE EMBS Conference on Neural Engineering, Kohala Coast, HI, USA, 2–5 May 2007; pp. 446–449. [CrossRef]

29. Shah, K.G.; Lee, K.Y.; Tolosa, V.; Tooker, A.; Felix, S.; Benett, W.; Pannu, S. Chronic, percutaneous connector for electrical recording and stimulation with microelectrode arrays. In Proceedings of the 36th Annual International Conference of the IEEE Engineering in Medicine and Biology Society, Chicago, IL, USA, 26–30 August 2014; pp. 5240–5243. [CrossRef]

30. Hoch, K.; Pothof, F.; Becker, F.; Paul, O.; Ruther, P. A Magnetic, micro-spring-suspended system for the safe electrical interconnection of neural implants. In Proceedings of the 31st IEEE International Conference on Micro Electro Mechanical Systems (MEMS), Belfast, UK, 21–25 January 2018; pp. 369–372. [CrossRef]

31. Kim, B.J.; Kuo, J.T.W.; Hara, S.A.; Lee, C.D.; Yu, L.; Gutierrez, C.A.; Hoang, T.Q.; Pikov, V.; Meng, E. 3D parylene sheath neural probe for chronic recordings. *J. Neural Eng.* **2013**, *10*, 045002. [CrossRef] [PubMed]

32. Herwik, S.; Paul, O.; Ruther, P. Ultrathin silicon chips of arbitrary shape by etching before grinding. *J. Microelectromech. Syst.* **2011**, *20*, 791–793. [CrossRef]

33. Pilkey, W.D. *Formulas for Stress, Strain, and Structural Matrices*, 2nd ed.; John Wiley & Sons, Inc.: Hoboken, NJ, USA, 2005; pp. 619–660. ISBN 0-471-03221-2.

34. Balke, H. *Einführung in Die Technische Mechanik: Kinetik*, 2nd ed.; Springer: Heidelberg, Germany, 2009; ISBN 978-3-540-89448-3.

35. Balke, H. *Einführung in Die Technische Mechanik: Festigkeitslehre*, 3rd ed.; Springer: Heidelberg, Germany, 2014; ISBN 978-3-642-40980-6.

36. Li, K.; Kasai, T.; Nakao, S.; Tanaka, H.; Ando, T.; Shikida, M.; Sato, K. A Method for measuring the fracture toughness of micrometer-sized single crystal silicon by tensile test. In Proceedings of the TRANSDUCERS '03 12th International Conference on Solid-State Sensors, Actuators and Microsystems, Boston, MA, USA, 8–12 June 2003; pp. 444–447. [CrossRef]
37. Petersen, K.E. Silicon as a Mechanical Material. *Proc. IEEE* **1982**, *70*, 420–457. [CrossRef]

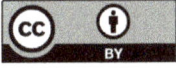

Communication

Genetic Modulation at the Neural Microelectrode Interface: Methods and Applications

Bailey M. Winter [1], Samuel R. Daniels [1], Joseph W. Salatino [1] and Erin K. Purcell [1,2,*]

[1] Department of Biomedical Engineering, Michigan State University, East Lansing, MI 48824, USA; winterb8@msu.edu (B.M.W.); danie276@msu.edu (S.R.D.); joeysal@msu.edu (J.W.S.)

[2] Department of Electrical and Computer Engineering, Michigan State University, East Lansing, MI 48824, USA

* Correspondence: epurcell@msu.edu; Tel.: +1-517-355-3867

Received: 3 August 2018; Accepted: 15 September 2018; Published: 20 September 2018

Abstract: The use of implanted microelectrode arrays (MEAs), in the brain, has enabled a greater understanding of neural function, and new treatments for neurodegenerative diseases and psychiatric disorders. Glial encapsulation of the device and the loss of neurons at the device-tissue interface are widely believed to reduce recording quality and limit the functional device-lifetime. The integration of microfluidic channels within MEAs enables the perturbation of the cellular pathways, through defined vector delivery. This provides new approaches to shed light on the underlying mechanisms of the reactive response and its contribution to device performance. In chronic settings, however, tissue ingrowth and biofouling can obstruct or damage the channel, preventing vector delivery. In this study, we describe methods of delivering vectors through chronically implanted, single-shank, "Michigan"-style microfluidic devices, 1–3 weeks, post-implantation. We explored and validated three different approaches for modifying gene expression at the device-tissue interface: viral-mediated overexpression, siRNA-enabled knockdown, and cre-dependent conditional expression. We observed a successful delivery of the vectors along the length of the MEA, where the observed expression varied, depending on the depth of the injury. The methods described are intended to enable vector delivery through microfluidic devices for a variety of potential applications; likewise, future design considerations are suggested for further improvements on the approach.

Keywords: microfluidic device; chronic implantation; gene modification

---

1. Introduction

An increasing prevalence of patients affected by neurodegenerative diseases and psychiatric disorders places an economic, social, and psychological burden on society [1–6]. In research settings, there has been a significant rise in the use of microelectrodes implanted in the brain to record neural activity and reveal the underlying mechanisms of these diseases. Moreover, brain-machine interfaces (BMIs) and closed-loop deep brain stimulation (DBS) are emerging applications of recording arrays, in preclinical and clinical trials [7–11]. However, their signal qualities are notoriously unstable and are prone to loss over time, which undermines the efficacy of decoding algorithms, the accuracy of data collection in basic science studies, and the detection of conditioning signals necessary to drive the closed-loop strategies [12–15]. The brain initiates a tissue response, following implantation, that is characterized by a progressive glial encapsulation and neuronal loss, which is widely believed to contribute to the diminished recording quality and signal loss [14,16,17]. However, despite recent findings, both, the nature of the relationship between the tissue response and recording quality, as well as the underlying mechanisms responsible, remain unclear [18].

In recent years, an increasingly complex view, of tissue response to neural implants, has emerged, where changes in the structure and function of the responding cell-types accompany well-known effects on cellular density (glial encapsulation and local loss of neurons). Recent evidence suggests that the local shifts in ion channel expression, synaptic transporter expression, and astrocyte subtype follow from a device implantation [14,19]. Additionally, Eles et al. noted new evidence that mechanical trauma accompanies prolonged, localized calcium influx, post-implantation [20]. For non-neuronal responses, a recent study employed a mouse bone marrow chimera model as an innovative approach to delineate the roles of resident microglia versus blood-derived macrophages, in determining the microelectrode performance. The study revealed that the knockout of CD14 from blood-derived macrophages improved the recording quality, over 16 weeks [21]. Further, new approaches using extracellular matrix-based intracortical arrays have reduced inflammatory responses, demonstrating the important role of acellular elements in modulating the tissue response [22,23]. While these findings provide insight on the fundamental mechanisms of the tissue response, they also illustrate the complexity of the device-tissue interactions and the significant unknowns that remain, with respect to the signaling pathways responsible.

Advances in the development of new genetic tools provide opportunities to identify the precise pathways of cellular responses, where devices are being designed and fabricated with increasingly sophisticated means of delivering the necessary reagents to the surrounding tissue. Multifunctional microelectrode arrays offer the ability to interrogate the cellular events surrounding the device, via electrical, chemical, and optical modes of stimulation [24–27], and integrated microfluidic channels permit the vector delivery for genetic modification of the local neural network [27,28]. The resulting upregulation or downregulation, of the specific signaling pathways, is a potentially powerful means of investigating the mechanisms of the tissue response. However, difficulties can arise in chronic settings, since biofouling and tissue ingrowth can compromise the patency of the infusion channel, making repeated dosing, and vector delivery at long-term time points, challenging [27,29,30].

Here, we present data illustrating a proof-of-principle for delivering vectors capable of modifying gene expressions (siRNA and viral vectors), via a functional microfluidic device capable of recording neural activity in the primary motor cortex of adult rats. By delivering reagents designed for gene knockdowns (BLOCK-iT^{TM} siRNA, Thermo Fischer, Waltham, MA, USA), overexpressions (AAV8-GFAP-mCherry, UNC Vector Core, Chapel Hill, NC, USA), and conditional expressions (AAV2-Cre-GFP, Vector Biolabs, Philadelphia, PA, USA), our results provide a methodology for the genetic modification, of the tissue response, at the neural-electrode interface.

2. Materials and Methods

2.1. Injection Protocol (In Vitro)

The workflow of the injection protocol developed is illustrated in Figure 1A. A custom 16-channel single shank microfluidic microelectrode array (Neuronexus, Ann Arbor, MI, USA) was pre-threaded with a 40 gauge SS316L wire (KidneyPuncher, Mesa, AZ, USA). Due to the slight bend in the microfluidic channel, near the electrical connector (Figure 1F), an infusion cannula (33 gauge internal cannula, C315LI/SPC PlasticsOne, Roanoke, VA, USA) was used as a guide for the wire insert. For initial in vitro testing and methods development, the MEA was inserted into a brain tissue phantom, consisting of a 0.6% agarose hydrogel, cast into a 10 cm cell culture petri dish, and was held in place using a hemostat and C-clamps (Figure 1B,C) [31]. Subsequently, the wire was inserted 1 mm past the tip of the MEA into the agarose medium, to clear the microfluidic channel and reduce the back pressure. To infuse, the infusion cannula was first attached to a 10 uL Hamilton syringe, with 7 cm silicon tubing (C313CT, PlasticsOne, Roanoke, VA, USA). Using a Quintessential Stereotaxic Injector (Stoelting, Gelsenkirchen, Germany), 4 µL of mineral oil was withdrawn at 0.1 µL/min, followed by 2 µL of air, and finally, 2 µL of saline, tinted with fast green (Electron Microscopy Sciences, Hatflied, PA, USA), at the same rate. Using hemostats, the cannula was carefully inserted into the microfluidic channel and glued in place. The saline was then infused into the agarose medium at a rate of 0.1 µL/min (a standard infusion rate for vector injection into brain tissue) [32].

2.2. Adapter Circuit

Due to the close proximity of the microfluidic channel, an adapter circuit was designed and fabricated to allow added clearance between the connector and the infusion channel, and facilitate the collection of neural recording data. Using the EAGLE schematic software (Autodesk, San Rafael, CA, USA), the circuit board was designed to extend the connection site 1 inch away from the device (fabricated by Gold Phoenix PCB, Wuhan, China) (Figure 1D,E). Electrical connectors (Omnetics, Minneapolis, MN, USA) with through-hole style leads were chosen for ease of assembly, and connection pads were determined based on manufacturer specifications.

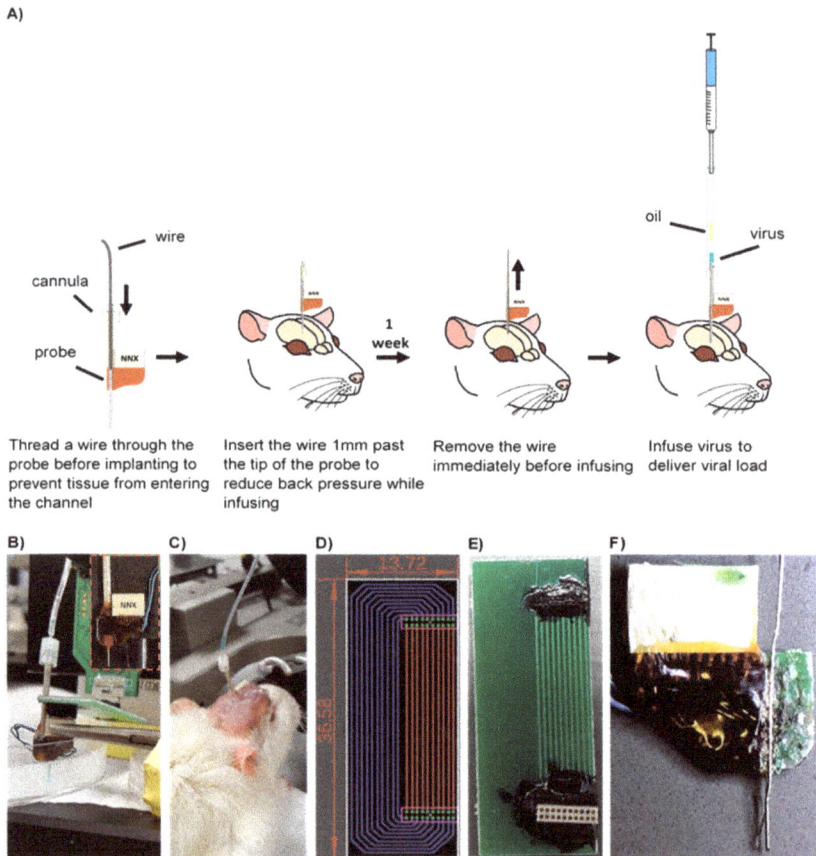

Figure 1. (**A**) Microfluidic device implantation and infusion protocol. (**B**) In vitro saline infusion into 0.6% agarose. Saline was tinted with fast green to confirm delivery. Inset displays the microfluidic device. (**C**) In vivo infusion of the AAV8 viral load. (**D**) Top view of the adapter board layout. Green circles indicate the plated through-holes through which the electrical connector (Omnetics, Minneapolis, MN, USA) leads were inserted. Electrical traces were placed on the top (red) and bottom (blue) to prevent traces from overlapping. Dimensions indicated in the figure are in millimeters. (**E**) Fabricated adapter board. (**F**) Cross section of a microfluidic probe. Red arrow indicates a slight bend in the microfluidic channel.

2.3. Surgical Procedure

For the conditional expression, we purchased a reporter rat strain from the National BioResource Project (Kyoto University, Kyoto, Japan) which enables high-resolution imaging of dendritic spines in ex vivo brain slices [33]. For the reporter strain, female Long Evans rats were generated with a floxed STOP tdTomato to allow conditional expression of the red fluorescent reporter, via viral delivery of Cre recombinase (4.0E12 GC/mL AAV2-Cre-GFP in 5% Glycerol in PBS, Vector Biolabs, Philadelphia, PA, USA). For overexpression and knockdown studies, adult male Sprague–Dawley rats (Charles River, Wilmington, MA, USA) were delivered an AAV vector, with a GFAP promoter and mCherry reporter (AAV8-GFAP-mCherry 2.7E12 virus molecules/mL in 350 nM NaCl and 5% D-Sorbitol in PBS, UNC Vector Core, Chapel Hill, NC, USA) and BLOCK-iT^{TM} siRNA (200 nM Invivofectamine-BLOCK-iT^{TM}-Complexation solution, Thermo Fisher, Waltham, MA, USA), respectively. Animals were unilaterally implanted in the motor cortex, using a commercially manufactured 16-channel single shank MEA, with a microfluidic channel (NeuroNexus, Ann Arbor, MI, USA) that was pre-threaded with a 40 gauge SS316L wire (KidneyPuncher, Mesa, AZ, USA), based on previously published methods that used single shank standard (non-microfluidic) Michigan arrays [19]. The majority of the implanted microfluidic devices were nonfunctional. All devices were modified so that the plastic tubing was ~2 cm long. Animals were anesthetized with ~2% isoflurane, throughout the surgery. Using a motorized drill, a 2 mm × 2 mm craniotomy was performed to expose the cortex (3 mm anterior, 2.5 mm lateral to bregma). The dura was resected and the MEA was implanted at a 2 mm depth, in the cortex. Subsequently, the wire was manually threaded and inserted ~1 mm past the tip of the MEA. A dental acrylic headcap, anchored by three bones screws, was used to support the MEA. Excess dental acrylic was used to attach the wire to the plastic tubing of the microfluidic channel. Bupivacaine was administered for topical analgesia, at the wound site, and meloxicam was administered for systemic analgesia, via an intraperitoneal injection during recovery. All surgical procedures were approved by the Michigan State University Animal Care and Use Committee (Project identification code AUF # 11/17-196-00).

2.4. Injection Protocol (In Vivo)

Animals were infused 1–3 weeks, post-implantation. Animals were anesthetized with ~2% isoflurane for the duration of the procedure. Oil, air and 2 µL of viral load were withdrawn, as described in the Injection Protocol section. The wire was removed from the microfluidic channel and the cannula was inserted, using hemostats, and was glued in place. The viral load was infused at 0.2–0.4 µL/min. For troubleshooting techniques, see Box 1.

Box 1. Troubleshooting techniques for in vivo infusions.

Troubleshooting Techniques
The channel became clogged
If the wire insert was pulled out, tissue could infiltrate and clog the microfluidic channel, preventing a successful infusion. In order to clear the channel, a new wire must be inserted; however, a blunt wire might not be able to pierce through the debris. Filing the tip of the wire to a point could help clear the debris from the channel and might require multiple attempts.
The plastic tubing broke off
The plastic tubing could be damaged or completely broken through contact with the environment, as the animal explored its cage. If the plastic tubing could be recovered from the enclosure, it could be reattached with super glue, immediately before infusion. If the tubing could not be recovered, a guide cannula (PlasticsOne, Roanoke, VA, USA) could be used as a substitute.
The microfluidic channel became damaged
If the plastic tubing was broken, the microfluidic channel could become damaged or could be removed, as well. If a portion of the microfluidic channel was still attached, the channel could be straightened out and reattached, or the plastic tubing could be replaced. If the microfluidic channel had broken off completely, the channel had to be reconstructed. First, it had to be ensured that the microfluidic channel was clear of debris. A cannula could be threaded with a wire insert, and inserted into the plastic tubing/guide cannula, until the ends were aligned. The wire should be extended far enough, past the opening, so that it could be easily manipulated. Using forceps, the wire could be guided into the microfluidic channel to align the cannula and plastic tubing/guide cannula. Super glue could be applied to the bottom of the plastic tubing/guide cannula to allow it to set. Finally, the cannula and wire insert could be removed.
The virus did not infuse
If the virus did not infuse, it was possible that the wire was not inserted far enough and the channel was blocked with tissue. A wire could be re-inserted through the channel until it extended approximately one millimeter past the end of the microfluidic channel. If the virus still did not infuse, the infusion rate was increased slightly, until successful.

2.5. Immunohistochemistry

Two to three weeks post-injection, animals were deeply anesthetized with an overdose of sodium pentobarbital, and transcardially perfused with 4% paraformaldehyde (PFA). Brains were extracted, stored in 4% PFA overnight and cryoembedded, following sucrose protection. Cryosections were collected at a 20 μm thickness and hydrated with PBS, prior to blocking in a 10% normal goat serum in PBS for 1 h. Tissue was subsequently incubated overnight, at 4 °C, with the mouse anti-glial fibrillary acidic protein (GFAP) (Cell Signaling Technology, Danvers, MA, USA). The following day, cryosections were rinsed with PBS and incubated with the goat anti-mouse IgG (H+L) Alexa Fluor 488 conjugate (1:200, Thermo Fisher Scientific, Waltham, MA, USA), for two hours, at room temperature. Finally, nuclei were counterstained with Hoechst and coverslipped with ProLong Gold antifade reagent (Fisher Scientific Company, Hampton, NH, USA). An Olympus Fluoview 1000 inverted confocal microscope was used to image samples with a 20× PlanFluor dry objective (0.5NA). For comparison, GFAP-stained tissue from "traditional" (non-microfluidic) single shank Michigan-style arrays, implanted in the motor cortex, was assessed using images collected during a previous study [34].

2.6. Image Analysis

All images were analyzed using a MATLAB script adapted from Kozai et al. [15] with modifications previously reported [19]. A hand-traced outline of the injury was used to define concentric 10 μm-thick bins. The average intensity of the fluorescent markers within each bin was calculated using the corners of the image as a reference. Bin intensity was normalized to the most distal bin. Results were assessed using a mixed model ANOVA and SPSS software (IBM, Chicago, IL, USA) as previously described [19].

2.7. Signal Processing

Neural recording data were acquired with a Tucker-Davis Technologies RZ2 system (Alchua, FL, USA) and processed using a MATLAB script. Wideband data was sampled at ~48 kHz, in isoflurane-anesthetized rats placed in a Faraday cage, and analyzed offline as described [34,35]. A combination of bandpass filtering and identification of threshold crossings (at 3.5 standard deviations from the mean of the sampling distribution) were used to collect and store 3 ms snippets, centered at the minimum of the recorded segment. Local field potentials (LFPs) were filtered between 1–100 Hz. LFP amplitude was calculated by multiplying the standard deviation of the signal by six, yielding 99.7% of the signal amplitude. Principal component analysis and fuzzy C-means clustering (membership index > 0.8) were performed to identify putative units, in combination with visual inspection of the mean waveforms. Common average referencing [36] was used to mitigate noise sources common to every electrode site (such as line noise and movement artifacts).

3. Results

3.1. Development of Injection Methods (In Vitro)

Optimal infusion methods were determined through trial and error in vitro, prior to implementation in vivo. The rate of withdrawal or infusion of each component (oil, air, and virus) was found to be a critical determinant of success for the overall procedure. When withdrawn at a rate higher than the optimum (0.1 μL/min), bubbles would form within the oil, preventing a successful infusion. Additionally, due to the viscosity of the oil, higher rates of withdrawal resulted in inaccuracies in the volume of oil collected. Subsequently, if the air was withdrawn at a higher rate, bubbles would form in the oil. Likewise, withdrawing the viral load at higher rates could result in withdrawal of air into the sample and an unsuccessful infusion.

3.2. Increased GFAP Expression Surrounding Microfluidic Devices

The inclusion of a microfluidic channel on the device necessarily increased the footprint of the implant. Given the evidence for a relationship between device architecture and tissue response [37,38], we explored the level of astrogliosis surrounding the microfluidic devices, in comparison to "traditional" single shank, silicon probes. Microfluidic devices created larger injuries compared to traditional devices, with average injury areas of 0.056 mm^2 and 0.004 mm^2, respectively (Figure 2A). Although the width of the microfluidic device was 185 μm, injury sizes were noticeably larger. Hoechst staining confirmed the absence of cells within the injury area (not shown). This exacerbated injury size could be due to the removal of the tissue that adhered to the device while extracting the brain. This larger injury size was accompanied by increased astrogliosis. Quantification of GFAP fluorescence surrounding microfluidic devices showed significantly elevated levels of GFAP expression ($p < 0.05$), up to 130 μm of the insertion site boundary (relative to the distal bin intensity values). Traditional devices showed a slightly more spatially restricted response, with significantly elevated levels of GFAP expression ($p < 0.05$) detected up to 100 μm from the device tract. Furthermore, a trend toward an overall elevation in GFAP expression was detected in microfluidic devices, in comparison to the traditional devices ($p < 0.1$) (Figure 2B). These results indicated that the larger footprint of the microfluidic device could slightly exacerbate the reactive astrogliosis.

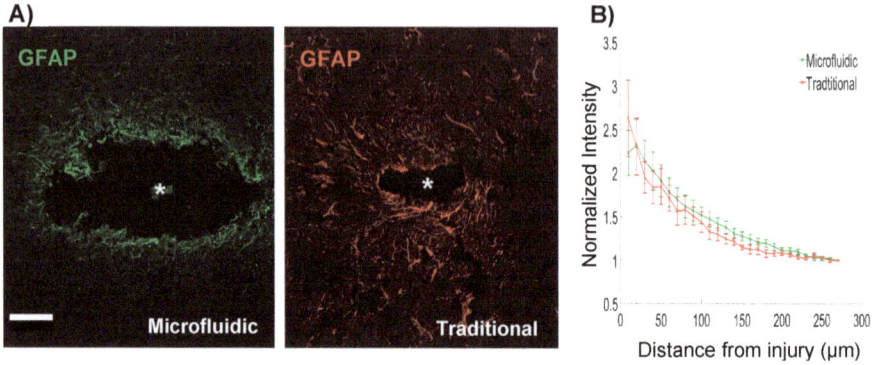

Figure 2. (**A**) GFAP staining surrounding microfluidic and traditional devices indicates astrogliosis and a larger injury footprint related to the microfluidic device. Scale bar = 100 μm. (**B**) Microfluidic devices show significantly elevated levels of GFAP expression within 130 μm of the injury, in comparison to the distal control values ($p < 0.05$). Traditional devices have a slightly more compact region of gliosis, with significantly elevated levels of GFAP within 100 μm ($p < 0.05$). * denotes injury center.

3.3. Signal Quality of Microfluidic Devices

We observed an initial increase in LFP amplitude one day, post-implantation, followed by a gradual decrease in the amplitude, before stabilizing at four weeks, post-implantation (Figure 3B). These observations follow a general trend of decreasing signal quality over time. Additionally, a cursory observation yielded limited identification of unit activity, with the units being detected only at 5 days, post-implantation (Figure 3A). While the sample size was limited, the observation confirms the ability to successfully detect unit activity with microfluidic devices, in a chronic setting.

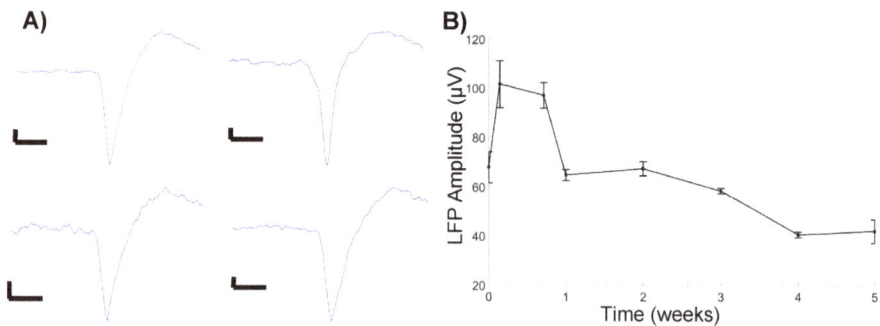

Figure 3. (**A**) Recorded units. All scale bars are 10 μV amplitude, 0.5 ms timescale. (**B**) Average LFP amplitude.

3.4. Microfluidic Devices Successfully Deliver Virus along the Length of the Injury

Animals were infused 1–3 weeks, post-implantation according to the methods developed in vitro. Some alterations to the infusion protocol developed in vitro were necessary to successfully deliver the viral load in vivo. An infusion rate of 0.1 μL/min proved insufficient to overcome the back pressure in an in vivo setting. Increasing the infusion rate to 0.2 μL/min was sufficient for most animals; however, variations between animals required infusion rates up to 0.4 μL/min for successful virus delivery.

Animals were sacrificed 2–3 weeks after infusing, and cryosections were imaged with an Olympus Fluoview 1000 confocal microscope to assess the expression of the infused virus. All successfully infused animals showed expression of the delivered fluorescent reporter surrounding the injury site (Figure 4). We observed a qualitative increase in the amount of expression, and diffusion of the vector at deeper sections of the injury, compared to the superficial sections. This pattern of dispersion is most likely due to the channel having a single opening at the tip of the probe.

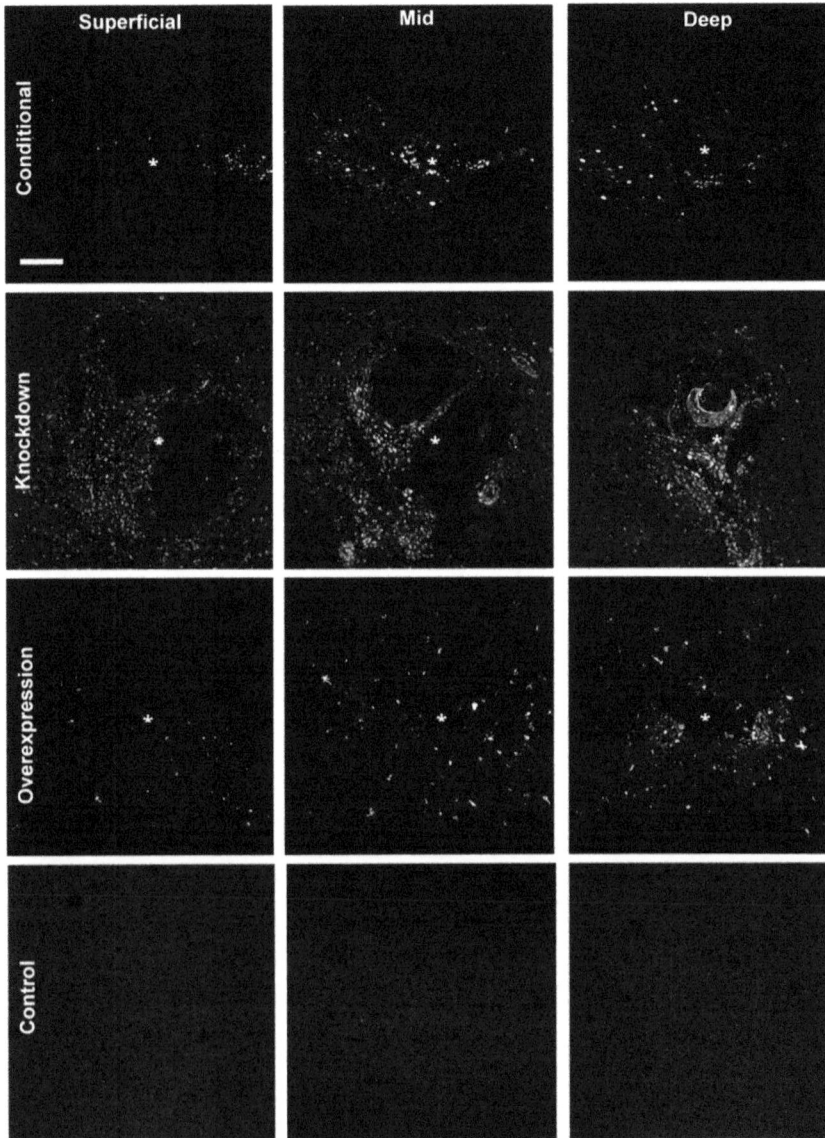

Figure 4. Spread of fluorescent reporter expression (appears white) of AAV8-GFAP-mCherry (overexpression), BLOCK-iT™ siRNA (knockdown), and AAV2-Cre-GFP (conditional) at superficial (~100–650 μm), mid (~750–1000 μm), and deep (~1100–1300 μm) sections of the injury. Reporter expression is spatially broader in deep sections of the injury (near the infusion tip) in comparison to more superficial sections. Control images were taken from the contralateral hemisphere; * denotes injury center. Scale bar = 100 μm.

4. Discussion

While it is widely believed that the biological response to implanted electrodes is intimately linked to their function [16,17], direct evidence for this relationship is surprisingly scarce. Multiple studies have explored correlations between a specific measure of recording quality (such as the number of units detected), impedance data, and/or an isolated metric of the biological response (for instance, local neuronal density) to gain insight into the association between functional characteristics and cellular responses. However, the variability in the outcomes reported in these studies underscores the complexity and multi-faceted nature of the underlying source(s) of recorded signal loss, interface instability, and shifting stimulation thresholds [18,39,40]. Likewise, while new device designs incorporate increasingly sophisticated features and materials [41], the relationship between each of these design features, the impacts on tissue response, and chronic device performance remain poorly characterized. The development of new tools and test beds, to understand the basic science governing tissue-device interactions, could provide a direct link between biological mechanisms and device function, ultimately delivering guiding principles for the design features necessary to enable improved tissue integration.

In the current study, we developed and validated methods to modify gene expression using multiple techniques (silencing, conditional expression, and overexpression). Each of these approaches provides a new "knob" to turn, to tune the biological response to devices in controlled ways, potentially providing a mechanistic link between observations of localized changes in gene and protein expression and device performance. This approach builds on previous work that has used drug-based strategies to modulate the biological response to electrodes, either through exacerbation or mitigation of effects, to explore the role of neuroinflammation in signal loss. For example, microelectrodes in animals administered lipopolysaccharide, a common pro-inflammatory stimulus, had a notably lower signal-to-noise ratio and fewer units detected, as compared to the control rats; whereas, anti-inflammatory drugs have been shown to decrease neuroinflammation and improve recording quality [17,42–45]. However, targeting specific signaling pathways, through a perturbation of the gene expression, may offer a more granular view of the key biological mechanisms mediating the neurotoxicity and inflammation that occur at the neural-electrode interface.

As more information on the genes differentially expressed at the device interface becomes available, new opportunities to identify relevant candidate pathways will emerge. Recent studies evaluating gene expression surrounding implanted devices noted an increased expression of GFAP, TNFα, NOS2, HMGB1, CD14, and numerous members of the IL gene family [46–48]. Additionally, Bennett et al. showed genes regulating tight junction and adherens junction proteins in the blood-brain barrier were downregulated, after 72 h, post-implantation [48]. Manipulation of gene expression, by upregulation or downregulation, could reveal potential breakthroughs in improving device function and integration in the brain. Further, Cre-recombinase allows an added layer of control of the local gene expression, by enabling the conditional knockout and genome editing [49].

While the approaches developed in this study were successful in the localized modulation of gene expression, several areas for future improvements were identified. The epoxy used to attach the plastic tubing to the probe was brittle and prone to cracking. This resulted in the potential loss of the plastic tubing during the natural exploratory behavior of the subject, ultimately leading to the microfluidic channel becoming damaged. A more flexible epoxy could reduce the likelihood of this issue. Additionally, the proximity of the microfluidic channel to the electrical connector necessitated the use of an adapter, in order to avoid damaging the channel, while recording the neural activity. While not affecting our ability to infuse, having a single opening at the tip of the probe resulted in an unequal distribution of the delivered virus, along the length of the probe. Alternative designs that enable more control over the distribution and location of viral delivery would be beneficial for applications that seek to perturb the environment, at specified sites, along the length of the probe.

Recent efforts in neural engineering have accentuated the need for understanding the basic science behind the biological mechanisms at the device interface. Next-generation device design is contingent on identifying these unknown device-tissue interactions. This work provides an approach to interrogate and understand the local environment around an implanted device, enabling new opportunities to investigate the tissue response to implants, and identify improved device designs.

Author Contributions: Conceptualization, E.K.P.; Methodology, B.M.W.; Formal Analysis, B.M.W.; Investigation, B.M.W., S.R.D. and J.W.S.; Writing-Original Draft Preparation, B.M.W., S.R.D. and E.K.P.; Writing-Review & Editing, B.M.W., S.R.D., J.W.S. and E.K.P.; Visualization, B.M.W.; Supervision, E.K.P.

Funding: This research was supported by the Department of Biomedical Engineering and the Department of Electrical and Computer Engineering at Michigan State University.

Acknowledgments: The authors thank Melinda K. Frame from Center for Advanced Microscopy for confocal training, and Takashi D. Y. Kozai and Zhannetta Gugel for the intensity profiling MATLAB script.

Conflicts of Interest: The authors declare no conflict of interest.

References

1. Dorsey, E.R.; Constantinescu, R.; Thompson, J.P.; Biglan, K.M.; Holloway, R.G.; Kieburtz, K.; Marshall, F.J.; Ravina, B.M.; Schifitto, G.; Siderowf, A.; et al. Projected number of people with Parkinson disease in the most populous nations, 2005 through 2030. *Neurology* **2007**, *68*, 384–386. [CrossRef] [PubMed]
2. Kowal, S.L.; Dall, T.M.; Chakrabarti, R.; Storm, M.V.; Jain, A. The current and projected economic burden of Parkinson's disease in the United States. *Mov. Disord.* **2013**, *28*, 311–318. [CrossRef] [PubMed]
3. Adelman, G.; Rane, S.G.; Villa, K.F. The cost burden of multiple sclerosis in the United States: A systematic review of the literature. *J. Med. Econ.* **2013**, *16*, 639–647. [CrossRef] [PubMed]
4. Greenberg, P.E.; Kessler, R.C.; Birnbaum, H.G.; Leong, S.A.; Lowe, S.W.; Berglund, P.A.A.; Corey-Lisle, P.K. The Economic Burden of Depression in the United States: How Did It Change Between 1990 and 2000? *J. Clin. Psychiatry* **2003**, *64*, 1465–1475. [CrossRef] [PubMed]
5. Arthur, K.C.; Calvo, A.; Price, T.R.; Geiger, J.T.; Chiò, A.; Traynor, B.J. Projected increase in amyotrophic lateral sclerosis from 2015 to 2040. *Nat. Commun.* **2016**, *7*, 12408. [CrossRef] [PubMed]
6. Wimo, A.; Jönsson, L.; Bond, J.; Prince, M.; Winblad, B.; Alzheimer Disease International. The worldwide economic impact of dementia 2010. *Alzheimer's Dement.* **2013**, *9*, 1–11.e3. [CrossRef] [PubMed]
7. Rosin, B.; Slovik, M.; Mitelman, R.; Rivlin-Etzion, M.; Haber, S.N.; Israel, Z.; Vaadia, E.; Bergman, H. Closed-Loop Deep Brain Stimulation Is Superior in Ameliorating Parkinsonism. *Neuron* **2011**, *72*, 370–384. [CrossRef] [PubMed]
8. Hascup, K.N.; Hascup, E.R.; Stephens, M.L.; Glaser, P.E.A.; Yoshitake, T.; Mathé, A.A.; Gerhardt, G.A.; Kehr, J. Resting glutamate levels and rapid glutamate transients in the prefrontal cortex of the Flinders Sensitive Line rat: A genetic rodent model of depression. *Neuropsychopharmacology* **2011**, *36*, 1769–1777. [CrossRef] [PubMed]
9. O'Doherty, J.E.; Lebedev, M.A.; Ifft, P.J.; Zhuang, K.Z.; Shokur, S.; Bleuler, H.; Nicolelis, M.A.L. Active tactile exploration using a brain-machine-brain interface. *Nature* **2011**, *479*, 228–231. [CrossRef] [PubMed]
10. Lebedev, M.A.; Nicolelis, M.A.L. Brain–machine interfaces: Past, present and future. *Trends Neurosci.* **2006**, *29*, 536–546. [CrossRef] [PubMed]
11. Ezzyat, Y.; Wanda, P.A.; Levy, D.F.; Kadel, A.; Aka, A.; Pedisich, I.; Sperling, M.R.; Sharan, A.D.; Lega, B.C.; Burks, A.; et al. Closed-loop stimulation of temporal cortex rescues functional networks and improves memory. *Nat. Commun.* **2018**, *9*, 365. [CrossRef] [PubMed]
12. Nolta, N.F.; Christensen, M.B.; Crane, P.D.; Skousen, J.L.; Tresco, P.A. BBB leakage, astrogliosis, and tissue loss correlate with silicon microelectrode array recording performance. *Biomaterials* **2015**, *53*, 753–762. [CrossRef] [PubMed]
13. McCreery, D.; Cogan, S.; Kane, S.; Pikov, V. Correlations between histology and neuronal activity recorded by microelectrodes implanted chronically in the cerebral cortex. *J. Neural Eng.* **2016**, *13*, 036012. [CrossRef] [PubMed]
14. Salatino, J.W.; Ludwig, K.A.; Kozai, T.D.Y.; Purcell, E.K. Glial responses to implanted electrodes in the brain. *Nat. Biomed. Eng.* **2017**, *1*, 862–877. [CrossRef]

15. Kozai, T.D.Y.; Li, X.; Bodily, L.M.; Caparosa, E.M.; Zenonos, G.A.; Carlisle, D.L.; Friedlander, R.M.; Cui, X.T. Effects of caspase-1 knockout on chronic neural recording quality and longevity: Insight into cellular and molecular mechanisms of the reactive tissue response. *Biomaterials* **2014**, *35*, 9620–9634. [CrossRef] [PubMed]

16. Kozai, T.D.Y.; Jaquins-Gerstl, A.S.; Vazquez, A.L.; Michael, A.C.; Cui, X.T. Brain Tissue Responses to Neural Implants Impact Signal Sensitivity and Intervention Strategies. *ACS Chem. Neurosci.* **2015**, *6*, 48–67. [CrossRef] [PubMed]

17. Jorfi, M.; Skousen, J.L.; Weder, C.; Capadona, J.R. Progress towards biocompatible intracortical microelectrodes for neural interfacing applications. *J. Neural Eng.* **2015**, *12*, 011001. [CrossRef] [PubMed]

18. Michelson, N.J.; Vazquez, A.L.; Eles, J.R.; Salatino, J.W.; Purcell, E.K.; Williams, J.J.; Cui, X.T.; Kozai, T.D.Y. Multi-scale, multi-modal analysis uncovers complex relationship at the brain tissue-implant neural interface: New emphasis on the biological interface. *J. Neural Eng.* **2018**, *15*, 033001. [CrossRef] [PubMed]

19. Salatino, J.W.; Winter, B.M.; Drazin, M.H.; Purcell, E.K. Functional remodeling of subtype-specific markers surrounding implanted neuroprostheses. *J. Neurophysiol.* **2017**, *118*, 194–202. [CrossRef] [PubMed]

20. Eles, J.R.; Vazquez, A.L.; Kozai, T.D.Y.; Cui, X.T. In vivo imaging of neuronal calcium during electrode implantation: Spatial and temporal mapping of damage and recovery. *Biomaterials* **2018**, *174*, 79–94. [CrossRef] [PubMed]

21. Bedell, H.W.; Hermann, J.K.; Ravikumar, M.; Lin, S.; Rein, A.; Li, X.; Molinich, E.; Smith, P.D.; Selkirk, S.M.; Miller, R.H.; et al. Targeting CD14 on blood derived cells improves intracortical microelectrode performance. *Biomaterials* **2018**, *163*, 163–173. [CrossRef] [PubMed]

22. Shen, W.; Karumbaiah, L.; Liu, X.; Saxena, T.; Chen, S.; Patkar, R.; Bellamkonda, R.V.; Allen, M.G. Extracellular matrix-based intracortical microelectrodes: Toward a microfabricated neural interface based on natural materials. *Microsyst. Nanoeng.* **2015**, *1*, 15010. [CrossRef]

23. Oakes, R.S.; Polei, M.D.; Skousen, J.L.; Tresco, P.A. An astrocyte derived extracellular matrix coating reduces astrogliosis surrounding chronically implanted microelectrode arrays in rat cortex. *Biomaterials* **2018**, *154*, 1–11. [CrossRef] [PubMed]

24. Canales, A.; Jia, X.; Froriep, U.P.; Koppes, R.A.; Tringides, C.M.; Selvidge, J.; Lu, C.; Hou, C.; Wei, L.; Fink, Y.; et al. Multifunctional fibers for simultaneous optical, electrical and chemical interrogation of neural circuits in vivo. *Nat. Biotechnol.* **2015**, *33*, 277–284. [CrossRef] [PubMed]

25. Seidl, K.; Spieth, S.; Herwik, S.; Steigert, J.; Zengerle, R.; Paul, O.; Ruther, P. In-plane silicon probes for simultaneous neural recording and drug delivery. *J. Micromech. Microeng.* **2010**, *20*, 105006. [CrossRef]

26. Anikeeva, P.; Andalman, A.S.; Witten, I.; Warden, M.; Goshen, I.; Grosenick, L.; Gunaydin, L.A.; Frank, L.M.; Deisseroth, K. Optetrode: A multichannel readout for optogenetic control in freely moving mice. *Nat. Neurosci.* **2011**, *15*, 163–170. [CrossRef] [PubMed]

27. Jeong, J.-W.; McCall, J.G.; Shin, G.; Zhang, Y.; Al-Hasani, R.; Kim, M.; Li, S.; Sim, J.Y.; Jang, K.-I.; Shi, Y.; et al. Wireless Optofluidic Systems for Programmable In Vivo Pharmacology and Optogenetics. *Cell* **2015**, *162*, 662–674. [CrossRef] [PubMed]

28. Jennings, J.H.; Stuber, G.D. Tools for Resolving Functional Activity and Connectivity within Intact Neural Circuits. *Curr. Biol.* **2014**, *24*, R41–R50. [CrossRef] [PubMed]

29. Sommakia, S.; Lee, H.C.; Gaire, J.; Otto, K.J. Materials approaches for modulating neural tissue responses to implanted microelectrodes through mechanical and biochemical means. *Curr. Opin. Solid State Mater. Sci.* **2014**, *18*, 319–328. [CrossRef] [PubMed]

30. Chen, R.; Canales, A.; Anikeeva, P. Neural recording and modulation technologies. *Nat. Rev. Mater.* **2017**, *2*, 16093. [CrossRef]

31. Chen, Z.-J.; Gillies, G.T.; Broaddus, W.C.; Prabhu, S.S.; Fillmore, H.; Mitchell, R.M.; Corwin, F.D.; Fatouros, P.P. A realistic brain tissue phantom for intraparenchymal infusion studies. *J. Neurosurg.* **2004**, *101*, 314–322. [CrossRef] [PubMed]

32. Cardin, J.A.; Carlén, M.; Meletis, K.; Knoblich, U.; Zhang, F.; Deisseroth, K.; Tsai, L.-H.; Moore, C.I. Targeted optogenetic stimulation and recording of neurons in vivo using cell-type-specific expression of Channelrhodopsin-2. *Nat. Protoc.* **2010**, *5*, 247–254. [CrossRef] [PubMed]

33. Igarashi, H.; Koizumi, K.; Kaneko, R.; Ikeda, K.; Egawa, R.; Yanagawa, Y.; Muramatsu, S.; Onimaru, H.; Ishizuka, T.; Yawo, H. A Novel Reporter Rat Strain That Conditionally Expresses the Bright Red Fluorescent Protein tdTomato. *PLoS ONE* **2016**, *11*, e0155687. [CrossRef] [PubMed]

34. Purcell, E.K.; Thompson, D.E.; Ludwig, K.A.; Kipke, D.R. Flavopiridol reduces the impedance of neural prostheses in vivo without affecting recording quality. *J. Neurosci. Methods* **2009**, *183*, 149–157. [CrossRef] [PubMed]

35. Ludwig, K.A.; Uram, J.D.; Yang, J.; Martin, D.C.; Kipke, D.R. Chronic neural recordings using silicon microelectrode arrays electrochemically deposited with a poly(3,4-ethylenedioxythiophene) (PEDOT) film. *J. Neural Eng.* **2006**, *3*, 59–70. [CrossRef] [PubMed]

36. Ludwig, K.A.; Miriani, R.M.; Langhals, N.B.; Joseph, M.D.; Anderson, D.J.; Kipke, D.R. Using a Common Average Reference to Improve Cortical Neuron Recordings from Microelectrode Arrays. *J. Neurophysiol.* **2009**, *101*, 1679–1689. [CrossRef] [PubMed]

37. Seymour, J.P.; Kipke, D.R. Neural probe design for reduced tissue encapsulation in CNS. *Biomaterials* **2007**, *28*, 3594–3607. [CrossRef] [PubMed]

38. Kozai, T.D.Y.; Langhals, N.B.; Patel, P.R.; Deng, X.; Zhang, H.; Smith, K.L.; Lahann, J.; Kotov, N.A.; Kipke, D.R. Ultrasmall implantable composite microelectrodes with bioactive surfaces for chronic neural interfaces. *Nat. Mater.* **2012**, *11*, 1065–1073. [CrossRef] [PubMed]

39. Kozai, T.D.Y.; Catt, K.; Li, X.; Gugel, Z.V.; Olafsson, V.T.; Vazquez, A.L.; Cui, X.T. Mechanical failure modes of chronically implanted planar silicon-based neural probes for laminar recording. *Biomaterials* **2015**, *37*, 25–39. [CrossRef] [PubMed]

40. Malaga, K.A.; Schroeder, K.E.; Patel, P.R.; Irwin, Z.T.; Thompson, D.E.; Bentley, J.N.; Lempka, S.F.; Chestek, C.A.; Patil, P.G. Data-driven model comparing the effects of glial scarring and interface interactions on chronic neural recordings in non-human primates. *J. Neural Eng.* **2016**, *13*, 16010–16024. [CrossRef] [PubMed]

41. Wellman, S.M.; Eles, J.R.; Ludwig, K.A.; Seymour, J.P.; Michelson, N.J.; McFadden, W.E.; Vazquez, A.L.; Kozai, T.D.Y. A Materials Roadmap to Functional Neural Interface Design. *Adv. Funct. Mater.* **2018**, *28*, 1701269. [CrossRef] [PubMed]

42. Kozai, T.D.Y.; Jaquins-Gerstl, A.S.; Vazquez, A.L.; Michael, A.C.; Cui, X.T. Dexamethasone retrodialysis attenuates microglial response to implanted probes in vivo. *Biomaterials* **2016**, *87*, 157–169. [CrossRef] [PubMed]

43. Rennaker, R.L.; Miller, J.; Tang, H.; Wilson, D.A. Minocycline increases quality and longevity of chronic neural recordings. *J. Neural Eng.* **2007**, *4*, L1–L5. [CrossRef] [PubMed]

44. Golabchi, A.; Wu, B.; Li, X.; Carlisle, D.L.; Kozai, T.D.Y.; Friedlander, R.M.; Cui, X.T. Melatonin improves quality and longevity of chronic neural recording. *Biomaterials* **2018**, *180*, 225–239. [CrossRef] [PubMed]

45. Potter, K.A.; Buck, A.C.; Self, W.K.; Callanan, M.E.; Sunil, S.; Capadona, J.R. The effect of resveratrol on neurodegeneration and blood brain barrier stability surrounding intracortical microelectrodes. *Biomaterials* **2013**, *34*, 7001–7015. [CrossRef] [PubMed]

46. Ereifej, E.S.; Smith, C.S.; Meade, S.M.; Chen, K.; Feng, H.; Capadona, J.R. The Neuroinflammatory Response to Nanopatterning Parallel Grooves into the Surface Structure of Intracortical Microelectrodes. *Adv. Funct. Mater.* **2018**, *28*, 1704420. [CrossRef]

47. Karumbaiah, L.; Saxena, T.; Carlson, D.; Patil, K.; Patkar, R.; Gaupp, E.A.; Betancur, M.; Stanley, G.B.; Carin, L.; Bellamkonda, R.V. Relationship between intracortical electrode design and chronic recording function. *Biomaterials* **2013**, *34*, 8061–8074. [CrossRef] [PubMed]

48. Bennett, C.; Samikkannu, M.; Mohammed, F.; Dietrich, W.D.; Rajguru, S.M.; Prasad, A. Blood brain barrier (BBB)-disruption in intracortical silicon microelectrode implants. *Biomaterials* **2018**, *164*, 1–10. [CrossRef] [PubMed]

49. Nagy, A. Cre recombinase: The universal reagent for genome tailoring. *Genesis* **2000**, *26*, 99–109. [CrossRef]

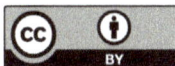

micromachines

MDPI

Review

Progress in the Field of Micro-Electrocorticography

Mehdi Shokoueinejad [1,2,†], Dong-Wook Park [3,4,†], Yei Hwan Jung [3], Sarah K. Brodnick [1],
Joseph Novello [1], Aaron Dingle [5], Kyle I. Swanson [2], Dong-Hyun Baek [1], Aaron J. Suminski [1,2],
Wendell B. Lake [2], Zhenqiang Ma [3,*] and Justin Williams [1,2,*]

[1] Department of Biomedical Engineering, University of Wisconsin-Madison, Madison, WI 53706, USA;
     mehdi.snm@bme.wisc.edu (M.S.); skkorinek@wisc.edu (S.K.B.); novello@wisc.edu (J.N.);
     wpvmqor@gmail.com (D.-H.B.); suminski@neurosurgery.wisc.edu (A.J.S.)
[2] Department of Neurosurgery, School of Medicine and Public Health, University of Wisconsin-Madison,
     Madison, WI 53792, USA; kiswanson@gmail.com (K.I.S.); lake@neurosurgery.wisc.edu (W.B.L.)
[3] Department of Electrical and Computer Engineering, University of Wisconsin-Madison,
     Madison, WI 53706, USA; dwpark31@uos.ac.kr (D.-W.P.); yhjung89@gmail.com (Y.H.J.)
[4] School of Electrical and Computer Engineering, University of Seoul, Seoul 02504, South Korea
[5] Division of Plastic and Reconstructive Surgery, Department of Surgery, University of Wisconsin-Madison,
     Madison, WI 53792, USA; dingle@surgery.wisc.edu
*   Correspondence: mazq@engr.wisc.edu (Z.M.); jwilliams@engr.wisc.edu (J.W.)
†   These authors contributed equally to this work.

Received: 9 December 2018; Accepted: 15 January 2019; Published: 17 January 2019

Abstract: Since the 1940s electrocorticography (ECoG) devices and, more recently, in the last
decade, micro-electrocorticography (μECoG) cortical electrode arrays were used for a wide set
of experimental and clinical applications, such as epilepsy localization and brain–computer interface
(BCI) technologies. Miniaturized implantable μECoG devices have the advantage of providing
greater-density neural signal acquisition and stimulation capabilities in a minimally invasive fashion.
An increased spatial resolution of the μECoG array will be useful for greater specificity diagnosis
and treatment of neuronal diseases and the advancement of basic neuroscience and BCI research.
In this review, recent achievements of ECoG and μECoG are discussed. The electrode configurations
and varying material choices used to design μECoG arrays are discussed, including advantages
and disadvantages of μECoG technology compared to electroencephalography (EEG), ECoG,
and intracortical electrode arrays. Electrode materials that are the primary focus include platinum,
iridium oxide, poly(3,4-ethylenedioxythiophene) (PEDOT), indium tin oxide (ITO), and graphene.
We discuss the biological immune response to μECoG devices compared to other electrode array types,
the role of μECoG in clinical pathology, and brain–computer interface technology. The information
presented in this review will be helpful to understand the current status, organize available
knowledge, and guide future clinical and research applications of μECoG technologies.

Keywords: electrocorticography; ECoG; micro-electrocorticography; μECoG; neural electrode
array; neural interfaces; electrophysiology; brain–computer interface; in vivo imaging; tissue
response; graphene

1. Introduction

Multichannel neural interfaces provide a direct communication pathway between the central
nervous system and the ex vivo environment. These front-end devices are critical tools that
enable breakthroughs in neuroscience research and the diagnosis/treatment of many neurological
disorders like epilepsy and stroke. Another exciting technology that makes use of these devices is a
brain–computer interface (BCI) or brain–machine interface (BMI). BCIs are restorative devices that
aim to replace functionality an individual lost to neural injury or disease, and they demonstrate the

variability and versatility of multichannel neural interfaces [1–4]. The methods of interfacing with the cerebral cortex and their corresponding electrodes can be mainly divided into four categories: external scalp recordings from electroencephalography (EEG), surface cortical recordings from electrocorticography (ECoG), surface cortical recordings from micro-electrocorticography (μECoG), and intracortical recordings from within the cortex and brain parenchyma using penetrating electrode arrays. Each type of neural interface methodology has its own advantages and disadvantages. EEG records neural signals through electrodes placed on the scalp. Due to its relative ease of use and non-invasive nature, EEG is a relatively well-known and commonly used method of acquiring neural signals. However, the information acquired from EEG is quite limited because the neural signal quality is diminished by the overlying tissues (i.e., scalp, soft tissues below the scalp, and bone) between the neuronal cells and the EEG electrodes. In contrast, ECoG electrodes are placed on the cerebral cortex, measuring local field potentials directly from the contact surface. This eliminates the attenuation/filtering of signals as they are transmitted through the skull and scalp, creating a more information-rich signal than EEG. However, conventional ECoG devices that are clinically available have an electrode site size of approximately 1 cm in diameter, which limits the spatial resolution of neural recording and stimulation [5].

Micro-ECoG electrode arrays utilize micro-scale electrodes with contact site diameters many orders of magnitude smaller than traditional clinical ECoG electrode sites and minimized inter-electrode spacing, allowing greater spatial resolution of the measured signals (Figure 1). Moreover, typical μECoG devices have ultrathin structure, thereby offering less invasive implantations [6]. Depending on the application, a μECoG device could have hundreds to thousands of electrode sites [7]. Lastly, intracortical electrode arrays can record individual action potentials from within the cortex or from deep brain regions. They give the most information-rich signal by recording individual action potentials in addition to intracortical local field potentials, but have the highest degree of invasiveness by penetrating into the tissue and eliciting an immune response to the foreign material. Among these device types, μECoG provides an appealing balance of information acquisition and spatial resolution with an acceptable degree of invasiveness (Figure 2). This article reviews the recent evolution of ECoG into μECoG, as well as the current direction these technologies are taking in the fields of engineering, neural interface research, and clinical medicine. Electrode array material choice is discussed, as is the role of ECoG and μECoG in the diagnosis and treatment of clinical disease pathologies, and current uses in BCI technologies, in addition to the host response to μECoG devices, in vivo imaging, and optical or electrical stimulation.

2. Evolution of ECoG into μECoG

Prior to the advent of μECoG, ECoG showed its advantages over EEG, providing greater temporal resolution than EEG, particularly regarding high gamma modulations (70–105 Hz) as the skull attenuates higher-frequency signals [5,8–12]. A gamma wave is a pattern of neural oscillation in humans or animals with a frequency between 25 and 100 Hz (and even above), although 40 Hz is typical. According to a popular theory, gamma oscillations are linked with high-level cognitive functions such as memory, attention, volitional movement, and conscious perception, which led to the theory that gamma activity plays a role in higher-level cortical processing [13,14]. Penfield was the first to describe the use of intraoperative ECoG to record localized abnormal neural activity in a seizure patient in 1947 [15]. Since this pioneering work, ECoG was used as a standard of care for clinical mapping of eloquent cortex prior to therapeutic resection of brain tissue.

ECoG rests on the surface of the cortex and is, by nature, less invasive than traditional intracortical microelectrodes by eliciting less of an immune response, and demonstrates better signal longevity [16–18]. ECoG BCIs concentrate on both restoring communication [19] and the control of prosthetic limbs [20,21]. ECoG devices further demonstrated their clinical applicability for BCI control with chronic implantation in animal models [22,23] and acute implantation in humans [21,24]. Most notably, Shimoda et al. demonstrated the signal stability and longevity of ECoG for decoding of continuous three-dimensional (3D) hand trajectories in non-human primates over several months [25]. Equally importantly, Breshears et al. demonstrated that pediatric brain signals for hand movement could be easily and accurately decoded using ECoG (70–99% accuracy with ~9 min training) [26]. Chronic ECoG implantation in humans is currently being investigated as a treatment/warning system for epilepsy with limited success [27]. Chronic BCI testing using ECoGs to control devices is limited, as most subjects are epilepsy patients fitted short-term with ECoG for diagnostic reasons, which are then recruited into research projects [11,28–30]. The major caveat to this model is that, within these small experimental groups, there is huge variability in patient age and health status, as well as the site and number of electrodes implanted [31]. High-density ECoG was also used to decode motor imagery of sign language gestures as an alternative mode of communication [29].

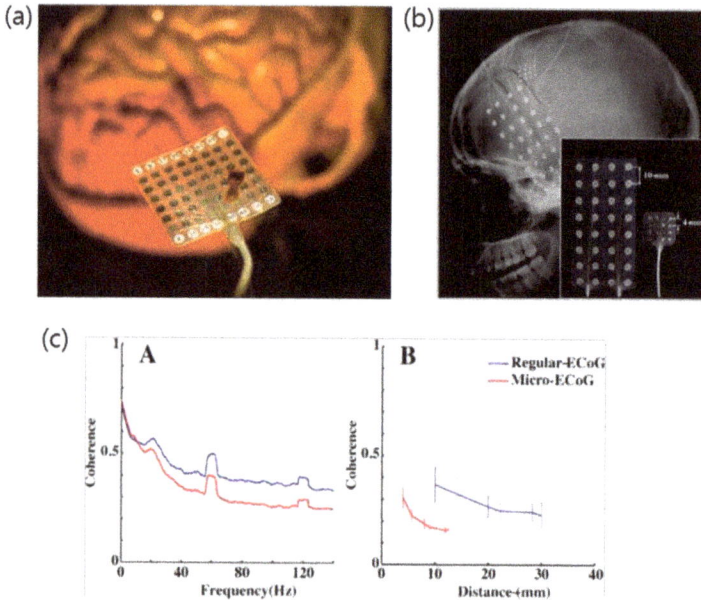

Figure 1. (**a**) Picture of a clinical electrocorticography (ECoG) grid underneath a micro-ECoG (μECoG) array. Side-by-side comparison of the regular macro-ECoG and μECoG arrays showing difference in electrode spacing. (**b**) X-ray image showing the implanted ECoG and μECoG electrode. (**c**) Coherence analysis to characterize independent neural signals recorded from both macro-ECoG and μECoG. This suggests μECoG offers higher spatial resolution for neural signal recording. (**a**) Photo was taken at Neural Interfaces Research (NITRO) lab at University of Wisconsin (UW) Madison; (**b**,**c**) reprinted with permission from Reference [6].

Micro-ECoG is becoming increasingly popular for its ability to provide higher temporal and spatial resolution than typical ECoG [6,17,32,33], often comparable to intracortical microelectrodes [33,34]. A major advantage is the smaller size of the electrode site, which allows for more precise and accurate readings and less invasive implantation than its ECoG predecessor [17,33,34]. The reduction in invasiveness predominantly refers both to the reduced size of the craniotomy required, as well as the amount of bulk material that is implanted, regardless of its implantation site. Bundy et al. suggested that μECoG should be implanted subdurally to avoid reduction in signal amplitude in humans [35], but μECoG arrays can also be implanted atop the dura with only a slight loss in signal quality. Chronic epidural μECoG implants for BCI control were successfully demonstrated in non-human primates [36]. Micro-ECoG was also applied to read local field potentials from below the cortical surface. By applying a sparse linear regression algorithm to μECoG readings,

Watanabe et al. demonstrated decoding of the hand trajectories in 3D space from depths of 0.2 to 3.2 mm, comparable to readings from more invasive microelectrode arrays [37]. Like ECoG, µECoG demonstrated applications for restoring communication and controlling prosthetic limbs. Kellis et al. demonstrated the effectiveness of µECoG to classify spoken words and distinguish between phonemes in humans [33,34]; however, these studies demonstrated limited success (<50% accuracy). The major caveat to decoding speech with µECoG relates to the spatiotemporal dynamics [30,38]. Speech involves a plethora of functional domains including motor, visual, auditory, and language domains in the high gamma range alone [30,36,38,39]. Brain activity becomes even more complex when the results are generated in real-life social settings, rather than the typical heavily controlled laboratory setting performing pre-determined tasks [28]. The continued research into decoding speech using both macro- and micro-ECoG is likely to be mutually beneficial. Alternatively, ECoG over the motor cortex is used for restoration of communication via BCI control of a computer cursor on a digital keyboard. Control of cursors on computers can be easily and rapidly learned with exceptional accuracy in both non-human primates [40] and humans [30,41]. Rouse et al. demonstrated that non-human primates could rapidly learn (days) to control velocity of a computer cursor with closed-loop recording of differential gamma-band amplitude (75–105 Hz) via µECoG [36].

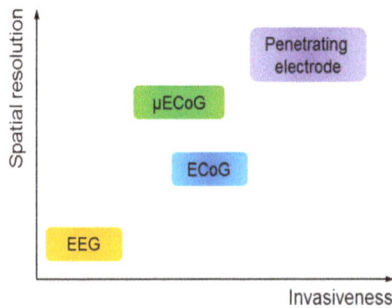

Figure 2. Spatial resolution versus invasiveness for various types of neural electrodes. Micro-ECoG has a balanced spatial resolution and invasiveness.

3. Micro-ECoG: Electrodes and Substrates

Each of the configurations mentioned above can utilize a wide variety of materials to obtain specific electrical recording types. These materials range from traditional biocompatible metals such as platinum, as well as new advances in the use of advanced two-dimensional materials such as graphene [42–44]. Not only do the materials themselves behave differently, but their properties can be further tunable via surface treatments or modifications. In this review, we categorize µECoG electrodes in terms of the electrode materials and review their usage.

3.1. Platinum

Platinum is a common material used in various applications of neural stimulation and recording due to its ability to resist corrosion and its long history of biocompatibility in the brain. This allows for long-term reliability of electrodes to be used in chronic studies [42]. Also, platinum is common in general microfabrication due to the ease of its fabrication process, which makes it readily amenable to most electrode construction protocols [43].

Furthermore, platinum is able to inject current into the brain through reversible reactions limiting damage or harm to the cortex. This current injection is achieved through a combination of Faradaic and double-layer charging, with the Faradaic component being the driving force under most neural stimulation conditions [43]. This Faradaic component is primarily from a displacement current component of the injected current achieved when the electrode is behaving as a capacitor.

These properties make platinum a viable material for use in many studies. One downside is that the materials are not transparent, which makes it impossible to do optical imaging of the cortex directly at the contact site [44,45]. Current uses for platinum electrodes include restoring or improving impairments in the visual, auditory, and somatosensory regions of the cortex through neural stimulations. With advances in technology throughout the field of neural engineering, improved platinum electrodes may show promise in prosthesis technology [42].

3.2. Sputtered Iridium Oxide

Iridium-oxide films are emerging as a technology in neural stimulation electrodes as a means to increase the electrode's ability to inject charge. These electrodes are able to inject charge via reversible reduction and oxidation between Ir^{3+}/Ir^{4+} valence states within the oxide film. By changing the thickness of the iridium-oxide layer, the electrical characteristics of the electrode can be tuned. This leads to a large variety of properties that can be obtained for the electrode [46].

One downside to iridium oxide is that it is more brittle compared to platinum, which prevents it from being used in flexible electrodes. This can prevent good contact with the cortical surface electrodes, as well as reduce the biocompatibility of the electrode due to the difference in the mechanical compliance of the electrode versus that of the brain tissue [43,45,47].

3.3. ITO

Indium tin oxide (ITO) is another potential candidate for transparent electrodes as it is used for commercial transparent electrodes in displays such as liquid crystal displays (LCDs) or active-matrix organic light-emitting diodes (AMOLEDs) [48,49]. Ledochowitsch et al. reported fabrication and characterization of a 49-channel ITO-based μECoG array [48]. Kwon et al. demonstrated an opto-μECoG array based on ITO epidural electrodes and integrated light-emitting diodes (LEDs) for optogenetics [49]. Due to the transparency of ITO (~80%), optical stimulation to brain tissue through the electrode was enabled. Kunori et al. demonstrated cortical electrical stimulation (CES) through ITO-based μECoG to investigate activation profiles of the cortex using a voltage-sensitive dye (Figure 3) [50]. CES is a technique that already reached clinical use in human patients through macro-ECoG devices. The implementation of CES through μECoG provides a useful tool in determining many of the effects that electrical stimulation has on the brain [51].

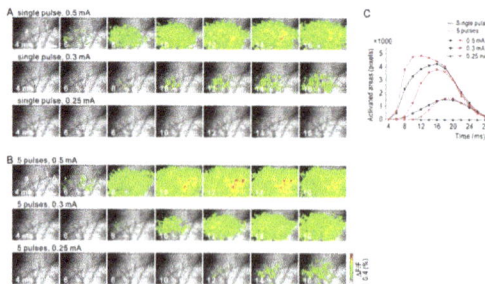

Figure 3. Anodic stimulation via indium tin oxide micro-ECoG. Neural activity captured via fluorescent voltage sensitive dye. (**A**) The white circle (a) indicates a clear electrode used for stimulation. Activation profiles captured after delivering single pulses of current intensity of 0.5, 0.3, and 0.25 mA. (**B**) Duplicate of experiment in (**A**) with a pulse train of five pulses at 500 Hz. (**C**) Comparison of spatial activation spreading due to different stimulation settings. The spatial extent of activity was evaluated by the number of pixels above threshold. A, anterior; L, lateral. Scale bar, 1.0 mm. Reprinted with permission from Reference [50].

However, in vivo studies with ITO electrode arrays are limited to acute animal experiments. In fact, the brittleness, limited transparency near ultraviolet (UV) light, and process dependency of ITO appear to be the limitations in terms of chronic in vivo studies and the compatibility of specific neural imaging modalities [49–51].

3.4. Graphene

In recent years, optical imaging of the cortical areas of the brain while recording the electrical activity through surface electrodes became possible [44,52–54]. This is due to the availability of conductive, optically transparent materials, unlike conventional metal-based conductive materials. Graphene's optically transparent nature and electrically conductive properties make it a good material for cortical electrode implementation. Graphene-based clear electrode arrays were used for a variety of optogenetic studies where light-evoked potentials could be measured on the same cortical areas that the light was administered [44]. Specifically, mouse species expressing light-sensitive proteins, either passed down genetically or through transfection, could undergo neuronal stimulation in the presence of certain wavelengths of light [55]. This makes clear µECoG appealing since it permits optical stimulation of the cortex directly below the recording site. This allows for more thorough probing of neural circuitry within the cortex, as well as other imaging modalities, simultaneously [44,54]. Generation of light-induced artefacts is one of the challenges in an integration of optical modalities with electrical recordings. However, this type of artefact could be minimized to enable cross-talk-free integration of two-photon microscopy, optogenetic stimulation, and cortical recordings in the same in vivo experiment [56].

In addition, graphene's mechanical compliance may help improve the long-term biocompatibility of the electrode. It is reported that graphene electrodes remain viable for chronic recording for extended time periods (70 days) [44].

In most cases, µECoG electrode electrical properties can be modeled by a constant phase element (Z_{CPE}), Warburg impedance (Z_W), charge transfer resistance (R_{CT}), and a solution resistance (R_S), as presented in Figure 4 [57]. Graphene's high transmittance and low electrical impedance make it a prime candidate for optically clear electrodes. According to Li et al. (2009), improved graphene development processes can make graphene sheets with low resistances. Similarly, graphene is able to achieve transmittances above 96% for single-layered graphene between the wavelengths of 400 nm and 1000 nm [58]. Park et al. characterized optical transparency of a four-layer graphene electrode at ~90% transmission over the ultraviolet-to-infrared spectrum, and demonstrated its utility for use in in vivo imaging and optogenetics (Figure 5) [44].

Graphene electrodes, like most electrodes, are electrically characterized with a resistive–capacitive model [54,59]. Therefore, as in all biological/electrical interfaces, resistance of the electrode changes with frequency. Typically, electrodes are characterized by this frequency response. Neural electrodes are also commonly characterized by their resistance at 1 kHz. [59] This is a common benchmark for neural electrodes due to the fact that the fundamental frequency of the neural action potential is at this frequency. While electrodes are typically characterized by their impedance at 1 kHz, this impedance can be quite variable, and ranges in vivo from approximately 50 kΩ to 1 MΩ [44,54,60], depending on the site size and material.

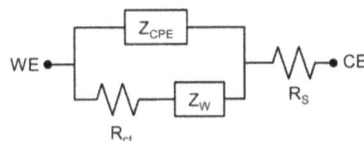

Figure 4. The representative equivalent model of a µECoG electrode. WE, working electrode; CE, counter electrode; Z_{CPE}, constant phase element; Z_W, Warburg impedance; R_{CT}, charge transfer resistance; R_S, solution resistance.

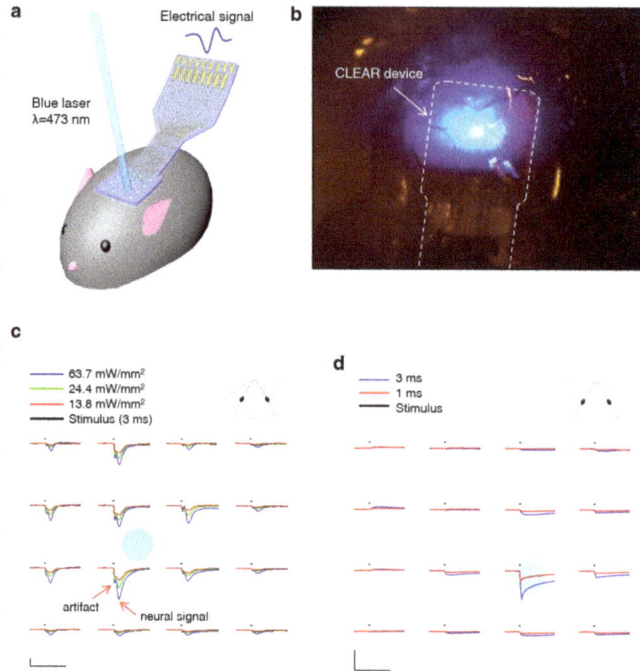

Figure 5. (**a**) Illustration depicting experimental ensemble combining optical stimulation with μECoG in a mouse model. (**b**) Optical illumination and stimulation spatially control over the mouse brain and μECoG via an optical fiber. (**c**) Spatial mapping of local field potentials obtained from a graphene μECoG throughout an optically evoked potential on the cortex of a channel rhodopsin positive mouse; *x*-scale bars represent 50 ms, *y*-scale bars represent 100 μV. (**d**) Post-mortem control depicting photo-electric artefact generated during blue-light optical stimulation; *x*-scale bar, 50 ms; *y*-scale bars, 100 μV. Reprinted with permission from Reference [44].

Previously reported μECoG devices are summarized in Table 1. For reference, penetrating electrode works are also summarized in Table 2.

Table 1. Comparison of different electrocorticography (ECoG) and micro-ECoG (μECoG) electrodes with regards to various parameters.

Layout	Substrate Materials	Recording Site Materials	Size/Impedance	Notes	Reference (Year)
2D planar array	Polyimide	Pt	1 mm² 1.5–5 kΩ	255 channels LFP and ECoG recording awake monkey for 4 months	[22] (2009)
2D planar array	Parylene C	Au-PEDOT:PSS	10 × 10 μm² 0.2 MΩ	LFP and ECoG recording in freely moving rat and humans	[61] (2015)
2D planar array	Parylene C	Graphene	Diameter: 150–200 μm, 100–600 kΩ	256 channels Transparency evoked potential by light (Optogenetics)(lifetime >70 days)	[44] (2014)
	Parylene C	Pt	Diameter: 150–200 μm 50–300 kΩ	(lifetime >70 days)	
2D planar array	Silicone rubber	Pt	-	SEP recording (μECoG) and stimulation	[62] (2011)

Table 1. *Cont.*

Layout	Substrate Materials	Recording Site Materials	Size/Impedance	Notes	Reference (Year)
2D planar array	Parylene C	Sputtered indium tin oxide (ITO)	49-channel (Pitch of 800 µm) 16-channel (Pitch of 200 µm)	Design, fabrication, and characterization	[48] (2011)
2D planar array	Parylene C	Sputtered indium tin oxide (ITO)	Diameter: 200 µm 100–200 kΩ	Optogenetics with integrated LEDs	[49] (2013)
2D planar array	Polyimide	Au-PEDOT	100 µm × 100 µm ~2.1 kΩ	recording from rat somatosensory cortex in vivo	[63] (2015)
2D planar array	Parylene C	PEDOT:PSS	10 × 10 µm 210–50 kΩ	Spike recording from surface (NeuroGrid),256 channel	[61] (2015)
2D planar array	Polyimide	Pt	300 × 300 µm^2 ~20 kΩ	Multiplexing with integrated transistors	[7] (2011)
2D planar array in a chamber system	Polyimide	Au	Diameter: 200 µm 24–45 kΩ	Electrographic seizures 124-channel µECoG and 32-channel microdrive, Multi-unit, LFP, µECoG comparison	[64] (2015)
2D planar array, perforated	Parylene C	Pt	Diameter: 200 µm	16 channel, optimizing vascular imaging.	[65] (2013)
2D planar array	Polyimide	Pt and Au	Diameter: 300 µm 5–10 kΩ	32-channel µECoG	[66] (2011)
2D planar array	Parylene C	Pt	Diameter: 200 µm<1000 kΩ	16 channel µECoG arrays, varying array footprint.	[67] (2014)
2D planar array	Silk	Au	30 electrodes	Mesh structure for conformal contact	[68] (2010)
2D planar array	Polyimide	Pt	360 channels each electrode 300 um × 300 um	Multiplexed using Si transistors	[7] (2011)
2D planar array	PLGA	Si	256 channels overall 3 cm × 3.5 cm	Bioresorbable	[69,70] (2016/2012)

2D, two-dimensional; Pt, platinum; Au, gold; Si, silicon; LED, light-emitting diode; LFP, local field potential; PLGA, poly(lactic-*co*-glycolic acid); PEDOT, poly(3,4-ethylenedioxythiophene); PSS, poly(styrenesulfonate); SEP, somatosensory evoked potential.

Table 2. Comparison of different penetrating electrodes with regards to various parameters.

Electrode Type	Layout	Substrate Materials	Recording Site Materials	Size/Impedance	Notes	Reference (Year)
Micro wire	3D array	N/A	Stainless	50 µm ×50 µm 64 channels	Primary auditory cortex (rat, ECoG recording)	[71] (2006)
	3D array	N/A	Stainless Or Tungsten	50 µm × 50 µm Teflon coated	Single cortical neurons (monkey)	[72] (2003)
	3D array	N/A	Tungsten	35 µm^2	Cerebral cortex (rat)	[73] (1999)
Michigan	Assembled 3D array	Si	Ir	100 µm^2, 2 MΩ	LFP	[74] (2000)
Michigan	Assembled 3D array	15 µm thickness of Si	Ir	177 µm^2, 0.72 MΩ 312 µm^2, 1.65 MΩ	Cerebral cortex (rat) Chronic recording (127 days)	[75] (2004)
Michigan	2D array	Si	PEDOT & Au	Gold, 9.1 MΩ PEDOT, 0.37 MΩ	Single unit implanted in layer V (rat)	[76] (2011)
Michigan	2D array	Si	PEDOT	-	PEDOT VS Carbon A new set of materials to make fundamental	[77] (2012)
Utah	10 × 10 3D array	Doped Si	Ti/Pt (50/240 nm)	Width 80 µm, length 1500 µm	Chronic single unit spikes in cortex Insulated with polyimide	[78] (1992)
Utah	10 × 10 3D array	Doped Si	Pt/Ir	100–300 kΩ	Tip exposed (500 µm) Cat auditory & visual cortex	[79] (1999)
Utah	10 × 10 3D array	Doped Si	Pt/Ir	1600 µm^2 100–750 kΩ	Tip exposed (40 µm) Primary motor cortex (M1, monkey)	[80] (2005)
Utah	10 × 10 3D array	Doped Si	Pt	125 kΩ 2 mC·cm^{-2}	Cortical stimulation/recording (>90 days in vitro)	[43] (2010)
		Doped Si	Sputtered iridium oxide film (SIROF)	6 kΩ 0.3 mC·cm^{-2}	Cortical stimulation/recording (>90 days in vitro)	
Utah	Unrestricted freedom in the 2D probe	300 µm thickness of Si	Ti/Au/Pt (30/200/100 nm)	1–2 MΩ	72 channels Recording LFP in layers 1, 2, and 3 for 15 days	[81] (2009)

3D, three-dimensional; Ir, iridium; Ti, titanium.

3.5. Bioresorbable Silicon

In clinical neurological monitoring involving μECoG with the abovementioned materials, a second surgical procedure for removal of the device is typically performed after the recording is over. Whether the implant is extensive or not, such a second procedure often adds cost and risk. In most cases, one to three weeks of recording is required. Ideally, a temporary monitoring system that can dissolve or disappear after the suggested period of implant time would eliminate such a second surgical procedure. Recent advances in silicon devices demonstrated bioresorbable forms of silicon sensors and electronics, where ultrathin silicon nanomembranes disappear after a certain period of time in fluids. For instance, a hydrolysis demonstration of block silicon nanomembrane (initial dimensions: 3 mm × 3 mm × 70 nm) in phosphate-buffered saline (PBS) at 37 °C suggests that a complete dissolution occurs after 12 days. It was also demonstrated that the constituent materials comprising such bioresorbable sensors and electronics are biocompatible, which is suitable for biomedical applications [70].

Precise recordings of brain signals from the cerebral cortex were achieved utilizing bioresorbable silicon electronics [69]. With an array of electrodes made of silicon nanomembranes mounted on bioresorbable poly(lactic-*co*-glycolic acid) (PLGA) substrate, the flexible μECoG device could achieve conformal contact with the cortex, owing to the ultrathin structure of the device. This technique of utilizing bioresorbable substrate was also demonstrated with traditional metal electrodes where the conformability of the electrodes was improved by eliminating the normal substrate, such as polyimide, and replacing it with bioresorbable silk [68]. Furthermore, sophisticated bioresorbable silicon μECoG arrays with actively multiplexed electronics involving silicon transistors were demonstrated for large array-based spatial mapping of cortical activity. The multiplexed electrode array using flexible silicon electronics was proven to achieve extremely high density (up to 25,600 channels) for precise mapping of the brain activity. Such a concept provides a robust foundation for bioresorbable implantable electrode technology, especially as the use of silicon aligns well with mature semiconductor manufacturing infrastructure [7].

Drawing from the Tables 1 and 2, a multitude of different studies can be formulated. Overall, the use of different materials within the microarrays is still up for debate, and wide varieties are still in testing. Additional materials such as graphene and poly(ethylenedioxythiphene) (PEDOT) were added to the traditional materials. These vary greatly from the traditional metallic electrodes in composition, but strive to imitate the electrical characteristics that are desirable [60]. In all cases, the general characteristics are known, but with each material having its own specific drawbacks. Overall, neuro-recording and stimulation are emerging fields, as a greater understanding of brain processes is required. Given this push, along with precise manufacturing techniques, the variety of implementation will go up. However, until long-term studies can be completed, the use of the original metallic electrode microarrays (Pt, Ir, and Tn) will remain the clinical standard.

4. Host Response to μECoG Devices

The brain has a unique and complex response to trauma that is heavily mediated by neurogenic inflammation. The complex inflammatory response to brain injury following trauma can be neuroprotective, but can also result in secondary injury, driving chronic neural injury. Neurogenic inflammation in response to trauma is beyond the scope of this review, and was best described elsewhere [47,82–84]. Of particular interest to this review is the chronic foreign body response (FBR), as implanted electrodes often incite an FBR, which can both affect the performance of implanted electrodes and the surrounding brain tissue itself [47,85,86].

Whilst host cells immediately respond to the surgical injury itself, the foreign body (electrode) induces chronic inflammation at the biotic–abiotic interface [47,87]. At the biotic–abiotic interface, microglia (resident immune cells of the central nervous system (CNS), analogous to macrophages in the rest of the body) become activated, undergo gliosis, and eventually encapsulate the implanted device [47]. The primary cause of this reaction is yet to be elucidated; however, the strongest evidence indicates that a mismatch between implanted materials and tissue compliance heavily mediates the activation of microglia, as demonstrated by several eloquent in vitro studies [88,89]. Increasing evidence demonstrates the importance of material properties on cell fate, including neural stem and progenitor cells, which holds implications for neural regeneration around the electrode site [90].

The most invasive electrodes, such as penetrating electrode arrays, cause the most trauma at the time of implant, and also elicit the greatest FBR response as a result of increased surface area between the implanted foreign body and the native tissue [85,86]. In contrast, less invasive devices, such as μECoG, are thought to generally elicit less of a response, demonstrated by greater electrode longevity [66,67,91].

Most commonly, implanted devices (particularly penetrating devices) become encapsulated in a glial scar similar to macrophage-induced fibrosis in other organs [92]. The foreign body response is dynamic, and considered an evolutionary survival mechanism to either remove or compartmentalize foreign objects (not self), preventing their interaction with surrounding tissues (self) as a means of self-preservation. The glial scar, astrocytes and microglia responding to a foreign body, can isolate the electrode from the desired neurons and insulate it from the rest of the cortex. This can lead to an increase in impedance, and make it harder for the electrode to record the electrical activity of the underlying tissue [47,59,85,86]. Astrocytes can be identified by increased expression of glial fibrillary acidic protein (GFAP) and vimentin [93,94]. Microglia are often identified by immunostaining for ionized calcium-binding adaptor molecule 1 (Iba1). Glial scars consist of an excess of extracellular matrix, including collagen IV and chondroitin sulfate proteoglycans [95]. The increase in inflammatory cell density and extracellular matrix deposition both lead to increased impedance and decreased recording capability [59].

Aside from the cellular elements of scarring, molecular elements such as proteins are known to adhere to the surface of recording sites (biofouling). These protein layers typically have no reactive impedance on signals below 5 MHz. Therefore, the buildup of protein can be modeled as an increase in series electrolytic resistance in the equivalent circuit. The electrode–electrolyte interface impedance is comparable to that of a high-pass filter, with larger impedances for low-frequency signals. This increase in electrolytic resistance increases the impedance for signals of all frequencies. This causes an upward shift in the virtual cutoff frequency, making the device more susceptible to noise at lower frequencies, and decreases the amplitude seen by the amplifier circuit, lowering the signal-to-noise ratio (SNR). Electrode design factors such as geometry, materials, and level of invasiveness all play important roles in the longevity of electrodes by reducing glial scar formation and biofouling. Providing open space as opposed to solid electrodes was shown to reduce scar formation [77,96]. Reducing invasiveness (μECoG vs. penetrating arrays) may also reduce scaring through reducing trauma, both to the parenchyma and the blood–brain barrier [67,87].

The host response can significantly affect the performance of the electrode. Typically, the implanted neural electrodes show a large increase in the impedance of the electrode after implantation for the first 7–10 days [44,59,65]. This is speculated to primarily be due to the host response to the implantation surgery rather than electrode degradation.

5. Role of ECoG and μECoG in Human Disease and BCI

The role of macro- and micro-ECoG for the clinical treatment of human patients is expanding. Seizure focus localization is the major traditional role for ECoG clinically [97,98]. Intraoperative ECoG can be used to identify abnormal interictal discharges as a proxy for the epileptic focus, but numerous constraints, especially limited time, make identification of a seizure focus in the operating room unreliable. Instead, temporarily implanted subdural ECoG arrays, often in conjunction with depth electrodes, provide longer-term monitoring, during which withdrawal of antiepileptic drugs and recording of multiple seizures can help localize the region of seizure onset [11,18,97].

In addition to localizing the source of seizures, ECoG can also be used to localize the eloquent cortex that must be spared during surgical resection. Traditionally, this is achieved with intraoperative mapping via bipolar cortical stimulation and identification of corresponding motor/sensory response or speech arrest, with ECoG arrays utilized to monitor for stimulation-induced after-discharges, which raise concern for stimulation-induced seizures. Performing eloquent cortex mapping with stimulation via an implanted ECoG array outside the operating room removes time constraints and results in a more detailed functional map. Cortical mapping using implanted ECoG arrays outside the operating room also negates the need for awake surgery, a key concern to maximize patient comfort especially for those patients unable to tolerate awake surgery [8,9,11,18,30,99,100].

The unpredictability of seizures is one of the sources of morbidity in epilepsy. If a patient has some warning of an impending seizure, they may be able to prepare for the event by making modifications to their physical environment or medication dosing. An implanted subdural ECoG array (NeuroVista, Seattle, WA, USA) linked to a subcutaneously implanted battery and telemetry unit that communicates with a patient advisory device was used to provide patients with an early warning of a possible impending seizure, with promising results reported in 2013 in an early feasibility human trial involving 15 patients [101].

The ability to detect impending seizure activity also opens the possibility of potentially interrupting that activity with direct responsive neurostimulation (RNS). In patients with seizure foci that are not amenable to surgical resection (e.g., foci involving the eloquent cortex or bilateral hippocampi), responsive neurostimulation (NeuroPace, Inc., Mountain View, CA, USA.) was shown in a randomized multicenter double-blinded controlled trial involving 191 patients to significantly decrease the frequency of partial-onset seizures, with a median reduction of 53% at two years. This system utilized either ECoG strip electrodes (1 × 4) or depth electrodes to provide continuous monitoring of electrical activity with subsequent stimulation based on specific abnormalities associated with seizure onset [102,103].

In an investigative fashion, subdural ECoG was used in humans to evaluate cortical activity surrounding areas of brain injury in patients with ischemic stroke, traumatic brain injury, and aneurysmal subarachnoid hemorrhage. These studies demonstrated frequent episodes of cortical spreading depolarization and depression around the area of injury and the resultant increased metabolic demand was associated with neurological worsening. It is uncertain at this time whether interventions based on detecting these episodes of cortical spreading depolarization or preventing them can be used to improve clinical outcomes [104–107].

Cortical stimulation via ECoG, coupled with rehabilitation therapy, was also postulated to aid functional recovery after stroke. Despite promising animal studies [57,108–113] and early human trials [114–117], a large multicenter randomized controlled human trial using a fully implanted epidural ECoG array and battery (Northstar Neuroscience, Inc, Seattle, WA, USA) to deliver continuous stimulation over an area of chronic infarct, combined with intensive therapy, failed to demonstrate clinically significant benefit [118,119].

The application of BCI for the control of prosthetic limbs exploded in the last decade, predominantly encouraged by the Defense Advanced Research Projects Agency's (DARPA) Revolutionizing Prosthetics Program [120]. Several groups demonstrated various applications for µECoG in the decoding of upper limb movements for control of prosthetics by humans, including virtual hand opening and closing [32], finger movements [6], and wrist movements [121]. Leuthardt et al. demonstrated that µECoG can be used to identify and separate motor movements in the wrist from <5 mm of motor cortex in humans [121], whilst Wang et al. showed that µECoG can be used by a patient with tetraplegia to control a cursor on a computer in both two and three dimensions [122]. Micro-ECoG is yet to be tested for the range of applications of its macro predecessor, such as for controlling the latest multifaceted, modular upper prosthetic limbs [123].

6. Discussion and Future Direction

The development of multichannel neural interfaces, including µECoG, allowed for great advances in understanding the link between neural activity and body function, as well as exploring the cause of neurological disorders such as epilepsy. Furthermore, these technologies enable the development of neuroprosthetic devices and therapies that hold tremendous potential to restore an individual's motor and sensory function that was lost to disease or traumatic injury. Due to its balance between invasiveness, spatial resolution, and biocompatibility, µECoG is a technology that is ideally placed to provide stable, reliable neural interfaces for years to come in both the research and clinical domains.

The use of µECoG in basic science and pre-clinical research gained significant momentum over the past decade especially for work exploring brain–computer interfaces and examining the viability of cortex following neural injury. However, µEcoG is still not the preferred method for recording cortical neural activity in the majority of neuroscience research, as it struggles to isolate the spiking activity of individual neurons, especially those from deeper cortical layers. The relationship between spiking activity in deeper cortical layers and the signal recorded by µECoG is an active area of research for many in vivo biophysical and computational modeling studies. We expect that results of these experiments could result in new techniques for localizing and predicting individual sources of neural activity leading to the greater usage of µECoG technology.

Despite the potential of µECoG alone, we see its greatest potential when used in concert with optical stimulation/imaging techniques to dissect the function of neural circuits. As we discussed above, the development of optically clear µECoG electrodes enables the simultaneous recording of cortical potentials and neural stimulation via optogenetic techniques (see Figure 5). More exciting is the combination of optically clear µECoG electrodes, advanced optical imaging modalities (i.e., multiphoton imaging and light sheet microscopy), and animal models with genetically encoded sensors offering the opportunity to interrogate structures located farther from the cortical surface. These techniques offer the ability to explore the relationship between electrophysiology, cellular metabolism, and vascular dynamics, which will be necessary to understand the etiology of many neural diseases like epilepsy.

Although µECoG shows great promise for clinical application, it has yet to reach widespread utilization in the diagnosis and treatment of human disease. The underwhelming use of µECoG in clinical settings stems from two factors. Firstly, there is currently no Food and Drug Administration (FDA)-approved device/indication for µECoG. While challenging, gaining the approval of regulators seems a matter of time given the similarity of µECoG with its technological cousin, ECoG. We expect that this obstacle will be overcome in the near future. Secondly, there is currently no pressing clinical need for µECoG, as current-generation ECoG technology satisfies today's clinical usage. For example, the use of ECoG in epilepsy patients drove much of what is currently known about the functional organization of the human cortex. We expect the use of µECoG to further push the boundaries established by conventional ECoG due to its ability to measure more detailed electrophysiological data, and the less invasive nature of µECoG has the potential expand the patient population appropriate for implanted devices. We believe that the application of µECoG for BCI will soon replace macro-ECoG as the new standard, due to its higher spatio-temporal resolution and reduced manufacturing limitations.

Aside from replacing current-generation ECoG with µECoG, new clinical indications requiring µECoG are on the horizon. Implanted devices, such as deep brain stimulation for movement disorders and responsive neurostimulation for the treatment of epilepsy, moved out of labs and are now standard-of-care treatment for thousands of patients. Micro-ECoG will most certainly be used to add closed-loop stimulation capabilities to the future generation of neuromodulation devices. Here, µECoG could provide a richer stream of electrophysiological information that will fine-tune decisions regarding when and where to initiate therapeutic stimulation. Furthermore, µECoG could most certainly be used to monitor neural signals in the first-generation clinical neuroprosthetic devices due to its relatively high spatial resolution and biocompatibility. However, the clinical viability of neuroprosthetic devices hinges on improvements in the wireless transmission of data and power, which will allow for a fully implantable form factor. We see a potentially bright future for µECoG technologies, one where many patients will see benefits from future generations of implanted neuromodulation and neuroprosthetic devices. The use and utility of µECoG is clearly ascending, as its core and supporting technologies are being refined and new applications are being imagined. Next-generation technologies could be catalyzed by the development of µECoG devices that are fully untethered from the external world and include all of the necessary electronics (i.e., data acquisition, power transmission, and communication) directly on the device [124–127]. Such developments will enable integrated neuroprosthetic and neuromodulation systems that will have the ability to function for the lifetime of the patient.

Author Contributions: M.S., D.-W.P., Z.M. and J.W. conceived and designed the review paper; M.S., D.-W.P., Y.H.J., S.K.B., J.N., A.D., K.I.S., D.-H.B., A.J.S., W.B.L., Z.M. and J.W. wrote the paper.

Acknowledgments: This work was sponsored in part by the Defense Advanced Research Projects Agency (DARPA) Biological Technology Office (BTO), under the auspices of Jack W. Judy and Douglas J. Weber as part of the Reliable Neural Technology Program, through the Space and Naval Warfare Systems Command (SPAWAR) System Center (SSC) Pacific grant no. N66001-12-C-4025 to Kevin J. Otto and Justin C. Williams. This work was also sponsored in part by the Army Research Office under grant W911NF-14-1-0652. The program manager is James Harvey and Joe X. Qiu (former). The work was also partly supported by the Basic Science Research Program through the National Research Foundation of Korea (NRF) funded by the Ministry of Science and ICT (grant no. 2018R1C1B6001529).

Conflicts of Interest: Multiple authors have financial or intellectual property interests in technologies that are described in this review or in the more general area of neuroengineering. J.C.W., D.-W.P., M.S., and Z.M. all have patents on technology described in this review. J.C.W. has an equity interest in NeuroOne Medical (Minnetonka, MN) and NeuroNexus (Ann Arbor, MI), companies that manufacture microfabricated electrode arrays for research and clinical applications.

References

1. Serruya, M.D.; Hatsopoulos, N.G.; Paninski, L.; Fellows, M.R.; Donoghue, J.P. Brain-machine interface: Instant neural control of a movement signal. *Nature* **2002**, *416*, 141–142. [CrossRef] [PubMed]

2. Carmena, J.M.; Lebedev, M.A.; Crist, R.E.; O'Doherty, J.E.; Santucci, D.M.; Dimitrov, D.F.; Patil, P.G.; Henriquez, C.S.; Nicolelis, M.A. Learning to control a brain–machine interface for reaching and grasping by primates. *PLoS Biol.* **2003**, *1*, e42. [CrossRef] [PubMed]

3. Hochberg, L.R.; Serruya, M.D.; Friehs, G.M.; Mukand, J.A.; Saleh, M.; Caplan, A.H.; Branner, A.; Chen, D.; Penn, R.D.; Donoghue, J.P. Neuronal ensemble control of prosthetic devices by a human with tetraplegia. *Nature* **2006**, *442*, 164. [CrossRef] [PubMed]

4. Collinger, J.L.; Wodlinger, B.; Downey, J.E.; Wang, W.; Tyler-Kabara, E.C.; Weber, D.J.; McMorland, A.J.; Velliste, M.; Boninger, M.L.; Schwartz, A.B. High-performance neuroprosthetic control by an individual with tetraplegia. *Lancet* **2013**, *381*, 557–564. [CrossRef]

5. Petroff, O.A.; Spencer, D.D.; Goncharova, I.I.; Zaveri, H.P. A comparison of the power spectral density of scalp EEG and subjacent electrocorticograms. *Clin. Neurophysiol.* **2016**, *127*, 1108–1112. [CrossRef] [PubMed]

6. Wang, W.; Degenhart, A.D.; Collinger, J.L.; Vinjamuri, R.; Sudre, G.P.; Adelson, P.D.; Holder, D.L.; Leuthardt, E.C.; Moran, D.W.; Boninger, M.L. Human motor cortical activity recorded with Micro-ECoG electrodes, during individual finger movements. In Proceedings of the 2009 Annual International Conference of the IEEE Engineering in Medicine and Biology Society, Minneapolis, MN, USA, 3–6 September 2009; pp. 586–589.

7. Viventi, J.; Kim, D.-H.; Vigeland, L.; Frechette, E.S.; Blanco, J.A.; Kim, Y.-S.; Avrin, A.E.; Tiruvadi, V.R.; Hwang, S.-W.; Vanleer, A.C. Flexible, foldable, actively multiplexed, high-density electrode array for mapping brain activity in vivo. *Nat. Neurosci.* **2011**, *14*, 1599–1605. [CrossRef]

8. Leuthardt, E.C.; Schalk, G.; Wolpaw, J.R.; Ojemann, J.G.; Moran, D.W. A brain–computer interface using electrocorticographic signals in humansThe authors declare that they have no competing financial interests. *J. Neural Eng.* **2004**, *1*, 63. [CrossRef]

9. Schalk, G.; Miller, K.; Anderson, N.; Wilson, J.; Smyth, M.; Ojemann, J.; Moran, D.; Wolpaw, J.; Leuthardt, E. Two-dimensional movement control using electrocorticographic signals in humans. *J. Neural Eng.* **2008**, *5*, 75. [CrossRef]

10. Towle, V.L.; Yoon, H.-A.; Castelle, M.; Edgar, J.C.; Biassou, N.M.; Frim, D.M.; Spire, J.-P.; Kohrman, M.H. ECoG gamma activity during a language task: Differentiating expressive and receptive speech areas. *Brain* **2008**, *131*, 2013–2027. [CrossRef]

11. Hill, N.J.; Gupta, D.; Brunner, P.; Gunduz, A.; Adamo, M.A.; Ritaccio, A.; Schalk, G. Recording human electrocorticographic (ECoG) signals for neuroscientific research and real-time functional cortical mapping. *J. Vis. Exp.* **2012**, *64*, e3993. [CrossRef]

12. Miran, S.; Akram, S.; Sheikhattar, A.; Simon, J.Z.; Zhang, T.; Babadi, B. Real-Time Tracking of Selective Auditory Attention From M/EEG: A Bayesian Filtering Approach. *Front. Neurosci.* **2018**, *12*, 262. [CrossRef] [PubMed]

13. Buzsaki, G. *Rhythms of the Brain*; Oxford University Press: Oxford, UK, 2006.

14. Ray, S.; Maunsell, J.H. Do gamma oscillations play a role in cerebral cortex? *Trends Cogn. Sci.* **2015**, *19*, 78–85. [CrossRef] [PubMed]

15. Penfield, W.; Steelman, H. The Treatment of Focal Epilepsy by Cortical Excision. *Ann. Surg.* **1947**, *126*, 740–761. [CrossRef]

16. Lycke, R.J.; Schendel, A.; Williams, J.C.; Otto, K.J. In vivo evaluation of a μECoG array for chronic stimulation. In Proceedings of the 2014 36th Annual International Conference of the IEEE Engineering in Medicine and Biology Society, Chicago, IL, USA, 26–30 August 2014; pp. 1294–1297.

17. Kellis, S.; Sorensen, L.; Darvas, F.; Sayres, C.; O'Neill, K.; Brown, R.B.; House, P.; Ojemann, J.; Greger, B. Multi-scale analysis of neural activity in humans: Implications for micro-scale electrocorticography. *Clin. Neurophysiol.* **2016**, *127*, 591–601. [CrossRef] [PubMed]

18. Schalk, G.; Kubanek, J.; Miller, K.; Anderson, N.; Leuthardt, E.; Ojemann, J.; Limbrick, D.; Moran, D.; Gerhardt, L.; Wolpaw, J. Decoding two-dimensional movement trajectories using electrocorticographic signals in humans. *J. Neural Eng.* **2007**, *4*, 264. [CrossRef] [PubMed]

19. Wang, G.; Zhang, J.; Hu, X.; Zhang, L.; Mao, L.; Jiang, X.; Liou, A.K.; Leak, R.K.; Gao, Y.; Chen, J. Microglia/macrophage polarization dynamics in white matter after traumatic brain injury. *J. Cereb. Blood Flow Metab.* **2013**, *33*, 1864–1874. [CrossRef] [PubMed]

20. Morishita, S.; Sato, K.; Watanabe, H.; Nishimura, Y.; Isa, T.; Kato, R.; Nakamura, T.; Yokoi, H. Brain-machine interface to control a prosthetic arm with monkey ECoGs during periodic movements. *Front. Neurosci.* **2014**, *8*, 417. [CrossRef]

21. Yanagisawa, T.; Hirata, M.; Saitoh, Y.; Goto, T.; Kishima, H.; Fukuma, R.; Yokoi, H.; Kamitani, Y.; Yoshimine, T. Real-time control of a prosthetic hand using human electrocorticography signals: Technical note. *J. Neurosurg.* **2011**, *114*, 1715–1722. [CrossRef]

22. Rubehn, B.; Bosman, C.; Oostenveld, R.; Fries, P.; Stieglitz, T. A MEMS-based flexible multichannel ECoG-electrode array. *J. Neural Eng.* **2009**, *6*, 036003. [CrossRef]

23. Chao, Z.C.; Nagasaka, Y.; Fujii, N. Long-term asynchronous decoding of arm motion using electrocorticographic signals in monkey. *Front. Neuroeng.* **2010**, *3*, 3. [CrossRef]

24. Yanagisawa, T.; Hirata, M.; Saitoh, Y.; Kishima, H.; Goto, T.; Fukuma, R.; Yokoi, H.; Kamitani, Y.; Yoshimine, T. Prosthetic arm control by paralyzed patients using electrocorticograms. *Neurosci. Res.* **2010**, *68*, e83. [CrossRef]

25. Shimoda, K.; Nagasaka, Y.; Chao, Z.C.; Fujii, N. Decoding continuous three-dimensional hand trajectories from epidural electrocorticographic signals in Japanese macaques. *J. Neural Eng.* **2012**, *9*, 036015. [CrossRef] [PubMed]

26. Breshears, J.D.; Gaona, C.M.; Roland, J.L.; Sharma, M.; Anderson, N.R.; Bundy, D.T.; Freudenburg, Z.V.; Smyth, M.D.; Zempel, J.; Limbrick, D.D. Decoding motor signals from the pediatric cortex: Implications for brain-computer interfaces in children. *Pediatrics* **2011**, *128*, e160–e168. [CrossRef] [PubMed]

27. Cook, M.J.; O'Brien, T.J.; Berkovic, S.F.; Murphy, M.; Morokoff, A.; Fabinyi, G.; D'Souza, W.; Yerra, R.; Archer, J.; Litewka, L. Prediction of seizure likelihood with a long-term, implanted seizure advisory system in patients with drug-resistant epilepsy: A first-in-man study. *Lancet Neurol.* **2013**, *12*, 563–571. [CrossRef]

28. Derix, J.; Iljina, O.; Schulze-Bonhage, A.; Aertsen, A.; Ball, T. "Doctor" or "darling"? Decoding the communication partner from ECoG of the anterior temporal lobe during non-experimental, real-life social interaction. *Front. Hum. Neurosci.* **2012**, *6*, 251. [CrossRef]

29. Bleichner, M.; Freudenburg, Z.; Jansma, J.; Aarnoutse, E.; Vansteensel, M.; Ramsey, N. Give me a sign: Decoding four complex hand gestures based on high-density ECoG. *Brain Struct. Funct.* **2016**, *221*, 203–216. [CrossRef]

30. Leuthardt, E.C.; Gaona, C.; Sharma, M.; Szrama, N.; Roland, J.; Freudenberg, Z.; Solis, J.; Breshears, J.; Schalk, G. Using the electrocorticographic speech network to control a brain–computer interface in humans. *J. Neural Eng.* **2011**, *8*, 036004. [CrossRef]
31. Felton, E.A.; Wilson, J.A.; Williams, J.C.; Garell, P.C. Electrocorticographically controlled brain-computer interfaces using motor and sensory imagery in patients with temporary subdural electrode implants: Report of four cases. *J. Neurosurg.* **2007**, *106*, 495–500. [CrossRef]
32. Vinjamuri, R.; Weber, D.; Degenhart, A.; Collinger, J.; Sudre, G.; Adelson, P.; Holder, D.; Boninger, M.L.; Schwartz, A.; Crammond, D. A fuzzy logic model for hand posture control using human cortical activity recorded by micro-ECoG electrodes. In Proceedings of the 2009 Annual International Conference of the IEEE Engineering in Medicine and Biology Society, Minneapolis, MN, USA, 3–6 September 2009; pp. 4339–4342.
33. Kellis, S.; Miller, K.; Thomson, K.; Brown, R.; House, P.; Greger, B. Decoding spoken words using local field potentials recorded from the cortical surface. *J. Neural Eng.* **2010**, *7*, 056007. [CrossRef]
34. Kellis, S.; Miller, K.; Thomson, K.; Brown, R.; House, P.; Greger, B. Classification of spoken words using surface local field potentials. In Proceedings of the 2010 Annual International Conference of the IEEE Engineering in Medicine and Biology, Buenos Aires, Argentina, 31 August–4 September 2010; pp. 3827–3830.
35. Bundy, D.T.; Zellmer, E.; Gaona, C.M.; Sharma, M.; Szrama, N.; Hacker, C.; Freudenburg, Z.V.; Daitch, A.; Moran, D.W.; Leuthardt, E.C. Characterization of the effects of the human dura on macro-and micro-electrocorticographic recordings. *J. Neural Eng.* **2014**, *11*, 016006. [CrossRef]
36. Rouse, A.G.; Williams, J.J.; Wheeler, J.J.; Moran, D.W. Cortical adaptation to a chronic micro-electrocorticographic brain computer interface. *J. Neurosci.* **2013**, *33*, 1326–1330. [CrossRef] [PubMed]
37. Watanabe, H.; Sato, M.-A.; Suzuki, T.; Nambu, A.; Nishimura, Y.; Kawato, M.; Isa, T. Reconstruction of movement-related intracortical activity from micro-electrocorticogram array signals in monkey primary motor cortex. *J. Neural Eng.* **2012**, *9*, 036006. [CrossRef] [PubMed]
38. Pei, X.; Leuthardt, E.C.; Gaona, C.M.; Brunner, P.; Wolpaw, J.R.; Schalk, G. Spatiotemporal dynamics of electrocorticographic high gamma activity during overt and covert word repetition. *Neuroimage* **2011**, *54*, 2960–2972. [CrossRef] [PubMed]
39. Price, C.J. The anatomy of language: Contributions from functional neuroimaging. *J. Anat.* **2000**, *197*, 335–359. [CrossRef] [PubMed]
40. Williams, J.J.; Rouse, A.G.; Thongpang, S.; Williams, J.C.; Moran, D.W. Differentiating closed-loop cortical intention from rest: Building an asynchronous electrocorticographic BCI. *J. Neural Eng.* **2013**, *10*, 046001. [CrossRef]
41. Krusienski, D.J.; Shih, J.J. Control of a visual keyboard using an electrocorticographic brain–computer interface. *Neurorehabil. Neural Repair* **2011**, *25*, 323–331. [CrossRef]
42. Weremfo, A.; Carter, P.; Hibbert, D.B.; Zhao, C. Investigating the interfacial properties of electrochemically roughened platinum electrodes for neural stimulation. *Langmuir* **2015**, *31*, 2593–2599. [CrossRef] [PubMed]
43. Negi, S.; Bhandari, R.; Rieth, L.; Solzbacher, F. In vitro comparison of sputtered iridium oxide and platinum-coated neural implantable microelectrode arrays. *Biomed. Mater.* **2010**, *5*, 015007. [CrossRef]
44. Park, D.-W.; Schendel, A.A.; Mikael, S.; Brodnick, S.K.; Richner, T.J.; Ness, J.P.; Hayat, M.R.; Atry, F.; Frye, S.T.; Pashaie, R. Graphene-based carbon-layered electrode array technology for neural imaging and optogenetic applications. *Nat. Commun.* **2014**, *5*, 5258. [CrossRef]
45. Richner, T.J.; Thongpang, S.; Brodnick, S.K.; Schendel, A.A.; Falk, R.W.; Krugner-Higby, L.A.; Pashaie, R.; Williams, J.C. Optogenetic micro-electrocorticography for modulating and localizing cerebral cortex activity. *J. Neural Eng.* **2014**, *11*, 016010. [CrossRef]
46. Cogan, S.F.; Plante, T.; Ehrlich, J. Sputtered iridium oxide films (SIROFs) for low-impedance neural stimulation and recording electrodes. In Proceedings of the 26th Annual International Conference of the IEEE Engineering in Medicine and Biology Society, IEMBS'04, San Francisco, CA, USA, 1–5 September 2004; pp. 4153–4156.
47. Polikov, V.S.; Tresco, P.A.; Reichert, W.M. Response of brain tissue to chronically implanted neural electrodes. *J. Neurosci. Methods* **2005**, *148*, 1–18. [CrossRef] [PubMed]
48. Ledochowitsch, P.; Olivero, E.; Blanche, T.; Maharbiz, M.M. A transparent µECoG array for simultaneous recording and optogenetic stimulation. In Proceedings of the 2011 Annual International Conference of the IEEE Engineering in Medicine and Biology Society, Boston, MA, USA, 30 August–3 September 2011; pp. 2937–2940.

49. Kwon, K.Y.; Sirowatka, B.; Weber, A.; Li, W. Opto-µECoG array: A hybrid neural interface with transparent µECoG electrode array and integrated LEDs for optogenetics. *IEEE Trans. Biomed. Circuits Syst.* **2013**, *7*, 593–600. [CrossRef] [PubMed]

50. Kunori, N.; Takashima, I. A transparent epidural electrode array for use in conjunction with optical imaging. *J. Neurosci. Methods* **2015**, *251*, 130–137. [CrossRef] [PubMed]

51. Johnson, L.; Wander, J.; Sarma, D.; Su, D.; Fetz, E.; Ojemann, J.G. Direct electrical stimulation of the somatosensory cortex in humans using electrocorticography electrodes: A qualitative and quantitative report. *J. Neural Eng.* **2013**, *10*, 036021. [CrossRef] [PubMed]

52. Kuzum, D.; Takano, H.; Shim, E.; Reed, J.C.; Juul, H.; Richardson, A.G.; de Vries, J.; Bink, H.; Dichter, M.A.; Lucas, T.H. Transparent and flexible low noise graphene electrodes for simultaneous electrophysiology and neuroimaging. *Nat. Commun.* **2014**, *5*, 5259. [CrossRef] [PubMed]

53. Park, D.-W.; Brodnick, S.K.; Ness, J.P.; Atry, F.; Krugner-Higby, L.; Sandberg, A.; Mikael, S.; Richner, T.J.; Novello, J.; Kim, H.; et al. Fabrication and utility of a transparent graphene neural electrode array for electrophysiology, in vivo imaging, and optogenetics. *Nat. Protoc.* **2016**, *11*, 2201. [CrossRef] [PubMed]

54. Park, D.-W.; Ness, J.P.; Brodnick, S.K.; Esquibel, C.; Novello, J.; Atry, F.; Baek, D.-H.; Kim, H.; Bong, J.; Swanson, K.I.; et al. Electrical Neural Stimulation and Simultaneous in Vivo Monitoring with Transparent Graphene Electrode Arrays Implanted in GCaMP6f Mice. *ACS Nano* **2018**, *12*, 148–157. [CrossRef]

55. Britt, J.P.; McDevitt, R.A.; Bonci, A. Use of channelrhodopsin for activation of CNS neurons. *Curr. Protoc. Neurosci.* **2012**, *58*, 2.16.1–2.16.19.

56. Thunemann, M.; Lu, Y.; Liu, X.; Kılıç, K.; Desjardins, M.; Vandenberghe, M.; Sadegh, S.; Saisan, P.A.; Cheng, Q.; Weldy, K.L.; et al. Deep 2-photon imaging and artifact-free optogenetics through transparent graphene microelectrode arrays. *Nat. Commun.* **2018**, *9*, 2035. [CrossRef]

57. Chang, W.H.; Kim, H.; Sun, W.; Kim, J.Y.; Shin, Y.-I.; Kim, Y.-H. Effects of extradural cortical stimulation on motor recovery in a rat model of subacute stroke. *Restor. Neurol. Neurosci.* **2015**, *33*, 589–596. [CrossRef]

58. Li, X.; Zhu, Y.; Cai, W.; Borysiak, M.; Han, B.; Chen, D.; Piner, R.D.; Colombo, L.; Ruoff, R.S. Transfer of large-area graphene films for high-performance transparent conductive electrodes. *Nano Lett.* **2009**, *9*, 4359–4363. [CrossRef] [PubMed]

59. Williams, J.C.; Hippensteel, J.A.; Dilgen, J.; Shain, W.; Kipke, D.R. Complex impedance spectroscopy for monitoring tissue responses to inserted neural implants. *J. Neural Eng.* **2007**, *4*, 410. [CrossRef] [PubMed]

60. Cogan, S.F. Neural stimulation and recording electrodes. *Annu. Rev. Biomed. Eng.* **2008**, *10*, 275–309. [CrossRef]

61. Khodagholy, D.; Gelinas, J.N.; Thesen, T.; Doyle, W.; Devinsky, O.; Malliaras, G.G.; Buzsáki, G. NeuroGrid: Recording action potentials from the surface of the brain. *Nat. Neurosci.* **2015**, *18*, 310–315. [CrossRef]

62. Gierthmuehlen, M.; Ball, T.; Henle, C.; Wang, X.; Rickert, J.; Raab, M.; Freiman, T.; Stieglitz, T.; Kaminsky, J. Evaluation of µECoG electrode arrays in the minipig: Experimental procedure and neurosurgical approach. *J. Neurosci. Methods* **2011**, *202*, 77–86. [CrossRef] [PubMed]

63. Castagnola, E.; Maiolo, L.; Maggiolini, E.; Minotti, A.; Marrani, M.; Maita, F.; Pecora, A.; Angotzi, G.N.; Ansaldo, A.; Boffini, M. PEDOT-CNT-coated low-impedance, ultra-flexible, and brain-conformable micro-ECoG arrays. *IEEE Trans. Neural Syst. Rehabil. Eng.* **2015**, *23*, 342–350. [CrossRef] [PubMed]

64. Orsborn, A.L.; Wang, C.; Chiang, K.; Maharbiz, M.M.; Viventi, J.; Pesaran, B. Semi-chronic chamber system for simultaneous subdural electrocorticography, local field potentials, and spike recordings. In Proceedings of the 2015 7th International IEEE/EMBS Conference on Neural Engineering (NER), Montpellier, France, 22–24 April 2015; pp. 398–401.

65. Schendel, A.A.; Thongpang, S.; Brodnick, S.K.; Richner, T.J.; Lindevig, B.D.; Krugner-Higby, L.; Williams, J.C. A cranial window imaging method for monitoring vascular growth around chronically implanted micro-ECoG devices. *J. Neurosci. Methods* **2013**, *218*, 121–130. [CrossRef]

66. Thongpang, S.; Richner, T.J.; Brodnick, S.K.; Schendel, A.; Kim, J.; Wilson, J.A.; Hippensteel, J.; Krugner-Higby, L.; Moran, D.; Ahmed, A.S. A micro-electrocorticography platform and deployment strategies for chronic BCI applications. *Clin. EEG Neurosci.* **2011**, *42*, 259–265. [CrossRef]

67. Schendel, A.A.; Nonte, M.W.; Vokoun, C.; Richner, T.J.; Brodnick, S.K.; Atry, F.; Frye, S.; Bostrom, P.; Pashaie, R.; Thongpang, S. The effect of micro-ECoG substrate footprint on the meningeal tissue response. *J. Neural Eng.* **2014**, *11*, 046011. [CrossRef] [PubMed]

68. Kim, D.-H.; Viventi, J.; Amsden, J.J.; Xiao, J.; Vigeland, L.; Kim, Y.-S.; Blanco, J.A.; Panilaitis, B.; Frechette, E.S.; Contreras, D. Dissolvable films of silk fibroin for ultrathin conformal bio-integrated electronics. *Nat. Mater.* **2010**, *9*, 511–517. [CrossRef]

69. Yu, K.J.; Kuzum, D.; Hwang, S.-W.; Kim, B.H.; Juul, H.; Kim, N.H.; Won, S.M.; Chiang, K.; Trumpis, M.; Richardson, A.G. Bioresorbable silicon electronics for transient spatiotemporal mapping of electrical activity from the cerebral cortex. *Nat. Mater.* **2016**, *15*, 782–791. [CrossRef] [PubMed]

70. Hwang, S.-W.; Tao, H.; Kim, D.-H.; Cheng, H.; Song, J.-K.; Rill, E.; Brenckle, M.A.; Panilaitis, B.; Won, S.M.; Kim, Y.-S. A physically transient form of silicon electronics. *Science* **2012**, *337*, 1640–1644. [CrossRef] [PubMed]

71. Tsytsarev, V.; Taketani, M.; Schottler, F.; Tanaka, S.; Hara, M. A new planar multielectrode array: Recording from a rat auditory cortex. *J. Neural Eng.* **2006**, *3*, 293. [CrossRef]

72. Nicolelis, M.A.; Dimitrov, D.; Carmena, J.M.; Crist, R.; Lehew, G.; Kralik, J.D.; Wise, S.P. Chronic, multisite, multielectrode recordings in macaque monkeys. *Proc. Natl. Acad. Sci. USA* **2003**, *100*, 11041–11046. [CrossRef] [PubMed]

73. Williams, J.C.; Rennaker, R.L.; Kipke, D.R. Long-term neural recording characteristics of wire microelectrode arrays implanted in cerebral cortex. *Brain Res. Protoc.* **1999**, *4*, 303–313. [CrossRef]

74. Bai, Q.; Wise, K.D.; Anderson, D.J. A high-yield microassembly structure for three-dimensional microelectrode arrays. *IEEE Trans. Biomed. Eng.* **2000**, *47*, 281–289. [PubMed]

75. Vetter, R.J.; Williams, J.C.; Hetke, J.F.; Nunamaker, E.A.; Kipke, D.R. Chronic neural recording using silicon-substrate microelectrode arrays implanted in cerebral cortex. *IEEE Trans. Biomed. Eng.* **2004**, *51*, 896–904. [CrossRef]

76. Ludwig, K.A.; Langhals, N.B.; Joseph, M.D.; Richardson-Burns, S.M.; Hendricks, J.L.; Kipke, D.R. Poly (3, 4-ethylenedioxythiophene)(PEDOT) polymer coatings facilitate smaller neural recording electrodes. *J. Neural Eng.* **2011**, *8*, 014001. [CrossRef]

77. Kozai, T.D.Y.; Langhals, N.B.; Patel, P.R.; Deng, X.; Zhang, H.; Smith, K.L.; Lahann, J.; Kotov, N.A.; Kipke, D.R. Ultrasmall implantable composite microelectrodes with bioactive surfaces for chronic neural interfaces. *Nat. Mater.* **2012**, *11*, 1065–1073. [CrossRef]

78. Jones, K.E.; Campbell, P.K.; Normann, R.A. A glass/silicon composite intracortical electrode array. *Ann. Biomed. Eng.* **1992**, *20*, 423–437. [CrossRef]

79. Normann, R.A.; Maynard, E.M.; Rousche, P.J.; Warren, D.J. A neural interface for a cortical vision prosthesis. *Vis. Res.* **1999**, *39*, 2577–2587. [CrossRef]

80. Suner, S.; Fellows, M.R.; Vargas-Irwin, C.; Nakata, G.K.; Donoghue, J.P. Reliability of signals from a chronically implanted, silicon-based electrode array in non-human primate primary motor cortex. *IEEE Trans. Neural Syst. Rehabil. Eng.* **2005**, *13*, 524–541. [CrossRef] [PubMed]

81. Herwik, S.; Kisban, S.; Aarts, A.; Seidl, K.; Girardeau, G.; Benchenane, K.; Zugaro, M.; Wiener, S.; Paul, O.; Neves, H. Fabrication technology for silicon-based microprobe arrays used in acute and sub-chronic neural recording. *J. Micromech. Microeng.* **2009**, *19*, 074008. [CrossRef]

82. Corps, K.N.; Roth, T.L.; McGavern, D.B. Inflammation and neuroprotection in traumatic brain injury. *JAMA Neurol.* **2015**, *72*, 355–362. [CrossRef] [PubMed]

83. Corrigan, F.; Mander, K.A.; Leonard, A.V.; Vink, R. Neurogenic inflammation after traumatic brain injury and its potentiation of classical inflammation. *J. Neuroinflamm.* **2016**, *13*, 264. [CrossRef]

84. Corrigan, F.; Vink, R.; Turner, R.J. Inflammation in acute CNS injury: A focus on the role of substance P. *Br. J. Pharmacol.* **2016**, *173*, 703–715. [CrossRef] [PubMed]

85. Leach, J.; Achyuta, A.K.H.; Murthy, S.K. Bridging the divide between neuroprosthetic design, tissue engineering and neurobiology. *Front. Neuroeng.* **2010**, *2*, 18. [CrossRef] [PubMed]

86. Richter, A.; Xie, Y.; Schumacher, A.; Löffler, S.; Kirch, R.D.; Al-Hasani, J.; Rapoport, D.H.; Kruse, C.; Moser, A.; Tronnier, V.; et al. A simple implantation method for flexible, multisite microelectrodes into rat brains. *Front. Neuroeng.* **2013**, *6*, 6. [CrossRef]

87. Jorfi, M.; Skousen, J.L.; Weder, C.; Capadona, J.R. Progress towards biocompatible intracortical microelectrodes for neural interfacing applications. *J. Neural Eng.* **2014**, *12*, 011001. [CrossRef]

88. Moshayedi, P.; Ng, G.; Kwok, J.C.; Yeo, G.S.; Bryant, C.E.; Fawcett, J.W.; Franze, K.; Guck, J. The relationship between glial cell mechanosensitivity and foreign body reactions in the central nervous system. *Biomaterials* **2014**, *35*, 3919–3925. [CrossRef]

89. Polikov, V.S.; Block, M.L.; Fellous, J.-M.; Hong, J.-S.; Reichert, W.M. In vitro model of glial scarring around neuroelectrodes chronically implanted in the CNS. *Biomaterials* **2006**, *27*, 5368–5376. [CrossRef] [PubMed]

90. Arulmoli, J.; Pathak, M.M.; McDonnell, L.P.; Nourse, J.L.; Tombola, F.; Earthman, J.C.; Flanagan, L.A. Static stretch affects neural stem cell differentiation in an extracellular matrix-dependent manner. *Sci. Rep.* **2015**, *5*, 8499. [CrossRef] [PubMed]

91. Reddy, C.G.; Reddy, G.G.; Kawasaki, H.; Oya, H.; Miller, L.E.; Howard III, M.A. Decoding movement-related cortical potentials from electrocorticography. *Neurosurg. Focus* **2009**, *27*, E11. [CrossRef] [PubMed]

92. Klopfleisch, R. Macrophage reaction against biomaterials in the mouse model–Phenotypes, functions and markers. *Acta Biomater.* **2016**, *43*, 3–13. [CrossRef] [PubMed]

93. Wang, K.; Bekar, L.K.; Furber, K.; Walz, W. Vimentin-expressing proximal reactive astrocytes correlate with migration rather than proliferation following focal brain injury. *Brain Res.* **2004**, *1024*, 193–202. [CrossRef] [PubMed]

94. Schouenborg, J.; Garwicz, M.; Danielsen, N. Reducing surface area while maintaining implant penetrating profile lowers the brain foreign body response to chronically implanted planar silicon microelectrode arrays. *Brain Mach. Interfaces Implic. Sci. Clin. Pract. Soc.* **2011**, *194*, 167.

95. Busch, S.A.; Silver, J. The role of extracellular matrix in CNS regeneration. *Curr. Opin. Neurobiol.* **2007**, *17*, 120–127. [CrossRef] [PubMed]

96. Seymour, J.P.; Kipke, D.R. Neural probe design for reduced tissue encapsulation in CNS. *Biomaterials* **2007**, *28*, 3594–3607. [CrossRef]

97. Goldring, S.; Gregorie, E.M. Surgical management of epilepsy using epidural recordings to localize the seizure focus: Review of 100 cases. *J. Neurosurg.* **1984**, *60*, 457–466. [CrossRef]

98. Goldring, S. A method for surgical management of focal epilepsy, especially as it relates to children. *J. Neurosurg.* **1978**, *49*, 344–356. [CrossRef]

99. Kubanek, J.; Miller, K.; Ojemann, J.; Wolpaw, J.; Schalk, G. Decoding flexion of individual fingers using electrocorticographic signals in humans. *J. Neural Eng.* **2009**, *6*, 066001. [CrossRef] [PubMed]

100. Schalk, G.; McFarland, D.J.; Hinterberger, T.; Birbaumer, N.; Wolpaw, J.R. BCI2000: A general-purpose brain-computer interface (BCI) system. *IEEE Trans. Biomed. Eng.* **2004**, *51*, 1034–1043. [CrossRef] [PubMed]

101. Cook, A.M.; Peppard, A.; Magnuson, B. Nutrition considerations in traumatic brain injury. *Nutr. Clin. Pract.* **2008**, *23*, 608–620. [CrossRef] [PubMed]

102. Heck, C.N.; King-Stephens, D.; Massey, A.D.; Nair, D.R.; Jobst, B.C.; Barkley, G.L.; Salanova, V.; Cole, A.J.; Smith, M.C.; Gwinn, R.P. Two-year seizure reduction in adults with medically intractable partial onset epilepsy treated with responsive neurostimulation: Final results of the RNS System Pivotal trial. *Epilepsia* **2014**, *55*, 432–441. [CrossRef] [PubMed]

103. Morrell, M.J. Responsive cortical stimulation for the treatment of medically intractable partial epilepsy. *Neurology* **2011**, *77*, 1295–1304. [CrossRef]

104. Dohmen, C.; Sakowitz, O.W.; Fabricius, M.; Bosche, B.; Reithmeier, T.; Ernestus, R.I.; Brinker, G.; Dreier, J.P.; Woitzik, J.; Strong, A.J. Spreading depolarizations occur in human ischemic stroke with high incidence. *Ann. Neurol.* **2008**, *63*, 720–728. [CrossRef]

105. Fabricius, M.; Fuhr, S.; Bhatia, R.; Boutelle, M.; Hashemi, P.; Strong, A.J.; Lauritzen, M. Cortical spreading depression and peri-infarct depolarization in acutely injured human cerebral cortex. *Brain* **2006**, *129*, 778–790. [CrossRef]

106. Fabricius, M.; Fuhr, S.; Willumsen, L.; Dreier, J.P.; Bhatia, R.; Boutelle, M.G.; Hartings, J.A.; Bullock, R.; Strong, A.J.; Lauritzen, M. Association of seizures with cortical spreading depression and peri-infarct depolarisations in the acutely injured human brain. *Clin. Neurophysiol.* **2008**, *119*, 1973–1984. [CrossRef]

107. Strong, A.J.; Fabricius, M.; Boutelle, M.G.; Hibbins, S.J.; Hopwood, S.E.; Jones, R.; Parkin, M.C.; Lauritzen, M. Spreading and synchronous depressions of cortical activity in acutely injured human brain. *Stroke* **2002**, *33*, 2738–2743. [CrossRef]

108. Baba, T.; Kameda, M.; Yasuhara, T.; Morimoto, T.; Kondo, A.; Shingo, T.; Tajiri, N.; Wang, F.; Miyoshi, Y.; Borlongan, C.V. Electrical stimulation of the cerebral cortex exerts antiapoptotic, angiogenic, and anti-inflammatory effects in ischemic stroke rats through phosphoinositide 3-kinase/Akt signaling pathway. *Stroke* **2009**, *40*, e598–e605. [CrossRef]

109. Kang, C.; Yang, C.-Y.; Kim, J.H.; Moon, S.-K.; Lee, S.; Park, S.-A.; Han, E.-H.; Zhang, L.-Q. The effect of continuous epidural electrical stimulation on neuronal proliferation in cerebral ischemic rats. *Ann. Rehabil. Med.* **2013**, *37*, 301–310. [CrossRef] [PubMed]

110. Kleim, J.A.; Bruneau, R.; VandenBerg, P.; MacDonald, E.; Mulrooney, R.; Pocock, D. Motor cortex stimulation enhances motor recovery and reduces peri-infarct dysfunction following ischemic insult. *Neurol. Res.* **2003**, *25*, 789–793. [CrossRef] [PubMed]

111. O'Bryant, A.J.; Adkins, D.L.; Sitko, A.A.; Combs, H.L.; Nordquist, S.K.; Jones, T.A. Enduring Poststroke Motor Functional Improvements by a Well-Timed Combination of Motor Rehabilitative Training and Cortical Stimulation in Rats. *Neurorehabil. Neural Repair* **2016**, *30*, 143–154. [CrossRef] [PubMed]

112. Plautz, E.J.; Barbay, S.; Frost, S.B.; Friel, K.M.; Dancause, N.; Zoubina, E.V.; Stowe, A.M.; Quaney, B.M.; Nudo, R.J. Post-infarct cortical plasticity and behavioral recovery using concurrent cortical stimulation and rehabilitative training: A feasibility study in primates. *Neurol. Res.* **2003**, *25*, 801–810. [CrossRef] [PubMed]

113. Teskey, G.C.; Flynn, C.; Goertzen, C.D.; Monfils, M.H.; Young, N.A. Cortical stimulation improves skilled forelimb use following a focal ischemic infarct in the rat. *Neurol. Res.* **2003**, *25*, 794–800. [CrossRef] [PubMed]

114. Brown, J.A.; Lutsep, H.L.; Weinand, M.; Cramer, S.C. Motor cortex stimulation for the enhancement of recovery from stroke: A prospective, multicenter safety study. *Neurosurgery* **2006**, *58*, 464–473. [CrossRef] [PubMed]

115. Brown, J.A.; Lutsep, H.; Cramer, S.C.; Weinand, M. Motor cortex stimulation for enhancement of recovery after stroke: Case report. *Neurol. Res.* **2003**, *25*, 815–818. [CrossRef]

116. Huang, M.; Harvey, R.L.; Stoykov, M.E.; Ruland, S.; Weinand, M.; Lowry, D.; Levy, R. Cortical stimulation for upper limb recovery following ischemic stroke: A small phase II pilot study of a fully implanted stimulator. *Top. Stroke Rehabil.* **2008**, *15*, 160–172. [CrossRef]

117. Levy, R.; Ruland, S.; Weinand, M.; Lowry, D.; Dafer, R.; Bakay, R. Cortical stimulation for the rehabilitation of patients with hemiparetic stroke: A multicenter feasibility study of safety and efficacy. *J. Neurosurg.* **2008**, *108*, 707–714. [CrossRef]

118. Levy, R.M.; Harvey, R.L.; Kissela, B.M.; Winstein, C.J.; Lutsep, H.L.; Parrish, T.B.; Cramer, S.C.; Venkatesan, L. Epidural Electrical Stimulation for Stroke Rehabilitation Results of the Prospective, Multicenter, Randomized, Single-Blinded Everest Trial. *Neurorehabil. Neural Repair* **2016**, *30*, 107–119. [CrossRef]

119. Plow, E.B.; Carey, J.R.; Nudo, R.J.; Pascual-Leone, A. Invasive cortical stimulation to promote recovery of function after stroke a critical appraisal. *Stroke* **2009**, *40*, 1926–1931. [CrossRef]

120. Miranda, R.A.; Casebeer, W.D.; Hein, A.M.; Judy, J.W.; Krotkov, E.P.; Laabs, T.L.; Manzo, J.E.; Pankratz, K.G.; Pratt, G.A.; Sanchez, J.C. DARPA-funded efforts in the development of novel brain–computer interface technologies. *J. Neurosci. Methods* **2015**, *244*, 52–67. [CrossRef] [PubMed]

121. Leuthardt, E.C.; Freudenberg, Z.; Bundy, D.; Roland, J. Microscale recording from human motor cortex: Implications for minimally invasive electrocorticographic brain-computer interfaces. *Neurosurg. Focus* **2009**, *27*, E10. [CrossRef] [PubMed]

122. Wang, W.; Collinger, J.L.; Degenhart, A.D.; Tyler-Kabara, E.C.; Schwartz, A.B.; Moran, D.W.; Weber, D.J.; Wodlinger, B.; Vinjamuri, R.K.; Ashmore, R.C. An electrocorticographic brain interface in an individual with tetraplegia. *PLoS One* **2013**, *8*, e55344. [CrossRef] [PubMed]

123. Fifer, M.S.; Acharya, S.; Benz, H.L.; Mollazadeh, M.; Crone, N.E.; Thakor, N.V. Towards electrocorticographic control of a dexterous upper limb prosthesis. *IEEE Pulse* **2012**, *3*, 38–42. [CrossRef]

124. Maharbiz, M.M.; Muller, R.; Alon, E.; Rabaey, J.M.; Carmena, J.M. Reliable Next-Generation Cortical Interfaces for Chronic Brain–Machine Interfaces and Neuroscience. *Proc. IEEE* **2017**, *105*, 73–82. [CrossRef]

125. Wang, F.; Zhang, X.; Shokoueinejad, M.; Iskandar, B.J.; Medow, J.E.; Webster, J.G. A Novel Intracranial Pressure Readout Circuit for Passive Wireless LC Sensor. *IEEE Trans. Biomed. Circuits Syst.* **2017**, *11*, 1123–1132. [CrossRef]

126. Iskandar, B.J.; Medow, J.; Luzzio, C.; Webster, J.G.; Maragheh, M.S.; Wang, F.; Zhang, X. Cerebrospinal-Fluid Shunt Valve System. U.S. Patent 15/473,126, 4 October 2018.

127. Ma, Z.; Williams, J.C.; Park, D.-W.; Schendel, A.A.; Mikael, S.T. Transparent and Flexible Neural Electrode Arrays. US Patent 9,861,288, 9 January 2018.

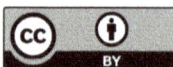

micromachines

MDPI

Review

Opportunities and Challenges for Single-Unit Recordings from Enteric Neurons in Awake Animals

Bradley B. Barth [1],*, **Hsin-I Huang [2]**, **Gianna E. Hammer [2] and Xiling Shen [1]**

[1] Department of Biomedical Engineering, Duke University, Durham, NC 27710, USA; xiling.shen@duke.edu
[2] Department of Immunology, Duke University, Durham, NC 27710, USA; hsin.i.huang@duke.edu (H.-I.H.); gianna.hammer@duke.edu (G.E.H.)
*   Correspondence: bradley.barth@duke.edu; Tel.: +1-919-684-8709

Received: 31 July 2018; Accepted: 23 August 2018; Published: 25 August 2018

Abstract: Advanced electrode designs have made single-unit neural recordings commonplace in modern neuroscience research. However, single-unit resolution remains out of reach for the intrinsic neurons of the gastrointestinal system. Single-unit recordings of the enteric (gut) nervous system have been conducted in anesthetized animal models and excised tissue, but there is a large physiological gap between awake and anesthetized animals, particularly for the enteric nervous system. Here, we describe the opportunity for advancing enteric neuroscience offered by single-unit recording capabilities in awake animals. We highlight the primary challenges to microelectrodes in the gastrointestinal system including structural, physiological, and signal quality challenges, and we provide design criteria recommendations for enteric microelectrodes.

Keywords: microelectrodes; in vivo electrophysiology; neural interfaces; enteric nervous system; conscious recording; electrode implantation

---

1. Introduction

The enteric nervous system is a subdivision of the peripheral, autonomic nervous system that resides in the gastrointestinal tract (Figure 1A–C). The small intestine alone has been estimated to contain more than 733,000 neurons in the mouse, 3.7 million neurons in the guinea-pig, and 88 million neurons in the sheep [1]. The human enteric nervous system is estimated to contain between 200 and 600 million neurons, roughly as many as the spinal cord [2]. For over a century, the enteric nervous system has been known to regulate gastrointestinal motility, and the circuitry controlling basic motor patterns is relatively well understood [3]. Pathologies of the enteric nervous system include functional and motility disorders, developmental disorders, and neurological disorders [4,5].

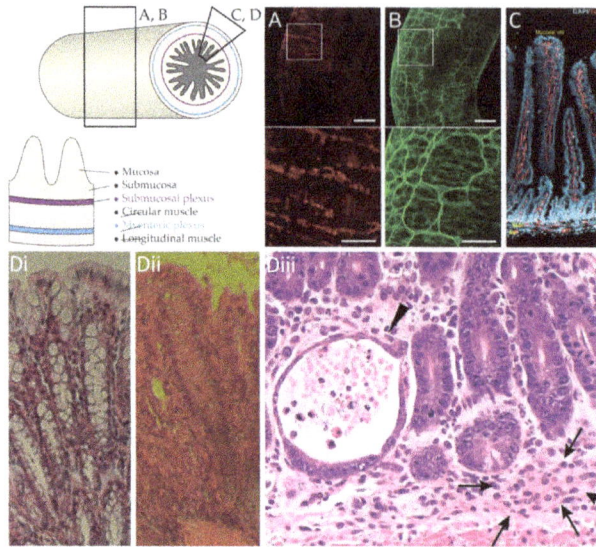

Figure 1. Anatomy of the enteric nervous system. A segment of the gastrointestinal tract and the anatomical tissue layers. Pan-neuronal marker HuC/D (**A**) and neuron tubulin marker Tuj-1 (**B**) imaged in whole intestinal tissue by light sheet microscopy, adapted from [6]; (**C**) Immunoreactive labelling of cell nuclei (DAPI, blue) and neuron tubulin (Tuj-1, red) in sections of the intestine, adapted from [7]; (**D**) Histology of (i) healthy colon; (ii) inflamed colon; and (iii) inflamed small intestine with crypt abscess (arrowhead) and granuloma (arrows).

Despite its size and importance, the enteric nervous system is under-examined compared to other systems in neuroscience. Our knowledge of enteric neuroscience remains antiquated compared to the central nervous system because of the lack of specialized tools and methods. For instance, it has been possible to record cortical neurons intracellularly in freely-moving animals [8], and calcium activity from populations of cortical neurons in head-fixed animals [9] for over a decade. In contrast, recordings from the enteric neurons have been conducted almost exclusively in excised tissue.

Classical enteric electrophysiology is conducted using flat-sheet preparations, a method that has remained largely unchanged for decades. As enteric neuroscience progresses, flat-sheet preparations are not sufficient to investigate the interactions of the enteric nervous system with other systems, including the gut-brain axis, neuro-immune crosstalk, interaction with microbiota, etc., in living systems. For proper context, our understanding of these systems will be enhanced by measurements in live animal models, which offer greater physiological fidelity and greater potential for translational research. However, technology for awake, single-unit recordings in the gastrointestinal system is underdeveloped.

Currently, in vivo neural recordings from the gastrointestinal tract must be conducted under anesthesia, presumably during acute, non-survival surgical procedures. Anesthesia and invasive surgical procedures greatly alter the physiology of the gastrointestinal environment, directly affecting neurotransmission and motility. To fully realize the advantages of in vivo enteric electrophysiology, neural recording and stimulation must be conducted in conscious animal models. Advancing neurogastroenterology with the tools for single-unit recordings in awake animal models demands new and innovative neural microelectrode technology.

First, we review the traditional methods for enteric electrophysiology, discussing ex vivo preparations and the limitations of anesthetized in vivo neural recordings. Secondly, we discuss the current challenges to single-unit recordings from enteric neurons in awake animal models, such as gastrointestinal pathophysiology (Figure 1D). Finally, we consider design criteria for novel enteric microelectrodes and potential applications of single-unit recordings from conscious animals and the potential synergy with other novel technologies.

2. Classical Methods for Enteric Electrophysiology

Electrophysiology in the enteric nervous system has largely been conducted in excised tissue (Figure 2). Excised tissue can be kept alive and functional for several hours, often with direct access to enteric ganglia. More complex preparations have been developed to capture neural activity with greater physiological relevance, such as suction electrodes for whole-organ recordings. Enteric neuron recordings are rarely conducted in vivo. In this section, we discuss the advantages and limitations of flat-sheet and whole-organ preparations, and the challenges of anesthetized recordings.

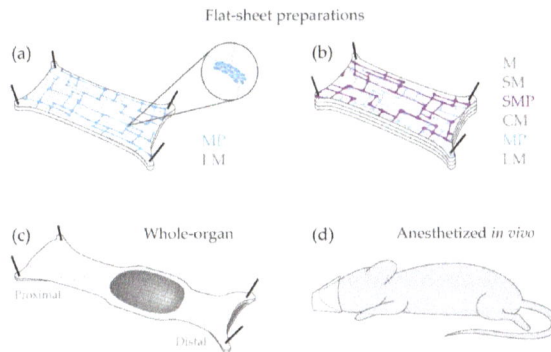

Figure 2. Classical methods for enteric electrophysiology. (**a**) Flat-sheet LMMP preparation; (**b**) Full-thickness flat-sheet preparation; (**c**) Whole-organ preparation; (**d**) Anesthetized in vivo preparation. M: mucosa, SM: submucosa, SMP: submucosal plexus, CM: circular muscle, MP: myenteric plexus, LM: longitudinal muscle.

2.1. Neural Recordings in Excised Tissue

Enteric neural recordings are most commonly conducted *ex vivo*, using flat-sheet preparations in organ baths. In these preparations, the gastrointestinal tract is dissected out, opened along the mesenteric border, and pinned flat in a Sylgard dish. The mucosa, submucosa, and circular muscle is frequently dissected away, leaving only the myenteric plexus attached to the longitudinal muscle (LMMP) [10]. The flat-sheet LMMP preparation was fundamental for the intracellular recordings that first classified electrophysiology in enteric neurons as S (Type 1) or AH (Type 2) neurons [11,12]. Although the electrophysiology classification system is less frequently used than neurochemical or functional classification [13,14], it is often used to characterize patient biopsies [15]. The primary advantage of this preparation is the accessibility of myenteric ganglia for pharmacological assays with extracellular recordings, patch clamp recordings, etc. [16]. However, the flat-sheet LMMP preparation has limited applications because the submucosal plexus, circular muscle, lamina propria, and epithelium have been dissected away. Therefore, this preparation is not suitable for examining the effect of intraluminal stimuli or communication with epithelial cells, resident immune cells, submucosal neurons, or circular muscle.

Alternatively, the full-thickness flat-sheet preparation maintains the connections to circular muscle, submucosal plexus, lamina propria, and epithelium. As a result, the full-thickness flat-sheet preparation is ideal for examining intraluminal stimuli and interactions between enteric neurons and the epithelium, resident immune cells, and smooth muscle. For example, Spencer and colleagues have revealed novel firing patterns in enteric neurons that drive coordinated smooth muscle response using the full-thickness flat-sheet preparations [17,18]. The full-thickness flat-sheet preparation is also advantageous for calcium imaging because it captures either plexus in a single imaging plane [19,20]. However, myenteric and submucosal neurons are enclosed within the smooth muscle layers and the lamina propria in the full-thickness flat preparation, making single-unit and intracellular recordings prohibitive in this preparation. A fundamental limitation of all flat-sheet preparations is the longitudinal incision along the mesenteric border. This incision disrupts the electrical syncytium, particularly in the circular muscle, and severs many circumferentially projecting fibers. Further, the flat-sheet preparation is not well equipped to propel luminal contents.

Gastrointestinal motility patterns are better examined in whole-organ preparations [21,22]. Whole-organ preparations maintain the intrinsic connections of the enteric nervous system, leaving the smooth muscle, lamina propria, and epithelial layers intact. Whole-organ preparations consist of intact segments of the gastrointestinal tract in organ baths, and they are well-suited for examining gastrointestinal motility patterns or intraluminal stimuli because the longitudinal and circular smooth muscles remain functional and intact. As with the full-thickness flat-sheet preparation, the enteric neurons in whole-organ preparations are inaccessible by classical electrophysiology methods. Suction electrodes on the serosal surface provide an alternate method by measuring smooth muscle activity in whole-organ and full-thickness flat-sheet preparations, but they are inadequate to describe enteric neural activity directly [23–25].

Neural recordings from excised tissue present a convenient platform for examining single-unit response under a variety of conditions and stimuli. However, several limitations exist for all excised tissue preparations, including, most notably, the lack of peripheral innervation and extrinsic circuitry. In some ex vivo preparations, peripheral fiber recordings are possible, but they lack extrinsic circuits in the central nervous system [26,27]. The limitations of ex vivo preparations can be addressed by studying the enteric nervous system in live animal models.

2.2. Challenges of Anesthetized Recordings from Enteric Neurons

Anesthesia allows for recordings from live animal models, which provide more physiologically-relevant conditions compared to excised tissue. Due to current technological limitations, flat-sheet preparations are better suited for single-unit recordings than anesthetized recordings. Additionally, anesthesia greatly changes gastrointestinal function, making results from anesthetized preparations difficult to interpret. We discuss two direct effects of various anesthetic agents on gastrointestinal function: the effect of anesthesia on various receptors of the enteric nervous system, and the effect of anesthesia on gastrointestinal motility.

First, several neuron species in the enteric nervous system act on receptors that are directly affected by various anesthetic agents. Here, we review the inhibiting and potentiating effects of common anesthetic agents on some of the primary receptor classes in the enteric nervous system: nicotinic cholinergic, P2X, 5-HT$_3$, N-methyl-D-aspartate (NMDA), α-amino-3-hydroxy-5-methyl-4-isoxazolepropionic acid (AMPA), gamma-Aminobutyric acid (GABA), and glycine receptors (Table 1). Agonists to these receptors are expressed by common neuron species in the myenteric ganglia and submucosal ganglia [13,28–30]. Although glutamate and glycine are less well-studied in enteric ganglia in comparison to acetylcholine, serotonin, and purinergic neurotransmitters, their role as enteric neurotransmitters are strongly supported by electrophysiological responses to pharmaceutical stimuli [30,31]. The receptor-specific responses for several forms of anesthesia have been reviewed by [32]. In addition to the direct effects of anesthesia, [33] have reported that common anesthetic agents (isoflurane, sevoflurane, ketamine, and urethane) modulate glutamate receptors, voltage-dependent calcium channels, and voltage-gated potassium channels, suggesting that anesthesia may have prolonged effects on neural activity.

Table 1. The effect of common anesthetic agents on various receptors of the enteric nervous system.

Neuron Species	Approximate Percentage	Affected Receptors	Inhibiting Anesthetic Agents	Potentiating Anesthetic Agents
Cholinergic	ChAT-positive neurons: ○ 80% of myenteric neurons [29,34,35] ○ 50% of submucosal neurons [29,34,35]	Neuronal nACh	Ketamine [36], pentobarbital [37], propofol [37], isoflurane [37,38], halothane [37,38], sevoflurane [37]	Urethane [39]
Purinergic	ATP-releasing neurons: ○ 2–25% of myenteric neurons [28,40] ○ 40–60% of submucosal neurons [28,40] ○ Other: Enteric glia (P2X$_7$) [41]	P2X$_2$	Sevoflurane [42]	-
		P2X$_3$	Pentobarbital [43]	-
		P2X$_4$	-	Propofol [44]
		P2X$_7$	-	Ketamine [45], propofol [45]
Serotinergic	5-HT-positive neurons: ○ 2% of myenteric neurons [13]	5-HT$_3$	Ketamine [46,47], pentobarbital [46], propofol [46]	Isoflurane [38,48], halothane [38,48]
Glutamatergic	NMDA-positive neurons: ○ Almost all myenteric neurons [30] ○ Almost all submucosal neurons [30]	NMDA	Ketamine [49], urethane [39], pentobarbital [50]	-
	AMPA-positive neurons: ○ 30–60% of myenteric neurons [30] ○ Almost all submucosal neurons [30]	AMPA	Urethane [39], pentobarbital [51], propofol [50]	-
	GABA$_A$-positive neurons: ○ 3–8% of myenteric and submucosal neurons [52,53]	GABA$_A$	-	Ketamine [54], urethane [39], pentobarbital [55,56], propofol [54,57], isoflurane [54,58], halothane [54,58]
Glycinergic	Glycine-responsive: ○ 57% of colonic myenteric neurons [31]	Glycine	-	Urethane [39], propofol [57], isoflurane [59], sevoflurane [59], halothane [59]

Secondly, commonly used anesthetic agents impair gastrointestinal motility. Here, we review the effects of commonly used injected and inhaled anesthetic agents (ketamine, urethane, pentobarbital, propofol, isoflurane, sevoflurane, and halothane) on gastrointestinal motility during anesthesia (Table 2). Generally, anesthetic agents have been shown to impair gastrointestinal motility by delaying gastric emptying or decreasing intestinal transit time.

In addition to the effects of anesthesia, invasive abdominal surgery has been shown to impair gastrointestinal motility. For example, human patients who have undergone laparotomy often experience motility disorders such as postoperative ileus or pseudo-obstruction [60,61]. In horses, surgery has been shown to disrupt gastrointestinal motility for 8 to 12 h [62]. Furthermore, complications during surgery can lead to acute acidosis, which has been shown to directly reduce gastrointestinal motility [63]. To mitigate the adverse effects of invasive surgery on gastrointestinal function, animals should be allowed to recover prior to neural recordings or other experiments.

Table 2. The effect of common anesthetic agents on gastrointestinal motility during anesthesia.

Anesthetic Agent	Route of Administration	Gastric Emptying	Intestinal Transit
Ketamine	Injection	Unaffected [64,65]	Unaffected/slight decrease [64–67]
Urethane	Injection	Decrease [68–71]	Decrease [68,69]
Pentobarbital	Injection	Decrease [70]	Dose-dependent increase/decrease [66]
Propofol	Injection	Decrease [72,73]	Slight decrease [66,67]
Isoflurane	Inhalation	Decrease [74,75]	Decrease [62,76]
Sevoflurane	Inhalation	Decrease [77]	Decrease [77,78]
Halothane	Inhalation	Decrease [79]	Decrease [79–81]

In summary, the flat-sheet preparation is a fundamental tool for enteric electrophysiology, and it will not be replaced by new technology. However, the versatility of ex vivo preparations are limited, and they lack the necessary context to examine more physiologically complex behaviors. Although anesthetized, in vivo animal models are more physiologically relevant, however, anesthesia and invasive surgery alter neurotransmission and impede gastrointestinal motility. Therefore, the effect of various anesthetic agents and sufficient recovery time should be considered in the design of experiments. Importantly, this demonstrates the potential advantages of conducting neural recordings in conscious animals, particularly for neurogastroenterology.

3. Challenges to Gastrointestinal Neuro-Electrophysiology in Conscious Animals

Recently, new technology has been developed for myo-electrophysiology in the gastrointestinal system of anesthetized animals and patients. L. K. Cheng and collaborators at the University of Auckland examine smooth muscle function and electrical slow wave, using methods originally developed by [82]. Arrays featuring multiple surface electrodes can be used to build spatiotemporal maps of slow wave propagation with high resolution in anesthetized animal models [83] and in patients during surgery [84]. In vivo myo-electrophysiology has led to an improved understanding of electrical slow wave activity in healthy and diseased models. Although high-resolution myo-electrophysiology has not yet reached conscious animals, it shows great promise, particularly for improved diagnosis of gut pathophysiology. Simultaneously, in vivo gastrointestinal neuro-electrophysiology remains largely out of reach, especially in awake animals. There are several barriers to in vivo gastrointestinal neuro-electrophysiology, most of which are not unique to the gastrointestinal environment, such as fibrosis and biofouling. In this section, we focus on the challenges that are greatly exacerbated in the gut.

We identified six key challenges to in vivo gastrointestinal neuro-electrophysiology across three categories: structural, physiological, and signal quality challenges (Table 3). The structural challenge is the movement of the gastrointestinal tract within the abdomen, worsened by the lack of accessible skeletal structures on which to mount a device. The two physiological challenges describe the risks of disrupting gastrointestinal function: the issue of ischemia and reperfusion, and maintaining gastrointestinal homeostasis. The three signal quality challenges are contamination from the electrical slow wave, smooth muscle action potentials, and artifact due to tissue movement.

Table 3. Key challenges to in vivo gastrointestinal neuro-electrophysiology.

Categories	Challenges
Structural	Large tissue displacements and no rigid structures on which to mount a device
Physiological	Ischemia and reperfusion injury Maintaining gastrointestinal homeostasis
Signal Quality	Electrical slow waves Smooth muscle action potentials Artifact due to tissue movement

3.1. Structural Challenges in Neurogastroenterology

Animal movement is problematic for all methods of awake electrophysiology; movement adds noise to the recording, damages the recording device, and harms the test subject. Generally, the effect of conscious movements on neural recordings can be mitigated in two ways: restraining the animal, such as head-fixed recordings, or minimizing aberrations in movement by fixing the recording device to the skeleton. Restrained recordings pose fewer movement-related problems than unrestrained (a.k.a. freely-behaving) recordings, but the restraint method may alter natural neural activity. For example, single-unit recordings from freely-moving rats led to the discovery of place cells in the hippocampus [85]. These methods have proven useful tools for probing the brain, and are adaptable for other systems; head-fixed preparations, for example, have led to spine-fixed recordings and spinal recordings in awake, moving rats [86,87]. However, these advancements have not led to similar innovation in enteric neuroscience because of unique movement-related challenges posed by the gastrointestinal environment.

Awake, single-unit recordings from enteric neurons are limited by structural challenges in the gastrointestinal system. First, there are no accessibly skeletal structures below the stomach on which to mount rigid devices, as used in brain and spine research. Additionally, enteric neurons are not fixed in place within the abdominal cavity. Enteric neurons are located within the wall of the gastrointestinal tract. In the gastrointestinal wall, smooth muscles drive macroscopic tissue motion in the form of stationary or propagating waves of contractions, known as segmentation and peristalsis, respectively. Smooth muscle contractions can induce tissue displacement several orders of magnitude greater than micromotions observed in the brain. For example, micromotions in the brain have been observed on the order of 10 to 100 µm in rats [88]. Meanwhile, maximum distension in the colon can deform the circular muscle up to 10 mm in guinea-pigs [89].

Movement-related challenges are amplified in the gastrointestinal system. Future implantable devices must consider the mechanical characteristics at the tissue, organ, and body scales. Such devices will likely combine flexible electrode arrays and interconnects, and rigid headstages mounted far from the recording site. Additionally, the inflammation and irritation caused by sutures or adhesives must be considered.

3.2. Disrupting Gastrointestinal Physiology

The gastrointestinal tract has evolved defense mechanisms that pose significant challenges for medical device implants, particularly neural microelectrodes. In addition to the foreign-body response associated with all medical implants, the gastrointestinal system poses unique challenges. Here, we discuss the general principles of maintaining homeostasis in the gastrointestinal tract and the potential challenges of intestinal injury caused by implanting neural microelectrodes. Intestinal injury and inflammation induced by resident immune responses and ischemia reperfusion injury pose challenges for enteric in vivo neuro-electrophysiology because they greatly alter the behavior of enteric neurons, enteric glial cells, and resident immune cells, and disrupt gastrointestinal function.

The mammalian intestine encounters trillions of innocuous foreign antigens, symbiotic microbes, and pathogens daily. The intestinal immune system is able to tolerate innocuous antigens and simultaneously respond to pathogens using three layers of regulation: physical barriers, antimicrobial reagents, and immune cells [90]. First, the intestine is covered by a single lining of intestinal epithelium cells, and specialized intestinal epithelium cells secrete mucus to protect the epithelium from microbiota [91,92]. Second, specialized intestinal epithelium cells also release antimicrobial compounds. For example, Paneth cells express antimicrobial peptides such as RegIIIγ and α-defensin to inhibit luminal microbe growth and colonization in intestine [93]. Third, antigen-presenting cells, including dendritic cells and macrophages, are responsible for immune surveillance and maintaining homeostasis. Intestinal dendritic cells make up the most complex dendritic cell populations in the body, and they are essential for establishing tolerance in the homeostatic environment by promoting regulatory T cells [94,95]. Gastrointestinal macrophages are unique; unlike most tissue-resident macrophages, which are yolk sac or embryo derived with self-renewal capacity, gastrointestinal macrophages are continuously replenished by circulating monocytes and are exquisitely sensitive to environmental stimuli [96,97]. Mature gastrointestinal macrophages maintain epithelial cell integrity, and limit bacteria-induced inflammatory responses by constantly secreting inhibitory cytokines and low levels of tumor necrosis factor (TNF), and engulfing penetrating bacteria via efficient phagocytosis, respectively [98,99]. The intestinal immune system carefully titrates the inflammatory response to innocuous antigens, symbiotic microbes, and pathogens, but it may be dysregulated by implanted neural microelectrodes.

Implanted neural microelectrodes in the intestine have the potential to cause severe intestinal inflammation by disrupting epithelial barrier function and activating antigen-presenting cells. First, epithelial barrier function is importance for homeostasis, and has been implicated in inflammatory bowel disease patients [100,101]. Breaking down epithelial cells in animal models, such as with dextran sulfate sodium or 2,4,6-trinitrobenzenesulfonic acid, has been shown to induce severe colitis and intestinal inflammation [102–105]. Barrier function can also be disrupted by ischemia reperfusion injury, a common gastrointestinal disease in which hypoxia-ischemia and reperfusion in the epithelium leads to epithelial cell death caused by enhanced reactive oxygen species production once blood flow is re-established in hypoxic regions [106,107]. Disrupted barrier function can lead to bacteria translocation and directly activate enteric neurons and glial cells that express innate pattern recognition receptors, such as toll-like receptors [108,109].

Additionally, intestinal inflammation may be induced by antigen-presenting cells in response to pathogens, translocated bacteria, or when they are dysregulated. For example, intestinal inflammation developed spontaneously in mice after knocking out A20, a nuclear factor kappa-light-chain-enhancer of activated B cells (NF-kB) signaling pathway inhibitor [110]. Distinct dendritic cells, pro-inflammatory monocytes, and pro-inflammatory macrophages promote the intestinal inflammation response, increase differentiation of pro-inflammatory monocytes and macrophages, and production of pro-inflammatory cytokines [111–114]. Chronic inflammation can mediate enteric neuron cell death, posing additional challenges to in vivo neuro-electrophysiology [115]. Neural microelectrode implants have the potential to disrupt homeostasis and barrier function, induce cell death and bacteria translocation, and lead to chronic inflammation.

3.3. Signal Quality

The signal-to-noise ratio of enteric neuro-electrophysiology will likely be contaminated by three main sources of noise specific to the gastrointestinal tract. First, electrical slow waves will introduce low-frequency noise. Second, action potentials from surrounding smooth muscle tissue will contribute high-frequency noise. Third, peristalsis and segmentation will create motion artifact, introducing additional high-frequency noise.

Electrical slow waves propagate through smooth muscle along the length of the gut, from esophagus to rectum, and they are driven by pacemaker cells known as interstitial cells of Cajal [116]. Populations of interstitial cells of Cajal vary along the length of the gut and occupy the myenteric, intramuscular, and submucosal layers and have individual pacemaker frequencies [117].

The pacemaker potentials conduct through the smooth muscle syncytium, generating electrical slow waves [118]. The smooth muscle layers directly border the myenteric and submucosal plexuses, and any recording from the plexus layers will contain signals from electrical slow waves [119]. The slow waves will contribute low-frequency noise, because they occur at 2–40 cycles per minute, depending on animal species and location along the gastrointestinal tract [29]. Therefore, high-pass filtering will remove most slow-wave noise from neural recordings.

Smooth muscle action potentials and motion artifact will contribute physiological noise to neural recordings at high frequencies. Smooth muscle fibers border the myenteric and submucosal plexuses, and recordings from the plexus layers will likely contain neural action potentials and muscle action potentials [120]. For single-unit recordings, it will be difficult to filter out muscle action potentials and claim with certainty that the spiking signals are of neural origin. Extracellular action potential shape analysis or template matching will likely be the most effective way to differentiate these signals [121].

Coincident with smooth muscle activity are macroscopic movements in gastrointestinal tissue, causing artifacts in electrical recordings. Motion artifact is a long-standing issue for gastrointestinal electrophysiology in excised tissue, and it continues to pose challenges for understanding electrical slow waves and characterizing smooth muscle action potentials [122,123]. In classical neuro-electrophysiology in excised tissue, slow waves, smooth muscle action potentials, and motion artifact can be blocked pharmacologically [15]. However, these sources of noise cannot be blocked during in vivo neuro-electrophysiology without disrupting gastrointestinal physiology. Instead, limiting these sources of noise during in vivo neural recordings may be achieved by improved implant design and various signal processing techniques.

4. Enteric Microelectrode Design Criteria

The gastrointestinal environment poses unique challenges that have slowed progress in enteric neuroscience. Novel neural microelectrodes designed specifically for the gut may overcome these unique challenges and provide access to single-unit activity for the first time. In this section, we suggest design criteria for enteric microelectrodes for awake, single-unit recordings. The design criteria target the six key challenges to in vivo gastrointestinal neuro-electrophysiology by focusing on: intrinsic material properties, extrinsic design parameters, and the implant procedure (Table 4).

Table 4. Enteric microelectrode design criteria for awake, single-unit recordings.

Design Criteria	Features
Material Properties	Low Young's modulus High elasticity
Design Parameters	Low cross-sectional area Tethered recording platform Multiple recording sites along the length of the shank
Implant Procedure	Implant along longitudinal axis Shallow insertion angle Undisturbed submucosa and epithelial layer

4.1. Intrinsic Material Properties

The gastrointestinal tract has high elasticity, and enteric microelectrodes will need to withstand large tissue displacements and strain without failure. Gastrointestinal tissues have an isotropic elastic modulus ranging from 0.3 kPa to 5 MPa depending on species and tissue segment [124]. For example, the rat distal colon and human small intestine have a Young's modulus as low as 0.3 kPa and 1.0 kPa, respectively [125]. The Young's modulus of the porcine and human rectum can reach up to 1.8 and 5.2 MPa, respectively, and the tissues can elongate up to 2.1 and 1.6 their original length before failure, respectively [126].

Due to the high elasticity of the gastrointestinal tract, enteric microelectrodes may benefit from flexible substrates with greater compliance and decreased bending stiffness [127]. Ultra-soft microwire electrodes, for example, have Young's modulus reportedly less than 1 MPa and may reduce the risk of intestinal injury [128]. Traditional microelectrodes such as monolithic silicon would be problematic due to their intrinsic stiffness, and would inevitably lead to increased cell death and pathophysiology [129]. Beyond the unique challenges of the gastrointestinal system, device characteristics such as electrical and insulative properties must also be considered. These material properties are discussed in detail by [130], and are summarized as: single-unit activity is better captured by low impedance and low surface area recording sites, with enough insulation to minimize parasitic capacitance.

4.2. Extrinsic Design Parameters

Extrinsic design parameters, such as probe geometry, electrode density, etc., can reduce the risk of disrupting gastrointestinal function and improve the signal-to-noise ratio of single-unit activity. First, enteric microelectrodes can increase flexibility with decreasing cross-sectional area, particularly probe thickness. For example, nanoelectronic thread electrodes are less than one-micron thick and "ultra-flexible"; the bending stiffness and mechanical interactions are on the order of cellular forces [131–133]. Ultrathin probes with a small cross-sectional area will be crucial to withstand the constant forces and movement within the gastrointestinal tract.

The macroscopic tissue movement in the gastrointestinal tract, and lack of nearby anchoring locations (i.e., skull, spine, etc.) pose additional challenges for enteric microelectrode design. The gastrointestinal environment will almost certainly demand a flexible tether between the anchored, transcutaneous connector and a recording platform [130]. The recording platform and enteric microelectrode must be anchored to the gastrointestinal wall without obstructing motility. Scaling up the mounting techniques from peripheral nerve interfaces, such as the spiral cuff [134] or locking-buckle cuff [135] are inappropriate, because they will prevent gastrointestinal distension and obstruct motility. Anchoring the recording platform with sutures through the serosa and muscular layers of the gastrointestinal wall will be less likely to obstruct the gastrointestinal tract and not directly disrupt barrier function [136–138].

Enteric microelectrodes should contain multiple recording sites along the length of the shank. To reach the myenteric plexus, the enteric microelectrode must penetrate the serosa and longitudinal muscle. Multiple recordings sites along the shank will allow a greater margin of error for probe depth and increase the likelihood of positioning a recording site near an enteric ganglion. The spacing between recording sites requires experimental optimization, and it will vary based on the insertion angle of the microelectrode. Importantly, multiple recording sites within the plexus layer will improve single-unit isolation [139]. Positioning additional recording sites in neighboring longitudinal or circular muscle layers may provide auxiliary physiological signals such as muscle action potentials or electrical slow wave activity. The additional recording sites and physiological signals could provide greater context for single-unit recordings or be used in signal processing techniques to increase the signal-to-noise ratio of single-unit recordings.

4.3. Implant Procedure

The implant procedure will greatly impact gastrointestinal physiology, and the procedure should be designed to reduce the risk of intestinal injury. A flexible microelectrode shank inserted into the gastrointestinal wall will be difficult to reliably position, and chronic macroscopic tissue motion will cause the electrode to drift over time, causing significant tissue damage [140,141]. To minimize the dimensions of tissue displacement relative to the probe, enteric microelectrodes should theoretically be implanted along the longitudinal axis, instead of the circumferential axis. However, this approach would be well-supported by experimental analysis.

Finally, enteric microelectrodes should be inserted at shallow angles relative to the serosa of the gastrointestinal wall. Microelectrodes should be designed to penetrate the longitudinal muscle layer without penetrating the submucosal layer. Piercing the epithelial layer or compromising barrier function will cause inflammation and sepsis [142]. Therefore the length of the microelectrodes and insertion angle should be designed specifically for the anatomy of the target species, because gastrointestinal dimensions scale across species [143].

5. Discussion

The available methods in enteric neuroscience are largely limited to excised tissue. While flat-sheet and whole-organ preparations are reliable tools to examine enteric neurophysiology, they are inadequate to study the interactions with the immune system, microbiota, extrinsic nervous system, etc. Anesthesia, on the other hand, modulates neurotransmission and impedes gastrointestinal motility, which confounds the interpretability of anesthetized in vivo recordings. Previously, we reported electrical activity from the enteric nervous system in anesthetized mouse, supported by simultaneous calcium imaging [144]. Although we observed increases in activity as expected with pharmacological stimulation and strong correlation with calcium activity, the source and robustness of the electrical activity remains disputed. This previous account demonstrates the challenges of anesthetized recordings, as well as the structural, physiological, and signal quality challenges in the gastrointestinal environment.

Single-unit recording capability from enteric neurons in awake animals has the potential to improve our understanding of the enteric nervous system, neurogastrointestinal function, and nutrition-mediated behavior. Single-unit resolution in awake animals will lead to computational models that better capture enteric neurophysiology which could guide future therapeutics [145,146]. Additionally, single-unit recordings pose great opportunities to synergize with advancements in other neurophysiology tools. Calcium imaging has been used reliably to monitor enteric neurons simultaneously in excised tissue [147,148] and anesthetized animals [144]. Furthermore, optogenetic stimulation and inhibition techniques have been adapted for enteric neurons [149], and have already been used to modulate motility in awake, freely-moving mice [150]. Additionally, neural microelectrodes designed for chronic, in vivo conditions have applications in electrical stimulation as an alternative to optogenetic stimulation.

6. Conclusions

In vivo electrophysiology in awake animals provides several opportunities and advantages over in vitro, ex vivo, and anesthetized in vivo recordings. Single-unit recordings from awake animals will require novel devices and methods to overcome the unique technical challenges posed by the gastrointestinal system. Importantly, single-unit recordings from awake animals have great potential to synergize with recent developments in optogenetics and in vivo imaging, but they will not completely replace traditional electrophysiology methods.

Author Contributions: B.B.B. conceptualized the content of this review, wrote the manuscript, and designed the figures; H.I.H. contributed to the challenges associated with gastrointestinal physiology; G.E.H. contributed to the design of the review; and X.S. assisted with the organization and design of the review.

Funding: This research was funded by the National Institutes of Health R35GM122465 and OT2OD023849, and the Defense Advanced Research Projects Agency N66001-15-2-4059.

Acknowledgments: The authors thank Dr. Laura Hale of Duke University for histological analysis.

Conflicts of Interest: The authors declare no conflict of interest.

References

1. Gabella, G. The number of neurons in the small intestine of mice, guinea-pigs and sheep. *Neuroscience* **1987**, *22*, 737–752. [CrossRef]
2. Furness, J.B.; Costa, M. Types of nerves in the enteric nervous system. *Neuroscience* **1980**, *5*, 235–252. (In English) [CrossRef]
3. Wood, J.D. Enteric nervous system: Reflexes, pattern generators and motility. *Curr. Opin. Gastroenterol.* **2008**, *24*, 149–158. (In English) [CrossRef] [PubMed]
4. Kapur, R.P. Developmental disorders of the enteric nervous system. *Gut* **2000**, *47*, iv81–iv83. [CrossRef] [PubMed]
5. Rao, M.; Gershon, M.D. The bowel and beyond: The enteric nervous system in neurological disorders. *Nat. Rev. Gastroenterol. Hepatol.* **2016**, *13*, 517–528. (In English) [CrossRef] [PubMed]
6. Neckel, P.H.; Mattheus, U.; Hirt, B.; Just, L.; Mack, A.F. Large-scale tissue clearing (pact): Technical evaluation and new perspectives in immunofluorescence, histology, and ultrastructure. *Sci. Rep.* **2016**, *6*, 34331. [CrossRef] [PubMed]
7. Hao, M.M.; Foong, J.P.; Bornstein, J.C.; Li, Z.L.; Berghe, P.V.; Boesmans, W. Enteric nervous system assembly: Functional integration within the developing gut. *Dev. Biol.* **2016**, *417*, 168–181. [CrossRef] [PubMed]
8. Lee, A.K.; Manns, I.D.; Sakmann, B.; Brecht, M. Whole-cell recordings in freely moving rats. *Neuron* **2006**, *51*, 399–407. [CrossRef] [PubMed]
9. Dombeck, D.A.; Khabbaz, A.N.; Collman, F.; Adelman, T.L.; Tank, D.W. Imaging large-scale neural activity with cellular resolution in awake, mobile mice. *Neuron* **2007**, *56*, 43–57. [CrossRef] [PubMed]
10. Ambache, N. Separation of the longitudinal muscle of the rabbit's ileum as a broad sheet. *J. Physiol.* **1954**, *125*, 53–55. (In English) [PubMed]
11. Nishi, S.; North, R.A. Intracellular recording from the myenteric plexus of the guinea-pig ileum. *J. Physiol.* **1973**, *231*, 471–491. [CrossRef] [PubMed]
12. Hirst, G.D.S.; Holman, M.E.; Spence, I. Two types of neurones in the myenteric plexus of duodenum in the guinea-pig. *J. Physiol.* **1974**, *236*, 303–326. [CrossRef] [PubMed]
13. Costa, M.; Brookes, S.J.; Steeled, P.A.; Gibbins, I.; Burcher, E.; Kandiah, C.J. Neurochemical classification of myenteric neurons in the guinea-pig ileum. *Neuroscience* **1996**, *75*, 949–967. [CrossRef]
14. Wood, J.D. Application of classification schemes to the enteric nervous system. *J. Auton. Nervous Syst.* **1994**, *48*, 17–29. [CrossRef]
15. Carbone, S.E.; Jovanovska, V.; Nurgali, K.; Brookes, S.J. Human enteric neurons: Morphological, electrophysiological, and neurochemical identification. *Neurogastroenterol. Motil. Off. J. Eur. Gastrointest. Motil. Soc.* **2014**, *26*, 1812–1816. (In English) [CrossRef] [PubMed]
16. Osorio, N.; Delmas, P. Patch clamp recording from enteric neurons in situ. *Nat. Protoc.* **2010**, *6*, 15–27. [CrossRef] [PubMed]
17. Spencer, N.J.; Hibberd, T.J.; Travis, L.; Wiklendt, L.; Costa, M.; Hu, H.; Brookes, S.J.; Wattchow, D.A.; Dinning, P.G.; Keating, D.J.; et al. Identification of a rhythmic firing pattern in the enteric nervous system that generates rhythmic electrical activity in smooth muscle. *J. Neurosci.* **2018**, *38*, 5507–5522. [CrossRef] [PubMed]
18. Spencer, N.J.; Hennig, G.W.; Dickson, E.; Smith, T.K. Synchronization of enteric neuronal firing during the murine colonic mmc. *J. Physiol.* **2005**, *564*, 829–847. [CrossRef] [PubMed]
19. Fried, D.E.; Gulbransen, B.D. In situ Ca^{2+} imaging of the enteric nervous system. *J. Vis. Exp. JoVE* **2015**, *52506*. [CrossRef]
20. Hibberd, T.J.; Travis, L.; Wiklendt, L.; Costa, M.; Brookes, S.J.H.; Hu, H.; Keating, D.J.; Spencer, N.J. Synaptic activation of putative sensory neurons by hexamethonium-sensitive nerve pathways in mouse colon. *Am. J. Physiol. Gastrointest. Liver Physiol.* **2018**, *314*, G53–G64. (In English) [CrossRef] [PubMed]
21. Hoffman, J.M.; Brooks, E.M.; Mawe, G.M. Gastrointestinal motility monitor (gimm). *J. Vis. Exp.* **2010**, *e2435*. [CrossRef] [PubMed]
22. Spencer, N.J.; Dinning, P.G.; Brookes, S.J.; Costa, M. Insights into the mechanisms underlying colonic motor patterns. *J. Physiol.* **2016**, *594*, 4099–4116. (In English) [CrossRef] [PubMed]
23. Bortoff, A. Configuration of intestinal slow waves obtained by monopolar recording techniques. *Am. J. Physiol.* **1967**, *213*, 157–162. (In English) [CrossRef] [PubMed]

24. Bozler, E. The action potentials of the stomach. *Am. J. Physiol. Leg. Content* **1945**, *144*, 693–700. [CrossRef]

25. Angeli, T.R.; Du, P.; Paskaranandavadivel, N.; Janssen, P.W.; Beyder, A.; Lentle, R.G.; Bissett, I.P.; Cheng, L.K.; O'grady, G. The bioelectrical basis and validity of gastrointestinal extracellular slow wave recordings. *J. Physiol.* **2013**, *591*, 4567–4579. (In English) [CrossRef] [PubMed]

26. Brierley, S.M.; Jones, R.C., III; Gebhart, G.F.; Blackshaw, L.A. Splanchnic and pelvic mechanosensory afferents signal different qualities of colonic stimuli in mice. *Gastroenterology* **2004**, *127*, 166–178. (In English) [CrossRef] [PubMed]

27. Buckley, M.M.; O'Malley, D. Development of an ex vivo method for multi-unit recording of microbiota-colonic-neural signaling in real time. *Front. Neurosci.* **2018**, *12*, 112. (In English) [CrossRef] [PubMed]

28. Castelucci, P.; Robbins, H.L.; Poole, D.P.; Furness, J.B. The distribution of purine P2X$_2$ receptors in the guinea-pig enteric nervous system. *Histochem. Cell Biol.* **2002**, *117*, 415–422. [CrossRef] [PubMed]

29. Furness, J.B.; Brown, A. (Eds.) *The Enteric Nervous System*; Blackwell Publishing: Malden, MA, USA, 2006; p. 288.

30. Liu, M.-T.; Rothstein, J.D.; Gershon, M.D.; Kirchgessner, A.L. Glutamatergic enteric neurons. *J. Neurosci.* **1997**, *17*, 4764–4784. [CrossRef] [PubMed]

31. Neunlist, M.; Michel, K.; Reiche, D.; Dobreva, G.; Huber, K.; Schemann, M. Glycine activates myenteric neurones in adult guinea-pigs. *J. Physiol.* **2001**, *536*, 727–739. [CrossRef] [PubMed]

32. Dilger, J.P. The effects of general anaesthetics on ligand-gated ion channels. *Br. J. Anaesth.* **2002**, *89*, 41–51. [CrossRef] [PubMed]

33. Kohtala, S.; Theilmann, W.; Suomi, T.; Wigren, H.K.; Porkka-Heiskanen, T.; Elo, L.L.; Rokka, A.; Rantamäki, T. Brief isoflurane anesthesia produces prominent phosphoproteomic changes in the adult mouse hippocampus. *ACS Chem. Neurosci.* **2016**, *7*, 749–756. [CrossRef] [PubMed]

34. Qu, Z.-D.; Thacker, M.; Castelucci, P.; Bagyanszki, M.; Epstein, M.L.; Furness, J.B. Immunohistochemical analysis of neuron types in the mouse small intestine. *Cell Tissue Res.* **2008**, *334*, 147–161. [CrossRef] [PubMed]

35. Erickson, C.S.; Lee, S.J.; Barlow-Anacker, A.J.; Druckenbrod, N.R.; Epstein, M.L.; Gosain, A. Appearance of cholinergic myenteric neurons during enteric nervous system development: Comparison of different chat fluorescent mouse reporter lines. *Neurogastroenterol. Motil. Off. J. Eur. Gastrointest. Motil. Soc.* **2014**, *26*, 874–884. [CrossRef] [PubMed]

36. Flood, P.; Krasowski, M.D. Intravenous anesthetics differentially modulate ligand-gated ion channels. *Anesthesiology* **2000**, *92*, 1418–1425. (In English) [CrossRef] [PubMed]

37. Violet, B.J.M.; Downie, D.L.; Nakisa, R.C.; Lieb, W.R.; Franks, N.P. Differential sensitivities of mammalian neuronal and muscle nicotinic acetylcholine receptors to general anesthetics. *Anesthesiology* **1997**, *86*, 866–874. [CrossRef] [PubMed]

38. Zhang, L.; Oz, M.; Stewart, R.R.; Peoples, R.W.; Weight, F.F. Volatile general anaesthetic actions on recombinant nach alpha 7, 5-ht3 and chimeric nach alpha 7-5-ht3 receptors expressed in xenopus oocytes. *Br. J. Pharmacol.* **1997**, *120*, 353–355. (In English) [CrossRef] [PubMed]

39. Hara, K.; Harris, R.A. The anesthetic mechanism of urethane: The effects on neurotransmitter-gated ion channels. *Anesth. Analg.* **2002**, *94*, 313–318. (In English) [PubMed]

40. Xiang, Z.; Burnstock, G. P2X$_2$ and P2X$_3$ purinoceptors in the rat enteric nervous system. *Histochem. Cell Biol.* **2004**, *121*, 169–179. [CrossRef] [PubMed]

41. Vanderwinden, J.-M.; Timmermans, J.-P.; Schiffmann, S.N. Glial cells, but not interstitial cells, express P2X$_7$, an ionotropic purinergic receptor, in rat gastrointestinal musculature. *Cell Tissue Res.* **2003**, *312*, 149–154. [CrossRef] [PubMed]

42. Masaki, E.; Kawamura, M.; Kato, F. Reduction by sevoflurane of adenosine 5′-triphosphate-activated inward current of locus coeruleus neurons in pontine slices of rats. *Brain Res.* **2001**, *921*, 226–232. [CrossRef]

43. Kitahara, S.; Yamashita, M.; Ikemoto, Y. Effects of ketamine and propofol on P2X receptors in dorsal root ganglion neurons of the rat. *J. Jpn. Dent. Soc. Anesthesiol.* **2003**, *31*, 11–16.

44. Tomioka, A.; Ueno, S.; Kohama, K.; Goto, F.; Inoue, K. Propofol potentiates ATP-activated currents of recombinant P2X$_4$ receptor channels expressed in human embryonic kidney 293 cells. *Neurosci. Lett.* **2000**, *284*, 167–170. (In English) [CrossRef]

45. Nakanishi, M.; Mori, T.; Nishikawa, K.; Sawada, M.; Kuno, M.; Asada, A. The effects of general anesthetics on P2X$_7$ and P2Y receptors in a rat microglial cell line. *Anesth. Analg.* **2007**, *104*, 1136–1144. [CrossRef] [PubMed]

46. Barann, M.; Göthert, M.; Fink, K.; Bönisch, H. Inhibition by anaesthetics of ^{14}C-guanidinium flux through the voltage-gated sodium channel and the cation channel of the 5-HT$_3$ receptor of N$_1$E$_{-115}$ neuroblastoma cells. *Naunyn Schmiedeberg's Arch. Pharmacol.* **1993**, *347*, 125–132. [CrossRef]

47. Emerit, M.B.; Riad, M.; Fattaccini, C.M.; Hamon, M. Characteristics of [^{14}C]guanidinium accumulation in NG 108-15 cell exposed to serotonin 5-HT$_3$ receptor ligands and substance P. *J. Neurochem.* **1993**, *60*, 2059–2067. [CrossRef] [PubMed]

48. Machu, T.K.; Harris, R.A. Alcohols and anesthetics enhance the function of 5-hydroxytryptamine3 receptors expressed in xenopus laevis oocytes. *J. Pharmacol. Exp. Ther.* **1994**, *271*, 898–905. (In English) [PubMed]

49. MacDonald, J.F.; Bartlett, M.C.; Mody, I.; Pahapill, P.; Reynolds, J.N.; Salter, M.W.; Schneiderman, J.H.; Pennefather, P.S. Actions of ketamine, phencyclidine and MK-801 on NMDA receptor currents in cultured mouse hippocampal neurones. *J. Physiol.* **1991**, *432*, 483–508. (In English) [CrossRef] [PubMed]

50. Dildy-Mayfield, J.E.; Eger, E.I., 2nd; Harris, R.A. Anesthetics produce subunit-selective actions on glutamate receptors. *J. Pharmacol. Exp. Ther.* **1996**, *276*, 1058–1065. (In English) [PubMed]

51. Marszalec, W.; Narahashi, T. Use-dependent pentobarbital block of kainate and quisqualate currents. *Brain Res.* **1993**, *608*, 7–15. [CrossRef]

52. Krantis, A.; Shabnavard, L.; Nichols, K.; De Blas, A.L.; Staines, W. Localization of gabaa receptor immunoreactivity in no synthase positive myenteric neurones. *J. Auton. Nervous Syst.* **1995**, *53*, 157–165. [CrossRef]

53. Krantis, A. Gaba in the mammalian enteric nervous system. *Physiology* **2000**, *15*, 284–290. [CrossRef]

54. Lin, L.H.; Chen, L.L.; Zirrolli, J.A.; Harris, R.A. General anesthetics potentiate gamma-aminobutyric acid actions on gamma-aminobutyric acida receptors expressed by xenopus oocytes: Lack of involvement of intracellular calcium. *J. Pharmacol. Exp. Ther.* **1992**, *263*, 569–578. (In English) [PubMed]

55. Wan, X.; Mathers, D.A.; Puil, E. Pentobarbital modulates intrinsic and gaba-receptor conductances in thalamocortical inhibition. *Neuroscience* **2003**, *121*, 947–958. (In English) [CrossRef] [PubMed]

56. Thompson, S.A.; Whiting, P.J.; Wafford, K.A. Barbiturate interactions at the human gabaa receptor: Dependence on receptor subunit combination. *Br. J. Pharmacol.* **1996**, *117*, 521–527. (In English) [CrossRef] [PubMed]

57. Hales, T.G.; Lambert, J.J. The actions of propofol on inhibitory amino acid receptors of bovine adrenomedullary chromaffin cells and rodent central neurones. *Br. J. Pharmacol.* **1991**, *104*, 619–628. [CrossRef] [PubMed]

58. Jones, M.V.; Brooks, P.A.; Harrison, N.L. Enhancement of gamma-aminobutyric acid-activated cl- currents in cultured rat hippocampal neurones by three volatile anaesthetics. *J. Physiol.* **1992**, *449*, 279–293. (In English) [CrossRef] [PubMed]

59. Downie, D.L.; Hall, A.C.; Lieb, W.R.; Franks, N.P. Effects of inhalational general anaesthetics on native glycine receptors in rat medullary neurones and recombinant glycine receptors in xenopus oocytes. *Br. J. Pharmacol.* **1996**, *118*, 493–502. [CrossRef] [PubMed]

60. Behm, B.; Stollman, N. Postoperative ileus: Etiologies and interventions. *Clin. Gastroenterol. Hepatol.* **2003**, *1*, 71–80. (In English) [CrossRef] [PubMed]

61. Wells, C.I.; O'Grady, G.; Bissett, I.P. Acute colonic pseudo-obstruction: A systematic review of aetiology and mechanisms. *World J. Gastroenterol.* **2017**, *23*, 5634–5644. [CrossRef] [PubMed]

62. Durongphongtorn, S.; McDonell, W.N.; Kerr, C.L.; Neto, F.J.; Mirakhur, K.K. Comparison of hemodynamic, clinicopathologic, and gastrointestinal motility effects and recovery characteristics of anesthesia with isoflurane and halothane in horses undergoing arthroscopic surgery. *Am. J. Vet. Res.* **2006**, *67*, 32–42. (In English) [CrossRef] [PubMed]

63. Tournadre, J.P.; Allaouichiche, B.; Malbert, C.H.; Chassard, D. Metabolic acidosis and respiratory acidosis impair gastro-pyloric motility in anesthetized pigs. *Anesth. Analg.* **2000**, *90*, 74–79. (In English) [CrossRef] [PubMed]

64. Grant, I.S.; Nimmo, W.S.; Clements, J.A. Lack of effect of ketamine analgesia on gastric-emptying in man. *Br. J. Anaesth.* **1981**, *53*, 1321–1323. (In English) [CrossRef] [PubMed]

65. Fass, J.; Bares, R.; Hermsdorf, V.; Schumpelick, V. Effects of intravenous ketamine on gastrointestinal motility in the dog. *Intensive Care Med.* **1995**, *21*, 584–589. [CrossRef] [PubMed]

66. Schreiber, D.; Klotz, M.; Laures, K.; Clasohm, J.; Bischof, M.; Schäfer, K.H. The mesenterially perfused rat small intestine: A versatile approach for pharmacological testings. *Ann. Anat. Anatomischer Anzeiger* **2014**, *196*, 158–166. [CrossRef] [PubMed]

67. Schnoor, J.; Unger, J.K.; Kochs, B.; Silny, J.; Rossaint, R. Effects of a single dose of ketamine on duodenal motility activity in pigs. *Can. Vet. J.* **2005**, *46*, 147–152. [PubMed]

68. Yuasa, H.; Watanabe, J. Influence of urethane anesthesia and abdominal surgery on gastrointestinal motility in rats. *Biol. Pharm. Bull.* **1994**, *17*, 1309–1312. [CrossRef] [PubMed]

69. Maggi, C.A.; Meli, A. Suitability of urethane anesthesia for physiopharmacological investigations. Part 3: Other systems and conclusions. *Experientia* **1986**, *42*, 531–537. [CrossRef] [PubMed]

70. Grundy, D. The effect of surgical anaesthesia on antral motility in the ferret. *Exp. Physiol.* **1990**, *75*, 701–708. [CrossRef] [PubMed]

71. Qualls-Creekmore, E.; Tong, M.; Holmes, G.M. Gastric emptying of enterally administered liquid meal in conscious rats and during sustained anaesthesia. *Neurogastroenterol. Motil. Off. J. Eur. Gastrointest. Motil. Soc.* **2010**, *22*, 181–185. (In English) [CrossRef] [PubMed]

72. Freye, E.; Sundermann, S.; Wilder-Smith, O.H.G. No inhibition of gastro-intestinal propulsion after propofol-or propofol/ketamine-N$_2$O/O$_2$ anaesthesia: A comparison of gastro-caecal transit after isoflurane anaesthesia. *Acta Anaesthesiol. Scand.* **1998**, *42*, 664–669. [CrossRef] [PubMed]

73. Lee, T.-L.; Ang, S.B.; Dambisya, Y.M.; Adaikan, G.P.; Lau, L.C. The effect of propofol on human gastric and colonic muscle contractions. *Anesth. Analg.* **1999**, *89*, 1246–1249. [CrossRef] [PubMed]

74. Anderson, D.L.; Bartholomeusz, F.D.; Kirkwood, I.D.; Chatterton, B.E. Liquid gastric emptying in the pig: Effect of concentration of inhaled isoflurane. *J. Nucl. Med. Off. Publ. Soc. Nucl. Med.* **2002**, *43*, 968–971. (In English)

75. Torjman, M.C.; Joseph, J.I.; Munsick, C.; Morishita, M.; Grunwald, Z. Effects of isoflurane on gastrointestinal motility after brief exposure in rats. *Int. J. Pharm.* **2005**, *294*, 65–71. [CrossRef] [PubMed]

76. Ailiani, A.C.; Neuberger, T.; Brasseur, J.G.; Banco, G.; Wang, Y.; Smith, N.B.; Webb, A.G. Quantifying the effects of inactin vs isoflurane anesthesia on gastrointestinal motility in rats using dynamic magnetic resonance imaging and spatio-temporal maps. *Neurogastroenterol. Motil. Off. J. Eur. Gastrointest. Motil. Soc.* **2014**, *26*, 1477–1486. (In English) [CrossRef] [PubMed]

77. Boscan, P.; Cochran, S.; Monnet, E.; Webb, C.; Twedt, D. Effect of prolonged general anesthesia with sevoflurane and laparoscopic surgery on gastric and small bowel propulsive motility and ph in dogs. *Vet. Anaesth. Analg.* **2014**, *41*, 73–81. (In English) [CrossRef] [PubMed]

78. Desmet, M.; Vander Cruyssen, P.; Pottel, H.; Carlier, S.; Devriendt, D.; Van Rooy, F.; De Corte, W. The influence of propofol and sevoflurane on intestinal motility during laparoscopic surgery. *Acta Anaesthesiol. Scand.* **2016**, *60*, 335–342. [CrossRef] [PubMed]

79. Schurizek, B.A.; Willacy, L.H.; Kraglund, K.; Juhl, B.; Andreasen, F. Effects of general anaesthesia with halothane on antroduodenal motility, ph and gastric emptying rate in man. *Br. J. Anaesth.* **1989**, *62*, 129–137. [CrossRef] [PubMed]

80. Marshall, M.S.F.N.; Pittinger, M.D.C.B.; Long, P.D.J.P. Effects of halothane on gastrointestinal motility. *Anesthesiology* **1961**, *22*, 363–366. [CrossRef] [PubMed]

81. Wright, J.W.; Healy, T.E.; Balfour, T.W.; Hardcastle, J.D. Effects of inhalation anaesthetic agents on the electrical and mechanical activity of the rat duodenum. *Br. J. Anaesth.* **1982**, *54*, 1223–1230. (In English) [CrossRef] [PubMed]

82. Lammers, W.J.; al-Kais, A.H.; Singh, S.A.; Arafat, K.H.; el-Sharkawy, T.Y. Multielectrode mapping of slow-wave activity in the isolated rabbit duodenum. *J. Appl. physiol.* **1993**, *74*, 1454–1461. (In English) [CrossRef] [PubMed]

83. Du, P.; O'Grady, G.; Egbuji, J.U.; Lammers, W.J.; Budgett, D.; Nielsen, P.; Windsor, J.A.; Pullan, A.J.; Cheng, L.K. High-resolution mapping of in vivo gastrointestinal slow wave activity using flexible printed circuit board electrodes: Methodology and validation. *Ann. Biomed. Eng.* **2009**, *37*, 839. [CrossRef] [PubMed]

84. Angeli, T.R.; O'Grady, G.; Vather, R.; Bissett, I.P.; Cheng, L.K. Intra-operative high-resolution mapping of slow wave propagation in the human jejunum: Feasibility and initial results. *Neurogastroenterol. Motil.* **2018**, *30*, e13310. [CrossRef] [PubMed]

85. O'Keefe, J.; Dostrovsky, J. The hippocampus as a spatial map. Preliminary evidence from unit activity in the freely-moving rat. *Brain Res.* **1971**, *34*, 171–175. [CrossRef]
86. Hadzipasic, M.; Ni, W.; Nagy, M.; Steenrod, N.; McGinley, M.J.; Kaushal, A.; Thomas, E.; McCormick, D.A.; Horwich, A.L. Reduced high-frequency motor neuron firing, emg fractionation, and gait variability in awake walking als mice. *Proc. Natl. Acad. Sci. USA* **2016**, *113*, E7600–E7609. [CrossRef] [PubMed]
87. Berg, R.W.; Chen, M.T.; Huang, H.C.; Hsiao, M.C.; Cheng, H. A method for unit recording in the lumbar spinal cord during locomotion of the conscious adult rat. *J. Neurosci. Methods* **2009**, *182*, 49–54. [CrossRef] [PubMed]
88. Aaron, G.; Jit, M. Brain micromotion around implants in the rodent somatosensory cortex. *J. Neural Eng.* **2006**, *3*, 189.
89. Smith, T.K.; Oliver, G.R.; Hennig, G.W.; O'Shea, D.M.; Berghe, P.V.; Kang, S.H.; Spencer, N.J. A smooth muscle tone-dependent stretch-activated migrating motor pattern in isolated guinea-pig distal colon. *J. Physiol.* **2003**, *551*, 955–969. [CrossRef] [PubMed]
90. Belkaid, Y.; Hand, T.W. Role of the microbiota in immunity and inflammation. *Cell* **2014**, *157*, 121–141. [CrossRef] [PubMed]
91. Hansson, G.C. Role of mucus layers in gut infection and inflammation. *Curr. Opin. Microbiol.* **2012**, *15*, 57–62. [CrossRef] [PubMed]
92. Van der Sluis, M.; De Koning, B.A.; De Bruijn, A.C.; Velcich, A.; Meijerink, J.P.; Van Goudoever, J.B.; Büller, H.A.; Dekker, J.; Van Seuningen, I.; Renes, I.B.; et al. Muc2-deficient mice spontaneously develop colitis, indicating that MUC2 is critical for colonic protection. *Gastroenterology* **2006**, *131*, 117–129. [CrossRef] [PubMed]
93. Bevins, C.L.; Salzman, N.H. Paneth cells, antimicrobial peptides and maintenance of intestinal homeostasis. *Nat. Rev. Microbiol.* **2011**, *9*, 356–368. [CrossRef] [PubMed]
94. Coombes, J.L.; Siddiqui, K.R.; Arancibia-Cárcamo, C.V.; Hall, J.; Sun, C.M.; Belkaid, Y.; Powrie, F.; et al. A functionally specialized population of mucosal CD103+ DCs induces Foxp3+ regulatory T cells via a TGF-β and retinoic acid-dependent mechanism. *J. Exp. Med.* **2007**, *204*, 1757–1764. [CrossRef] [PubMed]
95. Ruane, D.T.; Lavelle, E.C. The role of CD103+ dendritic cells in the intestinal mucosal immune system. *Front. Immunol.* **2011**, *2*, 25. [CrossRef] [PubMed]
96. Bain, C.C.; Bravo-Blas, A.; Scott, C.L.; Perdiguero, E.G.; Geissmann, F.; Henri, S.; Malissen, B.; Osborne, L.C.; Artis, D.; Mowat, A.M. Constant replenishment from circulating monocytes maintains the macrophage pool in the intestine of adult mice. *Nat. Immunol.* **2014**, *15*, 929–937. [CrossRef] [PubMed]
97. Tamoutounour, S.; Henri, S.; Lelouard, H.; de Bovis, B.; de Haar, C.; van der Woude, C.J.; Woltman, A.M.; Reyal, Y.; Bonnet, D.; Sichien, D.; et al. CD64 distinguishes macrophages from dendritic cells in the gut and reveals the th1-inducing role of mesenteric lymph node macrophages during colitis. *Eur. J. Immunol.* **2012**, *42*, 3150–3166. [CrossRef] [PubMed]
98. Cerovic, V.; Bain, C.C.; Mowat, A.M.; Milling, S.W. Intestinal macrophages and dendritic cells: What's the difference? *Trends Immunol.* **2014**, *35*, 270–277. [CrossRef] [PubMed]
99. Hadis, U.; Wahl, B.; Schulz, O.; Hardtke-Wolenski, M.; Schippers, A.; Wagner, N.; Müller, W.; Sparwasser, T.; Förster, R.; Pabst, O. Intestinal tolerance requires gut homing and expansion of Foxp3+ regulatory T cells in the lamina propria. *Immunity* **2011**, *34*, 237–246. [CrossRef] [PubMed]
100. Pastorelli, L.; De Salvo, C.; Mercado, J.R.; Vecchi, M.; Pizarro, T.T. Central role of the gut epithelial barrier in the pathogenesis of chronic intestinal inflammation: Lessons learned from animal models and human genetics. *Front. Immunol.* **2013**, *4*, 280. [CrossRef] [PubMed]
101. Pastorelli, L.; De Salvo, C.; Mercado, J.R.; Vecchi, M.; Pizarro, T.T. Genome-wide association study of ulcerative colitis identifies three new susceptibility loci, including the hnf4a region. *Nat. Genet.* **2009**, *41*, 1330–1334. [CrossRef]
102. Morris, G.P.; Beck, P.L.; Herridge, M.S.; Depew, W.T.; Szewczuk, M.R.; Wallace, J.L. Hapten-induced model of chronic inflammation and ulceration in the rat colon. *Gastroenterology* **1989**, *96*, 795–803. [CrossRef]
103. Okayasu, I.; Hatakeyama, S.; Yamada, M.; Ohkusa, T.; Inagaki, Y.; Nakaya, R. A novel method in the induction of reliable experimental acute and chronic ulcerative colitis in mice. *Gastroenterology* **1990**, *98*, 694–702. [CrossRef]
104. Poritz, L.S.; Garver, K.I.; Green, C.; Fitzpatrick, L.; Ruggiero, F.; Koltun, W.A. Loss of the tight junction protein ZO-1 in dextran sulfate sodium induced colitis. *J. Surg. Res.* **2007**, *140*, 12–19. [CrossRef] [PubMed]

105. Valatas, V.; Bamias, G.; Kolios, G. Experimental colitis models: Insights into the pathogenesis of inflammatory bowel disease and translational issues. *Eur. J. Pharmacol.* **2015**, *759*, 253–264. [CrossRef] [PubMed]
106. Grootjans, J.; Lenaerts, K.; Derikx, J.P.; Matthijsen, R.A.; de Bruïne, A.P.; van Bijnen, A.A.; van Dam, R.M.; Dejong, C.H.; Buurman, W.A. Human intestinal ischemia-reperfusion-induced inflammation characterized: Experiences from a new translational model. *Am. J. Pathol.* **2010**, *176*, 2283–2291. [CrossRef] [PubMed]
107. Gonzalez, L.M.; Moeser, A.J.; Blikslager, A.T. Animal models of ischemia-reperfusion-induced intestinal injury: Progress and promise for translational research. *Am. J. Physiol. Gastrointest. Liver Physiol.* **2015**, *308*, G63–G75. [CrossRef] [PubMed]
108. Veiga-Fernandes, H.; Mucida, D. Neuro-immune interactions at barrier surfaces. *Cell* **2016**, *165*, 801–811. [CrossRef] [PubMed]
109. Brun, P.; Giron, M.C.; Qesari, M.; Porzionato, A.; Caputi, V.; Zoppellaro, C.; Banzato, S.; Grillo, A.R.; Spagnol, L.; De Caro, R.; et al. Toll-like receptor 2 regulates intestinal inflammation by controlling integrity of the enteric nervous system. *Gastroenterology* **2013**, *145*, 1323–1333. [CrossRef] [PubMed]
110. Hammer, G.E.; Turer, E.E.; Taylor, K.E.; Fang, C.J.; Advincula, R.; Oshima, S.; Barrera, J.; Huang, E.J.; Hou, B.; Malynn, B.A.; et al. Expression of A20 by dendritic cells preserves immune homeostasis and prevents colitis and spondyloarthritis. *Nat. Immunol.* **2011**, *12*, 1184–1193. [CrossRef] [PubMed]
111. Liang, J.; Huang, H.I.; Benzatti, F.P.; Karlsson, A.B.; Zhang, J.J.; Youssef, N.; Ma, A.; Hale, L.P.; Hammer, G.E. Inflammatory Th1 and Th17 in the intestine are each driven by functionally specialized dendritic cells with distinct requirements for MyD88. *Cell Rep.* **2016**, *17*, 1330–1343. [CrossRef] [PubMed]
112. Rivollier, A.; He, J.; Kole, A.; Valatas, V.; Kelsall, B.L. Inflammation switches the differentiation program of ly6chi monocytes from antiinflammatory macrophages to inflammatory dendritic cells in the colon. *J. Exp. Med.* **2012**, *209*, 139–155. [CrossRef] [PubMed]
113. Bain, C.C.; Mowat, A.M. Macrophages in intestinal homeostasis and inflammation. *Immunol. Rev.* **2014**, *260*, 102–117. [CrossRef] [PubMed]
114. Bain, C.C.; Scott, C.L.; Uronen-Hansson, H.; Gudjonsson, S.; Jansson, O.; Grip, O.; Guilliams, M.; Malissen, B.; Agace, W.W.; Mowat, A.M. Resident and pro-inflammatory macrophages in the colon represent alternative context-dependent fates of the same Ly6C^{hi} monocyte precursors. *Mucosal. Immunol.* **2013**, *6*, 498–510. [CrossRef] [PubMed]
115. Gulbransen, B.D.; Bashashati, M.; Hirota, S.A.; Gui, X.; Roberts, J.A.; MacDonald, J.A.; Muruve, D.A.; McKay, D.M.; Beck, P.L.; Mawe, G.M.; et al. Activation of neuronal P2X$_7$ receptor-pannexin-1 mediates death of enteric neurons during colitis. *Nat. Med.* **2012**, *18*, 600–604. [CrossRef] [PubMed]
116. Sanders, K.M.; Ward, S.M.; Koh, S.D. Interstitial cells: Regulators of smooth muscle function. *Physiol. Rev.* **2014**, *94*, 859–907. [CrossRef] [PubMed]
117. Huizinga, J.D.; Martz, S.; Gil, V.; Wang, X.Y.; Jimenez, M.; Parsons, S. Two independent networks of interstitial cells of cajal work cooperatively with the enteric nervous system to create colonic motor patterns. *Front. Neurosci.* **2011**, *5*, 93. [CrossRef] [PubMed]
118. Sanders, K.M.; Kito, Y.; Hwang, S.J.; Ward, S.M. Regulation of gastrointestinal smooth muscle function by interstitial cells. *Physiology* **2016**, *31*, 316–326. [CrossRef] [PubMed]
119. Huizinga, J.D.; Thuneberg, L.; Klüppel, M.; Malysz, J.; Mikkelsen, H.B.; Bernstein, A. W/kit gene required for interstitial cells of cajal and for intestinal pacemaker activity. *Nature* **1995**, *373*, 347–349. (In English) [CrossRef] [PubMed]
120. Liu, L.W.; Huizinga, J.D. Canine colonic circular muscle generates action potentials without the pacemaker component. *Can. J. Physiol. Pharmacol.* **1994**, *72*, 70–81. (In English) [CrossRef] [PubMed]
121. Cao, Y.; Rakhilin, N.; Gordon, P.H.; Shen, X.; Kan, E.C. A real-time spike classification method based on dynamic time warping for extracellular enteric neural recording with large waveform variability. *J. Neurosci. Methods* **2016**, *261*, 97–109. (In English) [CrossRef] [PubMed]
122. Bayguinov, O.; Hennig, G.W.; Sanders, K.M. Movement based artifacts may contaminate extracellular electrical recordings from gi muscles. *Neurogastroenterol. Motil.* **2011**, *23*, 1029-e498. [CrossRef] [PubMed]
123. Sanders, K.M.; Ward, S.M.; Hennig, G.W. Problems with extracellular recording of electrical activity in gastrointestinal muscle. *Nat. Rev. Gastroenterol. Hepatol.* **2016**, *13*, 731–741. [CrossRef] [PubMed]
124. Stewart, D.C.; Rubiano, A.; Santisteban, M.M.; Shenoy, V.; Qi, Y.; Pepine, C.J.; Raizada, M.K.; Simmons, C.S. Hypertension-linked mechanical changes of rat gut. *Acta Biomater.* **2016**, *45*, 296–302. [CrossRef] [PubMed]

125. Stidham, R.W.; Xu, J.; Johnson, L.A.; Kim, K.; Moons, D.S.; McKenna, B.J.; Rubin, J.M.; Higgins, P.D. Ultrasound elasticity imaging for detecting intestinal fibrosis and inflammation in rats and humans with crohn's disease. *Gastroenterology* **2011**, *141*, 819–826. [CrossRef] [PubMed]

126. Christensen, M.B.; Oberg, K.; Wolchok, J.C. Tensile properties of the rectal and sigmoid colon: A comparative analysis of human and porcine tissue. *SpringerPlus* **2015**, *4*, 142. [CrossRef] [PubMed]

127. Lecomte, A.; Descamps, E.; Bergaud, C. A review on mechanical considerations for chronically-implanted neural probes. *J. Neural Eng.* **2017**, *15*, 031001. (In English) [CrossRef] [PubMed]

128. Du, Z.J.; Kolarcik, C.L.; Kozai, T.D.; Luebben, S.D.; Sapp, S.A.; Zheng, X.S.; Nabity, J.A.; Cui, X.T. Ultrasoft microwire neural electrodes improve chronic tissue integration. *Acta Biomater.* **2017**, *53*, 46–58. (In English) [CrossRef] [PubMed]

129. Seymour, J.P.; Kipke, D.R. Neural probe design for reduced tissue encapsulation in cns. *Biomaterials* **2007**, *28*, 3594–3607. (In English) [CrossRef] [PubMed]

130. Wellman, S.M.; Eles, J.R.; Ludwig, K.A.; Seymour, J.P.; Michelson, N.J.; McFadden, W.E.; Vazquez, A.L.; Kozai, T.D. A materials roadmap to functional neural interface design. *Adv. Funct. Mater.* **2018**, *28*, 1701269. [CrossRef] [PubMed]

131. Xie, C.; Liu, J.; Fu, T.M.; Dai, X.; Zhou, W.; Lieber, C.M. Three-dimensional macroporous nanoelectronic networks as minimally invasive brain probes. *Nat. Mater.* **2015**, *14*, 1286–1292. [CrossRef] [PubMed]

132. Luan, L.; Wei, X.; Zhao, Z.; Siegel, J.J.; Potnis, O.; Tuppen, C.A.; Lin, S.; Kazmi, S.; Fowler, R.A.; Holloway, S.; et al. Ultraflexible nanoelectronic probes form reliable, glial scar-free neural integration. *Sci. Adv.* **2017**, *3*, e1601966. (In English) [CrossRef] [PubMed]

133. Wei, X.; Luan, L.; Zhao, Z.; Li, X.; Zhu, H.; Potnis, O.; Xie, C. Nanofabricated ultraflexible electrode arrays for high-density intracortical recording. *Adv. Sci.* **2018**, *5*, 1700625. (In English) [CrossRef] [PubMed]

134. Naples, G.G.; Mortimer, J.T.; Scheiner, A.; Sweeney, J.D. A spiral nerve cuff electrode for peripheral nerve stimulation. *IEEE Trans. Biomed. Eng.* **1988**, *35*, 905–916. [CrossRef] [PubMed]

135. Cobo, A.M.; Boyajian, B.; Larson, C.; Schotten, K.; Pikov, V.; Meng, E. A parylene cuff electrode for peripheral nerve recording and drug delivery. In Proceeding of the 2017 IEEE 30th International Conference on Micro Electro Mechanical Systems (MEMS), Las Vegas, NV, USA, 22–26 January 2017; pp. 506–509.

136. Chen, J.D.; Schirmer, B.D.; McCallum, R.W. Serosal and cutaneous recordings of gastric myoelectrical activity in patients with gastroparesis. *Am. J. Physiol. Gastrointest. Liver Physiol.* **1994**, *266*, G90–G98. [CrossRef] [PubMed]

137. Li, X.; Hayes, J.; Peters, L.J.; Zhang, M.; Chen, J.D.Z. Electrical stimulation of small intestine using intraluminal ring electrodes. In Proceedings of the 20th Annual International Conference of the IEEE Engineering in Medicine and Biology Society. Vol.20 Biomedical Engineering Towards the Year 2000 and Beyond (Cat. No.98CH36286), Hong Kong, China, 1 November 1998; Volume 6, pp. 3230–3233.

138. Lin, X.; Hayes, J.; Peters, L.J.; Chen, J.D. Entrainment of intestinal slow waves with electrical stimulation using intraluminal electrodes. *Ann. Biomed. Eng.* **2000**, *28*, 582–587. (In English) [CrossRef] [PubMed]

139. Drake, K.L.; Wise, K.D.; Farraye, J.; Anderson, D.J.; BeMent, S.L. Performance of planar multisite microprobes in recording extracellular single-unit intracortical activity. *IEEE Trans. Biomed. Eng.* **1988**, *35*, 719–732. [CrossRef] [PubMed]

140. Biran, R.; Martin, D.C.; Tresco, P.A. Neuronal cell loss accompanies the brain tissue response to chronically implanted silicon microelectrode arrays. *Exp. Neurol.* **2005**, *195*, 115–126. (In English) [CrossRef] [PubMed]

141. Biran, R.; Martin, D.C.; Tresco, P.A. The brain tissue response to implanted silicon microelectrode arrays is increased when the device is tethered to the skull. *J. Biomed. Mater. Res. Part A* **2007**, *82A*, 169–178. [CrossRef] [PubMed]

142. Yoseph, B.P.; Klingensmith, N.J.; Liang, Z.; Breed, E.R.; Burd, E.M.; Mittal, R.; Dominguez, J.A.; Petrie, B.; Ford, M.L.; Coopersmith, C.M. Mechanisms of intestinal barrier dysfunction in sepsis. *Shock (Augusta, Ga.)* **2016**, *46*, 52–59. [CrossRef] [PubMed]

143. Kararli, T.T. Comparison of the gastrointestinal anatomy, physiology, and biochemistry of humans and commonly used laboratory animals. *Biopharm. Drug Dispos.* **1995**, *16*, 351–380. [CrossRef] [PubMed]

144. Rakhilin, N.; Barth, B.; Choi, J.; Munoz, N.L.; Kulkarni, S.; Jones, J.S.; Small, D.M.; Cheng, Y.-T.; Cao, Y.; LaVinka, C.; et al. Simultaneous optical and electrical in vivo analysis of the enteric nervous system. *Nat. Commun.* **2016**, *7*, 11800. [CrossRef] [PubMed]

145. Barth, B.B.; Henriquez, C.S.; Grill, W.M.; Shen, X. Electrical stimulation of gut motility guided by an in silico model. *J. Neural Eng.* **2017**, *14*, 066010. [CrossRef] [PubMed]

146. Barth, B.B.; Shen, X. Computational motility models of neurogastroenterology and neuromodulation. *Brain Res.* **2018**, *1693*, 174–179. (In English) [CrossRef] [PubMed]

147. Gulbransen, B.D. Emerging tools to study enteric neuromuscular function. *Am. J. Physiol. Gastrointest. Liver Physiol.* **2017**, *312*, G420–G426. [CrossRef] [PubMed]

148. Tack, J.; Smith, T.K. Calcium imaging of gut activity. *Neurogastroenterol. Motil.* **2004**, *16*, 86–95. [CrossRef] [PubMed]

149. Boesmans, W.; Hao, M.M.; Vanden Berghe, P. Optogenetic and chemogenetic techniques for neurogastroenterology. *Nat. Rev. Gastroenterol. Hepatol.* **2017**, *15*, 21–38. [CrossRef] [PubMed]

150. Hibberd, T.J.; Feng, J.; Luo, J.; Yang, P.; Samineni, V.K.; Gereau, R.W., 4th; Kelley, N.; Hu, H.; Spencer, N.J. Optogenetic induction of colonic motility in mice. *Gastroenterology* **2018**, *155*, 514–528. (In English) [CrossRef] [PubMed]

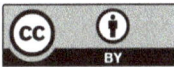

micromachines

MDPI

Perspective

The History and Horizons of Microscale Neural Interfaces

Takashi D. Y. Kozai [1,2,3,4,5]

1   Department of Bioengineering, University of Pittsburgh, Pittsburgh, PA 15261, USA; tdk18@pitt.edu
2   Center for the Neural Basis of Cognition, University of Pittsburgh, Pittsburgh, PA 15213, USA
3   Center for Neuroscience, University of Pittsburgh, Pittsburgh, PA 15261, USA
4   McGowan Institute of Regenerative Medicine, University of Pittsburgh, Pittsburgh, PA 15212, USA
5   NeuroTech Center, University of Pittsburgh Brain Institute, Pittsburgh, PA 15260, USA

Received: 7 August 2018; Accepted: 3 September 2018; Published: 6 September 2018

Abstract: Microscale neural technologies interface with the nervous system to record and stimulate brain tissue with high spatial and temporal resolution. These devices are being developed to understand the mechanisms that govern brain function, plasticity and cognitive learning, treat neurological diseases, or monitor and restore functions over the lifetime of the patient. Despite decades of use in basic research over days to months, and the growing prevalence of neuromodulation therapies, in many cases the lack of knowledge regarding the fundamental mechanisms driving activation has dramatically limited our ability to interpret data or fine-tune design parameters to improve long-term performance. While advances in materials, microfabrication techniques, packaging, and understanding of the nervous system has enabled tremendous innovation in the field of neural engineering, many challenges and opportunities remain at the frontiers of the neural interface in terms of both neurobiology and engineering. In this short-communication, we explore critical needs in the neural engineering field to overcome these challenges. Disentangling the complexities involved in the chronic neural interface problem requires simultaneous proficiency in multiple scientific and engineering disciplines. The critical component of advancing neural interface knowledge is to prepare the next wave of investigators who have simultaneous multi-disciplinary proficiencies with a diverse set of perspectives necessary to solve the chronic neural interface challenge.

Keywords: micromachine; neuroscience; biocompatibility; training; education; diversity; bias; BRAIN Initiative; multi-disciplinary; micro-electromechanical systems (MEMS)

1. Introduction

Neurotechnologies that are capable of stimulating or recording from a small population of neurons have revolutionized quality of life by enabling the deaf to hear [1,2], the blind to see [3,4], and the paralyzed to write, grasp, and walk [5–11]. The advancement of this technology has seen a dramatic growth over the past decade which has attracted additional attention and increasing promises of what these devices can accomplish to further improve quality of life. These neurotechnologies can range from implants that are inserted deep within the nervous system to non-invasive wearable technologies that generally have more limited capabilities. Key progress feeding into the growth of this field is the investment from major pharmaceutical and start-up companies to provide alternatives to drugs with side-effects as well as increased congressional and government support in developing and maintaining the infrastructural apparatus for technology development. In parallel, advancements in batteries, wireless recharging, miniaturization, sensors, computer chips, and advancements in decoding algorithms and machine learning promise potential for dramatic advances in the coming decades.

These neural interface technologies were originally employed as tools for basic science research in order to study how the brain works [12–15]. Basic science mapping experiments were carried out by using neural interfaces to electrically stimulate various regions of the brain or the nervous system and observing muscle twitches [16–20]. Mapping was also carried out in the opposite direction by applying sensory stimulation or driving motor activity and recording ionic currents from action potentials using microscale neural recording interfaces [21–23]. From these experiments, academic researchers discovered that specific functions of the nervous system were encoded in specific regions of the brain and nerve bundles [24–29]. Furthermore, they discovered that the frequency of action potentials recorded generally corresponded to the intensity of activity (sensation or muscle activation) [13–15,30,31]. These basic science discoveries have led to numerous neural interface applications from brain-computer interfaces that extract brain signals from paralyzed patients and allow them to control robotic limbs and computer cursors to electrical stimulation technologies that restore sensory function or treat Parkinson's tremors [2,3,5,7–9,11,32,33]. The present short-communication takes a brief glance at the history of the field as well as a wide-angle perspective of the emerging challenges and opportunities on the horizon along the frontier of neural engineering.

2. Brief History of Microscale Implantable Neural Technologies

Microscale neural interfaces were originally developed as research tools for academic investigation into the neural mechanisms that regulate attention, movement, and behavior [12]. Classically, these microscale interfaces have fallen into three categories: (1) microwire arrays (Figure 1a), (2) microfabricated planar arrays (Figure 1b), and (3) micromachined arrays (Figure 1c).

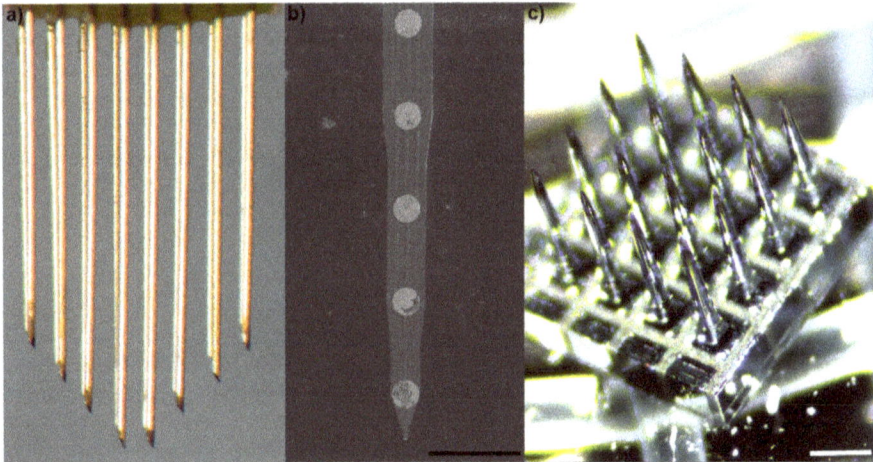

Figure 1. Classes of microscale implantable neural technologies: (**a**) 50 μm polyimide-insulated tungsten microwire with chiseled tips (Tucker–Davis Technologies, Alachua, FL, USA); (**b**) microfabricated silicon Michigan array with iridium electrode sites (NeuroNexus Technologies, Ann Arbor, MI, USA), scale = 100 μm; (**c**) macromachined boron-doped silicon array (Blackrock Microsystems, Salt Lake City, UT, USA), each needle is electrically separated at the base with glass. Scale = 400 μm.

Microwire electrodes have two key components: (1) a conductive core wires, and (2) an insulator such as glass, parylene, teflon, or polyimide. Generally, the insulation is exposed at the recording site at the tip. Sometimes, other electrode site materials are deposited on the tip of the wire, before insulation or after removal of the insulation from the tip, in order to improve the electrical properties of the microelectrode. These wires are typically manually assembled into bed of needle arrays with several different strategies employed to align the wires [34].

Microfabricated planar arrays are typically engineered through photolithography of silicon, metals, and polymers [35]. These arrays are generally microfabricated through layering of multiple conductive and non-conductive materials leading to a planar configuration. While early planar arrays were made from rigid silicon (such as the Michigan arrays), flexible configurations have been developed, including planar arrays that can be rolled, folded, or stacked into 3D configurations [36].

Micromachined arrays are similar to microwire arrays. Instead of assembling individual wires into an array, a block of silicon is micromachined into a pillar of needles [37]. Band-saws are used to mill large blocks of conductive (boron-doped) silicon into individual pillars. During the milling process, non-conductive glass is used to hold the pillars in a bed of needle configuration. Once the square pillars are etched into round pillars, the electrode tip material and insulation are deposited onto the array in a manner similar to microwires. Due to the band-saw micromachining process, it is much more difficult to develop arrays that have staggered configurations when compared to microwire arrays. However, it is much easier to precisely align all of the needles to have the same angle.

These three array technologies form the basic classes of implantable microscale neural interfaces; however, the diversity within these classes has dramatically increased in both functionality and application (Figure 2). Advances in materials and biomaterials, microfabrication techniques, and packaging have enabled a large breadth of distinct configurations over a wide range of design space parameters [36,38–57]. Still, it is crucial to recognize that optimizing one key parameter often leads to trade-offs on other critical parameters, and failure to maintain the functional domain in each of the crucial parameter spaces will lead to a non-functional device [36]. For example, while flexible polymer devices are hypothesized to reduce tissue inflammation and improve the electrode-tissue interface, the materials and designs behind these compliant devices typically result in more brittle implants, increased resistance and lower signal conductivity, higher impedance, greater shunt leakage, and enhancement of motion related electromagnetic artifacts [36,58]. A comprehensive examination of technical advances and trade-offs in microscale technology design space parameters has been covered in a separate review [36]. While much of the technological development of neural interfaces has focused on improving electrically stimulating and recording from central nervous system (CNS) targets, some recent advances have fundamentally altered the traditional limits of neural implants.

For example, optogenetics has dramatically altered the functionality of what once were exclusively electrical neural interfaces. Optogenetics includes transgenically expressing photon-gated ion channels called opsins in neuronal and non-neuronal cells whose cell activity are dependent on ion concentration [59]. Today, optogenetics also includes transgenically expressing fluorescent indicators into cells where the intensity level of the indicator changes based on the activity of the cells [60]. This is typically carried out by creating chimera proteins with a fluorescent protein, such as green fluorescent protein. The chimera is created such that the fluorescent protein is slightly denatured at rest. The other half of the chimera protein is designed to bind to key molecules of interest, such as calcium (released during action potentials) or glutamate [61–63]. The binding of the effector molecule leads to a conformation change in the binding site in the chimera, which rearranges the fluorescent protein into a conformation that allows the protein to fluoresce brightly, compared to the denatured state at rest. The adoption of optogenetic technology in the neuroscience community has motivated incorporation of waveguides as well as light-emitting and sensing diodes into microscale neural interfaces [36,40].

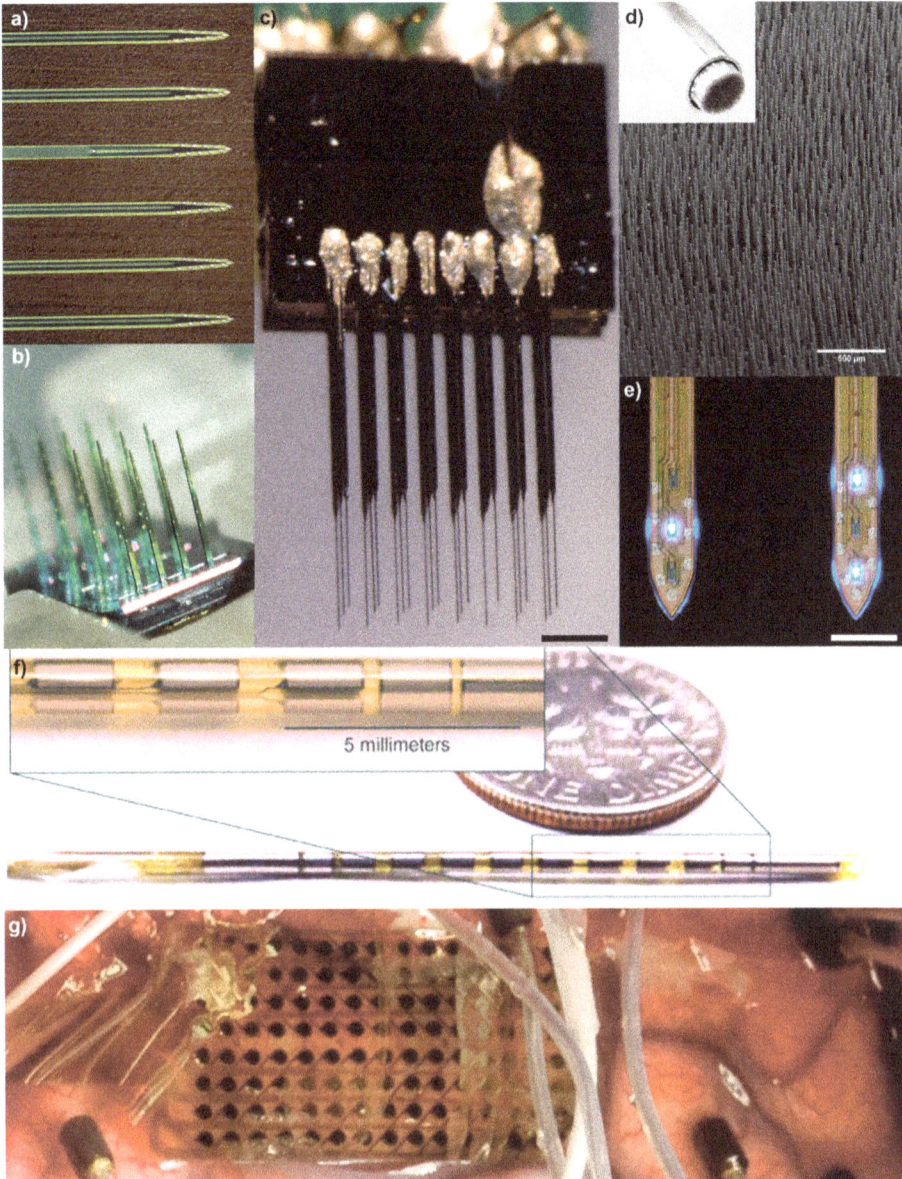

Figure 2. Advances in microscale neural interfaces: (**a**) 64-channel Buszaki Array (Neuronexus); (**b**) 128-channel Matrix Array (Neuronexus); (**c**) 24-channel ultra-small carbon fiber array on silicon stacks (courtesy of Paras Patel/Cynthia Chestek), scale = 100 μm; (**d**) high-density ultra-small microwire array (Paradromics Inc., San Jose, CA, USA), scale = 500 μm; (**e**) μLED silicon optoelectrode (courtesy of NeuroNex MINT Hub at University of Michigan, Ann Arbor, MI, USA (http://mint.engin.umich.edu)), scale = 100 μm; (**f**) a standard-sized 1.27 mm diameter Lawrence Livermore National Laboratories (LLNL) DBS-style penetrating probe constructed using microfabrication techniques, allowing for a higher-density of electrodes and avoiding typical hand-assembly techniques; and (**g**) A LNLL 128-channel microelectrocorticography (μECoG) array used for language mapping on awake patients. This 20-μm-thick flexible electrode array is constructed using thin-film polymers and metals and features 1.2 mm diameter electrodes.

Similarly, a better understanding of the nervous system and foreign body response in the central nervous system has motivated the development of peripheral nerve interfaces. The central nervous system (CNS) is separated from the rest of the body by the blood-brain barrier (BBB). It was once believed that the brain was "immune privileged". Today, this is understood to be an inaccurate dogma [64,65]. However, the inflammatory response and immune response that are triggered during surgical implantation of brain neural interfaces, as well as the threat of serious consequences from brain tissue infection along percutaneous connectors, have led investigators to search for less invasive neural interface approaches [66,67]. In parallel, new discoveries about the autonomic nervous system have led to the validation that modulating activity of peripheral nerves that feed into the brain can cause systemic physiological changes [24,25]. While early proof-of-concept studies utilized brain neural interfaces or modified brain neural interface technologies, interfacing with peripheral nerves requires dramatic differences in structure and design criteria compared to brain neural interfaces that are more suited to recording signals from neuronal cell bodies rather than axons.

Advancements in genetic engineering, biophysics, and a better understanding of functional connectivity and anatomy has opened up novel modalities for interfacing with the nervous system. In addition, as basic science understanding of the nervous system increases, it becomes possible to identify new targets for interfacing with the body and different aspects of physiology. Each new nervous system target requires a custom design in order to optimally interface with the nerve or neuron. This is especially true when interfacing the same peripheral physiological target across different animal models or different ages of the same model. Furthermore, it may be necessary, depending on the target, to consider "personalized device designs" similar to personalized medicine which accounts for person-to-person variability in clinical applications.

3. Challenges on the Horizon

Despite these numerous success stories, many challenges, and as a result, great opportunities remain unexplored [36,58,68]. There remains large variability in performance even between identical devices [69] due to both biological [58,67,70–72] and material integrity variance [73–75], even within the same subject [71,72]. Nevertheless, the field of neural engineering has reached a tipping point due to pioneers in neuroscience, technology development, and neurosurgery. Although many of the foundational components are primed for commercial growth of neural interfaces, there are still constraints in neural technology translation due to the unpredictability of discovery science. In addition, it remains highly risky to build a business plan around basic science breakthroughs. Therefore, big pharmaceutical companies have only recently started to gain confidence in foundational neural engineering science in order to invest in neurotechnology development. It is important to recognize that the considerable work necessary to advance the frontiers of neural interface science and lay the foundation for neural engineering had to come from tax-payers, government organizations (e.g., United States Department of Veterans Affairs (VA), Department of Defense (DoD), National Institute of Health (NIH), National Science Foundation (NSF)), and donors, rather than businesses. This foundational academic research is an educational and cultural process that is necessary but difficult to evaluate in terms of technology development due to the long time-scales between basic science discovery and developing technology applications [76]. However, because of the long time-scales, it is crucial to advocate for investing today, especially in order to avoid losing the tremendous academic, government, and industry momentum that has built up in the neural engineering field.

4. Need for the Science of Neural Engineering

Neural engineering is at crucial point, in which, unlike other established engineering industries, the basic scientific knowledge foundational for neural engineering is disproportionately incomplete. This limited understanding of the human brain shrouds undiscovered opportunities for advancement in neurotechnology. Biology is perhaps the most complex regulatory system known, and within biology, the nervous system is perhaps the most sophisticated control system that exists. As such, it is not possible to overpower biology with rudimentary physics and engineering. Instead, development of microscale neural interfaces requires a more challenging titration of increasing information bandwidth while minimizing injury and inflammation of the host tissue. Therefore, it is critical to continue advancing both technology development and neurobiology in parallel.

Currently, the advancement of neuroscience is limited by the current capabilities of neurotechnology tools. Similarly, the development of devices is limited by the inadequate understanding of which designs and parameter trade-offs need to be optimized in order to maximize the extraction of meaningful neural signals [36]. Due to the long-time scales between basic science research and development of technology applications, the neural engineering field has long experienced deep criticisms on the shortage of clinical applications and aiding patients. Today, greater emphasis in neural engineering is placed on clinical impact over basic science research. However, in order to dramatically advance neural engineering, it is necessary to advance the science of neural engineering. In other words, it is necessary to continue to invest in the development of technology and studies that are designed to expand scientific knowledge rather than for therapeutic applications [22,46,58,74,77–96], even when the market segment is currently too small to support commercialization.

For example, the standard Blackrock arrays have 400 μm shank pitch [97]. This is not because 400 μm is the optimal pitch to maximize signal detection or the optimal pitch to record from neighboring cortical columns. Studies in the hippocampus CA1 of rats showed that acutely the maximum recording radius of an extracellular electrode was 80–160 μm [98]. The 400 μm pitch was chosen because it was the width of the band-saw available at the time [37]. To this day, despite technological advancements that enable greater ranges of pitches, the physiologically optimal pitch for electrodes remains unknown. A major challenge for elucidating this optimal pitch is that it is necessary to evaluate a battery of different pitches individually. One might expect that a single design with a small pitch could easily allow oversampling to identify the optimal pitch for minimizing overlap. This would in theory identify the minimum pitch for enabling the densest recording configuration. However, the act of implanting the denser array leads to greater tissue strain, tissue response, and neurodegeneration, which ultimately alters the pattern of functional neurons around the implant [36,94].

The level of tissue response is also not limited to pitch, but also depends on the footprint of the probe, shape of tine, and surface chemistry of the interface, making it difficult to translate findings from one design to another [96,99]. Furthermore, there is an additional layer of complexity that is added due to the fact that the tissue response is dynamic and as a result, the optimal pitch is expected to also be dynamic over time [100,101]. The basic science discovery of identifying the optimal pitch has long-range impact on technology development. However, brain injury, neurodegeneration, neural regeneration, limited translatability across device designs, and immediate clinical impact and innovation is deemed to be too limited for current peer-review processes and commercial research.

Similarly, a major focus of research surrounding implantable neural interfaces are on neurons, implantable devices, and scar tissue around implants. However, rapidly growing evidence point to vasculature and glia as important regulators of neuronal health, network activity, and brain health [66,67,102–105]. Unfortunately, basic science studies aimed at understanding how glia and vascular dysfunction contribute to neural interface failure remain as long-range investments for improving neural interfaces and do not have immediate commercial value. These are only a few examples of many important topics that are critical to the overall advancement of the field, such as packaging (hermetic sealing) and glial-vascular interface technologies (as opposed to neural interface technologies) [36,68].

5. Need for Scientific and Engineering Convergence

Neural interface engineering requires a confluence of basic science, applied science, and engineering. For example, each anatomical target in the brain has distinct structures and circuit organization. Different brain regions are also composed of different structures of vascular network and different glial cell types as well as different ratios of neurons to glial cells. Even within neuronal cell-types, different regions of the nervous system are composed of uniquely diverse combination of excitatory and inhibitory neurons. This means that answering specific basic neuroscience questions can require technology designed for a specific target brain region and optimized to answer the specific question at hand. In other words, long-standing unanswered scientific questions could be better addressed by custom designs instead of a one-size-fits-all design. Unfortunately, from a financial point of view, a design that can only be applied to one specific experimental paradigm has limited commercial value due to a small and restricted market segment. Therefore, it is necessary to support academic infrastructures to accommodate technology development specifically designed to answer basic science questions.

The first steps to achieving this goal is that the engineers need to understand the anatomy, physiology, unintended consequences or "side-effects" of their designs, and the scientific principle behind the question their technology intended to answer. Similarly, scientists need to understand the limitations of materials, microfabrication techniques, failure modalities "in the field", and design-driven technology development. Scientists need to guide technology development to optimally answer scientific questions without adding confounding variables to their study. Because functional microscale neural interfaces require fine titration of design parameters that are interdependent on each other [36], it is necessary for scientists to understand how achieving one optimal parameter can break functionality of other interdependent parameters. Therefore, engineering scientists and scientific engineers are both necessary in advancing the frontiers of the nervous system and integrating the newly found discoveries into technologies that interface directly or indirectly with the nervous system. For clinical applications, additional specialists are necessary including clinicians, patients, and caregivers or other "end-users" that interact with individuals who receive the neurotechnology.

The development of neurotechnologies requires a convergence of multiple disciplinary backgrounds including electrical engineering, electrochemistry, mechanical engineering, computer science, physics, biochemistry, biomechanics, material science, optics, biomaterials, packaging, ergonomics, molecular and cellular neurobiology, clinical science, and health care services. This requires both a wide breadth of expertise as well as enough cross-training depth to be able to integrate multiple engineering and scientific fields as well as end-user needs. While it is necessary to draw on multiple disciplines in the form of teams, the delays of the feedback loop between team members are limited by the speed in which team-members can communicate with each other. A commonly sought strategy to shorten that loop is to house multiple expertise in a single mind. However, this requires considerable cross-training time and effort on behalf of the individual. Given the growing scientific knowledge and accelerated advancement of engineering, it is becoming increasingly demanding for an individual to be fully proficient in all relevant scientific, engineering, and clinical expertise. Therefore, it is crucial for neural engineers to form teams of engineers, scientists, clinicians, and end-users as well as develop efficient communication techniques to reach the next level of technology development. While an increasing number of labs and programs strive to achieve this integration of science and engineering, this requires substantial contribution from individuals to learn, incorporate, and pass on training.

In turn, this means that the critical challenge for neural interface education and training is in converging neurobiology and neural engineering. Biology and engineering are often taught divergently with minimal overlap instead of being taught in an integrated and convergent manner. The nervous system is one of the most sophisticated computational systems, whose neural network activity is tightly regulated by the neural vascular unit and glia. Therefore, it stands to reason, as engineers, that by understanding the mechansims of how neurons, glia, and the neurovascular units regulate the neural network, it will be possible to identify new targets and means for interfacing with the nervous system in order to treat and repair diseases and injuries. However, in order to achieve this, it is necessary to bring together a diverse set of expertise, perspectives, and problem solving approaches, but have the capability to rapidly communicate with a common set of neuroscience and neural engineering "language".

6. Need for Diversity

While the ultimate goal of the BRAIN Initiative (NSF, NIH, etc.) and commercial Bioelectronic Medicine (Galvani Bioelectronics (GSK and Verily), NeuraLink, Kernel, etc.) is to understand brain function and treat neurological and physiological disease via the nervous system, the critical hurdle is placed on unreliable neuroelectronic interfaces over relevant time scales and the limited understanding in the neural interfacing field [36,67,68,97,106–109]. Just as a diversity of expertise is necessary to develop the next-generation microscale neural interfaces, it is necessary to have a diversity of perspectives and problem-solving approaches. The consequence of lack of diversity translates into limited diversity of opinion and perspectives, the blind spread of popular dogma, and the quenching of minority views. For example, a prevailing hypothesis in the field is that flexible devices will out preform traditional stiff implants. While plenty of evidence suggests that tissue injury is reduced around softer biomaterials, 50 years of polymer microelectrode research and limited success support the unpopular view that flexible polymer implants suffer from higher electrical impedance, higher resistivity, lower material strengths, higher shunt capacitance, larger device sizes, and new delamination issues that result in poorer performance compared to traditional devices [36,58]. This demonstrates issues in diversity as emphasized by NSF, "*Diversity—of thought, perspective, and experience—is essential to achieving excellence in 21st century science and engineering research and education*" [110]. Multi-disciplinary training in science and engineering are necessary, as well as diversity in perspective to understand the underlying problem and diversity in the approach of solving the problem. It is crucial to recognize that diversity in perspective and approach often stem from diversity in cultural and socio-economic backgrounds.

This diversity in approach to understanding the underlying problem and approach to problem-solving are deeply entangled with cultural and social backgrounds [111]. One study showed that gender diversity is correlated to 41% higher productivity compared to all-female or all-male teams [112]. Another study found that companies were 15% more likely to gain financial returns for companies in the top quartile of gender diversity and 35% more likely for companies in the top quartile for racial/ethnic diversity [113]. These studies add to a growing body of research that demonstrates gender, cultural, and ethnic diversity improves productivity, medical research, and clinical outcomes [114–170]. While similar studies in neural interface engineering have not been carried out, evidence in other fields suggest a potential for growth in the field by addressing gender and ethnic diversity. In a multi-disciplinary field such as microscale neural interface engineering, it is important for teams to have a diverse multi-disciplinary portfolio of ideas, skills, interests, technical background, and cultural and social backgrounds [111].

Therefore, it is crucial to protect and nurture researchers and prospective-researchers of underrepresented minorities who have been the victims of biases. In a seminal study by Rosenthal and Fode [171], half of wild-type littermates were randomly labeled "smart rats" and researchers were asked to compare the performance of these "smart rats" he "discovered" against the other half of the litter. What he showed was that the "smart rats" significantly out-performed their littermate clones in maze-tasks. He further described the Experimenter Expectancy Effect in which the experimenter's bias leads to unconscious behavioral cues that in turn influence the behavioral outcome of the subject. While the potential of these clones should be statistically identical, the "normal rat" group did not reach their potential due to the interactions with the experimenter. Therefore, in promoting diversity, it is crucial to recognize the metrics, which are measures of past performance, do not represent future potential, in individuals who grew up in environments of bias including women, non-binary gender minorities, and ethnic minorities [172]. This further extends to the fact that "equal opportunity" cannot equate "equal distribution" until such time that all implicit biases are eliminated [172]. Similarly, multiple studies have demonstrated that affirmative action admittees with lower incoming scores have a higher predisposition to success [173–175]. Therefore, it is necessary to provide for underrepresented minorities to counter the history of bias, facilitate reaching their full potential, and contribute to the diverse perspectives and problem-solving approaches necessary to address the multifaceted challenges surrounding neural interfaces.

7. Conclusions

Microscale neural interfaces have demonstrated great potential in basic neuroscience research and clinical neuroprosthetics. While these early results have generated enormous enthusiasm, limitations, and challenges in reliability and large performance variability remain. In other words, there is much more to be explored and discovered at the frontiers of microscale neural interfaces. Pioneers that are advancing these frontiers will be better positioned with cross-training in microfabrication/biomaterials engineering and neurobiology/neuroscience, as well as assembling teams with a diverse set of technical expertise as well as culture backgrounds. This is because fundamental basic science research is an academic and cultural process, and as greater cultural diversity is intermingled into this process, richer and deeper discoveries will be generated.

Funding: TDYK was financially supported by NIH National Institute of Neurological Disorders and Stroke (Grant R01NS062019, R01NS094396, R01NS089688, R21NS108098) and DARPA-BAA-16-09-NESD-FP-001.

Acknowledgments: The author would like to thank James R. Eles and Kip A. Ludwig for valuable input and discussion. In addition, the author would like to thank Victor Rush, Tucker-Davis Technologies, Rio Vetter, NeuroNexus, Rajmohan Bhandari, Sandeep Negi, Blackrock Microsystems, Paras R. Patel, Cynthia Chestek, Matthew Angle, Yifan Kong, Paradromic Inc., John Seymour, Euisik Yoon, NeuroNex MINT Hub, Razi-ul Haque, Shivshankar Sundaram, Lawrence Livermore National Laboratories, and Eddie Change at UCSF for devices or images of arrays.

Conflicts of Interest: The author declares no financial, political, or ethnic conflict of interest. Specifically, based on a reviewer's comment, the author points out that Asian men do not fall under the category of underrepresented minorities.

References

1. House, L.R. Cochlear implant: The beginning. *Laryngoscope* **1987**, *97 Pt 1*, 996–997.
2. House, W.F. Cochlear implants. *Ann. Otol. Rhinol. Laryngol.* **1976**, *85 Pt 2* (Suppl. 27), 1–93. [CrossRef]
3. Dobelle, W.H.; Mladejovsky, M.G.; Girvin, J.P. Artifical vision for the blind: Electrical stimulation of visual cortex offers hope for a functional prosthesis. *Science* **1974**, *183*, 440–444. [CrossRef] [PubMed]
4. Dobelle, W.; Mladejovsky, M. Phosphenes produced by electrical stimulation of human occipital cortex, and their application to the development of a prosthesis for the blind. *J. Physiol.* **1974**, *243*, 553–576. [CrossRef] [PubMed]
5. Wodlinger, B.; Downey, J.E.; Tyler-Kabara, E.C.; Schwartz, A.B.; Boninger, M.L.; Collinger, J.L. Ten-dimensional anthropomorphic arm control in a human brain-machine interface: Difficulties, solutions, and limitations. *J. Neural Eng.* **2015**, *12*, 016011. [CrossRef] [PubMed]
6. Wang, W.; Collinger, J.L.; Degenhart, A.D.; Tyler-Kabara, E.C.; Schwartz, A.B.; Moran, D.W.; Weber, D.J.; Wodlinger, B.; Vinjamuri, R.K.; Ashmore, R.C.; et al. An electrocorticographic brain interface in an individual with tetraplegia. *PLoS ONE* **2013**, *8*, e55344. [CrossRef] [PubMed]
7. Collinger, J.L.; Wodlinger, B.; Downey, J.E.; Wang, W.; Tyler-Kabara, E.C.; Weber, D.J.; McMorland, A.J.; Velliste, M.; Boninger, M.L.; Schwartz, A.B. High-performance neuroprosthetic control by an individual with tetraplegia. *Lancet* **2013**, *381*, 557–564. [CrossRef]
8. Hochberg, L.R.; Bacher, D.; Jarosiewicz, B.; Masse, N.Y.; Simeral, J.D.; Vogel, J.; Haddadin, S.; Liu, J.; Cash, S.S.; van der Smagt, P.; et al. Reach and grasp by people with tetraplegia using a neurally controlled robotic arm. *Nature* **2012**, *485*, 372–375. [CrossRef] [PubMed]
9. Hochberg, L.R.; Serruya, M.D.; Friehs, G.M.; Mukand, J.A.; Saleh, M.; Caplan, A.H.; Branner, A.; Chen, D.; Penn, R.D.; Donoghue, J.P. Neuronal ensemble control of prosthetic devices by a human with tetraplegia. *Nature* **2006**, *442*, 164–171. [CrossRef] [PubMed]

10. Cushing, H. A note upon the faradic stimulation of the postcentral gyrus in conscious patients. *Brain* **1909**, *32*, 44–53. [CrossRef]

11. Flesher, S.N.; Collinger, J.L.; Foldes, S.T.; Weiss, J.M.; Downey, J.E.; Tyler-Kabara, E.C.; Bensmaia, S.J.; Schwartz, A.B.; Boninger, M.L.; Gaunt, R.A. Intracortical microstimulation of human somatosensory cortex. *Sci. Transl. Med.* **2016**, *8*, 361ra141. [CrossRef] [PubMed]

12. Strumwasser, F. Long-term recording' from single neurons in brain of unrestrained mammals. *Science* **1958**, *127*, 469–470. [CrossRef] [PubMed]

13. Kipke, D.R.; Shain, W.; Buzsaki, G.; Fetz, E.; Henderson, J.M.; Hetke, J.F.; Schalk, G. Advanced neurotechnologies for chronic neural interfaces: New horizons and clinical opportunities. *J. Neurosci.* **2008**, *28*, 11830–11838. [CrossRef] [PubMed]

14. Schwartz, A.B.; Cui, X.T.; Weber, D.J.; Moran, D.W. Brain-controlled interfaces: Movement restoration with neural prosthetics. *Neuron* **2006**, *52*, 205–220. [CrossRef] [PubMed]

15. Giancoli, D.C. *Physics: Principles with Applications*; Prentice Hall: Upper Saddle River, NJ, USA, 1998.

16. Galvani, L.; Aldini, G. *Aloysii Galvani... De Viribus Electricitatis in Motu Musculari Commentarius cum ioannis Aldini Dissertatione et notis. Accesserunt Epistolæ ad Animalis Electricitatis Theoriam Pertinentes*; Apud Societatem Typographicam: Paris, France, 1792.

17. Galvani, L. *D Viribus Electricitatis in Motu Musculari: Commentarius*; Bologna: Tip; Istituto delle Scienze: Bologna, Italy, 1791; p. 58.

18. Du Bois-Reymond, E.H. Untersuchungen über Thierische Elektricität. *Anal. Phys.* **1884**, *151*, 463–464. [CrossRef]

19. Fritsch, G.; Hitzig, E. Ueber die elektrische Erregbarkeit des Grosshirns. *Arch. Anat. Physiol. Wiss. Medizin.* **1870**, *37*, 300–332.

20. Volta, A. XVII. On the electricity excited by the mere contact of conducting substances of different kinds. In a letter from Mr. Alexander Volta, FRS Professor of Natural Philosophy in the University of Pavia, to the Rt. Hon. Sir Joseph Banks, Bart. KBPR S. *Philos. Trans. R. Soc. Lond.* **1800**, *90*, 403–431. [CrossRef]

21. Dow, B.M.; Vautin, R.G.; Bauer, R. The mapping of visual space onto foveal striate cortex in the macaque monkey. *J. Neurosci.* **1985**, *5*, 890–902. [CrossRef] [PubMed]

22. Iordanova, B.; Vazquez, A.L.; Kozai, T.D.Y.; Fukuda, M.; Kim, S.G. Optogenetic investigation of the variable neurovascular coupling along the interhemispheric circuits. *J. Cereb. Blood Flow Metab.* **2018**, *38*, 627–640. [CrossRef] [PubMed]

23. Stecker, M. Factors Affecting Stimulus Artifact: Solution Factors. *EC Neurol.* **2017**, *5*, 52–61.

24. Ben-Menachem, E. Vagus-nerve stimulation for the treatment of epilepsy. *Lancet Neurol.* **2002**, *1*, 477–482. [CrossRef]

25. Kahn, A. Motion artifacts and streaming potentials in relation to biological electrodes. In Proceedings of the Dig 6th International Conference Medical Electronics and Biological Engineering, Tokyo, Japan, 22–27 August 1965; Volume 112, pp. 562–563.

26. Espinosa, J.; Aiello, M.T.; Naritoku, D.K. Revision and removal of stimulating electrodes following long-term therapy with the vagus nerve stimulator. *Surg. Neurol.* **1999**, *51*, 659–664. [CrossRef]

27. Penry, J.K.; Dean, J.C. Prevention of intractable partial seizures by intermittent vagal stimulation in humans: Preliminary results. *Epilepsia* **1990**, *31* (Suppl. 2), S40–S43. [CrossRef]

28. Rutecki, P. Anatomical, physiological, and theoretical basis for the antiepileptic effect of vagus nerve stimulation. *Epilepsia* **1990**, *31* (Suppl. 2), S1–S6. [CrossRef]

29. Brindley, G.S.; Lewin, W.S. The sensations produced by electrical stimulation of the visual cortex. *J. Physiol.* **1968**, *196*, 479–493. [CrossRef] [PubMed]

30. Schwartz, A.B. Cortical neural prosthetics. *Annu. Rev. Neurosci.* **2004**, *27*, 487–507. [CrossRef] [PubMed]

31. Paralikar, K.; Rao, C.; Clement, R.S. Automated reduction of non-neuronal signals from intra-cortical microwire array recordings by use of correlation technique. In Proceedings of the 30th Annual International Conference of the IEEE EMBS 2008 Engineering in Medicine and Biology Society, Vancouver, BC, Canada, 21–24 August 2008; pp. 46–49.

32. Agnesi, F.; Muralidharan, A.; Baker, K.B.; Vitek, J.L.; Johnson, M.D. Fidelity of frequency and phase entrainment of circuit-level spike activity during DBS. *J. Neurophysiol.* **2015**, *114*, 825–834. [CrossRef] [PubMed]

33. Collinger, J.L.; Kryger, M.A.; Barbara, R.; Betler, T.; Bowsher, K.; Brown, E.H.; Clanton, S.T.; Degenhart, A.D.; Foldes, S.T.; Gaunt, R.A.; et al. Collaborative approach in the development of high-performance brain-computer interfaces for a neuroprosthetic arm: Translation from animal models to human control. *Clin. Transl. Sci.* **2014**, *7*, 52–59. [CrossRef] [PubMed]

34. Schmidt, E.; McIntosh, J.; Bak, M. Long-term implants of Parylene-C coated microelectrodes. *Med. Biol. Eng. Comput.* **1988**, *26*, 96–101. [CrossRef] [PubMed]

35. Drake, K.L.; Wise, K.D.; Farraye, J.; Anderson, D.J.; BeMent, S.L. Performance of planar multisite microprobes in recording extracellular single-unit intracortical activity. *IEEE Trans. Biomed. Eng.* **1988**, *35*, 719–732. [CrossRef] [PubMed]

36. Wellman, S.M.; Eles, J.R.; Ludwig, K.A.; Seymour, J.P.; Michelson, N.J.; McFadden, W.E.; Vazquez, A.L.; Kozai, T.D. A Materials Roadmap to Functional Neural Interface Design. *Adv. Funct. Mater.* **2018**, *28*, 201701269. [CrossRef] [PubMed]

37. Campbell, P.K.; Jones, K.E.; Huber, R.J.; Horch, K.W.; Normann, R.A. A silicon-based, three-dimensional neural interface: Manufacturing processes for an intracortical electrode array. *IEEE Trans. Biomed. Eng.* **1991**, *38*, 758–768. [CrossRef] [PubMed]

38. Patel, P.R.; Zhang, H.; Robbins, M.T.; Nofar, J.B.; Marshall, S.P.; Kobylarek, M.J.; Kozai, T.D.Y.; Kotov, N.A.; Chestek, C.A. Chronic In Vivo Stability Assessment of Carbon Fiber Microelectrode Arrays. *J. Neural Eng.* **2016**, *13*, 066002. [CrossRef] [PubMed]

39. Patel, P.R.; Na, K.; Zhang, H.; Kozai, T.D.Y.; Kotov, N.A.; Yoon, E.; Chestek, C.A. Insertion of linear 8.4 mu m diameter 16 channel carbon fiber electrode arrays for single unit recordings. *J. Neural Eng.* **2015**, *12*. [CrossRef] [PubMed]

40. Mendrela, A.E.; Kim, K.; English, D.; McKenzie, S.; Seymour, J.P.; Buzsáki, G.; Yoon, E. A High-Resolution Opto-Electrophysiology System With a Miniature Integrated Headstage. *IEEE Trans. Biomed. Circuits Syst.* **2018**. [CrossRef] [PubMed]

41. Seymour, J.P.; Wu, F.; Wise, K.D.; Yoon, E. State-of-the-art MEMS and microsystem tools for brain research. *Microsyst. Nanoeng.* **2017**, *3*, 16066. [CrossRef]

42. Kampasi, K.; Stark, E.; Seymour, J.; Na, K.; Winful, H.G.; Buzsáki, G.; Wise, K.D.; Yoon, E. Fiberless multicolor neural optoelectrode for in vivo circuit analysis. *Sci. Rep.* **2016**, *6*, 30961. [CrossRef] [PubMed]

43. Seymour, E.Ç.; Freedman, D.S.; Gökkavas, M.; Özbay, E.; Sahin, M.; Ünlü, M.S. Improved selectivity from a wavelength addressable device for wireless stimulation of neural tissue. *Front. Neuroeng.* **2014**, *7*, 5. [CrossRef] [PubMed]

44. Khurram, A.; Seymour, J.P. Investigation of the photoelectrochemical effect in optoelectrodes and potential uses for implantable electrode characterization. In Proceedings of the 2013 35th Annual International Conference of the IEEE Engineering in Medicine and Biology Society (EMBC), Osaka, Japan, 3–7 July 2013; pp. 3032–3035.

45. Seymour, J.P.; Langhals, N.B.; Anderson, D.J.; Kipke, D.R. Novel multi-sided, microelectrode arrays for implantable neural applications. *Biomed. Microdevices* **2011**. [CrossRef] [PubMed]

46. Eles, J.R.; Vazquez, A.L.; Snyder, N.R.; Lagenaur, C.F.; Murphy, M.C.; Kozai, T.D.Y.; Cui, X.T. Neuroadhesive L1 coating attenuates acute microglial attachment to neural electrodes as revealed by live two-photon microscopy. *Biomaterials* **2017**, *113*, 279–292. [CrossRef] [PubMed]

47. Du, Z.J.; Kolarcik, C.L.; Kozai, T.D.Y.; Luebben, S.D.; Sapp, S.A.; Zheng, X.S.; Nabity, J.A.; Cui, X.T. Ultrasoft microwire neural electrodes improve chronic tissue integration. *Acta Biomater.* **2017**. [CrossRef] [PubMed]

48. Khilwani, R.; Gilgunn, P.J.; Kozai, T.D.Y.; Ong, X.C.; Korkmaz, E.; Gunalan, P.K.; Cui, X.T.; Fedder, G.K.; Ozdoganlar, O.B. Ultra-miniature ultra-compliant neural probes with dissolvable delivery needles: Design, fabrication and characterization. *Biomed. Microdevices* **2016**, *18*, 97. [CrossRef] [PubMed]

49. Kozai, T.D.Y.; Catt, K.; Du, Z.; Na, K.; Srivannavit, O.; Haque, R.-U.M.; Seymour, J.; Wise, K.D.; Yoon, E.; Cui, X.T. Chronic In Vivo Evaluation of PEDOT/CNT for Stable Neural Recordings. *IEEE Trans. Bio-Med. Eng.* **2016**, *63*, 111–119. [CrossRef] [PubMed]

50. Kolarcik, C.L.; Luebben, S.D.; Sapp, S.A.; Hanner, J.; Snyder, N.; Kozai, T.D.Y.; Chang, E.; Nabity, J.A.; Nabity, S.; Lagenaur, C.F.; et al. Elastomeric and soft conducting microwires for implantable neural interfaces. *Soft Matter* **2015**, *11*, 4847–4861. [CrossRef] [PubMed]

51. Alba, N.A.; Du, Z.J.; Catt, K.A.; Kozai, T.D.Y.; Cui, X.T. In vivo electrochemical analysis of a PEDOT/MWCNT neural electrode coating. *Biosensors* **2015**, *5*, 618–646. [CrossRef] [PubMed]

52. Kolarcik, C.L.; Catt, K.; Rost, E.; Albrecht, I.N.; Bourbeau, D.; Du, Z.; Kozai, T.D.Y.; Luo, X.; Weber, D.J.; Cui, X.T. Evaluation of poly(3,4-ethylenedioxythiophene)/carbon nanotube neural electrode coatings for stimulation in the dorsal root ganglion. *J. Neural Eng.* **2015**, *12*, 016008. [CrossRef] [PubMed]

53. Kozai, T.D.Y.; Alba, N.A.; Zhang, H.; Kotov, N.A.; Gaunt, R.A.; Cui, X.T. Nanostructured Coatings for Improved Charge Delivery to Neurons. In *Nanotechnology and Neuroscience: Nano-electronic, Photonic and Mechanical Neuronal Interfacing*; De Vittorio, M., Martiradonna, L., Assad, J., Eds.; Springer: New York, NY, USA, 2014; pp. 71–134.

54. Gilgunn, P.J.K.R.; Kozai, T.D.Y.; Weber, D.J.; Cui, X.T.; Erdos, G.; Ozdoganlar, O.B.; Fedder, G.K. An ultra-compliant, scalable neural probes with molded biodissolvable delivery vehicle. In Proceedings of the 2012 IEEE 25th International Conference on Micro Electro Mechanical Systems (MEMS), Paris, France, 29 January–2 Febuary 2012; Volume 2012, pp. 56–59.

55. Kozai, T.D.Y.; Kipke, D.R. Insertion shuttle with carboxyl terminated self-assembled monolayer coatings for implanting flexible polymer neural probes in the brain. *J. Neurosci. Methods* **2009**, *184*, 199–205. [CrossRef] [PubMed]

56. Escamilla-Mackert, T.; Langhals, N.B.; Kozai, T.D.Y.; Kipke, D.R. Insertion of a three dimensional silicon microelectrode assembly through a thick meningeal membrane. *Conf. Proc. IEEE Eng. Med. Biol. Soc.* **2009**, *2009*, 1616–1618. [PubMed]

57. Kozai, T.D.Y.; Jaquins-gerstl, A.S.; Vazquez, A.L.; Michael, A.C.; Cui, X.T. Dexamethasone retrodialysis attenuates microglial response to implanted probes in vivo. *Biomaterials* **2016**, *87*, 157–169. [CrossRef] [PubMed]

58. Michelson, N.J.; Vazquez, A.L.; Eles, J.R.; Salatino, J.W.; Purcell, E.K.; Williams, J.J.; Cui, X.T.; Kozai, T.D.Y. Multi-scale, multi-modal analysis uncovers complex relationship at the brain tissue-implant neural interface: New Emphasis on the Biological Interface. *J. Neural Eng.* **2018**, *15*. [CrossRef] [PubMed]

59. Boyden, E.S.; Zhang, F.; Bamberg, E.; Nagel, G.; Deisseroth, K. Millisecond-timescale, genetically targeted optical control of neural activity. *Nat. Neurosci.* **2005**, *8*, 1263. [CrossRef] [PubMed]

60. Tian, L.; Hires, S.A.; Mao, T.; Huber, D.; Chiappe, M.E.; Chalasani, S.H.; Petreanu, L.; Akerboom, J.; McKinney, S.A.; Schreiter, E.R.; et al. Imaging neural activity in worms, flies and mice with improved GCaMP calcium indicators. *Nat. Methods* **2009**, *6*, 875–881. [CrossRef] [PubMed]

61. Dana, H.; Chen, T.W.; Hu, A.; Shields, B.C.; Guo, C.; Looger, L.L.; Kim, D.S.; Svoboda, K. Thy1-GCaMP6 transgenic mice for neuronal population imaging in vivo. *PLoS ONE* **2014**, *9*, e108697. [CrossRef] [PubMed]

62. Chen, Q.; Cichon, J.; Wang, W.; Qiu, L.; Lee, S.-J.; Campbell, N.R.; DeStefino, N.; Goard, M.J.; Fu, Z.; Yasuda, R.; et al. Imaging Neural Activity Using Thy1-GCaMP Transgenic Mice. *Neuron* **2012**, *76*, 297–308. [CrossRef] [PubMed]

63. Xie, Y.; Chan, A.W.; McGirr, A.; Xue, S.; Xiao, D.; Zeng, H.; Murphy, T.H. Resolution of high-frequency mesoscale intracortical maps using the genetically encoded glutamate sensor iGluSnFR. *J. Neurosci.* **2016**, *36*, 1261–1272. [CrossRef] [PubMed]

64. Louveau, A.; Harris, T.H.; Kipnis, J. Revisiting the mechanisms of CNS immune privilege. *Trends Immunol.* **2015**, *36*, 569–577. [CrossRef] [PubMed]

65. Carson, M.J.; Doose, J.M.; Melchior, B.; Schmid, C.D.; Ploix, C.C. CNS immune privilege: Hiding in plain sight. *Immunol. Rev.* **2006**, *213*, 48–65. [CrossRef] [PubMed]

66. Wellman, S.M.; Kozai, T.D.Y. Understanding the Inflammatory Tissue Reaction to Brain Implants to Improve Neurochemical Sensing Performance. *ACS Chem. Neurosci.* **2017**. [CrossRef] [PubMed]

67. Kozai, T.D.Y.; Jaquins-Gerstl, A.; Vazquez, A.L.; Michael, A.C.; Cui, X.T. Brain Tissue Responses to Neural Implants Impact Signal Sensitivity and Intervention Strategies. *ACS Chem. Neurosci.* **2015**, *6*, 48–67. [CrossRef] [PubMed]

68. Salatino, J.W.; Ludwig, K.A.; Kozai, T.D.Y.; Purcell, E.K. Glial responses to implanted electrodes in the brain. *Nat. BME* **2017**, *1*, 862–877. [CrossRef]

69. Williams, J.C.; Rennaker, R.L.; Kipke, D.R. Long-term neural recording characteristics of wire microelectrode arrays implanted in cerebral cortex. *Brain Res. Brain Res. Protoc.* **1999**, *4*, 303–313. [CrossRef]

70. Bedell, H.W.; Hermann, J.K.; Ravikumar, M.; Lin, S.; Rein, A.; Li, X.; Molinich, E.; Smith, P.D.; Selkirk, S.M.; Miller, R.H.; et al. Targeting CD14 on blood derived cells improves intracortical microelectrode performance. *Biomaterials* **2018**, *163*, 163–173. [CrossRef] [PubMed]

71. Rousche, P.J.; Normann, R.A. Chronic recording capability of the Utah Intracortical Electrode Array in cat sensory cortex. *J. Neurosci. Methods* **1998**, *82*, 1–15. [CrossRef]

72. Kozai, T.D.Y.; Marzullo, T.C.; Hooi, F.; Langhals, N.B.; Majewska, A.K.; Brown, E.B.; Kipke, D.R. Reduction of neurovascular damage resulting from microelectrode insertion into the cerebral cortex using in vivo two-photon mapping. *J. Neural Eng.* **2010**, *7*, 046011. [CrossRef] [PubMed]

73. Kozai, T.D.Y.; Catt, K.; Li, X.; Gugel, Z.V.; Olafsson, V.T.; Vazquez, A.L.; Cui, X.T. Mechanical failure modes of chronically implanted planar silicon-based neural probes for laminar recording. *Biomaterials* **2015**, *37*, 25–39. [CrossRef] [PubMed]

74. Prasad, A.; Xue, Q.S.; Dieme, R.; Sankar, V.; Mayrand, R.C.; Nishida, T.; Streit, W.J.; Sanchez, J.C. Abiotic-biotic characterization of Pt/Ir microelectrode arrays in chronic implants. *Front. Neuroeng.* **2014**, *7*, 2. [CrossRef] [PubMed]

75. Barrese, J.C.; Rao, N.; Paroo, K.; Triebwasser, C.; Vargas-Irwin, C.; Franquemont, L.; Donoghue, J.P. Failure mode analysis of silicon-based intracortical microelectrode arrays in non-human primates. *J. Neural Eng.* **2013**, *10*, 066014. [CrossRef] [PubMed]

76. Wilson, R.R. Congress' Joint Committee on Atomic Energy. In *Authorizing Legislation for FY 1970*; Congress of the United States: Washington, DC, USA, 1969.

77. Michelson, N.J.; Islam, R.; Vazquez, A.L.; Ludwig, K.A.; Kozai, T.D.Y. Calcium activation of frequency dependent temporally phasic, localized, and dense population of cortical neurons by continuous electrical stimulation. *BioRxiv* **2018**. [CrossRef]

78. Michelson, N.J.; Kozai, T.D.Y. Isoflurane and Ketamine Differentially Influence Spontaneous and Evoked Laminar Electrophysiology in Mouse V1. *J. Neurophysiol.* **2018**. [CrossRef] [PubMed]

79. Wellman, S.M.; Kozai, T.D.Y. In vivo spatiotemporal dynamics of NG2 glia activity caused by neural electrode implantation. *Biomaterials* **2018**, *164*, 121–133. [CrossRef] [PubMed]

80. Eles, J.; Vazquez, A.; Kozai, T.; Cui, X. In vivo imaging of neuronal calcium during electrode implantation: Spatial and temporal mapping of damage and recovery. *Biomaterials* **2018**. [CrossRef] [PubMed]

81. Kozai, T.D.Y.; Eles, J.R.; Vazquez, A.L.; Cui, X.T. Two-photon imaging of chronically implanted neural electrodes: Sealing methods and new insights. *J. Neurosci. Methods* **2016**, *256*, 46–55. [CrossRef] [PubMed]

82. Kozai, T.D.Y.; Du, Z.; Gugel, Z.V.; Smith, M.A.; Chase, S.M.; Bodily, L.M.; Caparosa, E.M.; Friedlander, R.M.; Cui, X.T. Comprehensive chronic laminar single-unit, multi-unit, and local field potential recording performance with planar single shank electrode arrays. *J. Neurosci. Methods* **2015**, *242*, 15–40. [CrossRef] [PubMed]

83. Kozai, T.D.Y.; Li, X.; Bodily, L.M.; Caparosa, E.M.; Zenonos, G.A.; Carlisle, D.L.; Friedlander, R.M.; Cui, X.T. Effects of caspase-1 knockout on chronic neural recording quality and longevity: Insight into cellular and molecular mechanisms of the reactive tissue response. *Biomaterials* **2014**, *35*, 9620–9634. [CrossRef] [PubMed]

84. Kozai, T.D.Y.; Vazquez, A.L.; Weaver, C.L.; Kim, S.-G.; Cui, X.T. In vivo two-photon microscopy reveals immediate microglial reaction to implantation of microelectrode through extension of processes. *J. Neural Eng.* **2012**, *9*, 066001–066001. [CrossRef] [PubMed]

85. Golabchi, A.; Wu, B.; Li, X.; Carlisle, D.L.; Kozai, T.D.Y.; Friedlander, R.M.; Cui, X.T. Melatonin improves quality and longevity of chronic neural recording. *Biomaterials* **2018**, *180*, 225–239. [CrossRef] [PubMed]

86. Prasad, A.; Xue, Q.-S.; Sankar, V.; Nishida, T.; Shaw, G.; Streit, W.J.; Sanchez, J.C. Comprehensive characterization and failure modes of tungsten microwire arrays in chronic neural implants. *J. Neural Eng.* **2012**, *9*, 056015. [CrossRef] [PubMed]

87. Hermann, J.K.; Ravikumar, M.; Shoffstall, A.; Ereifej, E.S.; Kovach, K.; Chang, J.; Soffer, A.; Wong, C.T.; Srivastava, V.; Smith, P.; et al. Inhibition of the cluster of differentiation 14 innate immunity pathway with IAXO-101 improves chronic microelectrode performance. *J. Neural Eng.* **2017**. [CrossRef] [PubMed]

88. Ravikumar, M.; Sunil, S.; Black, J.; Barkauskas, D.S.; Haung, A.Y.; Miller, R.H.; Selkirk, S.M.; Capadona, J.R. The roles of blood-derived macrophages and resident microglia in the neuroinflammatory response to implanted intracortical microelectrodes. *Biomaterials* **2014**, *35*, 8049–8064. [CrossRef] [PubMed]

89. Nolta, N.F.; Christensen, M.B.; Crane, P.D.; Skousen, J.L.; Tresco, P.A. BBB leakage, astrogliosis, and tissue loss correlate with silicon microelectrode array recording performance. *Biomaterials* **2015**, *53*, 753–762. [CrossRef] [PubMed]

90. Biran, R.; Martin, D.C.; Tresco, P.A. The brain tissue response to implanted silicon microelectrode arrays is increased when the device is tethered to the skull. *J. Biomed. Mater. Res. A* **2007**, *82*, 169–178. [CrossRef] [PubMed]

91. Saxena, T.; Karumbaiah, L.; Gaupp, E.A.; Patkar, R.; Patil, K.; Betancur, M.; Stanley, G.B.; Bellamkonda, R.V. The impact of chronic blood-brain barrier breach on intracortical electrode function. *Biomaterials* **2013**. [CrossRef] [PubMed]

92. Karumbaiah, L.; Saxena, T.; Carlson, D.; Patil, K.; Patkar, R.; Gaupp, E.A.; Betancur, M.; Stanley, G.B.; Carin, L.; Bellamkonda, R.V. Relationship between intracortical electrode design and chronic recording function. *Biomaterials* **2013**, *34*, 8061–8074. [CrossRef] [PubMed]

93. Karumbaiah, L.; Norman, S.E.; Rajan, N.B.; Anand, S.; Saxena, T.; Betancur, M.; Patkar, R.; Bellamkonda, R.V. The upregulation of specific interleukin (IL) receptor antagonists and paradoxical enhancement of neuronal apoptosis due to electrode induced strain and brain micromotion. *Biomaterials* **2012**, *33*, 5983–5996. [CrossRef] [PubMed]

94. McConnell, G.C.; Rees, H.D.; Levey, A.I.; Gutekunst, C.A.; Gross, R.E.; Bellamkonda, R.V. Implanted neural electrodes cause chronic, local inflammation that is correlated with local neurodegeneration. *J. Neural Eng.* **2009**, *6*, 56003. [CrossRef] [PubMed]

95. Purcell, E.K.; Seymour, J.P.; Yandamuri, S.; Kipke, D.R. In vivo evaluation of a neural stem cell-seeded prosthesis. *J. Neural Eng.* **2009**, *6*, 026005. [CrossRef] [PubMed]

96. Seymour, J.P.; Kipke, D.R. Neural probe design for reduced tissue encapsulation in CNS. *Biomaterials* **2007**, *28*, 3594–3607. [CrossRef] [PubMed]

97. Cody, P.A.; Eles, J.R.; Lagenaur, C.F.; Kozai, T.D.; Cui, X.T. Unique electrophysiological and impedance signatures between encapsulation types: An analysis of biological Utah array failure and benefit of a biomimetic coating in a rat model. *Biomaterials* **2018**, *161*, 117–128. [CrossRef] [PubMed]

98. Henze, D.A.; Borhegyi, Z.; Csicsvari, J.; Mamiya, A.; Harris, K.D.; Buzsaki, G. Intracellular features predicted by extracellular recordings in the hippocampus in vivo. *J. Neurophysiol.* **2000**, *84*, 390–400. [CrossRef] [PubMed]

99. Kozai, T.D.Y.; Langhals, N.B.; Patel, P.R.; Deng, X.; Zhang, H.; Smith, K.L.; Lahann, J.; Kotov, N.A.; Kipke, D.R. Ultrasmall implantable composite microelectrodes with bioactive surfaces for chronic neural interfaces. *Nat. Mater.* **2012**, *11*, 1065–1073. [CrossRef] [PubMed]

100. Kozai, T.D.Y.; Gugel, Z.; Li, X.; Gilgunn, P.J.; Khilwani, R.; Ozdoganlar, O.B.; Fedder, G.K.; Weber, D.J.; Cui, X.T. Chronic tissue response to carboxymethyl cellulose based dissolvable insertion needle for ultra-small neural probes. *Biomaterials* **2014**, *35*, 9255–9268. [CrossRef] [PubMed]

101. Potter, K.A.; Buck, A.C.; Self, W.K.; Capadona, J.R. Stab injury and device implantation within the brain results in inversely multiphasic neuroinflammatory and neurodegenerative responses. *J. Neural Eng.* **2012**, *9*, 046020. [CrossRef] [PubMed]

102. Montagne, A.; Nikolakopoulou, A.M.; Zhao, Z.; Sagare, A.P.; Si, G.; Lazic, D.; Barnes, S.R.; Daianu, M.; Ramanathan, A.; Go, A. Pericyte degeneration causes white matter dysfunction in the mouse central nervous system. *Nat. Med.* **2018**, *24*, 326. [CrossRef] [PubMed]

103. Wang, F.; Yang, Y.-J.; Yang, N.; Chen, X.-J.; Huang, N.-X.; Zhang, J.; Wu, Y.; Liu, Z.; Gao, X.; Li, T. Enhancing Oligodendrocyte Myelination Rescues Synaptic Loss and Improves Functional Recovery after Chronic Hypoxia. *Neuron* **2018**. [CrossRef] [PubMed]

104. Gorelick, P.B.; Scuteri, A.; Black, S.E.; DeCarli, C.; Greenberg, S.M.; Iadecola, C.; Launer, L.J.; Laurent, S.; Lopez, O.L.; Nyenhuis, D. Vascular contributions to cognitive impairment and dementia: A statement for healthcare professionals from the American Heart Association/American Stroke Association. *Stroke* **2011**, *42*, 2672–2713. [CrossRef] [PubMed]

105. Wellman, S.M.; Cambi, F.; Kozai, T.D.Y. The role of oligodendrocytes and their progenitors on neural interface technology: A novel perspective on tissue regeneration and repair. *Biomaterials* **2018**. [CrossRef] [PubMed]

106. Ward, M.P.; Rajdev, P.; Ellison, C.; Irazoqui, P.P. Toward a comparison of microelectrodes for acute and chronic recordings. *Brain Res.* **2009**, *1282*, 183–200. [CrossRef] [PubMed]

107. Tresco, P.A.; Winslow, B.D. The challenge of integrating devices into the central nervous system. *Crit. Rev. Biomed. Eng.* **2011**, *39*, 29–44. [CrossRef] [PubMed]

108. Liu, X.; McCreery, D.B.; Bullara, L.A.; Agnew, W.F. Evaluation of the stability of intracortical microelectrode arrays. *IEEE Trans. Neural Syst. Rehabil. Eng.* **2006**, *14*, 91–100. [CrossRef] [PubMed]

109. Liu, X.; McCreery, D.B.; Carter, R.R.; Bullara, L.A.; Yuen, T.G.; Agnew, W.F. Stability of the interface between neural tissue and chronically implanted intracortical microelectrodes. *IEEE Trans. Rehabil. Eng.* **1999**, *7*, 315–326. [PubMed]

110. Córdova, F.A. *Dear Colleague Letter: NSF INCLUDES (Inclusion across the Nation of Communities of Learners of Underrepresented Discoverers in Engineering and Science)*; National Science Foundation: Alexandria, VA, USA, 2016.

111. Orfield, G. *Diversity Challenged: Evidence on the Impact of Affirmative Action*; ERIC: New York, NY, USA, 2001.

112. Ellison, S.F.; Mullin, W.P. Diversity, social goods provision, and performance in the firm. *J. Econ. Manag. Strategy* **2014**, *23*, 465–481. [CrossRef]

113. Hunt, V.; Layton, D.; Prince, S. *Diversity Matters*; McKinsey & Company: New York, NY, USA, 2015.

114. Cox, T.H.; Lobel, S.A.; McLeod, P.L. Effects of ethnic group cultural differences on cooperative and competitive behavior on a group task. *Acad. Manag. J.* **1991**, *34*, 827–847.

115. Miller, T.; del Carmen Triana, M. Demographic diversity in the boardroom: Mediators of the board diversity–firm performance relationship. *J. Manag. Stud.* **2009**, *46*, 755–786. [CrossRef]

116. Richard, O.C.; Murthi, B.S.; Ismail, K. The impact of racial diversity on intermediate and long-term performance: The moderating role of environmental context. *Strateg. Manag. J.* **2007**, *28*, 1213–1233. [CrossRef]

117. Buttner, E.H.; Lowe, K.B.; Billings-Harris, L. The challenge of increasing minority-group professional representation in the United States: Intriguing findings. *Int. J. Hum. Resour. Manag.* **2009**, *20*, 771–789. [CrossRef]

118. Athey, S.; Avery, C.; Zemsky, P. Mentoring and diversity. *Am. Econ. Rev.* **2000**, *90*, 765–786. [CrossRef]

119. Hong, L.; Page, S.E. Groups of diverse problem solvers can outperform groups of high-ability problem solvers. *Proc. Natl. Acad. Sci. USA* **2004**, *101*, 16385–16389. [CrossRef] [PubMed]

120. Hoffman, L.R.; Maier, N.R. Quality and acceptance of problem solutions by members of homogeneous and heterogeneous groups. *J. Abnorm. Soc. Psychol.* **1961**, *62*, 401. [CrossRef] [PubMed]

121. McLeod, P.L.; Lobel, S.A.; Cox, T.H., Jr. Ethnic diversity and creativity in small groups. *Small Group Res.* **1996**, *27*, 248–264. [CrossRef]

122. Herring, C. Does diversity pay: Race, gender, and the business case for diversity. *Am. Sociol. Rev.* **2009**, *74*, 208–224. [CrossRef]

123. Grossman, G.M.; Maggi, G. Diversity and trade. *Am. Econ. Rev.* **2000**, *90*, 1255–1275. [CrossRef]

124. Jones, J.R.; Wilson, D.C.; Jones, P. Toward Achieving the "Beloved Community" in the Workplace: Lessons for Applied Business Research and Practice From the Teachings of Martin Luther King Jr. *Bus. Soc.* **2008**, *47*, 457–483. [CrossRef]

125. Watson, W.E.; Kumar, K.; Michaelsen, L.K. Cultural diversity's impact on interaction process and performance: Comparing homogeneous and diverse task groups. *Acad. Manag. J.* **1993**, *36*, 590–602.

126. Ostrom, E. The Difference: How the Power of Diversity Creates Better Groups, Firms, Schools, and Societies. By Page Scott E. Princeton: Princeton University Press, 2007. 448p. $27.95 cloth, $19.95 paper. *Perspect. Politics* **2008**, *6*, 828–829. [CrossRef]

127. Bristow, L.R.; Butler, A.S.; Smedley, B.D. *In the Nation's Compelling Interest: Ensuring Diversity in the Health-Care Workforce*; National Academies Press: Washington, DC, USA, 2004.

128. Antonio, A.L.; Chang, M.J.; Hakuta, K.; Kenny, D.A.; Levin, S.; Milem, J.F. Effects of racial diversity on complex thinking in college students. *Psychol. Sci.* **2004**, *15*, 507–510. [CrossRef] [PubMed]

129. Ruhe, J.; Eatman, J. Effects of racial composition on small work groups. *Small Group Behav.* **1977**, *8*, 479–486. [CrossRef]

130. Watson, W.E.; Kumar, K. Differences in decision making regarding risk taking: A comparison of culturally diverse and culturally homogeneous task groups. *Int. J. Int. Relat.* **1992**, *16*, 53–65. [CrossRef]

131. Copeland, L. Valuing Diversity, Part 1: Making the Most of Cultural Differences at the Workplace. *Personnel* **1988**, *65*, 52–54.

132. Cox, T., Jr. *Creating the Multicultural Organization: A Strategy for Capturing the Power of Diversity*; Jossey-Bass: San Francisco, CA, USA, 2001.

133. Cox, T., Jr. The multicultural organization. *Acad. Manag. Perspect.* **1991**, *5*, 34–47. [CrossRef]

134. Cox, T.H.; Blake, S. Managing cultural diversity: Implications for organizational competitiveness. *Acad. Manag. Perspect.* **1991**, *5*, 45–56. [CrossRef]

135. Maznevski, M.L. Understanding our differences: Performance in decision-making groups with diverse members. *Hum. Relat.* **1994**, *47*, 531–552. [CrossRef]
136. Mohammed, S.; Angell, L.C. Surface-and deep-level diversity in workgroups: Examining the moderating effects of team orientation and team process on relationship conflict. *J. Organ. Behav.* **2004**, *25*, 1015–1039. [CrossRef]
137. Richard, O.; McMillan, A.; Chadwick, K.; Dwyer, S. Employing an innovation strategy in racially diverse workforces: Effects on firm performance. *Group Organ. Manag.* **2003**, *28*, 107–126. [CrossRef]
138. Thomas, D.A. Diversity as strategy. *Harv. Bus. Rev.* **2004**, *82*, 98–98. [PubMed]
139. Johnson, N.L. Science of CI: Resources for change. In *Collective Intelligence: Creating a Prosperous World at Peace*; CreateSpace Independent Publishing Platform: Scotts Valley, CA, USA, 2008; pp. 265–274.
140. Johnson, N.L.; Watkins, J.H. The Where-How of Leadership Emergence (WHOLE) Landscape: Charting Emergent Collective Leadership. 2009. Available online: https://papers.ssrn.com/sol3/papers.cfm?abstract_id=1516618 (accessed on 26 Aug 2018).
141. Whitla, D.K.; Orfield, G.; Silen, W.; Teperow, C.; Howard, C.; Reede, J. Educational benefits of diversity in medical school: A survey of students. *Acad. Med.* **2003**, *78*, 460–466. [CrossRef] [PubMed]
142. Lakhan, S.E. Diversification of US medical schools via affirmative action implementation. *BMC Med. Educ.* **2003**, *3*, 6. [CrossRef] [PubMed]
143. Reichert, W.M. A Success Story: Recruiting & Retaining Underrepresented Minority Doctoral Students in Biomedical Engineering. *Lib. Educ.* **2006**, *92*, 52–55.
144. Rabinowitz, H.K.; Diamond, J.J.; Veloski, J.J.; Gayle, J.A. The impact of multiple predictors on generalist physicians' care of underserved populations. *Am. J. Public Health* **2000**, *90*, 1225. [PubMed]
145. Saha, S.; Taggart, S.H.; Komaromy, M.; Bindman, A.B. Do patients choose physicians of their own race? *Health Aff.* **2000**, *19*, 76–83. [CrossRef] [PubMed]
146. Traylor, A.H.; Schmittdiel, J.A.; Uratsu, C.S.; Mangione, C.M.; Subramanian, U. Adherence to cardiovascular disease medications: Does patient-provider race/ethnicity and language concordance matter? *J. Gen. Intern. Med.* **2010**, *25*, 1172–1177. [CrossRef] [PubMed]
147. Noah, B.A. The participation of underrepresented minorities in clinical research. *Am. J. Law Med.* **2003**, *29*, 221. [PubMed]
148. Saha, S.; Shipman, S.A. Race-neutral versus race-conscious workforce policy to improve access to care. *Health Aff.* **2008**, *27*, 234–245. [CrossRef] [PubMed]
149. Kim, M.J.; Holm, K.; Gerard, P.; McElmurry, B.; Foreman, M.; Poslusny, S.; Dallas, C. Bridges to the doctorate: Mentored transition to successful completion of doctoral study for underrepresented minorities in nursing science. *Nurs. Outlook* **2009**, *57*, 166–171. [CrossRef] [PubMed]
150. Magnus, S.A.; Mick, S.S. Medical schools, affirmative action, and the neglected role of social class. *Am. J. Public Health* **2000**, *90*, 1197. [PubMed]
151. Shaya, F.T.; Gbarayor, C.M. The case for cultural competence in health professions education. *Am. J. Pharm. Educ.* **2006**, *70*, 124. [CrossRef] [PubMed]
152. Komaromy, M.; Grumbach, K.; Drake, M.; Vranizan, K.; Lurie, N.; Keane, D.; Bindman, A.B. The role of black and Hispanic physicians in providing health care for underserved populations. *N. Engl. J. Med.* **1996**, *334*, 1305–1310. [CrossRef] [PubMed]
153. Guiton, G.; Chang, M.J.; Wilkerson, L. Student body diversity: Relationship to medical students' experiences and attitudes. *Acad. Med.* **2007**, *82*, S85–S88. [CrossRef] [PubMed]
154. Mitchell, D.A.; Lassiter, S.L. Addressing health care disparities and increasing workforce diversity: The next step for the dental, medical, and public health professions. *Am. J. Public Health* **2006**, *96*, 2093–2097. [CrossRef] [PubMed]
155. Stoddard, J.J.; Back, M.R.; Brotherton, S.E. The respective racial and ethnic diversity of US pediatricians and American children. *Pediatrics* **2000**, *105*, 27–31. [CrossRef] [PubMed]
156. Okunseri, C.; Bajorunaite, R.; Abena, A.; Self, K.; Iacopino, A.M.; Flores, G. Racial/ethnic disparities in the acceptance of Medicaid patients in dental practices. *J. Public Health Dent.* **2008**, *68*, 149–153. [CrossRef] [PubMed]
157. Friedemann, M.-L.; Pagan-Coss, H.; Mayorga, C. The workings of a multicultural research team. *J. Transcult. Nurs.* **2008**, *19*, 266–273. [CrossRef] [PubMed]

158. Ginther, D.K.; Schaffer, W.T.; Schnell, J.; Masimore, B.; Liu, F.; Haak, L.L.; Kington, R.S. Diversity in Academic Biomedicine: An Evaluation of Education and Career Outcomes with Implications for Policy. 2009. Available online: https://core.ac.uk/download/pdf/6268557.pdf (accessed on 26 Aug 2018).

159. Brown, T.T.; Scheffler, R.M.; Tom, S.E.; Schulman, K.A. Does the Market Value Racial and Ethnic Concordance in Physician–Patient Relationships? *Health Serv. Res.* **2007**, *42*, 706–726. [CrossRef] [PubMed]

160. Teal, C.R.; Street, R.L. Critical elements of culturally competent communication in the medical encounter: A review and model. *Soc. Sci. Med.* **2009**, *68*, 533–543. [CrossRef] [PubMed]

161. Grumbach, K.; Coffman, J.M.; Young, J.Q.; Vranizan, K.; Blick, N. Physician supply and medical education in California. A comparison with national trends. *West. J. Med.* **1998**, *168*, 412. [PubMed]

162. Katz, R.V.; Kegeles, S.S.; Kressin, N.R.; Green, B.L.; James, S.A.; Wang, M.Q.; Russell, S.L.; Claudio, C. Awareness of the Tuskegee Syphilis Study and the US presidential apology and their influence on minority participation in biomedical research. *Am. J. Public Health* **2008**, *98*, 1137–1142. [CrossRef] [PubMed]

163. Philips, B.; Mahan, J.; Perry, R. Minority recruitment to the health professions: A matched comparison six-year follow-up. *J. Med. Educ.* **1981**, *56*, 742–747. [CrossRef] [PubMed]

164. Thomson, W.A.; Ferry, P.G.; King, J.E.; Martinez-Wedig, C.; Michael, L.H. Increasing access to medical education for students from medically underserved communities: One program's success. *Acad. Med.* **2003**, *78*, 454–459. [CrossRef] [PubMed]

165. Saha, S.; Guiton, G.; Wimmers, P.F.; Wilkerson, L. Student body racial and ethnic composition and diversity-related outcomes in US medical schools. *JAMA* **2008**, *300*, 1135–1145. [CrossRef] [PubMed]

166. Daley, S.; Wingard, D.L.; Reznik, V. Improving the retention of underrepresented minority faculty in academic medicine. *J. Natl. Med. Assoc.* **2006**, *98*, 1435. [PubMed]

167. Thom, D.H.; Tirado, M.D.; Woon, T.L.; McBride, M.R. Development and evaluation of a cultural competency training curriculum. *BMC Med. Educ.* **2006**, *6*, 38. [CrossRef] [PubMed]

168. Pohlhaus, J.R.; Jiang, H.; Wagner, R.M.; Schaffer, W.T.; Pinn, V.W. Sex differences in application, success, and funding rates for NIH extramural programs. *Acad. Med.* **2011**, *86*, 759. [CrossRef] [PubMed]

169. Tabak, L.A.; Collins, F.S. Weaving a richer tapestry in biomedical science. *Science* **2011**, *333*, 940–941. [CrossRef] [PubMed]

170. Heggeness, M.L.; Evans, L.; Pohlhaus, J.R.; Mills, S.L. Measuring diversity of the National Institutes of Health-funded workforce. *Acad. Med.* **2016**, *91*, 1164. [CrossRef] [PubMed]

171. Rosenthal, R.; Fode, K.L. The effect of experimenter bias on the performance of the albino rat. *Syst. Res. Behav. Sci.* **1963**, *8*, 183–189. [CrossRef]

172. Sowell, T. *Affirmative Action around the World: An Empirical Study*; Yale University Press: New Haven, CT, USA, 2004.

173. Massey, D.S.; Mooney, M. The effects of America's three affirmative action programs on academic performance. *Soc. Prob.* **2007**, *54*, 99–117. [CrossRef]

174. Sander, R.H. A systemic analysis of affirmative action in American law schools. *Stan. Law Rev.* **2004**, *57*, 367.

175. Holzer, H.; Neumark, D. Assessing affirmative action. *J. Econ. Lit.* **2000**, *38*, 483–568. [CrossRef]

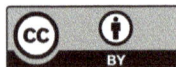

MDPI

St. Alban-Anlage 66

4052 Basel

Switzerland

Tel. +41 61 683 77 34

Fax +41 61 302 89 18

www.mdpi.com

Micromachines Editorial Office

E-mail: micromachines@mdpi.com

www.mdpi.com/journal/micromachines

www.ingramcontent.com/pod-product-compliance
Lightning Source LLC
Chambersburg PA
CBHW051709210326
41597CB00032B/5420